MORRIS HEPATOMAS
Mechanisms of Regulation

ADVANCES IN EXPERIMENTAL MEDICINE AND BIOLOGY

Recent Volumes in this Series

MORRIS HEPATOMAS
Mechanisms of Regulation

Edited by
Harold P. Morris
and Wayne E. Criss

Department of Biochemistry and
Howard Cancer Research Center
Howard University Medical School
Washington, D.C.

Springer Science+Business Media, LLC

Library of Congress Cataloging in Publication Data

Hepatoma Symposium, 6th, Washington, D. C., 1977.
   Morris hepatomas.

   (Advances in experimental medicine and biology; v. 92)
   "Based on the proceedings of the Sixth Biennial Hepatoma Symposium held in Washington,
D. C., May 22–24, 1977."
   Bibliography: p.
   Includes index.
   1. Hepatoma—Congresses. 2. Oncology, Experimental—Congresses. 3. Diseases—Animal
models—Congresses. I. Morris, Harold Paul, 1900-   II. Criss, Wayne E. III. Title. IV.
Series.
RC280.L5H47 1977   616.9'94'36   77-13136
ISBN 978-1-4615-8854-2   ISBN 978-1-4615-8852-8 (eBook)
DOI 10.1007/978-1-4615-8852-8

Based on the proceedings of the Sixth Biennial Hepatoma Symposium
held in Washington, D.C., May 22–24, 1977

© 1978 Springer Science+Business Media New York
Originally published by Plenum Press, New York 1978
Softcover reprint of the hardcover 1st edition 1978

Preface

In 1960, Dr. Van R. Potter and Dr. Henry Pitot (at McCardle Laboratory in Madison, Wisconsin), Dr. Tetsuo Ono (then at McCardle Laboratory and now at the Japanese Foundation for Cancer Research in Tokyo, Japan) and Dr. Harold P. Morris (then at the National Cancer Institute and now at Howard University, Washington, D.C.) decided that an experimental cancer model would be an invaluable tool to examine neoplastic changes in cells. Since they were studying the various highly specific metabolic processes which are unique to liver tissues, they determined that a transplantable liver cancer model would be the ideal system to work with. This system would provide for comparison of normal liver tissue of the non-tumor bearing animal, the tumor bearing animal's (host) liver and the liver cancer. Dr. Morris undertook a series of rat studies employing several chemicals known to cause liver cancer. Soon the first Morris hepatomas (#3683, 3924A, 5123) were being studied by several labs. During the next 18 years, Dr. Morris developed and transplanted numerous strains of hepatomas of which no two were identical. These tumors ranged from the very slowly-growing, highly differentiated cancer tissues, e.g., 9618A which is a diploid tumor containing glycogen and a "nearly normal" complement of enzymes, to a large group of rapidly-growing, poorly differentiated cancer tissues, e.g., 3924A and 9618A2 (latter being derived from 9618A) both of which are heteroploid and have lost almost all of their complement of enzymes which carry out the differentiated functions of liver tissue. This spectrum of cancer tissues has been and is now being utilized by hundreds of laboratories located all over the world. It has provided cancer researchers with a stable population of cancer cells for examining every parameter of molecular and cellular functioning. The spectrum of Morris hepatoma has provided us up to now with the most complete understanding possible of cancer tissues in action. We now know more about the "typical" cancer tissue, from the hundreds of reports on the Morris hepatomas, than from any other single cancer model system.

The present book represents the first attempt to accumulate and review our knowledge about cancer as gained during the last two decades from studying the Morris hepatomas. It provides the reader

with a beautiful example of the open sharing of scientific ideas and
concepts and it elegantly demonstrates how the devoted cooperation
among scientists can truly yield highly synergistic results. It gives
a clearer picture of the origin, evolution, and demise of cancer
theories. And it also provides the reader with a distinct preview of
new cancer theories which may now be present on the horizon.

We wish to sincerely thank the several hundred scientists,
students and technicians who over the many years have worked with and
searched out the now classical metabolism of cancer tissues, as gained
from studies of the Morris hepatomas. We wish to gratefully acknow-
ledge the key people involved in the daily induction, transplantation and management of the many strains of Morris hepatomas:
Billy P. Wagner (Dr. Morris' assistant at NCI for 17 years),
Charity M. Jackson (Dr. Morris' assistant at Howard University for
the last 10 years), Louise Lawson, Debra Richardson, Martha Mosley,
Dr. David Meranze, and Dr. Leonard Slaughter. We wish also to express our sincere appreciation to Nur Bilge Criss for her assistance
in reviewing, editing, typing and proofing this book.

All senior authors were supported, in part, by USPHS Grant
10429.

Contents

SECTION II:
NUCLEAR COMPOSITION

SECTION III:
REGULATIONS OF NUCLEAR FUNCTIONING

SECTION IV:
INTRACELLULAR ORGANELLES AND MEMBRANES

CONTENTS

SECTION V:
REGULATION OF CYTOPLASMIC FUNCTIONING

HISTORICAL DEVELOPMENT OF TRANSPLANTABLE HEPATOMAS

Harold P. Morris and Lynnard J. Slaughter

Departments of Biochemistry and Pathology
Howard University, College of Medicine
Washington, D.C.   20059

One of the criteria considered important as a test of malignancy of tumors that developed following the ingestion of chemical carcinogens was transplantability of the neoplasm. A stock of rats was available in early 1940 at N.I.H. that had been obtained by Dr. Carl Vogetlin from Dr. Carl Cori who was then at the Institute of Malignant Diseases in Buffalo, New York. The stock of rats of Wistar Institute origin was designated Buffalo rats and was maintained at the National Institute of Health as the principle stock rat available for experimental work at the Institute. These animals had been pen bred for more than ten years after they were received around 1930. Inbreeding was begun from this stock of rats in the early 1940's. Some difficulty occurred in the early stages of the inbreeding program because of sterility among mated pairs. After several years of inbreeding effective brother to sister mating was successfully practiced. In some cases the inbreeding was father to daughter or son to mother. After a few years no difficulty was encountered in the raising of offspring from such close inbreeding. It was not until several years later, however, in the early 50's that successful transplantation of induced tumors was successful into this inbred strain of rats.   N-2-fluorenylacetamide (2-FAA) was modified by the addition of a second acetyl group on the nitrogen in the two position to form N-2-fluorenyldiacetamide (2-FdiAA) (11). This compound enhanced carcinogenic activity toward the rat liver. This effect differs by sex and was further modified by sex hormones (12). Liver tumors developed rapidly in normal male rats but its carcinogenic activity was almost completely inhibited in the female rat and in the castrated male rat receiving in addition to the carcinogen, diethylstilbestrol. Experiments with the feeding of FdiAA will be found in Table 1. The carcinogen in the diet was ingested by the rats continuously for different periods,

1

Table One
N-2-Fluorenyldiacetamide (FdiAA)

Animal Strain and Tumor No.	Sex	Time on carcinogen (weeks)	Percent FdiAA in diet (diet no.)	Body Weight Initial (gm)	Body Weight Final (gm)	With-out carcinogen (weeks)	Total carcinogen intake (mg)	Total carcinogen take/100 gm avg. body wt. (mg)	Size[a] of tumor (cm)	Total primary no.	Date first trans-fers	Histologic Characteri-zation[b]
ACI 9098	M	16.7	0.015[c] (272)	169	220	41	130	62		7	8-14-64	HD,WD[d,c]
ACI 9108	M	25.7	0.015[c] (272)	171	244	13	193	90	6.7	9	4-2-64	WD[d,e]
ACI 9121	M	30.7	0.015[c] (272)	230	270	15	300	113	2.5	9	5-14-64	WD G[d,e]
Buffalo 9523	M	41.0	0.012[c] (222A)	270	370	0	424	129		11	2-3-65	CC[d], PDTC[c]
ACI 3683	M	4.7	0.050[c] (231)	155	175	62[f]	118			338	6-7-51	PD[g,h]
ACI 3924A	F[i]	16.0	0.050[i] (143a)	153	132	32	321		4.0	223	1-15-51	PD[g,h]

a Size: sum of two measurements.
b WD well differentiated; HD highly differentiated; PD poorly differentiated; G glycogen; CC cholangiocarcinoma; PDTC poorly differentiated trabecular carcinoma.
c Continuous ingestion
d Reuber, personal communication.
e Meranze, personal communication.

f On diet 231 without FdiAA for 10 days; on diet 214a for 62 weeks.
g (21).
h (22).
i Castrated testosterone (18).
j Continuous ingestion for 2 weeks; then alternately, 1 week on carcinogen, 1 week without carcinogen.
k (15).

sixteen weeks for tumor 9098; twenty-five weeks for tumor 9108; thirty weeks for tumor 9121 and forty-one weeks for tumor 9523. Table 1 shows that a level of 0.015% of FdiAA in the diet for the first three tumors listed in Table 1 resulted in liver tumors of HD, WD, and WD. In addition, tumor 9121 contained some glycogen. The tumor 9523 ingested the carcinogen for forty-one weeks and this tumor was classified as CC and PDTC. Tumors 3683 and 3924A ingested FdiAA at a level of 0.050 percent. At this high level of carcinogen intake the tumors were rapidly growing, poorly or undifferentiated carcinomas. These latter two tumors were originally transplanted in 1951. They have been transplanted continuously since that date. The WD and HD tumors arose in rats ingesting lesser amounts of the carcinogen than tumor 9523. It is believed that a high level of the carcinogen in the diets is a contributing factor in the development of PD tumors. Although the length of time the animals received the carcinogen at the higher dietary level is also an important factor affecting the degree of differentiation. Other inducing agents used-Table 2.

An experiment was started in 1954 designated our experiment No. 288[1]. The carcinogen used in the diet in this experiment was N-(2-fluorenyl)phthalamic acid (2-FPA) (16-17). This carcinogen containing diet was fed to a group of female rats for ten months at which time they were placed on the same diet without the carcinogen. Twelve of the rats were sacrificed 8-1/2 months later. These rats had multiple raised dark red nodules scattered throughout the liver. At sacrifice grossly a large tumor nodule was observed on the left lobe in animal 5123[2], the other liver lobes of rat 5123 also had multiple nodules. The large tumor nodule approximately 2cm in diameter in rat 5123 was selected for transplantation because of its large size and deep red color, the same color as the host liver. Three rats were originally given inoculations of minced tumor tissue using a 12-gauge trocar. Small pieces of the primary neoplasm were used. All subsequent transfers were made in a similar fashion. All three inoculations grew in the three new hosts of the Buffalo inbred strain. After 16 transfers in 4 years sublines A,B,C and D were established from tumor 5123.

[1] Diet 222-A was composed of the following constituents by weight, in grams:commercial casein, 3.00; edible grade skim-milk powder, 22.75; whole wheat meal (hard spring), 60.52; brewer's dehydrated debittered yeast, 1.00; whole-liver powder 1.00; sodium chloride, 1.40; ferric citrate, 0.13; cod-liver oil, 2.00; corn oil, 8.20.

[2] It was the original intent of the author to maintain consecutive numbers for each rat in all experiments from 1-10,000 so that there would be no duplication. The first experiment of 288 was carried out with animals numbered in the 5100 series. Our series of transplantable hepatomas were based on four digit numbers until we reached 9633 at which time we reverted back to animal number one. Some

Table Two
Inducing Agents

		No. Tumor lines/agent
1	N-2-fluorenyldiacetamid (N-2-FdiAA)	17
2	(N2-FPA)N-2-fluorenylphthalamic acid	12
3	(2-(4'CH$_3$)BAF)2-(4'methyl)benzoylamino-fluorene	4
4	(ENAF)2-ethylnitrosaminofluorene	None
5	[2,7-FAA(F$_6$)]N,N'-2,7-fluorenylenebis-2,2,2-trifluoroacetamide	None
6	(2,7-FdiSA)Fluorenyl-2,7-disuccinoamic acid	4
7	(2,4,6-TMA) 2,4,6 Trimethylaniline	2
8	(4'F-4BAA)4'fluoro-4-biphenylacetamide	3
9	N-F-2 Nicotinamide	1
10	Aflatoxin B$_1$	5
		48

Three tumors in ACI strain rats listed in Table 1 - 9098, 9108 and 9121 were subsequently reported by (19) (20) to be diploid tumors. These animals ingested FdiAA in their diet at a level of 0.015% for different periods of time ranging from 16-30 weeks as pointed out above. In a later experiment the same regimen was followed in efforts to develop additional diploid tumors in the Buffalo strain rat. The animals in this second experiment were fed the FdiAA containing diet at a level of 0.015% for a period of 6 months and autopsies were performed on these animals at various periods after taking them off the diet. In a series of 24 male Buffalo strain rats we autopsied 5 rats when death appeared imminent. Several tumor nodules were transplanted 5-6 months after removal of the carcinogen from the diet. We obtained 6 transplantable tumors from these animals. Many of the tumor nodules did not grow after transplanting them in a new host. These tumors except for one animal developed very slow growing transplantable tumors. They have been transplanted from June 1967 to the present time and have been transplanted from 19-23 generations. All of the animals developed lung metastases and all the tumors are well to highly differentiated hepatomas. So far, we have been unable to characterize the chromosomes in these tumors because they have not been studied in female rats where they often do not grow and the ones that have been examined show only the normal diploid chromosome complex (of the host). Some of the biological and biochemical properties of these tumors have been described by other investigators which are outlined as follows: (2-8, 10, 13-19, 22-23 and 25). Some of these biochemical properties are of great interest. The average growth rate of these hepatomas between 1973 and 1976 as measured by caliper in two dimensions at the time of sacrifice of the tumor bearing rat show reasonably stable growth rate over this 3 year period (Fig 1), except for tumor 28A which had a somewhat faster growth rate in '76 than was found for this tumor line in 1973. The reasonable stability of the growth rate over a 3 year period gives investigators confidence in using these tumors in repeat experiments of a given study, that they could expect to obtain similar results if their experiments were repeated or could expect to get consistent results for continuation experiments (Fig. 1).

In another experiment male Buffalo strain rats were fed 0.015% FdiAA in diet 222A continuously for 6 months and maintained on the diet without the carcinogen until death appeared imminent. We obtained transplantable tumors in this series of experiment as follows: 28A, 38B, 39A, 44 and 47C. These tumor lines with the exception of 38B were all well to highly differentiated hepatocellular

2 (continued)...of our later tumors therefore were numbered from 1-66. Not all animals however, in any one experiment developed transplantable tumors.

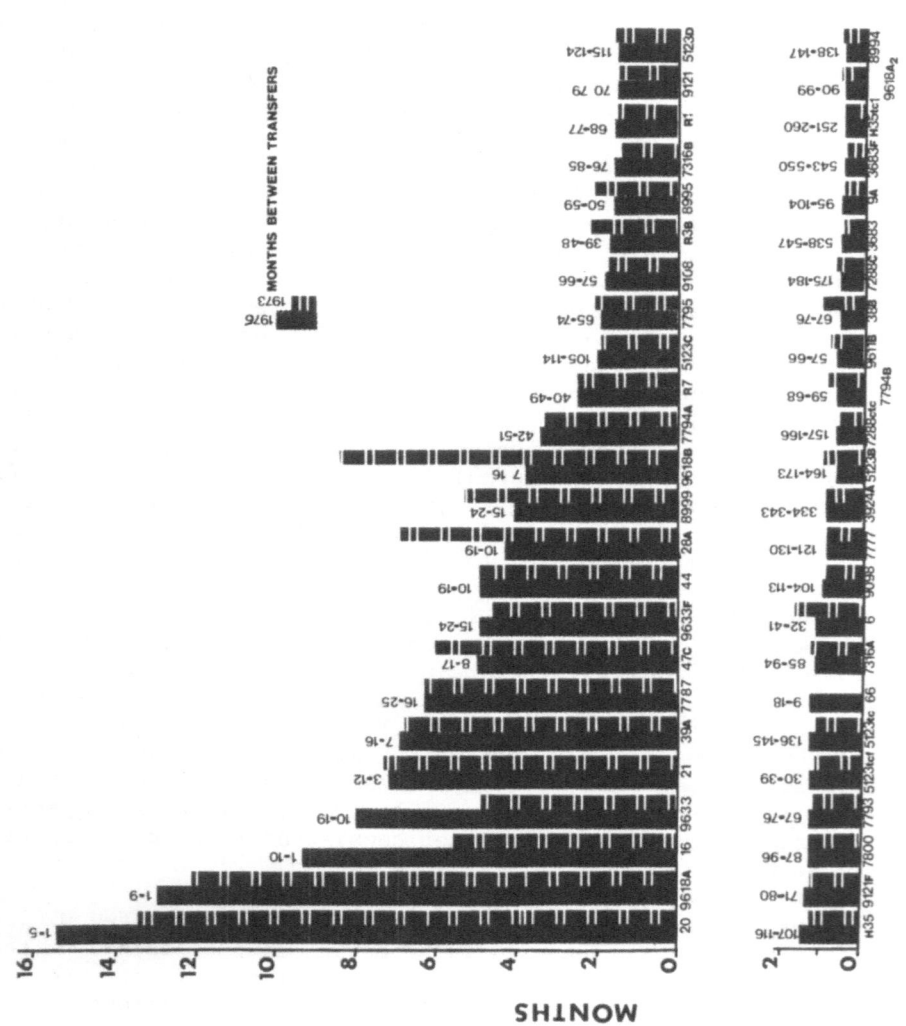

Text Figure 1

This figure lists a double column for each tumor line representing the growth in months of these tumors between 1973 and 1976 as
described in the legend. The growth of the tumors was obtained by
measuring in 2 dimensions tumor or tumors in each rat used for trans-
ferring the tumors to the next generation. The growth rate is expressed in months on the ordinate. The left hand column of each
pair represents the average growth in 1976 and the right hand column
represents the average growth rate in 1973. The numbers at the
bottom of each double column represents the tumor line used in computing average tumor growth. The numbers at the top of the 1976
column of each tumor line represents the generations used in obtaining the average growth of that tumor line. The tumors are
arranged from left to right, top of the figure and from left to
right on the bottom part of the figure. A total of 48 tumor lines
are presented in this figure. The slowest growing tumor is in the
top part of the figure on the left hand side of the chart. It may
be noted that the slowest growing tumors were slower growing in
1976 than they were in 1973. A few intermediate growth rate tumors
were slower growing in 1973 than in 1976. Most of the rapidly growing tumors showed little if any difference in their average growth
rates between 1973 and 1976. By this method of estimating the growth
rate it will be noted that most of the tumors have shown little
variation in their growth rate between 1973 and 1976 except as noted
above. An average of 10 generations has been selected for obtaining
the average tumor growth for all tumor lines for both periods except
in the very slowest growing tumors where less than 10 generations
were available for computing the average growth rate.

carcinomas and slowly growing. The purpose of this experiment
was an effort to produce diploid tumors in the Buffalo strain rat.
So far, we have not been successful in karyotyping the chromosome
spread in these latest tumor lines because we get a normal female
host cell type chromosome picture when the tumor is grown in the
opposite sex and we cannot be sure that the chromosomes came from
the tumor. We have previously described three tumor lines which
were produced in the CLI strain rat fed a diet containing the same
level of FdiAA (15). It is hoped that some of these latest described tumor lines will have a diploid number of chromosomes and
a normal karyotype.

Table Three
Transplantable Hepatomas in Buff M
Rats Ingesting Aflatoxin B_1, 1.5 ppm.
Started 6/17/66

Tumor	Date of Sacrifice	Transplant Generations	Last Date Transferred	Avg. Months	Histological Type Primary
5	12/12/67	10	4/23/69	1.7	WDAC
5L	9/3/68	8	4/23/69	1.0	___
9A	12/12/67	141	4/28/77	0.8	WDTH
16	12/12/67	12	8/5/76	9.0	WDTH
21	9/22/67	16	1/6/77	7.2	WDTH
6	9/28/67	52	3/31/77	2.1	WDTH
8	12/12/67	2	10/4/68	5.5	WDTH
20	12/12/67	8	11/4/76	13.3	WDTH

WDAC Well-differentiated adenocarcinoma
WDTH Well-differentiated trabecular hepatoma

We express out thanks to Dr. G.N. Wogan for the aflatoxin B_1
used in this experiment.

One of the most potent carcinogens which we have employed to
produce transplantable hepatomas has been aflatoxin B_1 produced by
Aspergillus flavus (9). Seven transplantable liver tumors have
been produced by feeding Buffalo strain male rats a diet containing
1.5 ppm of aflatoxin B_1. These experiments were started in June
1966 and the animals were fed a diet containing the aflatoxin B_1 for

four periods each of four weeks with rest periods of one week
between each period in which no carcinogen was included in the diet.
We recorded a total intake per rat of 1.8 to 2.8 mg. of aflatoxin
B_1. After a period of 15-18 months the rats were sacrificed.
Multiple hepatomas were present in all the rats at the time of
autopsy. One primary tumor which grew when transplanted was diagnosed histologically as a well-differentiated adenocarcinoma.
The first generation transplant of this tumor (#5) was diagnosed
as a poorly differentiated cholangiocarcinoma. It metastasized
extensively to the lung and was carried for 10 generations from
12-12-67 to 4-23-69. In the second transfer a lung nodule was
also transplanted and it was carried from 9-3-68 thru 4-23-69. The
original tumor was listed as tumor No. 5 and its metastises 5L
(L=lung). Both tumors were found to be quite unsatisfactory and
both were discontinued on 4-23-69. Six other transplantable hepatomas were obtained from this experiment. Five are still in our
spectrum (9). Four of these tumors as illustrated in Table 3 were
slow to very slow growing well differentiated trabecular carcinomas.
Over a period of about 10 years three of these transplantable hepatomas have been extremely slow growing. Tumor 20 and tumor 21
during this period have been transplanted 8 and 16 times respectively. The other tumor number 16 has been transplanted 12 times during
the same interval. These 3 tumors are among the slowest growing
tumors in our entire spectrum. Two of these primary tumors induced
by B_1 were found by Weinhouse (personal communication) to be devoid
of glucokinase. Tumor number 5 had an extremely high hexokinase
activity characteristic of some of these aflatoxin induced transplantable hepatomas (25) (1) fed a higher intake of aflatoxin B_1
for a period of 16 weeks. The incident of liver tumors was approximately the same in the livers in both sexes. In their experiment
the tumors developed 67-70 weeks after the start of the experiment.

    A histological comparison of primary tumor 5123 tumor, the 15th
transfer generation of 5123 and the 119th transfer generation of
5123C (5123C is a tumor line established in the 16th generation from
5123 and designated with the letter C), the primary tumor line 44,
the first transfer generation of tumor 44, and the 20th transfer
generation of tumor 44; and the primary tumor number 21; the histological characterization of these tumors was made to see if morho-
logical or histological changes could be detected during the period
in which these tumors have been maintained in our laboratory. The
histological descriptions of these tumor lines are found in figures
2-17 with the descriptive lesions described for each tumor line in
each generation including the primaries and the several transfer
generations.

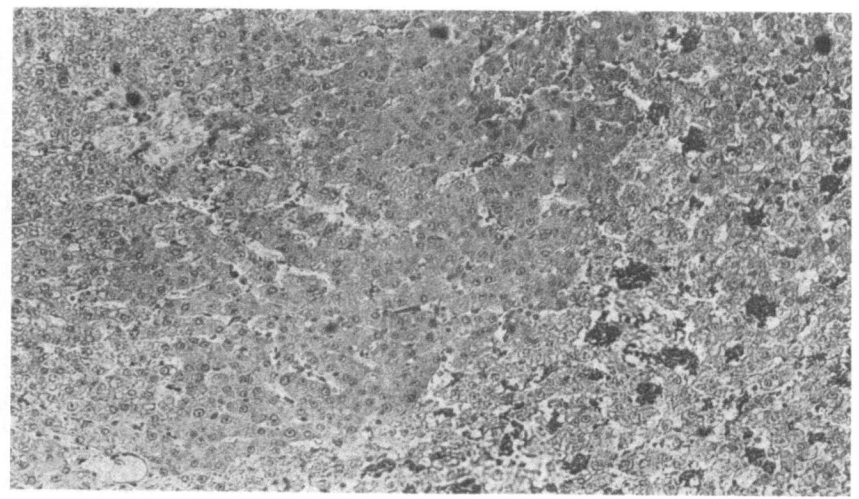

Figure 2
5123. Primary. Photomicrograph of a section of liver that
contains a nodule of hepatoma cells (right half of photograph).
The adjacent hepatic tissue is congested and degenerative, X 164.
(Figures 2-17 reduced 10% for reproduction).

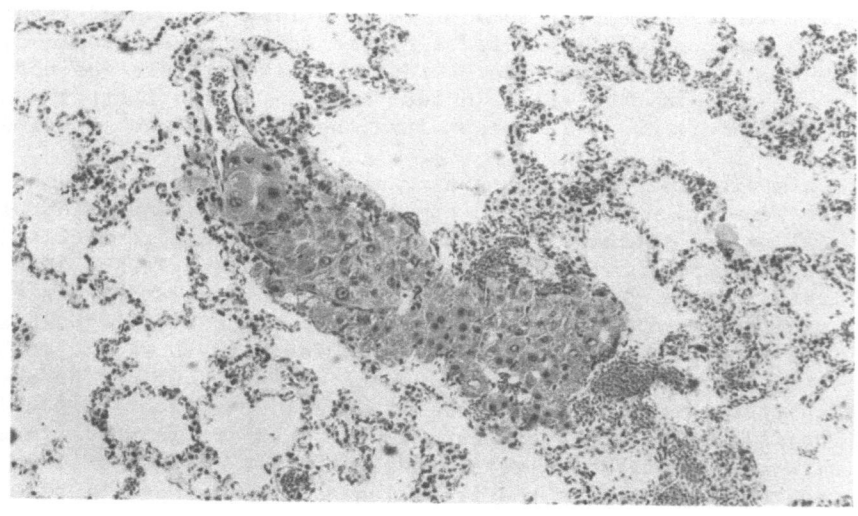

Figure 3
5123. Primary. Photomicrograph of a hepatoma cellular pulmonary
vascular thrombus, X 164.

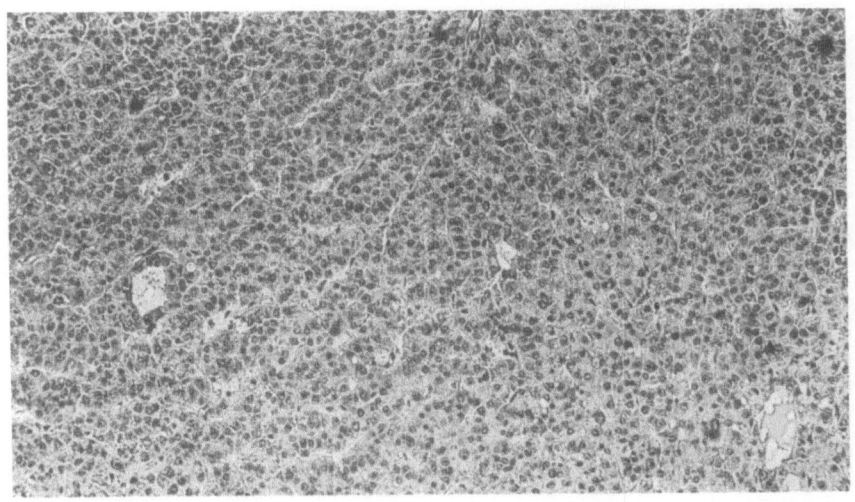

Figure 4
5123. 15. Photomicrograph of a solid sheet of cords of hepatoma cells in which there are several proteinceous fluid filled
cysts. The cysts are lined by hepatoma cells, X 164.

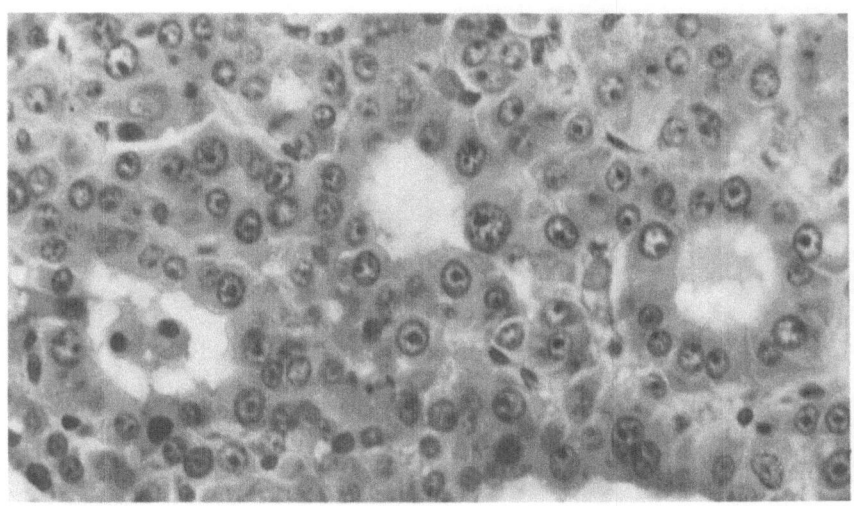

Figure 5
5123. 15. Photomicrograph of hepatoma 5123 (same as in Fig. 4)
is composed of uniform well differentiated cells. Note that some
hepatoma cells have a ductal configuration, X660.

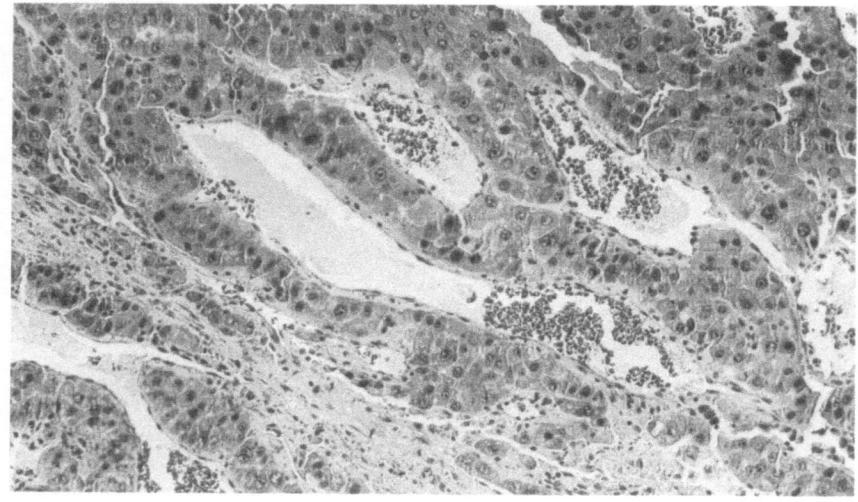

Figure 6
5123. 119. Photomicrograph of broad cords of hepatoma cells
that are separated by partially blood filled vascular channels and
a band of fibrous tissue, X164.

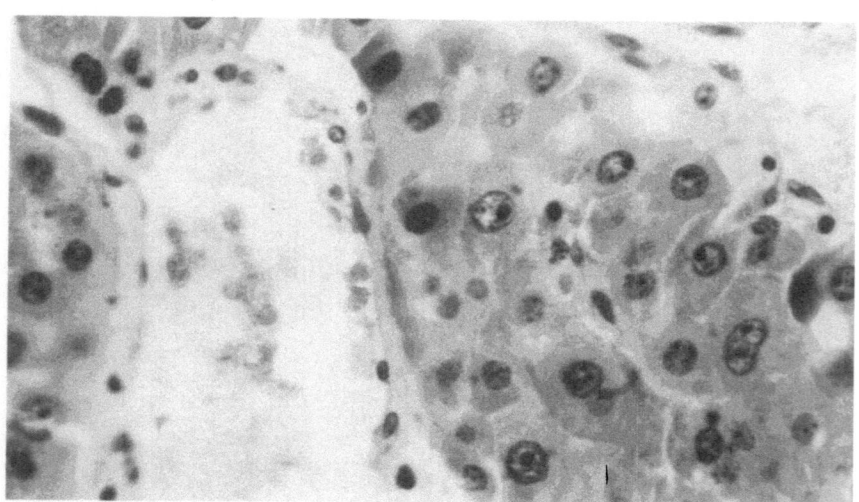

Figure 7
5123. 119. Photomicrograph of a hepatoma that is composed of
well differentiated hepatoma cells which are moderately plemorphic
and well vascularized, X 660.

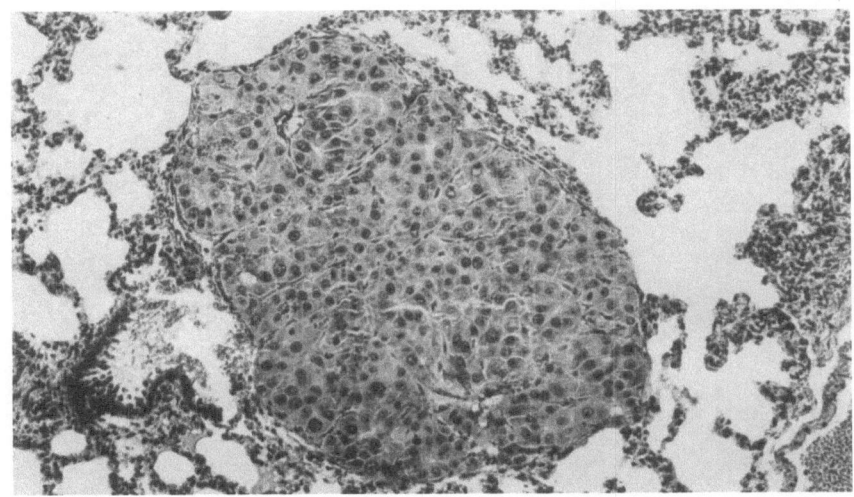

Figure 8
5123. 119. Photomicrograph of a hepatoma cellular metastasis
in the peribronchiolar region of the lung, X 164.

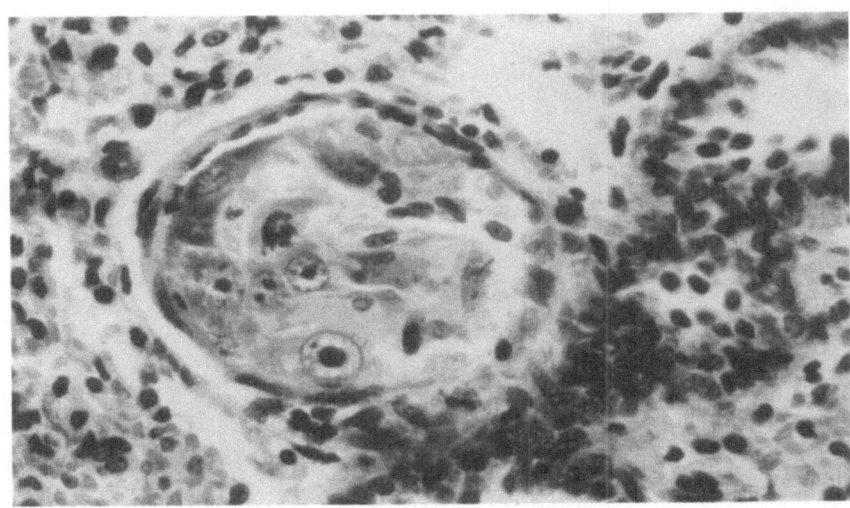

Figure 9
5123. 119. Photomicrograph of a hepatoma cell thrombus that is
occluding and invading the wall of a pulmonary peribronchiolar
blood vessel, X 660.

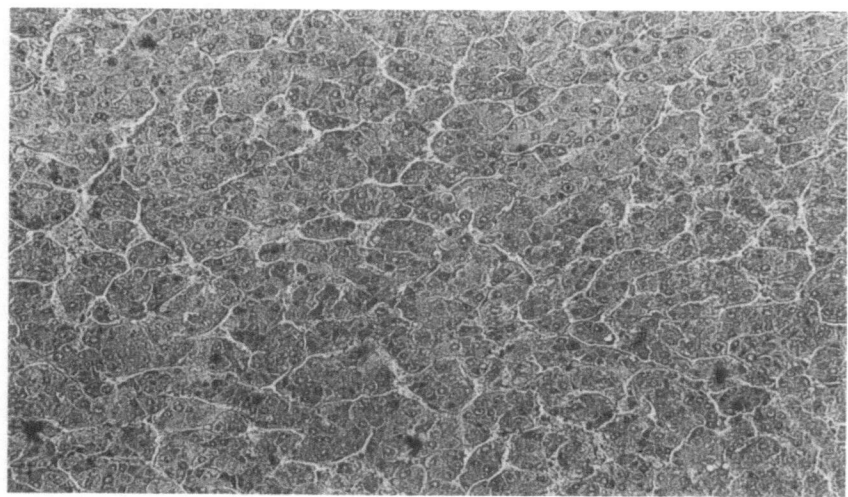

Figure 10
44. Primary. Photomicrograph of a solid compact sheet of
broad short cords and nests of hepatoma cells that are separated
by vascular channels which are partially filled with red blood
cells, X 164.

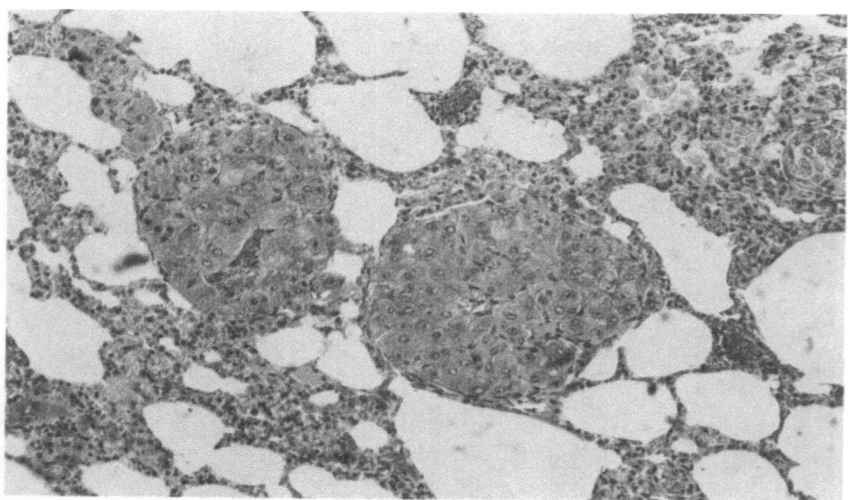

Figure 11
44. Primary. Photomicrograph of several hepatoma cellular
metastases that have replaced portions of the pulmonary septa,
X 164.

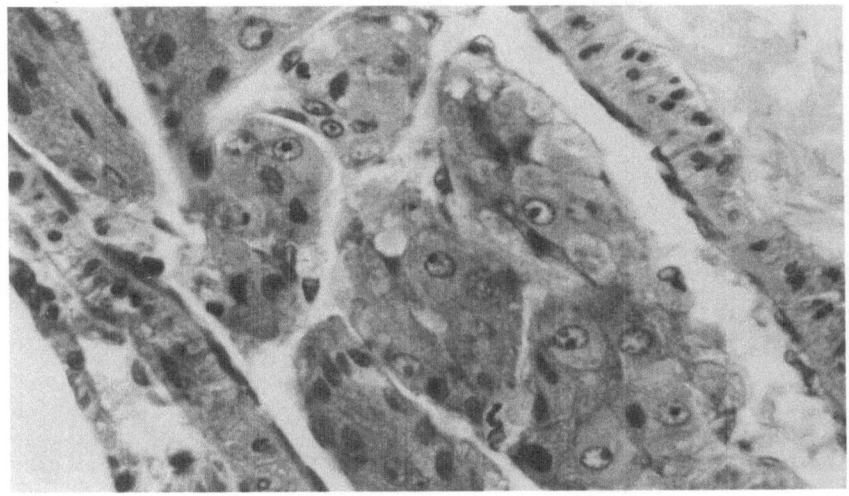

Figure 12
44. Primary. Photomicrograph of pulmonary vessel that is
partially occluded by hepatoma cellular emboli, X 660.

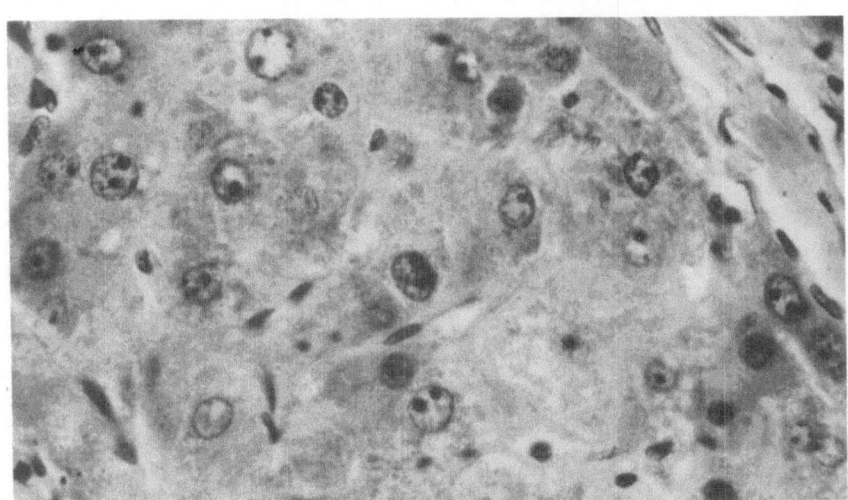

Figure 13
44. 1. Photomicrograph of a hepatoma that is composed of well
differentiated cells that have abundant granular cytoplasm. The
tumor is partially circumscribed by fibrous tissue, X 660.

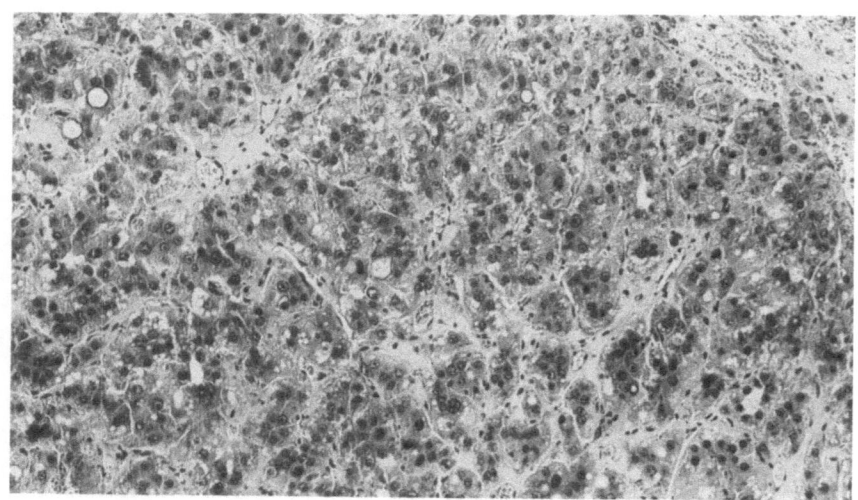

Figure 14
44. 20. Photomicrograph of a hepatoma that is composed of
compact solid nests and irregular disrupted cords of cells.   Some
tumor cells have single or multiple clear cytoplasmic vascuoles.
The cords and nests of cells are separated by vascular channels
and maturing collagen, X 164.

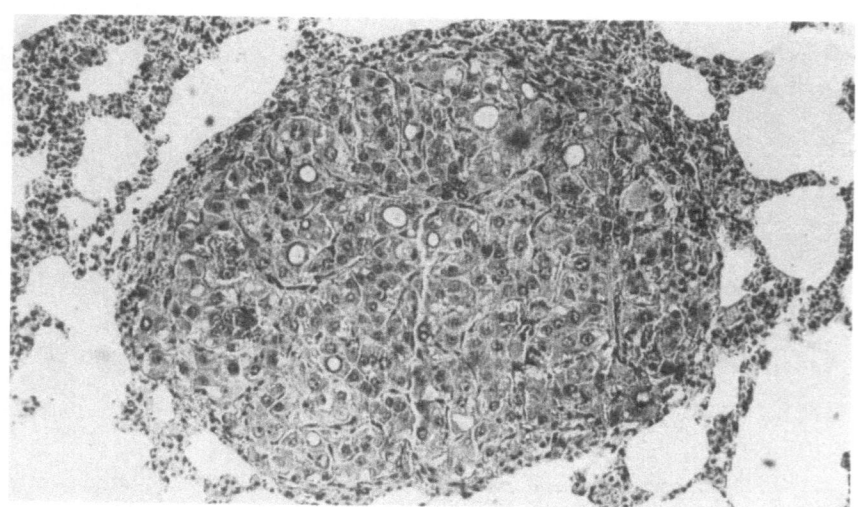

Figure 15
44. 20. Photomicrograph of hepatoma cellular metastatic nodule
that has replaced a portion of the pulmonary septa, X 164.

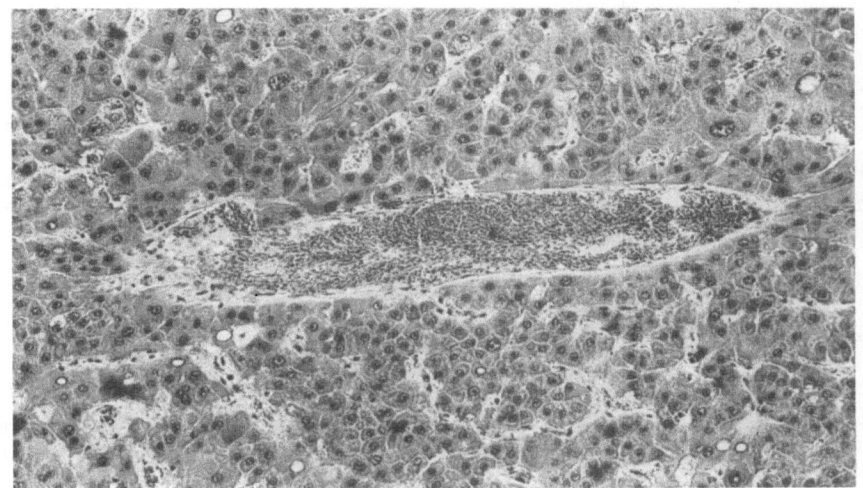

Figure 16
21. Primary. Photomicrograph of a hepatoma that is composed
of a solid sheet of short cords and compact nests of cells. The
cords and nests of cells are separated by vascular channels containing red blood cells. A large blood vessel filled with red
blood cells is present in the center of the photograph, X 164.

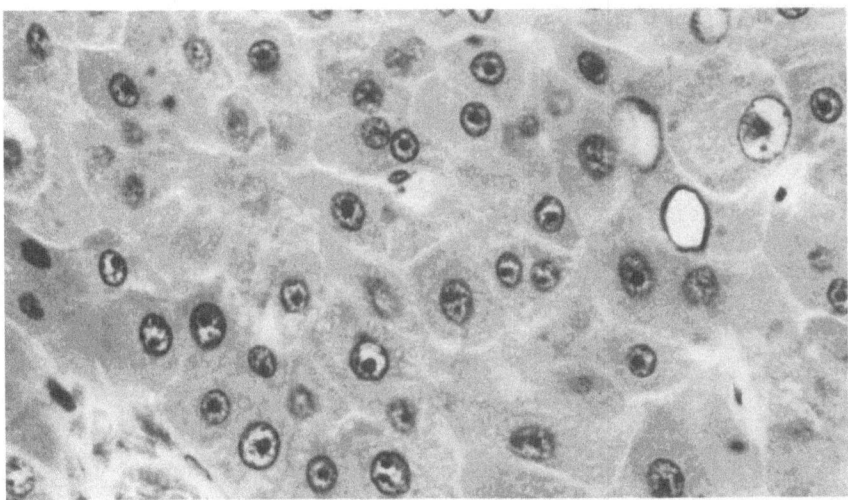

Figure 17
21. Primary. Photomicrograph of a hepatoma that is composed of
uniform well differentiated hepatoma cells, X660.

REFERENCES

1. Barnes, J.M. and Butler, W.H. Nature, 202 (1964) 1016.

2. Kavi, E. and Morris, H.P. In: Advances in Enzyme Regulations, G. Weber (ed). Pergamon Press, Oxford, 14 (1976) pp. 139-162.

3. Morris, H.P. In: Handbuch der allgemeinen Pathologie, Sechster Band Geschwulste, Tumors III, Siebenter Teil, E. Grundmann (ed). Springer-Verlag, New York (1975) pp. 277-334.

4. Morris, H.P. J. Natl. Cancer Inst. 15 (1955) 1535.

5. Morris, H.P. In: Progress in Experimental Tumor Reserach, New York, Karger, Basel, 3 (1963) pp. 370-411.

6. Morris, H.P. In: Advances in Cancer Research, S. Weinhouse and A. Haddow (eds). Academic Press, New York 9 (1965) pp. 227-302.

7. Morris, H.P., Dyer, H.M, Wagner, B.P., Miyaji, H. and Rechcigl, M. In: Advances in Enzyme Regulations, G. Weber (ed). Pergamon Press, New York 2 (1964) pp. 321-333.

8. Morris, H.P. In: Gann Monograph 1, H.P. Morris and O. Hayaishi (eds). Japan: The Japanese Foundation for Cancer Res. and the Japanese Cancer Assoc., (1966) pp. 1-10.

9. Morris, H.P. In: Metabolic Aspects of Food Safety, F.J.C. Roe (ed), (1970) pp. 309-327.

10. Morris, H.P. and Eyestone, W.H. J. Natl. Cancer Inst. 13 (1953) 1139.

11. Morris, H.P., Dubnik, C.S. and Johnson, J.M. J. Natl. Cancer Inst. 10, (1950) 1201.

12. Morris, H.P. and Firminger, H.I. J. Natl. Cancer Inst. 16 (1956) 927.

13. Morris, H.P. and Meranze, D.R. In: Recent Results in Cancer Research, E. Grundmann (ed). Springer-Verlag, New York 44 (1974) pp.103-114.

14. Morris, H.P., Meranze, D.R. and Miyaji, H. In: Proc. Vth Qudrennial Int'l Conf. on Cancer, L. Severi (ed), Perugia, Italy (1974) pp. 955-966.

15. Miyaji, H., Morris, H.P. and Wagner, B.P. In: Methods in Cancer Research, H. Busch (ed). Academic Press, New York IV(1968) p. 153.

16. Morris, H.P. and Wagner, B.P. In: Methods In Cancer Reserach, H. Busch (ed). Academic Press, New York IV (1968) pp. 125-152.

17. Morris, H.P., Sidransky, H., Wagner, B.P. and Dyer, H.M. Cancer Res. 20 (1960) 1252.

18. Morris, H.P., Velat, C.A., Wagner, B.P., Dahlgard, M. and Ray, F.E. J. Natl. Cancer Inst. 24 (1960) 149.

19. Morris, H.P. and Wagner, B.P. Acta Unio Intern. Contra. Cancrum. 20 (1964) 1364.

20. Nowell, P.C. and Morris, H.P. Cancer Res. 29 (1969) 969.

21. Nowell, P.C., Morris, H.P. and Potter, V.R. Cancer Res. 27 (1967) 1565.

22. Odashima, S. and Morris, H.P. In: Gann Monograph 1, H.P. Morris, and O. Hyaishi (eds). (1966) pp. 55-64.

23. Reuber, M.D. In: Gann Monograph 1, H.P. Morris and O. Hyaishi (eds). (1966) pp. 43-54.

24. Sidransky, H., Wagner, B.P. and Morris, H.P. J. Natl. Cancer Inst. 26 (1961) 151.

25. Weber, G. In: Morris Hepatomas-Mechanisms of Regulation, H.P. Morris and W.E. Criss (eds). Plenum Press, New York (1977).

CONTRIBUTION OF THE MORRIS HEPATOMAS TO THE BIOCHEMISTRY OF CANCER – ESTABLISHMENT OF THE PHENOTYPIC HETEROGENEITY OF NEOPLASMS IN VIVO

Henry C. Pitot and James Cardelli

The McArdle Laboratory for Cancer Research
Departments of Oncology and Pathology
University of Wisconsin Medical School
Madison, Wisconsin   53706

SUMMARY

Studies on the biochemistry of the Morris hepatomas have demonstrated that concepts of cancer held prior to 1960 which included that of Warburg on the glycolysis of tumors, Greenstein on the convergence of tumors and various aspects of the deletion hypothesis do not apply to a number of these hepatocellular carcinomas. Extensive investigations of the Morris hepatomas have been unable to demonstrate any single, unqiue biochemical characteristic of all of these hepatomas. Rather one can say that mechanisms regulating the expression of genetic information are defective in a variety of ways in this series of neoplasms, with no hepatoma exhibiting completely normal responses to the environment in vivo. This abnormal regulation of genetic expression extends to the expression of fetal isozymes as well.

In accord with the varieties of abnormalities in the regulation of genetic expression, one may say that the Morris hepatomas exemplify to the greatest extent yet found, the phenotypic individuality of each neoplasm and neoplastic line. Such biochemical heterogeneity has also been seen in a number of other experimental and human neoplasms of varied tissue origin. Recent studies in hepatocarcinogenesis from this and other laboratories has demonstrated that phenotypic heterogeneity may occur at the earliest stage in the development of hepatocellular carcinomas, further establishing phenotypic heterogeneity as the ubiquitous biochemical characteristic of neoplasms in vivo.

INTRODUCTION

Biochemical Concepts of Neoplasia In Vivo - Pre 1960

Almost half a century has now elapsed since the publication of
Otto Warburg's treatise on the metabolism of tumors (59). During
this time many studies on the biochemistry of cancer have come and
gone. Since Warburg many investigators have searched for a ubiquitous biochemical characteristic of cancer. The late Jesse Greenstein
in the second edition of his "Biochemistry of Cancer" (16) summarized
most of the available knowledge of the biomedical characteristics of
neoplastic cells which had been accumulated up to the middle of this
century.

Greenstein's approach to the search for the biochemical unique-
ness of cancer was developed on a background of a wider breadth of
biochemical knowledge than that available to Warburg. Greenstein
was acutely aware of the biology of the organism and the fact that
the various tissues of the animal were not only morphologically
unique,but his morphology resulted in or from a unique biochemistry
of the tissue itself. With this knowledge Greenstein demonstrated
that a variety of normal mouse tissues each exhibited a characteristic pattern of levels of 10 different enzymes (17). In modern ter-
minology one may say that each of the tissues studied exhibited a
distinct phenotype. On the other hand a variety of neoplasms arising
from a number of these various tissues exhibited a relatively uniform
enzyme pattern of phenotype with the exception of one tumor, an osteo-
genic sarcoma, which exhibited very high levels of phosphatases. Thus
Greenstein's extension of the Warburg hypothesis stated that not only
did all neoplasms exhibit a relatively higher rate of glycolysis, but
also that all neoplasms tended toward an expression of the same or
similar enzymatic patterns. In other words the phenotypes of experimental neoplasms were converging towards a similar ubiquitous state
of biochemical equilibrium.

While Greenstein was working on the experiments from which he
formulated this theory of convergence, the Millers at the McArdle
laboratory demonstrated that neoplasms arising in animals fed carcinogenic azo dyes (28) or those tumors occurring in the skin after treatment with benzpyrene (27) exhibited a loss of the ability of the proteins of the neoplasms to bind the carcinogen to such macromolecules
in a covalent manner. Later these investigators formulated the deletion hypothesis of oncogenesis on the basis of these findings (29).
In simplest terms, the Millers suggested that the carcinogen inter-
acted with key macromolecules, presumably proteins (the molecular
biology of the genetic material was not understood when the deletion
hypothesis was first formulated) and by some mechanism these key macromolecules, likely proteins, were eliminated from the cell thus resulting in the derangement of growth and biochemical phenotype. Later

Potter (47) brought the deletion hypothesis into contemporary biochemical thinking by relating it to the genetic material, DNA,
suggesting, on the basis of his own and other experiments, that the
action of the carcinogen resulted in the deletion of certain enzymes,
especially those not necessary for or antagonistic to cellular replication and anabolism (47).

Thus in 1959 the biochemical concept of neoplasia consisted of
three principal characteristics.

1) The neoplastic cell exhibited a defective respiration and
an increased rate of glycolysis (Warburg).

2) All neoplastic cells tended to converge on a similar biochemical phenotype (Greenstein).

3) Neoplastic cells resulting from chemical carcinogenesis exhibited a loss of proteins with both known and unknown functions, especially of enzymes related to catabolic cellular functions (Miller
and Miller; Potter). It was at this time the Morris hepatomas made
their appearance in cancer research.

Biochemical Concepts of Neoplasia In Vivo - Post 1960

Although in 1959 our understanding of the biochemistry of cancer
was, as summarized above, generally accepted, experimental oncologists
were not unanimously in support of these concepts. In 1956 Weinhouse
(61) disagreed with the basic concepts of Warburg as a critical biochemical characteristic of neoplasia. In 1959, studies by Pitot (35)
demonstrated that both primary and transplanted rat hepatomas differed in their morphology as well as their biochemistry. In the latter
instance several hepatomas exhibited the presence of catabolic enzymes
which were absent from hepatomas (exemplified by the transplantable
Novikoff hepatoma) studied as models in support of the enzyme deletion
hypothesis, In retrospect these findings, which played a role leading
to the definitive biochemical investigations of a number of highly differentiated hepatocellular carcinomas, were a corroboration of earlier
data described in Greenstein's book (28, 45).

From 1960 on a number of transplanted hepatocellular carcinomas
were shown to differ dramatically from the vast majority of hepatomas
studied up until that time in that their biochemical characteristics
were quite similar to those seen in normal liver (36, 49, 50). In a
summary of the biochemical characteristics of the first of the Morris
hepatomas to be investigated, the 5123, Pitot (39) pointed out a
number of the biochemical characteristics of this neoplasm which had
been uncovered during the first four years that it was investigated.
Particularly in relation to our discussion, the following points were
noted.

1)   The Morris hepatoma 5123 exhibited no aerobic glycolysis (1).

2)   The hepatoma bound hepatocarcinogens to its proteins
although at a somewhat lower level than that seen in liver and this
hepatoma possessed the characteristic protein which bound the dye and
had reportedly been absent from previous hepatomas investigated.

3)   The Morris hepatoma 5123 exhibited a biochemical phenotype,
i.e. a qualitative enzymatic pattern essentially identical to that
seen in normal liver.

Therefore within only a couple of years and the intense investigation of a relatively few neoplasms from one tissue, liver, the
entire background and basis of the biochemistry of neoplasia up to
that time was severely shaken if not eliminated. Although the biochemical concepts of neoplasia prior to 1960 continued to occupy the
studies of some oncologists, it was clear that a new theoretical
framework on which to plan rational experiments designed to delienate
molecular mechanisms of the neoplastic transformation in vivo was
necessary. The time had come to relate the pathology or biology of
neoplasia to our attempts to understand its molecular basis.

MAIN BODY

The Pathobiology of Neoplasia - Its Relationship to Molecular
Mechanisms

Studies of the pathology, pathogenesis and natural history of
neoplasia in man and lower animals have occupied physicians and
scientists for more than 100 years. Greenstein recognized the importance of understanding the biology of neoplasia before undertaking
an investigation of its molecular characteristics. In actual fact
however, even today the biology of neoplasia is not understood or
even considered in depth by many investigators studying it molecular
mechanisms. Even the definition of the disease entity in its simplest form becomes an essential guide to mechanistic experiments.
Such was clearly the case with the Morris transplanted hepatocellular
carcinomas, malignant neoplasms by biologic criteria but nonconforming
to the biochemical concepts of neoplasia at that time.

"A neoplasm is a relatively autonomous growth of tissue (38)".

This general definition modified from Ewing emphasizes the operational characteristic of neoplasms, their growth, and the fact that
they arise in tissues. Most critical to this and any definition of
neoplasia is the phrase "relative autonomy" or its equivalent. As has
been pointed out by this laboratory (38) as well as that of others (50)
relative autonomy may be equated with the regulation of the expression
of the genetic information inherent in the cell. Normal cells obey a

relatively limited and strict pattern of response to their environment while neoplastic cells in one way or another do not obey the same regulatory pattern as the cells from which they arose. This fact and the advances in biochemical knowledge, especially in the area of the regulation of genetic expression, led investigators to study the biochemistry of "relative autonomy".

The autonomy of Ewing's definition, which was intially formulated prior to 1940, was based on the biological observations of altered control in neoplasm dating back to the last century. In 1957 Burnet expressed the biological feature of "relative autonomy" in his writings (9). In 1959 Pitot described experiments using both primary and transplanted hepatocellular carcinomas in which the environmental regulation of the level of tryptophan oxygenase (then termed tryptophan peroxidase) was absent or abnormal in the neoplasms compared to liver (34). Later studies confirmed and extended these investigations both with this enzyme and with other enzymes as well (6, 7, 31, 42, 44). Since the early 1960's when these investigations were intially published, numerous examples of the "relative autonomy" of enzymes in the Morris hepatomas have been described. A partial list of such enzymes may be seen in Table 1.

The abnormalities in the environmental regulation of the enzymes listed in Table 1 are not all in the same direction. These control mechanisms are absent or markedly decreased in perhaps the majority of the enzymes listed. On the other hand some enzymes show a greater than normal environmental response to specific stimuli. Examples of this are seen in the case of tyrosine aminotransferase in the Morris 5123 hepatoma (37), glutamine synthetase in response to cortisone administration in several Morris hepatomas (65, 66) and a marked increase in histidase and urocanase activity in the H-35 hepatoma in animals given choline, methionine and vitamine B_{12} (33). In some hepatomas under certain conditions the response of an enzyme to specific environmental regulation may be considered as near normal such as may be seen with several of the microsomal mixed function oxygenases (53) and tyrosine aminotransferase (37). However, it should be noted that not all of the Morris hepatomas exhibit all of the defects noted in Table 1. Rather the rule is that the defective mechanisms controlling these enzymes appear to differ in different neoplasms to the degree that no two neoplasms are identical but rather that each neoplasm is phenotypically unique. This was first exemplified by the studies of Bottomley et al. (7) who demonstrated that the environmental regulation of threonine dehydratase and glucose-6-phosphate dehydrogenase were reciprocal one to the other, i.e. when one enzyme was high the other was low and vice versa. However, in a variety of Morris hepatomas virtually all neoplasms exhibited no environmental regulation of these two enzymes although the constitutive levels in the tumors were found to coincide with at least one reciprocal value pair in normal liver with the exception of the Morris 7800 hepatoma. Later studies by Potter et al.

Table One

Enzymes Exhibiting Abnormalities in their Environmental Regulation in Morris Hepatomas
in vivo

Acetyl Coenzyme A Carboxylase	(25)
Aminolevulinate Synthetase	(5)
Arginase	(69)
Arginosuccinate Synthetase	(69)
Citrate Cleavage Enzyme	(53)
Cytochrome p450	(30)
Fatty Acid Synthetase	(25)
Ferritin	(24)
Glucokinase	(65)
Glucose-6-phosphate dehydrogenase	(7,31,51,53)
Glutamine Aminotransferase	(68)
Glutamine Synthetase	(68)
α Gylcerophosphate Dehydrogenase	(20)
Histidase	(34)
HMG Coenzyme A Reductase	(15,59)
Microsomal Mixed Function Oxygenases	(18,56)
Ornithine Aminotransferase	(51)
Ornithine Decarboxylase	(32)
Pyruvate Kinase	(10,12)
Stearyl Coenzyme A Desaturase	(22)
Threonine Serine Dehydratase	(6,7,51,53)

Table One (Continued)

Tryptophan Oxygenase	(44)
Thymine furacil Reductase	(31)
Thymidine kinase	(51)
Tyrosine Aminotransferase	(38,51,53)
Urocanase	(34)

(50) extended investigations to a measure of four different enzymes under three environmental conditions in 9 Morris hepatomas. No two neoplasms exhibited the same degree of regulation of the four enzymes with the variation extending from a complete lack of control to a "hyper" control of the level of the enzyme in question.

Despite this tremendous degree of heterogeneity, Siperstein and his associates have published extensive data indicating that the feedback regulation of cholesterol biosynthesis probably through HMG-coenzyme A reductase was uniformly absent in all hepatomas, whether transplanted or primary, human or animal (56). However, recent studies by Goldfarb (personal communication) has indicated that certain primary hepatomas do retain this regulatory mechanism. Beirne and Watson (3) recently demonstrated an absence of the cholesterol feedback on HMG-coenzyme A reductase in a hepatoma in vivo but its presence when this hepatoma is grown in vitro. This raises the question of the significance of the absence of cholesterol feedback on HMG-coenzyme A reductase in hepatomas seen in vivo. On the other hand the failure of the induction of ornithine aminotransferase in cells in culture (42) indicates that other regulatory mechanisms efective in Morris hepatomas in vivo may also be seen when tested in vitro. Ultimately when methods are available it will be important to determine which control mechanism defective in neoplasms growing in vivo may also be exhibited in those same neoplasms explanted to tissue culture. On the other hand the delicate host-tumor relationships which exist in the abnormal regulation of several enzymes in Morris hepatomas in vivo are clearly much more meaningful in relation to the natural history of the neoplasm in the host animal than the correction of such defects when the neoplasm is maintained in cells culture. Thus, in attempting to determine the molecular characteristics unique to the neoplastic hepatoma cell, one must consider the cell in many different environments.

The Phenotypic Heterogeneity of Neoplasms As Exemplified by the Morris Hepatomas

From the brief outline of information available to date, one may therefore make the statement that a large number of mechanisms regulating the absolute levels of enzymes in vivo are defective when compared with regulatory mechanisms exhibited by normal liver in vivo. Furthermore it is possible to make the generalization that biochemical mechanisms regulating the expression of genetic information in the Morris hepatomas are defective in some manner in all such neoplasms. However, unlike the concepts of Warburg, Greenstein and others, there is no single control mechanism defective in all hepatomas which could be said to be characteristic of the neoplastic state. Rather it is evident from the available data that (61) even the expression of fetal isozymes, an extreme example of the abnormalities of the regulation of genetic expression seen in experimental hepatomas, are not uniformly controlled in all neoplasms (63). These latter areas are covered in other chapters of this text and thus will not be considered further here.

Although the Morris hepatomas are not the only neoplasms exhibiting phenotypic heterogeneity they best exemplify this ubiquitous biochemical characteristic of neoplasia. Table 2 lists examples of phenotypic heterogeneity seen in other biological types of neoplasms.

Michael Potter and his associates have pioneered the studies of proteins produced by a series of mouse myelomas, demonstrating that the protein produced by each neoplasm is unique to that tumor (47). Such a phenomenon had actually already been known in the case of human myelomas. Hilf and his associates have also demonstrated that in a series of primary and transplanted mammary carcinomas of the rat each neoplasm or neoplastic line is biochemically unique with respect both to its set of quantitative enzyme levels and the environmental mechanisms regulating the level of these enzymes in these neoplasms (19). Several studies (2, 23) have shown that both the isozymic content and the level of amino acid metabolizing enzymes in human renal cell carcinomas vary between different primary neoplasms. Wollman (65) demonstrated considerable variation in ^{131}I uptake in a series of experimental thyroid neoplasms. Both the patterns of the isozymes of aldolase (21) and the activities of enzymes of glycolysis and the TCA cycle (58, 59) differ among different neoplasms of the central nervous system. In this instance, however, the morphologic variation of neoplasms in the central nervous system is also considerable, and thus one may question whether the enzymic variation is actually a result of different cells of origin of the neoplasms. Primary and transplanted mouse hepatomas also exhibit considerable variation in their biochemical phenotypes (8, 53). The example of phenotypic heterogeneity seen in acute leukemia is that of the activity of deoxycytidylate deaminase in human leukemia (4).

Thus it is clear that the Morris hepatomas are not the only series of neoplasms of a specific biological origin which exhibit a wide degree of biochemical heterogeneity. Rather as we learn more of the biochemistry of neoplasms in vivo it would appear that there is no single biochemical phenotype or characteristic unique to all neoplasms or even to all neoplasms of one biological origin. Rather the biochemical characteristic of neoplasia in vivo is its extreme phenotypic heterogeneity. As we have seen earlier (3) whether such phenotypic heterogeneity is characteristic of neoplastic cells when isolated from the host remains to be seen. In part the extreme phenotypic heterogeneity noted in neoplasms may be the result of a delicate host-tumor relationship which magnifies a subtle difference in the regulation of genetic expression between neoplastic cells and their normal tissues of origin.

<u>Table Two</u>

<u>Examples of Phenotypic Heterogeneity Seen in
Neoplasm</u>+

	<u>Ref</u>
Myelomas	(24,49)
Mammary Carcinomas	(19)
Renal Carcinomas	(2,23)
Thyroid neoplasms	(67)
Brain Tumors	(21,60,21)
Primary Mouse Hepatomas	(8,55)
Acute Leukemia	(4)

+ See text for further details.

INTERPRETATION

Implications of Phenotypic Heterogeneity in the Natural History and Molecular Mechanisms of the Origin of Neoplasia

If phenotypic heterogeneity is the biochemical characteristic of all neoplasms, a major question arises as to whether or not such biochemical heterogeneity is merely the result of the natural history of neoplasia. On the basis of the biochemistry of the Morris hepatomas both the Warburg and Greenstein hypotheses are likely the result of tumor progression as suggested by Foulds (13). Therefore, if biochemical heterogeneity were the result of tumor progression, one would expect early neoplastic, or so called "pre-neoplastic" lesions, to exhibit little or no phenotypic heterogeneity. As has been pointed out from this laboratory earlier this does not seem to be so (46).

In 1968 Frudrich-Freska and his associates demonstrated the production of glucose-6-phosphate dehydrogenase deficient "islands" of hepatic tissue following administration of diethylnitrosamine (14). Later studies by these and other workers (52) demonstrated the likely precursor relationship of such "islands" to hepatocellular carcinoma. Recent experiments in our laboratory (41) modeled after those of Scherer and Emmelot (57) and Perano et al.(33) have shown that such "islands" are biochemically heterogenous with respect to three different enzymes. Therefore, although experiments have not been carried out as yet to follow the progression of these enzyme altered foci completely to hepatic neoplasms, the evidence to date strongly argues that even in the earliest identifiable cellular population which gives rise to neoplasms, phenotypic heterogeneity is already evident. Therefore biochemical variation does not appear to be a function of tumor progression but rather may be characteristically seen in the earliest cellular populations leading to biologic malignancy.

While it is not the purpose of this paper to discuss at length potential mechanisms of phenotypic heterogeneity seen in neoplasms our previous studies have suggested that such heterogeneity, at least in liver neoplasms, may reflect alterations in messenger RNA template stability (40). We have postulated that messenger RNA template stability itself may be a result of the interaction of messenger RNA molecules directly with the surface of intracellular membranes. The stabilization of messenger RNA may be mediated through the interaction of proteins on the surface of the membrane. Such a postulation suggests that this may be true as noted in Figure 1. This figure shows SDS polyarcylamide gel electrophoretograms of protein associated with polysoma mRNA of liver and three Morris hepatomas. The molecular weights of the pricipal proteins are noted in the upper pattern and it can be seen that two of these proteins, those having a molecular weight of 73,000 and 52,000 are relatively constant in amount between liver and

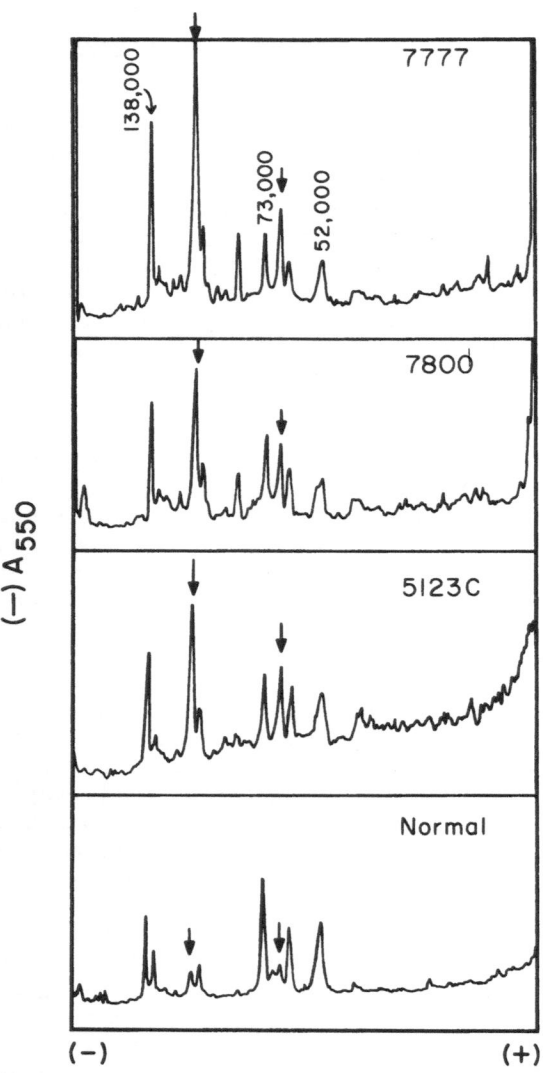

Figure 1
Gel electrophoresis of Oligo (dT)-cellulose Isolated Free
Polysomal mRNP. Free polysomal mRNP eluted from columns with a
formamide containing buffer were precipitated overnight with ethanol.
Pellets were dissolved in sample buffer and aliquots were subjected
to SDS polyacrylamide gel electrophoresis, After staining with
coomassie Blue gels were scanned at 550 nonometers.

the three hepatomas. However, differences in the protein patterns of the hepatomas themselves can be discerned. The significance of this data which shows that there may be differences in the types of protein bound to messenger RNAs in hepatomas when compared to mRNA bound proteins in normal liver remains uncertain. These proteins may be involved in some aspect of mRNA metabolism including its degredation but the exact mechanism by which they act remains to be determined. Conceivably these proteins affect the phenotypic heterogeneity seen in Morris hepatomas.

REFERENCES

1. Aisenberg, A.C. and Morris, H.P. Nature, 91 (1961) 1314.

2. Allegri, G., Benassi, C.A., Boccu, E., DeNadai, A. and
    Perissinotto, B. Biritsh J. of Cancer 19 (1965) 754.

3. Beirne, O.R. and Watson, J.A. Proc. Natl. Acad. Sci. U.S.A.
    73 (1976) 2735.

4. Bernengo, M.G. and Pegoraro. Eur. J. of Cancer 12 (1976) 611.

5. Bonkowsky, H.L., Tschudy, D.P., Collins, A. and Doherty, J.M.
    J. Natl. Cancer Inst. 50 (1973) 1215.

6. Bottomley, R.H., Pitot, H.C. and Morris, H.P. Cancer Res. 23
    (1963) 392.

7. Bottomley, R.H., Pitot, H.C., Potter, V.R. and Morris, H.P.
    Cancer Res. 23 (1963) 400.

8. Bresnick, E., Mayfiled, E.D., Liebelt, A.G. and Liebelt, R.A.
    Cancer Res. 31 (1971) 743.

9. Burnet, M. British Med. J 1 (1957) 779.

10. Campadelli-Fiume, G., Della Corte, D. and Stirpe, F. Biochem.
    J. 118 (1970) 195.

11. Cho, Y.S., Pitot, H.C. and Morris, H.P. Cancer Res. 24 (1964) 52.

12. Criss, W.E., and Morris, H.P. Cancer Res. 31 (1971) 1879.

13. Foulds, L. Cancer Res. 25 (1965) 1339.

14. Freidrich-Freska, H., Papadopulu, G. and Gossner, W. Zeitschrift
    Kreboforschung, 72 (1969) 240.

15. Goldfarb, S. and Pitot, H.C. Cancer Res. 24 (1964) 52.

16. Greenstein, J.P. Biochemistry of Cancer. New York. Academic
    Press, 1954.

17. Greenstein, J.P. Cancer Res. 16 (1956) 641.

18. Hart, L.B., Adamson, R.H., Morris, H.P. and Fouts, J.R. J. Pharm.
    and Exper. Therapeutics, 149 (1965) 7.

19. Hilf, R., Goldenberg, H., Gruenstein, M., Meranz, D.R. and

Schimkin, M.B. Cancer Res. 30 (1970) 1223.

20. Hunt, S.M., Osnos, M.and Rivlin, R.S. Cancer Res. 30 (1970) 1764.

21. Kumanishi, T., Iku, T.A. and Yamamoto, T. Acta Neuropath. (Berlin) 16 (1970) 220.

22. Lee, T.C., Stephens, N. and Snyder, F. Cancer Res. 30 (1970) 1764.

23. Li, J.J., Li, S.A., Klein, L.A. and Villee, C.A. In: Isozymes, C.L. Markerd (ed). Academic Press, New York, 3 (1975) 837.

24. Linder, M., Munro, H.N. and Morris, H.P. Cancer Res. 30 (1970) 2231.

25. Magerus, P.W., Jacobs, R. and Smith, M.B. J. Biol. Chem. 243 (1968) 3588.

26. McIntrire K.R. and Potter, M. J. Natl. Cancer Inst. 33 (1964) 631.

27. Miller, E.C. Cancer Res. LL (1951) 100.

28. Miller, E.C. and Miller, J.A. Cancer Res. 7 (1947) 468.

29. Miller, J.A. and Miller, E.C. Adv. in Cancer Res. 1 (1953) 340.

30. Miyake, Y., Gaylor, J.L. and Morris, H.P. J. Biol. Chem. 249 (1974) 1980.

31. Ono, T., Potter, V.R., Pitot, H.C. and Morris, H.P. Cancer Res. 23 (1964) 385.

32. Pariza, M.W., Yanagi, S., Gurr, J.A., Morris, H.P. and Potter, V.R. Life Sciences 19 (1976) 1553.

33. Perano, C., Fry, R.J.M., Staffeldt, E. and Kisieleski, W.E. Cancer Res. 33 (1974) 2701.

34. Petri, W.A., Poirier L.A. and Morris, H.P. Biochem. Biophys. Acta, 321 (1973) 681.

35. Pitot, H.C. Bultn. Tulane Univ. Med. Fac. 19 (1959) 17.

36. Pitot, H.C. Studies on the Control of Protein Synthesis in Normal and Neoplastic Rat Liver; Ph.D. Thesis, Tulane Univ. New Orleans, 1959.

37. Pitot, H.C. Cancer Res. 20 (1960) 1262.

38. Pitot, H.C. Adv. in Enzyme Reg. 1 (1962) 309.

39. Pitot, H.C. Cancer Res. 23 (1963) 1474.

40. Pitot, H.C. Acta Union Internatl. Cont. Can. 20 (1964) 919.

41. Pitot, H.C. J. Natl. Cancer Inst. 53 (1974) 905.

42. Pitot, H.C. Amer. J. Pathol., in the press.

43. Pitot, H.C. and Jost, J.P. J. Natl. Cancer Inst. Mono. 26 (1967) 145.

44. Pitot, H.C. and Morris, H.P. Cancer Res. 21 (1961) 1009.

45. Pitot, H.C., Cardell, J. Long, B. and McLaughlin, C. In: Control Mechanisms in Cancer, W.E. Criss, T. Ono and J.R. Saline (eds). Raven Press, New York, (1976) p. 329.

46. Pitot, H.C., Peraino, C., Bottomley, R.H. and Morris, H.P. Cancer Res. 23 (1963) 135.

47. Pitot, H.C., Potter, V.R. and Morris, H.P. Cancer Res. 23 (1964) 385.

48. Pitot, H.C., Shires, T.K., Moyer, G. and Garrett, C.T. In: The Molecular Biology of Cancer, H. Busch (ed). Academic Press, New York (1974) p. 523.

49. Potter, M. J. Exper. Med. 115 (1962) 339.

50. Potter, V.R. Federation Proc. 17 (1958) 691.

51. Potter, V.R. Gebert, R.A., Pitot, H.C., Peraino, C., Lamar, C., Lesher, S. and Morris, H.P. Cancer Res. 26 (1966) 1547.

52. Potter, V.R., Pitot, H.C., Ono, T. and Morris, H.P. Cancer Res. 20 (1960) 1255.

53. Potter, V.R., Watanabe, M., Pitot, H.C. and Morris, H.P. Cancer Res. 29 (1969) 55.

54. Rabes, H.M., Scholze, P. and Jantsch, B. Cancer Res. 32 (1972) 2577.

55. Reynolds, R.D., Potter, V.R., Pitot, H.C. and Reuber, M.D. Cancer Res. 31 (1971) 808.

56. Rogers, L.A., Morris, H.P. and Fouts, J.R. J. Phar. Exper.

Therapeutics, 157 (1967) 227.

57. Scherer, E. and Emmelot, P. Cancer Res. 36 (1976) 2544.

58. Shatton, J.B., Morris, H.P. and Weinhouse, S. Cancer Res. 29 (1969) 1161.

59. Siperstein, M.D., Gude, A.M. and Morris, H.P. Proc. Natl. Acad. Sci. U.S.A. 86 (1971) 315.

60. Viale, G.L. Acta Neurochirurgica, 20 (1969) 263.

61. Viale, G.L. Acta Neurochirurgica, 20 (1969) 273.

62. Warburg, O. Metabolism of Tumors. Arnold Constable, London, 1930.

63. Weber, G. In: The Molecular Biology of Cancer. H. Busch (ed). Academic Press, New York (1974) p. 487.

64. Weinhouse, S. Science, 124 (1956) 267.

65. Weinhouse, S. Federation Proc. 32 (1973) 2162.

66. Williamson, D.H., Krebs, A.J., Stubbs, M., Page, M.A., Morris, H.P. and Weber, G. Cancer Res. 30 (1970) 2049.

67. Wollman, S.H. Recent Progress in Hormone Res. 15 (1963) 579.

68. Wu, C. and Morris, H.P. Cancer Res. 30 (1970) 2675.

69. Wu, C., Bauer, J.M. and Morris, H.P. Cancer Res. 31 (1971) 12.

THE MORRIS HEPATOMAS AS MODELS FOR STUDIES OF GENE EXPRESSION IN NEOPLASIA[1]

Jennie B. Shatton and Sidney Weinhouse

The Fels Research Institute and the Department of
Biochemistry
Temple University School of Medicine
Philadelphia, Pennsylvania 19140

It would be difficult to exaggerate the impact of the Morris hepatomas on contemporary cancer research. For nearly two decades this series of chemically-induced, transplantable rat liver neoplasms has been a favored experimental model system for a wide range of approaches to the understanding of the neoplastic process. The large volume of research publications, reviews and symposia that have focused on the Morris hepatomas (48, 49, 50, 54, 81, 83) attest to their importance for large segments of cancer biology. One area in particular, that of tumor enzymology and metabolism, has exploited the Morris hepatomas to great advantage. It has become evident that the Morris hepatomas, derived from a single cell type, the parenchymal cell of the liver, can exhibit an astonishing range of biological properties such as growth rate, morphology, and chromosome number. Underlying and paralleling these is an equally broad range of enzymic and metabolic activities (48, 49, 50, 54, 81, 83). This diversity of behavior has been both a challange and unprecendented opportunity for revealing molecular mechanisms responsible for neoplastic behavior. From a comprehensive study of a wide range of Morris hepatomas Weber (81), in enunciating what he has termed the Molecular Correlation Concept, pointed out that their wide range of growth rates is accompanied by and is probably determined by variations in the relative activities of so-called anabolic and catabolic enzymes.

It is equally striking that variations in growth rate, differentiation and metabolism of the Morris hepatomas are associated with marked changes in isozyme composition, that expand, amplify, and add functional significance to a growing recognition of a common thread, interwoven through the literature of experimental and clinical cancer; namely, that neoplasia involves abnormalities of gene expression, manifested phenotypically by mis-programming of protein synthesis.

Before proceeding to describe these isozyme alterations, it will be desirable to explain what isozymes are. In 1959 Markert and Moller (43) discovered that enzymes can exist in multimolecular forms, thus adding new dimensions to our knowledge of enzyme regulation. The term isozyme or isoenzyme is generally restricted to different gene products; those with different primary structures, as contrasted with modifications of an enzyme protein such as may be achieved by phosphorylation, adenylation, partial proteolysis, etc. An illustrative example is lactate dehydrogenase, which occurs as two distinct protein subunits. The active form of the enzyme is a tetramer, which may consist of the same subunits, or different combinations of the two subunits; e.g., M_4, M_3H, M_2H_2, MH_3, and H_4. The M (muscle) and H (heart) subunits have different primary structures and regulatory and kinetic properties, and the hybrid forms act as mixtures of the two. Each tissue has its distinctive pattern of isozyme composition, presumably determined by selective gene activation, although other factors, such as differential rates of destruction may also play a part.

Since Markert's original discovery, the number of enzymes known to exist in isozymic forms has multiplied exponentially (44), and it has become increasingly recognized that the isozyme composition of a tissue is of great functional importance. This is particularly true of the liver, which has a unique pattern of isozymes, reflecting the many unique biochemical functions of this organ. To cite a few examples of isozymes unique to liver, there are hepatic forms of hexokinase, aldolase, pyruvate kinase, phosphorylase, and tyrosine aminotransferase (37). These are geared kinetically for specific hepatic functions; and in keeping with the role of the liver in maintaining metabolic hemeostasis, the activity levels of many of these isozymes are under the control of hormones. Other isozymes of the enzymes, which occur in non-hepatic tissues, are either low or absent in the normal adult liver.

Isozyme Alteration in Hepatomas

Studies conducted by ourselves and others (13, 54, 60, 83) using the Morris hepatomas or other similar liver neoplasms have made it clear that in liver tumors this pattern of isozyme composition is altered. The degree of alteration depends on the growth rate and the degree of differentiation. The general pattern of alteration, as revealed by studies on a wide spectrum of hepatomas, is depicted in Figure 1. In the most highly differentiated, slow-growing tumors (to which the name "minimal deviation" aptly applies) the isozyme pattern is close to that of the normal adult liver, with a preponderance of the liver type isozymes. These hepatomas also may carry out certain liver functions, such as glycogen storage,

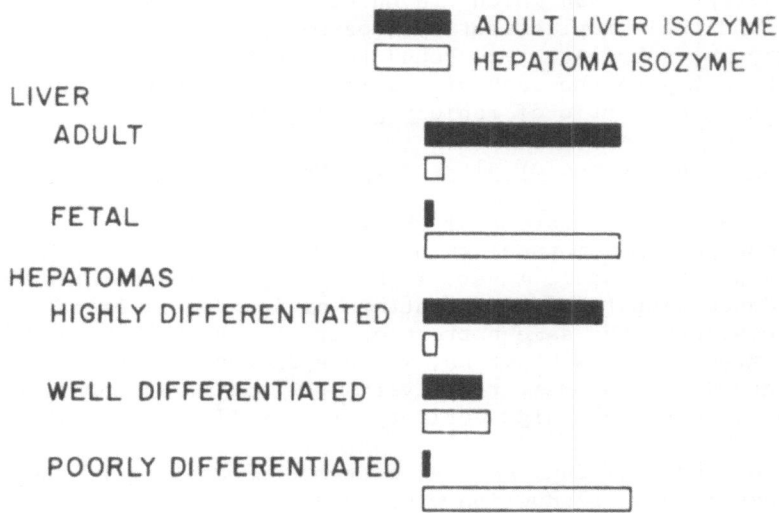

Figure 1
Isozyme patterns typical of a series of enzymes in fetal and adult livers and various hepatomas of the rat. The lengths of the solid bars (liver isozyme) and open bars (hepatoma isozyme) denote relative activities, but are not meant to represent exact quantitative relationships.

(40) ketone body production (8), urea synthesis (39), etc., thus revealing that the retention of liver function in the highly differentiated, slow-growing hepatomas has an underlying molecular foundation in the retention of liver type isozymes.

With decreased differentiation and more rapid growth rate there is a progressive loss of the liver type isozymes, and with further loss of differentiation and rapid growth, a dramatic switch occurs. The liver type isozymes disappear and are replaced by high activities of the non-hepatic isozymes. In view of the differences in their kinetic properties, it is evident that the loss of those liver-type isozymes that are geared for physiological functions in hepatic metabolism, and which are under host dietary and hormonal control, and their replacement by isozymes geared only for efficient utilization of substrates, is bound to result in altered metabolism, and may be a key to the lack of host control and unbridled growth that are characteristic of rapidly growing tumors.

Functional Significance of Altered Isozymes Composition

A striking illustration of the functional importance of isozyme alterations in tumor metabolism has emerged from studies on pyruvate kinase. In normal adult liver, Type I isozyme predominates (Fig 2). In accordance with the general pattern of isozyme alteration in the Morris hepatomas, the same pattern occurs in the highly differentiated, slow-growing 9618A hepatoma, whereas in the poorly differentiated, rapidly growing hepatomas, the liver type isozyme is completely replaced by an extremely high activity of Type III isozyme (18).

One of the striking features of tumor metabolism is their high rate of lactic acid production when incubated in vitro with glucose in an oxygen atmosphere. This process was termed aerobic glycolysis by the famous biochemist, Otto Warburg, and was regarded by him as the key to the cause and possibly the cure of this disease (78, 79). The significance of this phenomenon has been a cause celebre and a subject of much controversy (80, 84, 85). A possible explanation of the high aerobic glycolysis of tumors has come from studies on the Morris hepatomas. The early observations of Aisenberg and Morris (3) and Weber, et al.(82) revealed that the well-differentiated, so-called "minimal deviation" hepatomas had a low aerobic glycolysis and thus differed strikingly from virtually all other tumors, including the rapidly growing, poorly differentiated Morris hepatomas. This divergence in aerobic glycolysis obviously parallels the divergence in pyruvate kinase, as shown in Figure 2, and there is a good reason to believe that the latter may be causal to the former. It was suggested many years ago that glycolysis is held in check by competition between respiration and glycolysis for common substrates (36, 42). Since pyruvate kinase competes with the respiratory system of oxidative phosphorylation for the common substrate, ADP, this enzyme appeared

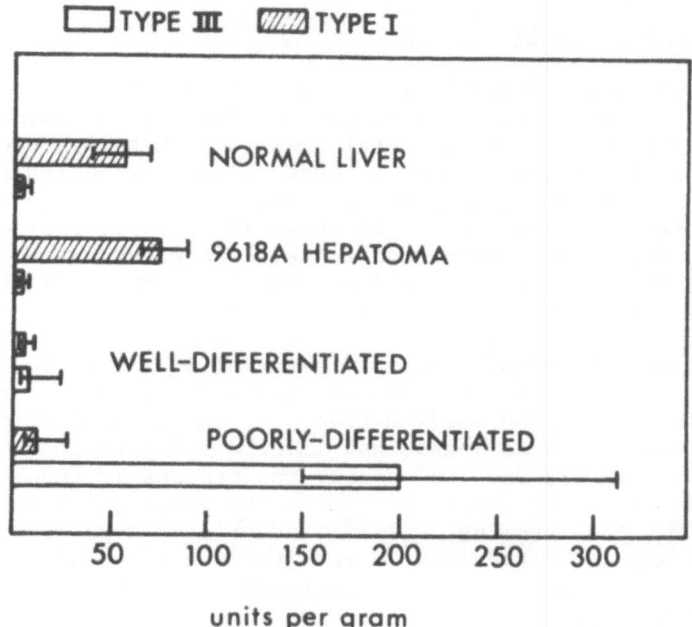

Figure 2
Isozyme pattern of pyruvate kinase in normal adult liver, and various hepatomas of the rat. Shaded bars denote the liver isozyme, pyruvate kinase 1; and open bars denote the hepatoma isozyme, pyruvate kinase 111.

to be a plausible candidate for a determining role in glycolysis of
tumors. In experiments in which glycolytic and respiratory activities were manipulated by varying the relative activities of pyruvate
kinase and mitochondrial respiration, confirmation was obtained for
a rate-determining role of pyruvate kinase in the aerobic glycolysis
of tumors (29, 30). The Morris hepatomas therefore indicate to us
that high aerobic glycolysis is not a sine qua non of cancer, but
rather is associated with a late stage of de-differentiation, accompanied by a marked rise in the activity of a particular isozyme
of pyruvate kinase.

Fetal Isozyme Expression

An extraordinary feature of isozyme alteration in tumors is
that many of the non-hepatic isozymes that replace the liver forms
in hepatomas are also found in fetal tissues. This is a property
of great potential significance, because of the already large and
growing literature pointing to fetal expression of other proteins
in a wide variety of neoplasms. As shown in Table 1, the switch
of isozyme expression in hepatomas to fetal forms occurs with many
enzymes, and there is every likelihood that many more will be discovered with further exploration of other enzymes.

The common pattern of isozyme alteration during differentiation,
and its reversal in cancer is illustrated in Figure 3. A primordial
isozyme characterizes the early embryo. As embryonic development
proceeds, tissues such as muscle and liver develop their own distinctive sets of isozymes. In cancer, the process is reversed. The
reversal does not necessarily occur with the neoplastic transformation, since the slow-growing, well-differentiated hepatomas retain
liver type isozymes. It evidently results from a stepwise process
and reaches the end-point of complete reversion only with loss of
differentiation.

Studies of Fishman and his collaborators have uncovered some
particularly interesting examples of alteration of isozyme composition
associated with fetal and placental expression of alkaline phosphatases in human tumors, including cells in culture (20, 21). Following their initial discovery of a heat-stable placental isozyme in
various human tumors, this enzyme and its numerous variants have
become the subject of much clinical and experimental study (22, 23).

Expression of Fetal Antigens in Cancer

The resurgence of fetal isozymes in cancer has its most striking
parallel in cancer immunology. It has been observed that antigens
present in adult tissues of origin are lost in the neoplastic transformation, and new antigens appear that are not present in the adult,
but may have been present in fetal tissue (1). Baldwin has documented

Table One

Enzymes Expressed as Fetal Isozymes in Liver Neoplasia

		Reference No.
1.	Glucose-ATP phosphotransferase	65
2.	Aldolase	2,61,62
3.	Pyruvate kinase	18,62,63
4.	Glycogen phosphorylase	59
5.	Adenylate kinase	14
6.	Thymidine kinase	53
7.	Alkaline phosphatase	20
8.	Branched-chain amino acid aminotransferase	34
9.	Glutathione- γ-glutamylpeptidotransferase	19
10.	Alcohol dehydrogenase	11
11.	Creatine kinase	64

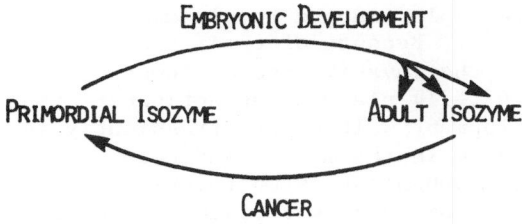

Figure 3
Schematic diagram of isozyme differentiation during normal
embryonic development and its reversal in cancer.

the presence of embryonal antigens in experimental, chemically induced hepatomas (7) and Stonehill and Bendich (70) made similar
observations for a large series of mouse neoplasms. A variety of
liver tumors of the human produce α-fetoglobulin, a protein synthesized in fetal liver and other embryonal tissues (1); and many
human tumors of the gastrointestinal tract produce a glycoprotein
synthesized normally by cells of the fetal, but not the adult digestive system. This protein, termed carcinoembryonic antigen is
being studied intensively as a possible diagnostic aid in human
cancer (27, 28). The literaure on oncofetal gene expression has
become too vast for adequate coverage here, and the reader is referred to several recent comprehensive reviews for more detailed
discussion of its wide occurrance and significance (1, 5, 6, 23,
28, 33).

Fetal Expression and Other Proteins

     Fetal expression in neoplasia is by no means restricted to
enzymes or antigens as such. A variety of human tumors including
HeLa cells have isoferritins, (an iron storage protein), that differ
from the ferritins in normal adult human liver, but share electrophoretic properties with fetal liver isoferritins (15). Ferritins
also appear in animal tumors and cultured cells (58) and can be
detected by radioimmunoassay in serum, thus offering some promise
of clinical significance (52).

     According to Yeoman et al.(86) a chromatin glycoprotein, which
can be detected by double diffusion immunoprecipitation in fetal,
but not in adult rat liver, not in adult kidney or heart, was also
present in the Novikoff hepatoma and the Walker carcinoma. These
ordinarily repressed proteins are alleged to play key roles in cell
growth and division; and their expression in cancer, in the absence
of the controls that keep them in check during normal embryonic
development, may be a key to the neoplastic state.

     An especially exciting example of fetal gene expression in
cancer is the occurrance in transformed cells in culture of proteases which convert plasminogen to plasmin; the so-called plasminogen activators (75). Because of their proteolytic activity they
may play a role in the invasiveness of tumor cells. According to
Sherman, et al. (67, 71) plasminogen activator appears very early
in embryonic development. It occurs transiently in the trophoblast
and parietal endoderm in the mouse, and peaks between the 7th and
9th days when the trophoblast is most invasive. The enzyme activity
appears also in embryoid bodies derived from embryonal carcinoma
cells, but disappears when the embryoid bodies are induced to undergo differentiation to a teratocarcinoma (72).

Ectopic Synthesis of Polypeptide Hormones

One of the most dramatic examples of misplaced protein synthesis in cancer is the bizarre production of polypeptide hormones by numerous non-endocrine neoplasms. Tumors of lung, prostate, kidney, stomach, liver and other organs produce a wide variety of such substances (32), and there is good basis for the belief that ectopic hormone production may also be embryonic in origin. Nathanson and Hall (51) pointed to the common embryonic origin of the pituitary and lung in the endoderm, and suggest that the production of pituitary hormones by lung tumors is a reflection of this common embryonic ancestry.

Levine and Metz (41) have classified most of the hormone-producing tumors in two groups. The tissues involved, and the hormones that may be produced by their tumors are listed in Table 2. Tumors of Group 1 arise from cells which originate from the endoderm and mesoderm. Evidently cancers derived from a wide range of tissues can express potentialities possessed by cells from which these tissues originated during normal embryonic development.

Cancer Disorder of Differentiation

The characterization of cancer as a disorder of differentiation raises a number of questions; and as so often happens in unresolved scientific inquiries, one question leads to others. One of these un-resolved questions concerns the nature of the disorder in cancer. Various terms have been used to describe the phenomenon of fetal gene expression; for example, retrodifferentiation (76), retro-genetic expression (70), derepressive de-differentiation (27), oncofetal expression (22) and blocked ontogeny (57). These words, which describe a general phenomenon attributable to many different experimental and clinical observations, do not convey any implica-tions of mechanism. We know that cancer cells are never totally de-differentiated, nor do they ever reach a stage approaching that of the adult tissúe. Thus the range of differentiation of cancer cells represents only a minor segment of a broader spectrum dis-played by normal tissue. Loss of differentiation in cancer, moreover, does not represent simply a reversal of the orderly phased sequences of normal embryonic development, but is rather a disordered process, aptly described by Matsushima, et al. (45) as dis-differentiation.

Nature of the Cell Target for Neoplasia

One of the baffling enigmas of cancer is that we cannot yet identify a specific cell type that is the target of the transforming agent in vivo. Three possibilities may be envisioned: (a) a fully differentiated cell is transformed, the immediately or in subsequent cell divisions undergoes de-differentiation; (b) an undifferentiat-

Table Two
Human Tumors and Polypeptide Hormone Expression (41)

Tumors of Group I
Major Tumors

Foregut carcinoid
Oat cell carcinoma
Islet cell tumors
Pancreatic and biliary ducts
Thyroid medullary carcinoma
Malignant epithelial thymoma

Hormones

Insulin	Gastrin
Calcitonin	Glucagon
ACTH	Secretin
MSH	Vasopressin

Tumors of Group II
Major Tumors

Hepatoma	Vascular
Cholangioma	Connective tissue and meso-dermal
Wilms	Reticuloendothelial
Hypernephroma	Lung (except oat cell)
Adrenal cortical	Gastrointestinal
Non-germinal gonadal	Melanoma

Hormones

Parathormone	Growth hormone
Erythropoietin	Insulin-like
Gonatotropin	Renin
Placental lactogen	Thyrotropin
Prolactin	

ed stem cell is transformed, then undergoes incomplete and aberrant differentiation; (c) a cell in mid-transition is transformed and becomes locked into a state of incomplete differentiation. Uriel (76) has marshalled impressive arguments for a reversion in cancer from a differentiated cell, pointing out that retrodifferentiation is a common adaptive response to cell injury, without necessarily involving metaplasia. The best studied example is the liver regeneration following hepatectomy. Accompanying this process are transient expressions of fetal antigens and isozymes (77); and an early, marked increase of template activity of chromatin, presumably in preparation for synthesis of products of genes ordinarily suppressed (26, 46). Retrodifferentiation also occurs in liver injury due to administration of hepatotoxic chemicals such as carbon tetrachloride, ethionine, etc. and is commonly seen early after carcinogen administration in the liver destined to neoplasia.

In contrast with these transient effects, the retrodifferentiation observed in cancer is generally, with a few outstanding exceptions permanent, and in fact is progressive. Tumors that are originally well-differentiated invariably undergo, with successive cell divisions, stepwise de-differentiation accompanied by a series of alterations toward loss of tissue-specific enzymes, antigens, drug and hormone responsiveness, aneuloidy, etc. This process, termed progression by Foulds (24), is common to both experimental and human tumors, and represents probably the strongest evidence for the view that the neoplastic transformation occurs in a differentiated cell. Over 30 years ago Greenstein (31) on the basis of assays of many enzymes, stated that tumors of the most diverse cells origins converge in their natural history to a common cell type, in which the tumors resemble each other more closely than they resemble their tissues of origin. This obviously represents the biochemical counterpart of the tendency for tumors to undergo progressive de-differentiation with successive cell divisions. From data provided by Harold Morris, it is clear that although many of the Morris hepatomas have remained stable over many years, some also have undergone progressively decreased differentiation with increased growth rate, as they have been successively transplanted over the years. That a mature hepatocyte is a direct precursor of the hepatoma cell may be inferred from the fact that liver neoplasia by chemicals is preceded by a reversible pre-neoplastic stage consisting of clusters of hepatocytes that are well-differentiated by histologic and enzymatic criteria (17).

An opposite viewpoint is championed by Pierce (55, 56), who has suggested a modern version of the original Cohnheim "embryonic rest" hypothesis (12). Since cancer has to arise in cells capable of mitosis, Pierce proposed that the mitotically active stem cell is the precursor of the cancer cell and is the target for the neoplastic transformation. Such transformed cells are assumed to give rise to the apparently de-differentiated tumor by an abortive or incomplete dif-

ferentiation. This hypothesis is supported by experiments with a
mouse testicular teratocarcinoma, a highly malignant tumor that
consists of both undifferentiated cells and portions that are differentiated to the degree of producing disordered collections of
bone, brain, cartilage, etc.; and with a rat squamous cell carcinoma
which also consists of differentiated and undifferentiated elements.
With each tumor type he demonstrated that the undifferentiated
malignant cell had the capability to undergo differentiation to
yield the differentiated tumor.

Other examples of re-differentiation of tumor cells are not
uncommon. In rare instances the human neuroblastoma will re-
differentiate to fully mature ganglion cells which no longer exhibit neoplastic properties (16). The erythroleukemia produced by
the Friend virus can be made to produce hemoglobin by treatment
with dimethyl sulfoxide and other agents (25). According to Silagi
and Bruce (68) a highly malignant mouse melanoma cell line may be
caused to exhibit phenotypic properties of normal cells by treatment with 5-bromodeoxyuridine. Cyclic 3'5'-adenosine monophosphate
also brings about a quasi reversion of cultured cancer cells to expression of untransformed phenotype (66), and cells transformed by
temperature-sensitive mutants of the Rous sarcoma virus can oscillate
between the normal and transformed phenotype by manipulation of the
temperature (73).

The third possibility, that cells in mid-transition between the
stem cell and the differentiated hepatocyte may undergo transformation, also requires consideration despite the lack of any experimental evidence. In view of the wide diversity of tumor differentiation,
such an event would require either that all cells have the potential
for transformation, and that the cell once transformed, may diverge
in either direction. Indeed, primary or early generation transplanted
hepatomas are likely to consist of several cell types differing in
histology, cell organization and morphology (17), suggesting either
that the hepatoma arise from multiple foci or that progeny cells can
differentiate or de-differentiate.

Cancer a Genetic or Epigenetic Process

The prevailing opinion regards the triggering event in cancer as
a somatic mutation. Admittedly, this viewpoint has compelling support.
The most obvious target, indeed the only target that can explain the
heritability of cancer is DNA. Overwhelmingly supportive evidence has
come from a host of studies that point to DNA as the common site of the
carcinogenic action of viruses, radiation and chemicals. Additional
support has come from the close correspondence between carcinogenicity
and mutagenicity as revealed by studies with microbial systems, introduced originally by Ames (4). There is also no doubt that genetic
abnormalities predispose to human cancer (38).

On the other hand, the mis-programming of protein synthesis in cancer points to aberrations of transcription or translation rather than mutation, and it is significant in this connection that the mis-programmed proteins are not new proteins. In fact, there has never appeared in cancer a protein unique to the neo-plastic state, thus arguing against a mutation of structural genes. These findings support and extend previous evidence for an epi-genetic causation. Braun (9, 10), has described experiments clear-ly demonstrating that plant neoplasms, grown in culture for many generations, can be induced to develop into whole plants, which flower and bear fertile seed. In experiments by McKinnell et al. (47) nuclei from the Lucke tumor of the frog, induced by a Herpes type virus, when inserted into an enucleated frog egg, leads to normal fertilization and development to fully functioning tadpoles of the nuclear genetic strain. This observation demonstrates not only the integrity of the tumor genome for normal differentiation, but also establishes a role of the cytoplasm in regulation of the expression of the neoplastic state.

Another striking illustration of the totipotency of the tumor genome was provided recently by Illmensee and Mintz (35). These investigators demonstrated that when single cells are taken from the embryoid bodies of a teratocarcinoma growing as an ascites tumor, and are inserted into blastocysts of a genetically marked mouse, progeny can develop normally, with no trace of cancer. Such mice, fathered by a tumor cell have genetic traits of the mouse from which the tumor was derived.

Molecular Basis of Abnormalities of Gene Expression

A central problem in development is the molecular mechanism by which the expression of specific genes is allocated to the various tissues, and is maintained with a high degree of fidelity throughout life. The same question concerns the way this mechanism is apparently reversed in cancer. The foregoing paragraphs reveal that by whatever functional means of protein identification that are employed, enzy-matic, immunological or hormonal, there occurs in cancer a massive alteration in protein composition. Apparently the rigid selective mechanisms of gene regulation that operate to maintain the differen-tiated state in normal, adult tissues become "unlocked", thus result-ing both in an inactivation of genes normally expressed, and an activation of genes that were expressed during embryonic development. This alteration in the programming of protein synthesis undoubtedly contributes to the many metabolic aberrations in cancer, and probably provides an underlying basis for their unrestrained growth, their un-responsiveness to signals of the host, the wide diversity of pheno-types, and their invasiveness.

It is an article of faith in biology that all cells of an

organism contain the same complement of genes. There is a relatively simple and elegant mechanism for selective gene expression
operating in the bacterial cell. In such primitive systems there
are linear arrays of regulatory and structural genes on the genome.
Protein synthesis normally is repressed by a protein coded by a
regulatory gene. There is an interplay between the repressor and
co-repressors or inducers, which influences the binding of the repressor to the genome, and thereby determines whether a particular
messenger RNA will be transcribed. Similar regulatory systems presumably operate in higher animals; and beautiful examples of hormonal substrate control of enzyme synthesis are known in both normal
and neoplastic cells (37, 77).

A higher level of gene regulation must operate however, in
normal, adult differentiated tissue, where all but a minuscule
portion of the genome is repressed. The end-result of normal
embryonic development of organs is a tightly and rigidly fixed
pattern of genetic expression which is essentially irreversible
throughout adult life. It is just such higher mechanisms, which
determine the organ specificity of gene activity, which appear to
be circumvented in cancer. Although we do not yet understand how
these mechanisms operate, they also may involve a highly structured
system of regulatory and structural genes, acting together with highly specific repressor or inducer proteins (74). One can envision
that such a rigid system requires a precise topographic arrangement
of regulatory and structural genes, and that this might be disturbed
in the neoplastic transformation. With oncogenic viruses, this
could occur by integration of all or part of the viral DNA at strategic sites in the host cell genome. With radiation or chemicals,
this might occur either directly, by displacement or mutation of regulatory genes; or indirectly, by errors in their structure or placement introduced during repair of DNA damage.

The significance of the mis-programming of gene expression in
cancer remains to be determined. Are we dealing with an intrinsic
feature of neoplasia or merely an accompaniment of the lack of control
of cell proliferation? There is little doubt however, that these
alterations contribute to the characteristic abnormal behavior of the
neoplastic cell. Several examples have been cited as to how alterations of isozyme expression may lead to metabolic abnormalities. The
ectopic production of polypeptide hormones by human tumors often
creates hormonal imbalances, leading to metabolic abnormalities that
transcend the effects of the tumor itself. It is likely that many
other abnormalities of protein synthesis remain to be discovered.
Our present knowledge thus may be only the tip of an iceberg. Abnormalities in nuclear proteins could affect cell replication as well
as transcription. Changes of cell surface proteins could lead to
alterations in the antigen structure of the cell, rendering it unrec-
ognizable to immune systems; to changes in transport of nutrients;
to loss of appropriate receptors, leading to unresponsiveness to

drugs, hormones, etc.; and to impairment of those mechanisms whereby signals generated at the cell membrane are transmitted to the nuclear machinery for protein synthesis and cell proliferation.

Obviously, we need to know much more about normal differentiation before we can understand the disorder of differentiation that may well lie at the heart of the cancer problem. Basic knowledge of the biology of the cell and its regulation is our most pressing need.

1 Experimental work of the authors was supported by grants from the National Cancer Institute, CA-10916, CA-12227, and from the American Cancer Society, BC-74.

The aid of Albert Williams and David Meranze is acknowledged with deep appreciation. Most of the work of the authors quoted here was conducted in collaboration with Harold P. Morris.

REFERENCES

1. Abelev, G.I. Adv. Cancer Res. 14 (1971) 295.

2. Adelman,R.C., Morris, H.P. and Weinhouse, S. Cancer Res. 27
    (1967) 2408.

3. Aisenberg, A.C. and Morris, H.P. Nature 191 (1961) 1314.

4. Ames, B.N., Lees, F.D. and Durston, W.E. Proc. Natl. Acad. Sci.
    70 (1973) 782.

5. Anderson, N.G. and Coggin, J.H. Models of Differentiation, retro-
    gression and cancer. Proc. ist Conference on embryonic and fetal
    antigens in cancer. Oak Ridge National Laboratory (1971) p. 7

6. Anderson, N.G. and Coggin, J.H. Cancer Res. 36 (1976) 3384.

7. Baldwin,R.W. Adv. in Cancer Res. 18 (1973) 1.

8. Bloch-Frankenthal,L., Langan, J. Morris, H.P. and Weinhouse S.
    Cancer Res. 25 (1965) 732.

9. Braun, A. In: Cancer, A Comprehensive Treatise. F.F. Becker
    (ed). Plenum Press, New York and London, 4 (1975) pp. 411-28.

10. Braun, A. In: Cancer, A Comprehensive Treatise, F.F. Becker
    (ed). Plenum Press, New York and London, 3 (1975) pp. 3-20.

11. Cederbaum, A.I. and Rubin, E. Cancer Res. 36 (1976) 2274.

12. Cohnheim, J. Lectures in General Pathology (Transl. by A.B.
    McKee), New Sydenham Society, London, 11 (1889) 789.

13. Criss, W.E., Cancer Res. 31 (1971) 1523.

14. Criss, W.E., Litwack, G., Morris, H.P. and Weinhouse, S. Cancer
    Res. 30 (1970) 370.

15. Drysdale, J.W. and Alpert E., Ann. N.Y. Acad. Sci. 259 (1975)
    427.

16. Everson, T.C. and Cole, W.H. Spontaneous regression of Cancer,
    Saunders, Philadelphia (1966).

17. Farber, E. In: Metabolic Alterations in Cancer, W.J. Whelan and
    J. Schultz (eds). North Holland Publ. Co., Amsterdam (1970)
    pp. 314-34.

18. Farina, F.A., Shatton, J.B., Morris, H.P. and Weinhouse, S.
    Cancer Res. 34 (1974) 1439.

19. Fiala, S. and Fiala, A.E. Experientia, 26 (1970) 889.

20. Fishman, W.H. Am. J. Med. 56 (1974) 617.

21. Fishman, W.H., Nishiyama, T., Rule, A., Green, S., Inglis, N.R.
    and Fishman, L. In: Onco-developmental Gene Expression,
    W.H. Fihman and S. Sell (eds). Academic Press, New York, (1976)
    pp. 165-72.

22. Fishman, W.H. and Singer, R.M. Ann. N.Y. Acad. Sci. 259 (1975)
    261.

23. Fishman, W.H. and S. Sell (eds). Cancer Res. 36 (1976) 4205.

24. Foulds, L. Neoplastic Development. Academic Press, New York
    (1969).

25. Friend, C., Scher, W., Holland, J.G. and Sato, T. Proc. Natl.
    Acad. Sci., U.S.A. 378 (1971) 68.

26. Gerrard, W.T. and Bonner, J. J. Biol. Chem. 249 (1974) 5570.

27. Gold, P. Prog. Exptl. Tumor Res. 14 (1971) 43.

28. Goldenberg, D.M. Current Topics in Pathology Springer-Verlag,
    Berlin, Heidelberg, (1979) pp. 290-342.

29. Gosalvez, M., Perez-Garcia, J. and Weinhouse, S. Eur. J. Biochem.
    46 (1974) 133.

30. Gosalvez, M., Lopez-Alarcon, L., Garcia-Suarez, S., Montalvo, A.
    and Weinhouse, S. Eur. J. Biochem. 55 (1975) 315.

31. Greenstein, J.P. Biochemsitry of Cancer, Academic Press, New
    York (1947) 328.

32. Hall, T.C. Ann. N.Y. Acad. Sci. 230 (1974) 1.

33. Hirai, H. and Alpert, E. (eds). Ann. N.Y. Acad. Sci. 259 (1975)1.

34. Ichihara, A. Ann. N.Y. Acad. Sci. 259 (1975) 347.

35. Illmensee, K. and Mintz, B. Proc. Natl. Acad. Sci. 73 (1976) 549.

36. Johnson, M.J. Science, 94 (1941) 200.

37. Knox, W.E. Enzyme Patterns in Fetal, Adult and Neoplastic Rat Tissues, S. Krager AG, Basel (1972).

38. Knudsen, A.G. Adv. Cancer Res. 17 (1973) 317.

39. Lawson, D., Paik, W.K., Morris, H.P. and Weinhouse, S. Cancer Res. 37 (1977) 850.

40. Lea, M.A., Murphy, P. and Morris, H.P. Cancer Res. 32 (1972) 61.

41. Levine, R.J. and Metz, S.A. Ann. N.Y. Acad. Sci. 230 (1974) 533.

42. Lynen, F. Ann. Chem. 546 (1941) 120.

43. Markert, C.L. and Moller, F. Proc. Natl. Acad. Sci. U.S.A. 45 (1959) 753.

44. Markert, C.L. (ed). Isozymes, Academic Press, New York, 4 (1975).

45. Matsushima,T., Kawake, S., Shibuya, M. and Sugimura, T. Biochem. Biophys. Res. Comm. 30 (1968) 565.

46. Mayfield, J.E. and Bonner, J. Proc. Natl. Acad. Sci. 69 (1972) 7.

47. McKinnell, R.G., Deggins, B.A. and Labat, D.D. Science 165 (1969) 394.

48. Morris, H.P. In: Handbuch der Allgemeinen Pathologie, Springer-Verlag, Berlin, Heidelberg, New York, 1 (1975) pp. 277-334.

49. Morris, H.P. Adv. Cancer Res. 9 (1965) 227.

50. Morris, H.P. and Wagner, B.P. In: Methods in Cancer Research, H. Busch (ed). Academic Press, New York, 4 (1968) pp. 125-152.

51. Nathanson, L. and Hall, T.C. Ann. N.Y. Acad. Sci. 230 (1974) 367.

52. Niitsu, Y., Kohgo, Y., Yokota, M. and Urushizaki, I. Ann. N.Y. Acad. Sci. 259 (1975) 450.

53. Ohashi, M. and Taguchi, T. Cancer Res. 36 (1976) 2216.

54. Ono, T. and Weinhouse, S. (eds). Isozymes and Enzyme Regulation in Cancer, Gann Mono. Univ. Tokyo Press, Tokyo, 13 (1972).

55. Pierce, G.B. In: Current Topics in Cellular Biology,A.A. Moscona and A. Mongoy (eds). Academic Press, New York, (1967) 223.

56. Pierce, G.B. Fed. Proc. 29 (1970) 1248.

57. Potter, V.R. In: <u>Environmentally-induced Metabolic Oscillations as a Challange to Tumor Autonomy</u>, Miami Winter Symposium, North Holland Publ. Co., Amsterdam 2 (1970) pp. 291-313.

58. Richter, G.W. and Lee, J.K.C. Cancer Res. 30 (1970) 880.

59. Sato, K., Morris, H.P. and Weinhouse, S. Cancer Res. 33 (1973) 724.

60. Schapira, F. Adv. in Cancer Res. 18 (1972) 77.

61. Schapira, F., Dreyfus, J.C. and Schapira, G. Nature, 200 (1963) 995.

62. Schapira, F., Reuber, M.D. and Hatzfeld, A. Biochem. Biophys. Res. Comm. 40 (1970) 321.

63. Schapira, F. and Gregori, C. Compt. Rend. 272 (1971) 1169.

64. Schapira, F., Micheau, C. and Junien, C. Rev. Eur. Etudes. Clin. et Biol. 17 (1972) 896.

65. Shatton, J.B., Morris, H.P. and Weinhouse, S. Cancer Res. 29 (1969) 1161.

66. Sheppard, J.R. Nature, New Biol. 236 (1972) 14.

67. Sherman, M.I., Strickland, S. and Reich, E. Cancer Res. 36 (1976) 4208.

68. Silagi, S. and Bruce, S.A. Proc. Natl. Acad. Sci. U.S.A. 66 (1970) 72.

69. Stolbach, L.L., Fishman, W.H. and Krant, M.J. N. Eng. J. Med. 281 (1969) 757.

70. Stonehill, E.H. and Bendich, A. Nature, 228 (1970) 370.

71. Strickland, S., Reich, E. and Sherman, M.I. Cell, 9 (1976) 231.

72. Topp, W., Hall, J.D., Marsden, M., Teresky, A.K., Rifkin, D., Levine, A.J. and Pollack, R. Cancer Res. 36 (1976) 4217.

73. Toyoshima, K. and Vogt, P.K. Virology, 39 (1969) 930.

74. Tsanev, R. and Sendov, B.L. J. Theoretical Biol. 30 (1971) 337.

75. Unkeless, J.C., Tobias, A., Ossowski, L., Quigley, J.P., Rifkin, D.B. and Reich, E. J. Exp. Med. 137 (1973) 85.

76. Uriel, J. Cancer Res. 36 (1976) 4269.

77. Walker, P.R. and Potter, V.R. Adv. in Enzyme Red. 10 (1972) 339.

78. Warburg, O. The Metabolism of Tumors, Arnold Constable, London (1930).

79. Warburg, O. Science, 123 (1956) 309.

80. Warburg, O. Science, 124 (1956) 269.

81. Weber, G. In: The Molecular Biology of Cancer, H. Busch (ed). Academic Press, New York (1974) pp. 487-521.

82. Weber, G., Banerjee, G. and Morris, H.P. Cancer Res. 21 (1961) 933.

83. Weinhouse, S. Cancer Res. 32 (1972) 20007.

84. Weinhouse, S. Respiration, Glycolysis and Enzyme Alterations in Liver Neoplasms. Miami Winter Symposium, North Holland Publ. Co., Amsterdam, 2 (1970) pp. 462-480.

85. Weinhouse, S. Z. Krebs. 87 (1976) 115.

86. Yeoman, L.D., Jordan, J.J., Busch, R.K., Taylor, C.W., Savage, H.E. and Busch, H. Proc. Natl. Acad. Sci. 73 (1976) 3258.

HORMONAL INDUCTION OF ENZYME FUNCTIONS, CYCLIC AMP LEVELS AND AIB

TRANSPORT IN MORRIS HEPATOMAS AND IN NORMAL LIVER SYSTEMS

Van Rensselaer Potter

McArdle Laboratory for Cancer Research
The University of Wisconsin Medical Center
Madison, Wisconsin 53706

I. INTRODUCTION

   A. Cancer as Regulatory Dysfunction

   In a chapter on the "Biochemistry of Cancer"(57) I quoted F.F.
Becker (6, p.v) "...despite these advances...one major problem
exists...As we noted earlier, the problem is our inability to define the malignant cell" (Italics by Becker). In contrast I noted
that H.C. Pitot (44, p.145) had reiterated his earlier view "...
the fact still remains that the most significant biological and
biochemical distinctions defining the neoplastic phenomenon are the
abnormalities seen in the regulation of gene expression".

   In attempting to understand this seeming discrepancy in outlook
I commented that "Underlying the Becker position is the fundamental
issue of diversity among individual cancers. This diversity is so
great that it is probable that no two autochthonous cancers are exactly alike. Yet, despite the diversity our intellects are impelled
to seek an underlying unity. It is possible that Becker is right in
the sense that there is no malignant cell archetype while Pitot is
right in the sense that all malignant cells have in common the feature that they no longer are subject to the orchestrated controls
that enable each organism to respond to changes in the environment by
regulating gene expression in its component cells." (Italics added).

   The concept that normal cells are governed by orchestrated controls that enable them to respond to changes in their environment by
regulating gene expression in the vast array of component cells in
the tissues that make up the total organism is an important one.

The key word is orchestrated and I can think of no real substitute
for it.   The story of <u>Mechanisms of Regulation</u> as studied in the
Morris hepatomas is probably the strongest available evidence that
can be generalized to support the view that malignant cells are no
longer subject to the <u>orchestrated</u> <u>controls</u> that make a normal multi-
cellular organism possible.   In other words, cancer is a problem in
regulatory dysfunction, which in this case results in a failure to
orchestrate the available repertoire of gene capabilities in a manner
appropriate to the whole organism at any given time.   We can separate
the problem into two categories: regulatory dysfunction may involve
alterations in regulatory DNA sequences that control transcription of
structrual genes or it may involve alterations in structural genes
for regulatory proteins.   The latter include receptor proteins, transport systems, protein kinases, and many other protein modifying proteins.

That regulatory dysfunction is the epitome of the definition of
malignancy is further emphasized by Donald F.H. Wallach in his book
"Membrane Molecular Biology of Neoplastic Cells" (85, p.1) in which
two of his four "critical features" in cancer, namely, biologic autonomy and asocial cell behavior, are the features that change cell
proliferation, invasion, and metastasis into malignant processes.
The word autonomy must not be misinterpreted.   As so beautifully illustrated by the Morris hepatomas, a cancer cell can never be completely autonomous - it merely has to be autonomous <u>enough</u>.   Further
indication of how unity is brought into diversity by the concept of
normal orchestration and cancer dissonance is illustrated in George
Klein's Foreword to the Wallach book (85, p.xviii) in which he at-
tributes the concept of neoplasia as a membrane disease to Wallach:
"The thought that neoplasia is essentially a 'membrane disease' has
been raised by Wallach at an early stage and with force.   It is an
exciting thought, because the cell membrane is an almost compulsory
transfer point for the action of growth controlling signals.   Changes
in critically important membrane sites, or, as Wallach puts it, the
alteration of concerted membrane behavior by oncogenic agents may bring
the free-wheeling of the cell cycle recognized as neoplastic growth."
Again we must mention, as the Morris hepatomas have taught us, some
tumors are less free-wheeling than others, but all are deviant with
respect to one or more of the orchestrated controls, a view that is
compatible with the various ways of looking at the cancer problem:
whether we look at cancer as a "membrane disease" (85), as a "disease
of differentiation" (41), as "altered gene expression" (44, 90), as
"blocked ontogeny" (64) or as "retrodifferentiation" (80, p.21),
studies of nutrient transport systems and their mechanisms of regulation are of paramount interest.   Thus Holley (23) expressed the view
of many in the statement "The primary cause of tumor growth is the
increased concentration of critical nutrients inside the cell." The
search for <u>a</u> critical nutrient has continued unabated for a number of
years and has led to studies involving glucose, 2-deoxyglucose, 3-0-

methyl glucose, natural amino acids, amino acid analogs, nucleosides, cations, phosphate and special molecules, as detailed in a recent symposium on "Cellular Regulation of Transport and Uptake of Nutrients" introduced by H.M. Kalckar (28). No studies on Morris hepatomas were reported at that conference although we reported studies on aminoisobutyric acid (AIB) transport and its hormonal regulation in primary cultures of rat liver cells (31) as part of our program for comparing Morris hepatomas and normal rat liver systems. In the book by Wallach, the only studies on amino acid transport that are mentioned (85, pp.312-315) are on Ehrlich ascites cells in vivo, in cultured "transformed" cells, in cultured HTC hepatoma cells (1, 71) and on Morris hepatomas in vivo, the latter all reported from our laboratory (3, 19, 70, 74, 76). In recent reports Holley (24, 25) has indicated that there may not be a single critical nutrient that would be the key to all malignant growth, but rather that a number of known and unknown nutrients and hormones (serum factors) may be transported in combinations and to varying extents so that growth is limited by critical factors that differ from one neoplasm to another.

In considering cancer as a "membrane disease" it is clear that membrane function includes (a) transport, (b) secretion, and (c) signal reception and transduction by cell surface receptors. Nearly every type of regulatory dysfunction can be expected in one neoplasm or another (85, pp.497-505) and many are known for Morris hepatomas. The only studies on transport of amino acids in these hepatomas appear to be those that we have reported, for which the conclusions will be reviewed. We are not aware of any transport studies on glucose or its analogs or of other nutrients in Morris hepatomas. Such studies would contribute greatly to the multiple factor concept expressed by Holley (24, 25).

Studies on regulatory dysfunction in the case of protein secretion in the case of Morris hepatomas are available in the case of albumin and alpha fetoprotein.

Regulatory dysfunction in the case of membrane receptors and signal transduction has also been reported for the Morris hepatomas. Thus, the availability of a variety of Morris hepatomas has provided a fertile field for the study of all 3 major types of regulatory membrane dysfunction although the exploration has barely begun.

B. Studies on Morris Hepatomas

Our studies on Morris hepatomas began in collaboration with Pitot, Ono and Morris in 1960 with a series entitled "The Comparative Enzymology and Cell Origin of Rat Hepatomas", in which certain marker enzymes or properties were studied in animals without special environmental controls (62). These studies evolved into a series on "Metabolic Adaptations in Rat Hepatoma" in which changing enzyme

levels due to dietary changes were evaluated on a time scale in
days (48). By 1966 the in vivo studies had moved to a time scale
of hourly changes in metabolic functions in hepatomas from animals
on controlled feeding and lighting schedules employing semi-synthetic
diets in which the protein/carbohydrate ratio was varied over a
wide range. These studies were reported under some variant of the
title "Systematic Oscillations in Metabolic Functions in Liver and
Hepatomas from Rats Adapted to Controlled Feeding Schedules" (59, 60).
In 1968 we reported our first study on amino acid transport under
controlled environmental and dietary conditions in liver and hepatomas in vivo (2, 4). By 1969 enzyme induction as affected by hydrocortisone, glucagon, and adrenalectomy superimposed on the naturally
occurring systematic oscillations in liver and hepatomas were under
study (3, 87). Also in 1969 "The Importance of Studies on Fetal Tissues" was emphasized (54) and the concept of "Oncogeny as Blocked
Ontogeny" was stated. Quantitation of fetal and adult isoenzymes
followed (64, 83). In 1971 concurrent measurements of cyclic AMP and
amino acid transport in vivo were begun under controlled conditions
of feeding and lighting and hormone administration (17, 18). These
studies were the forerunners of similar concurrent measurements carried out subsequently using primary cultures of adult rat liver parenchymal cells (37). In 1964 our first report on enzyme induction in a
hepatoma in tissue culture had appeared (46) and 1972 a "Workshop on
Liver Cell Culture" was convened (56). In 1974 our first report appeared on "Primary Monolayer Cultures of Isolated Rat Liver Parenchymal Cells Suitable for the Study of the Regulation of Enzyme Synthesis" (8).

In 1977 our first report appeared on the production of slowly
growing autochthonous hepatomas comparable to the least altered
Morris hepatomas (29) using minimal initiating doses of acetylaminofluorene followed by 0.05% phenobarbital according to the Peraino
protocol (40).

C. The 3-Dimensional Program

Thus the 3-dimensional framework of a program intended to un-
cover the nature of regulatory dysfunction in chemically-induced hepatomas of the minimal deviation type, provided in great quantity and
in diverse lines by the efforts of Dr. Harold Morris, now clearly
emerges. To be seen in its totality one must envision the components
of each dimension in detail and it will follow that any given research
report can be seen as occupying one or more niches in the 3D structure.
The first dimension is the category labeled "Cell System". This includes control liver of all kinds, fetal, neonatal, regenerating, pre-
neoplastic and host liver in vivo. Also included are in vitro cultures
of liver and hepatoma cells from various sources. The hepatoma cells
for comparison include all of the transplantable Morris livers as well
as autochthonous hepatomas.

The second dimension is labeled "Parameters Under Study".
Quantitation of more than one parameter is essential in order to
detect coordinate inductions or repressions. Transport functions
include those for amino acids, glucose and nucleosides among others.
Metabolic functions need to be examined in terms of the balance between anabolic and catabolic reactions (34, 53, 72, 73, 89). Regulatory functions need to be studied in terms of cyclic nucleotides,
cyclases, protein kinases, other protein modifiers, and nutrient
transports.

The third dimension can be labeled "Environmental Variables".
Control of this approach is essential if the nature of the regulatory
dysfunction in cancer cells is to be understood, and there are far
too few studies other than our own that have systematically varied
dietary composition, periods of light and darkness, periods of food
availability, and hormone status (ablation or supplementation), while
examining chosen parameters in three or more Morris hepatomas. It is
apparent that in a 3-D framework as here described, the number of
cubicles (projects) runs into thousands, and many are as yet unoccupi-
ed. Nevertheless, largely owing to the efforts of Dr. Morris, it can
be stated without reservation that the availability of diverse but in-
ternally consistent hepatoma lines provides the operational foundation
on which the entire 3D structure rests.

D. The Theoretical Framework

Meanwhile the theoretical basis for interpreting the experiments
has been developing rapidly (5, 44, 57, 80, 91). The orchestration
of normal cellular function can be seen as a coordinated series of
rapid inductions or derepressions of transcription by steroid hormones
and other as yet unknown agents to produce messenger RNA. Translation
of mRNA to form proteins is modulated by the polypeptide hormones and
the proteins are in turn subject to degradation, activation or inactivation by other proteins. Adaptation to the environment occurs on
an hourly basis merely in the course of a normal 24-hour day. The
occurrence of enzyme and transport proteins with short half-lives and
with inactive and active forms provides a factual background that must
be considered in looking for subtle departures from the orchestration
that marks normal organismic function. The Morris hepatomas provide
a spectrum of deviations from the responses that can be elicited from
normal liver cells. They contain normal enzymes (according to available evidence) and they give many normal responses, but they reveal
their character by the holistic test: from the standpoint of the
whole organism, one or more responses are inappropriate to the situation. The studies to be mentioned need to be considered from the
overall standpoint of "orchestration".

II. RESULTS

A. Naturally Occurring Enzyme Levels in Hepatomas and in Normal

Liver

     The first publication (62) from this laboratory that employed
Morris hepatomas appeared in 1960 and resulted from earlier expressions of dissatisfaction with the use of the Novikoff hepatomas as
the sole representative of the category "hepatoma" in comparison
with normal liver (49, 50). At the same time, Dr. Henry Pitot was
at Tulane University also searching for additional hepatomas for
biochemical studies and he brought the Dunning hepatoma to my attention when he came to my group as a postdoctoral fellow in 1959.
We found that dCMP deaminase was elevated in fetal liver, in Novikoff
hepatoma, and in precancerous liver, but nearly absent in adult liver
and in Dunning LC18 transplantable hepatoma (47). This finding, plus
an earlier study in 1945 helped formulate the blocked ontogeny theory
of cancer, which was not formally expressed until about 10 years later. More importantly, it showed that wide variations in phenotypic
expression could be observed with only two hepatomas. The search was
on to find more hepatomas that were available in transplantable form.
An appeal to Dr. H.P. Morris met with a prompt response, and hepatomas 3683, 3924A and 5123 were soon in our hands. Our first report
came in 1960, when both Dr. Henry Pitot and Dr. Tetsuo Ono were in my
laboratory (62). Ten different hepatoma types were surveyed for dCMP
deaminase and for thymine degradation. The deaminase was viewed as a
fetal liver enzyme retained by bile duct epthelilum and by the Novikoff hepatoma, Morris 3683, and Morris 3924A but not Morris 5123,
Dunning LC18, or adult liver. Thymine degradation was missing in the
Novikoff and Dunning hepatomas but present in the Morris 5123 hepatoma and in adult liver. Thus on the basis of both of the enzymes
studied, hepatoma 5123 was unique in resembling adult liver, and loss
of thymine degradation could no longer be regarded as an essential
"deletion" for transformation. This report led to the formulation of
the minimal deviation concept (51, 52) and to the search for other
hepatomas that resembled No. 5123. We were concerned that No. 5123
would be lost through progression and called Dr. Morris by telephone
on the day the thymine results were obtained, advising him to set up
parallel transplant lines A, B, C and D. This was done and a subsequent (1967) study of karyotypes showed that indeed the resulting
four lines had developed different numbers of chromosomes (33).

     With hepatoma 5123 still the tumor of major interest, further in-
dications of its resemblance to normal liver were obtained. Pitot (43)
compared it with several other hepatomas and showed that it resembled
normal liver with respect to glucose-6-phosphatase, glutamate dehydrogenase, choline oxidase and that it had moderate levels of tryptophan
peroxidase (pyrrolase) and abnormally high levels of threonine dehydrase. He expressed the view that Morris hepatomas 5123 "offers perhaps the best system, at present, for the elucidation of any alterations in enzymatic and controlling mechanisms between the normal and
malignant cell. Whether or not any difference that is found between the

two can be generalized to other hepatomas must await careful experimental investigation." (Subsequently other hepatoma lines
showed properties that are even closer to normal liver.)

B. Metabolic Adaptations in Morris Hepatoma 5123 (1960-1963)

With the above thought in mind, and with the knowledge that
certain enzymes are quite variable in normal liver due to variations
in diet or to hormone administration, coupled to the fact that hepatoma 5123 had an abnormally high level of threonine dehydrase (43)
we embarked on what has been one of the unique contributions from
the McArdle laboratory: the comparison of the metabolic adaptation
capability of the Morris hepatomas with normal liver based on concepts jointly held with Pitot (42, 29, 58).

The first report (48, paper I) was carried out with only Morris
hepatoma 5123 because other "minimal deviation" hepatomas were not
yet available. The basic plan involved adaptation to either high
protein (91% casein) or low protein (2% casein) diets, followed by
a shift to the alternative diet, with killings at 0, 4, 7 and 11 days
(48). (Later work in 1966 and subsequent years involved additional
levels of dietary protein, additional enzymes and additional hepatoma
lines, with several killings within a 24 hour period, see below).
Both host livers and control (non-tumor-bearing) livers were analyzed
in addition to hepatoma 5123, and the report covered serine and
threonine dehydrases (now understood to be the same enzyme) and tryptophan peroxidase (pyrrolase). The most striking outcome was the
very high levels of serine and threonine dehydrase in hepatoma 5123
whether the diet contained 2% or 91% casein, in contrast to control
liver which responded to either diet within three days, to give low
levels of enzyme on low protein intake and high levels of enzyme on
high levels of protein intake, i.e. appropriate "orchestration".

Additional studies were carried out by Pitot with hepatoma 5123
concentrating on tryptophan pyrrolase and tyrosine aminotransferase
(6, paper II). Adrenalectomized animals were included, as well as
animals given cortisone. Tyrosine aminotransferase was elevated in
the hepatomas compared to host liver, was reduced in adrenalectomized
animals and elevated by cortisone. The conclusion was drawn that
"certain inducible enzymes are repressed in the tumor, and certain
repressible enzymes are derepressed". (Subsequent work has supported
and expanded this conclusion).

In 1961 Potter and Ono reported additional studies on metabolic
adaptation in hepatoma 5123 at an historic symposium on Cellular Regulatory Mechanisms (61) at which Monod and Jacob presented their much
quoted paper on Teleonomic Mechanism in Cellular Metabolism, Growth
and Differentiation, (61, p.389). We studied glucose-6-phosphate dehydrogenase (G6P-DH) in particular and emphasized the use of "metabolic

transitions" to test the operation of feedback controls in hepatoma
compared with liver. We employed the "Tepperman protocol" because
it had been shown that animals fed after a 3 day fast responded with
a remarkable increase in glucose-6-phosphate dehydrogenase that resulted in a striking"overshoot" with a maximum at 3 days, followed
by a slow return to normal over a period of a week or more. In hepatoma 5123 there was almost no change in G6P-DH in either the fasting,
refeeding, or late period and the same was true of the host liver.
Concomitant measurements for threonine dehydrase showed that the
high levels in 5123C tripled in the fasting period, declined to the
original value during the refeeding period while host liver remained
at low values throughout. Thus the tumor responded to the manipulation with one enzyme but not in the case of G6P-DH.

In the first paper in the Metabolic Adaptation series (48) it
was possible to examine results in terms of the adaptation response
of normal liver and the non-adaptative response of hepatoma 5123,
because the enzymes were "amino acid catabolizing" in response to increases in dietary protein. The 1961 report (61) showed an optimum
protein level for the response of glucose-6-phosphate dehydrogenase
in normal liver following a 3 day fast, and a lack of response in
hepatoma 5123. Paper III (35) gave further consideration to this enzyme using samples from the earlier study (48) plus additional experiments. The G6P-dehydrogenase was measured along with pyrimidine
reductases, in both male and female hosts. For the latter enzymes,
the control livers showed increased levels on high protein and decreased levels on low protein diets. Host livers showed muted responses, and 5123 hepatoma showed no response in either direction.
Although in female rats the reductases in the hepatoma showed much
greater activity than in male rats, striking sex differences were
seen in the response of G6P-dehydrogenase to a high protein diet,
and it was surprising to note that while control liver in female rats
greatly exceeded control liver in male rats, the hepatoma initial
values and responses were just the opposite: in males, hepatoma (725
units) exceeded controls (214 units) while in females, controls (639
units) exceeded hepatomas (346 units). (The primary hepatoma 5123
was in a female (33)). From these data it appears that a generalization that hepatoma 5123 has elevated levels of G6P-DH compared to
normal liver would seem to be secure on the basis of data from male
hosts, only to be upset by data from female hosts. The only universal
rule seems to be regulatory dysfunction.

C. Metabolic Adaptations in Additional Morris Hepatomas (1963 and
Later).

By 1962 several new Morris hepatomas had become available and
could be compared with each other (45). Paper IV by Bottomley, Pitot
and Morris (9) reported on threonine and serine dehydratase from 7
new lines numbered 7288C through 7800. This report was the first in-

dication for the generalization that the Morris hepatomas tend to
be insensitive to dietary adaptation. While host and control livers
had low activity for the 2 enzymes on chow diet and much higher activity on a high protein diet, any given hepatoma was high, medium
or low on either diet.

The earlier studies on G6P-DH were now combined with the above
measurements (10, paper V). Further evidence for regulatory dysfunction was obtained. In normal liver, high levels of dietary protein results in high levels of threonine dehydrase and a lowered
level of G6P-DH. However, in various tumors the reciprocal relationship seems to be independent of the diet and characteristic of the
tumor line. (Later studies seem to indicate that this may be correlated with amino acid transport capability, see below).

A comparative study of several Morris hepatomas which had become available were carried out on alternative pyrimidine pathways
in "five frames of reference", with the statement "Included are
several alternative pathways which are of particular interest, because the ratio of anabolic to catabolic pathways for a given substrate can be calculated for liver and for the tumors" (34). This
approach (53, 72, 73) has been employed by Weber in relation to the
growth rate of the Morris hepatomas. (See Weber papers in Volume
I of Advances in Enzyme Regulation, 1963 (89) and in subsequent
volumes up to the present). Our paper on pyrimidine pathways is an
important statement of our view that "Correlations of growth rate
with enzyme pattern cannot be made with a series of two unrelated
tumors, and in a larger series it seems inevitable that, in the progression of slowly growing minimal deviation hepatomas to rapidly
growing multiple-deviation hepatomas, the various stages in the progression might involve one sequence of deletions in one progression
and another sequence of deletions to give an equally rapid growth
rate in the multiple-deviation hepatoma at an advanced stage of
another progression." In general, the results were in support of
the concept that anabolic enzymes increase and catabolic enzymes decrease with growth rate but the data indicate a less than perfect
correlation. In other words, the concept is correct in principle
but not in detail.

D. Systematic Metabolic Oscillations on Controlled Feeding
Schedules (From 1966)

The first report (60) on rapid metabolic changes in the Morris
hepatomas involved No. 7793, a well-differentiated hepatoma with a
transfer time of 1.8 months (77) and 45 chromosomes, originally induced in a female Buffalo rat with the weak carcinogen N-2-fluorenyl-
phthalamic acid (33) and subsequently characterized as producing
only the lowest levels of alphafetoprotein in the serum of host rats
(77). The protocol was the most complicated ever used and was sub-

sequently somewhat simplified. In this original protocol "Hepatoma-
bearing rats were divided among 20 experimental groups testing all
possible combinations of 5 levels of dietary protein and 4 different
times in the 24-hour day. Casein was fed at levels of 0, 12, 30, 60
and 90% with glucose as the other variable. Lighting was 6 A.M. to
6 P.M. and animals were killed at 06:00, 12:00, 18:00 and 24:00"(60).
The tumors grew very slowly in this experiment and weighed only 3 to
6 grams when the animals were killed 149 days after transplantation.
The animals were thoroughly adapted to the diets, which they received
for 44 days prior to killing although less time would be required.
Radioactive thymidine was administered one hour before killing and
incorporation into DNA in hepatomas and host livers was measured.
The hepatomas showed a marked daily oscillation in rate of incorporation in all dietary groups. The maximum occurred at the dark to
light transition as in regenerating and growing rat liver (27) indicating some response to host controls, but at a rate 10 to 100X
that of host liver, indicating "inappropriate" DNA synthesis since
the organism did not call upon host liver cells to divide. Concomitant assays for thymidine kinase revealed highest levels at 6 A.M. to
12:00 noon and lowest levels at 6 P.M. which was also the minimum for
thymidine incorporation in vivo. Glycogen was measured in host liver
and showed a marked daily oscillation with levels inversely proportional to dietary protein (i.e. proportional to dietary carbohydrate).
Three dimensional graphs were presented for hepatoma and host liver
with dietary protein on the Y-axis, time of day on the X-axis and enzyme activity on the Z-axis. Enzymes measured were ornithine transaminase (OAT), serine dehydratase (SDH), tyrosine aminotransferase
(TAT), glucose-6-phosphate dehydrogenase, and thymidine kinase. The
data were also presented as 2-dimensional charts, with either dietary
protein or time of day as abscissa. The results presented in this
study were fully substantiated in subsequent reports and extended to
a number of Morris hepatomas. They demonstrated a picture of regulatory dysfunction that is not available from any other source despite the fact that the report is over 10 years old.

The response of each enzyme to diet and time of day, relative to
host liver, was unique, yet the overall conclusion can be plainly
stated. For serine dehydrase, tyrosine aminotransferase and ornithine
aminotransferase, host liver activity plotted against dietary protein
showed a nearly linear proportionality, with high values at high protein levels and low activity at low protein levels, but each enzyme
had a different intercept at the low end of the protein scale. Thus
at 0% protein, the curve for TAT activity had an intercept on the ordinate, the curve for OAT activity was essentially a straight line
through the origin and the curve for SDH had an intercept on the abscissa at about 20% dietary protein. The significant point to be
made is that hepatoma 7793 showed high levels of activity at the lowest levels of dietary protein greatly exceeding liver activity by 10-
100 fold while at high levels of protein the hepatoma values were
either equal to or lower than the values for liver.

With respect to time of day, this report was the first to note the rapid diurnal changes in tyrosine aminotransferase with peak values at midnight according to the protocol employed, in which midnight came at 6 hours after food dishes were replaced in the cages. Because of the rapid increase in the activity of this enzyme in relation to darkness and onset of feeding, we subsequently employed an "inverted" lighting schedule with darkness from 9 A.M. to 9 P.M. and with food available for only the first 8 hours of darkness ("8+16" protocol) and more recently for only the first 2 hours of darkness ("2+22"protocol) (93). In the latter case the rats are first trained to the 8+16 protocol and then shifted to the 2+22 schedule and caged individually.

The marked oscillation in TAT with time of day in hepatoma 7793 was correlated with feeding and host liver maxima only at the two highest levels of protein, while at the two lowest levels of protein the peak in hepatoma occurred 12 hours after feeding and greatly exceeded host liver values at all time points. In subsequent work with other hepatomas the time point for minimal TAT activity in host or control liver on the 8+16 schedule was at the end of the 16 hour period without food, and hepatomas with high maxima did not show decreases to the minimal values seen in host or control liver.

Based on the 1966 findings, extensive applications of the protocol were carried out with control liver (26, 59, 86, 93) and with a series of Morris hepatomas (65, 67, 87, 88) with most of the work based on the 8+16 protocol. A survey of 6 diploid and 3 other Morris hepatomas was carried out with 3 levels of dietary casein, 12, 30 and 60% (67) omitting the extremes of 0% and 90% employed in the earlier (60) study. More animals and more frequent samplings were employed to establish the time course of the changes in normal liver. Thus in normal controls on an inverted light schedule with darkness for 12 hours and food availability for 8 hours from 9 A.M. 3 animals per diet were killed at 9, 10, 11, 15, 17 and 21 hours. Tyrosine aminotransferase showed a peak at 1500 hours on each diet, proportional to protein content, while at 9:00 A.M. the starting values were all at the same low level regardless of the diet composition. Serine dehydratase was almost zero activity on 12% protein, with strong activity on 30% protein and with activity on 60% protein showing a twofold increase over the 30% level. All values for SDH were independent of time of day, in contrast to TAT. Glucose-6-phosphate dehydrogenase, citrate cleavage enzyme, glucose-6-phosphatase, glycogen, and plasma corticosterone were also determined. The latter peaked at the end of the period without food and declined from 9 A.M. to 9 P.M. during feeding in the dark.

Based on the 6 time points above, the original 20 experimental groups (60) were streamlined down to 3 time points (9:00, 15:00 and 21:00) and 3 diets (12%, 30% and 60% casein) and 3 rats per group, to

give 9 experimental groups for each hepatoma studied. With 3 rats
per group each hepatoma line required 27 rats, with host liver and
hepatoma studied in six parameters by Dr. Minro Watanabe.

Hepatomas studied were 5123C, 9108, 7794B, 7800, 9633, 9098,
7794A and 9618A (67). Of these all were diploid except 9108 (42-
43 chromosomes), 7794B (44 chromosomes) and 5123C (90-96 chromosomes)
(33). In agreement with the indications from the earlier experiment
with hepatoma 7793, all of the hepatomas showed a marked tendency to
be less responsive to decreases in dietary protein than normal or
host liver, with nearly identical values at the 3 levels of protein
in some cases. The report cannot be summarized because of the differences in detail shown by each hepatoma line but the consistency
of the data is established by the comparison of data from animals
on different diets. An important feature of the report is the comparison of all the host livers with normal control liver. Certain
hepatomas produced marked changes in levels of certain enzymes in
host liver while others did not.

Of considerable interest are the data on glucose-6-phosphate
dehydrogenase. Whereas in normal liver this enzyme activity is proportional to dietary carbohydrate, in the hepatomas the enzyme decreased at the higher levels of carbohydrate and increased at the
higher levels of protein. All of the host livers deviated considerably from normal liver, some above and some below. Hepatomas 5123C,
9121 and 7794B had less than normal amounts of the enzyme on a 12%
protein diet but higher amounts on a 60% protein diet. An earlier
report dealt with the reciprocal relationship between glucose-6-
phosphate dehydrogenase and serine dehydratase (10). With the data
in the 1969 report (67) we now had data from 27 rats for each hepatoma
and could show the correlation at 3 levels of dietary protein (Chart
10B in 67).

From all considerations hepatoma 9618A emerged as the hepatoma
that was least deviated in comparison with normal liver (65), but
even this hepatoma lacked many features seen in adult liver (see
below). Among the 10 hepatomas studied in terms of diet and daily
variations (60, 65, 67, 87) No. 9618A was the only one to exhibit substantial levels of citrate cleavage enzyme, although the relationship
to protein reversed that seen in normal liver. At 12, 30 and 60% dietary protein normal liver had 400, 316 and 159 units of the enzyme,
host liver had 221, 214 and 168 units, and hepatoma 9618A had 193,
283 and 262 units, respectively. Thus the hepatoma was below normal
at 12% protein and above normal at 60% protein. No. 9618A was also
the only hepatoma in the series that contained substantial levels of
glycogen (2% at 9 A.M., 3% at 9 P.M., on 60% protein diet) (65). This
hepatoma has also been shown to have glucokinase levels in the same
range as normal adult liver by Shatton, Morris and Weinhouse (78), who
showed that most Morris hepatomas contain very little or none of this

enzyme, while all contained hexokinase. (They found 2 other hepatomas with near normal levels of glucokinase, 7787 and 9618B).

Hepatoma 9618A was studied in greater detail in 29 animals
over a period of 450 days (88). Previous data (65, 67) were confirmed and extended. Tyrosine aminotransferase and serine dehydratase were reduced to only 1 to 5 percent of host or control liver
values and were accordingly near zero at all levels of dietary protein. The deficiency in serine dehydratase was also noted in hepatomas 9633, 7794A, 9121, and 9098 all of which had low but significant levels of TAT (67). These relative values for TAT and SDH are
believed to be secondary and to reflect the effects of the amino
acid pool on translation of the respective mRNA's. At 12% dietary
protein normal liver has TAT activity equivalent to about 1/3 the
maximal value at 60 to 90% dietary protein, whereas at 12% dietary
protein SDH is essentially zero. Corresponding to this differential,
considering those hepatomas that have TAT values (at all protein
levels) equivalent to or less than the values for normal liver at
12% dietary protein, it can be seen that they have zero values for
SDH (at all protein levels) corresponding to the zero value for SDH
in normal liver at 12% protein.

The zero levels for TAT and SDH in hepatoma 9618A match the
value for <u>newborn</u> normal rat liver, in which the enzymes are induced
within 24 hours after birth by endogenous glucagon under conditions
of hypoglycemia (68). By administering glucagon following hydrocortisone (3, 87) or at more effective doses (69) we were able to
induce the previously non-inducible TAT in hepatoma 9618A to essentially normal liver levels, thereby proving that the hepatoma possessed the structural gene for TAT but was unable to express it at
any level of dietary protein. In the same animals however, SDH remained unexpressed under conditions that induced TAT. The induction
of TAT was correlated with an increase in amino acid transport (see
below). The behavior of TAT and SDH in hepatoma 9618A emphasizes
the broader aspects of the "minimal deviation" concept (51): in
comparing the Morris hepatomas with normal rat liver it is essential
to examine the entire spectrum of "normal" liver from birth to old
age and in the various stages in regeneration: under basal conditions, with dietary alteration, and in response to hormonal or other
organismic signals. Thus 9618A has glucokinase, pyruvate kinase I,
citrate cleavage enzyme, and glycogen levels in the adult liver range,
but lacks tyrosine amino transferase and serine dehydratase making it
comparable to newborn rat liver in these two respects. But just as
newborn rat liver can respond to hormonal stimulation by increasing
TAT, so also can the 9618A hepatoma. In recent experiments we have
demonstrated that serine dehydrase responds more slowly than TAT to
dietary changes (93) and it would be interesting to see if SDH in
9618A would respond to glucagon stimulation if continued for 2 or 3
days.

The minimal deviation concept must be examined in the context
of the blocked ontogeny hypothesis, according to which various
sequences of transitory gene expressions exist and can be blocked
at points equivalent to various points in the time scale of normal
development. Thus hepatoma 9618A has developed to the adult level
on the glucokinase sequence (which is expressed at about 15 days
after birth) (81) but remains at the newborn level for TAT and SDH.

As suggested earlier, there is a remarkable insensitivity to
the levels of dietary protein and carbohydrate in the 10 hepatomas
studied and the enzymes that are exquisitely sensitive to dietary
protein in normal liver are almost unaffected in the hepatomas,
although each has its own characteristic level of enzyme activity
at all levels of protein. It is as if the hepatomas with the higher
"locked in" level of TAT could ignore the lower levels of dietary
protein by virtue of their ability to concentrate aminoacids from
the blood. Data relevant to this idea are in the next section.

E.   Amino Acid Transport (From 1968)

The first experiments on amino acid transport in the Morris hepatomas were carried out in our laboratory by Dr. Earl F. Baril,
just at the time that the controlled feeding experiments (previous
section) were being standardized. Using radioactive cycloleucine
Baril found (2, 4) that animals fed ad libitum showed no consistent
pattern of distribution ratio between liver and blood but that in
animals trained to an "8+16" protocol there was a daily oscillation
in the liver/blood ratio. It was soon found that amino-isobutyric
acid (AIB, which can also be seen as alphamethylalanine) was concentrated to higher distribution ratios than cycloleucine. In the
earliest report, at the Third Kettering Symposium (4), Baril's data
on AIB were compared with Dr. Watanabe's data on TAT and a straight
line correlation was shown to exist for 4 hepatomas 9618A, 9633,
7800, and 5123C, with AIB ratios of 8, 19, 41 and 152 correlating
with TAT values of 23, 114, 173, and 824. Although the AIB ratios
were exaggerated by an unresolved calculation factor, the relative
values are valid (75). In the first detailed report on radioactive
AIB transport in Morris hepatomas (3) the technique led to an expression of the equilibrium distribution ratio between tissue and blood
on the day following a single injection, since it had been established that uptake was rapid, excretion was slow, no conversion to CO_2
or protein occurred, and distribution ratios on the day after injection oscillated in a fairly reproducible manner in animals on controlled feeding schedules. In this report hepatomas 5123C, 7800,
9633 and 9618A were studied with respect to AIB distribution ratios
on 12%, 30%, and 60% dietary protein, at different times of day
(08:00 and 14:30 just prior to onset of feeding and after 6 hours of
food intake), and with concurrent hydrocortisone and glucagon injections (see below). Assays on livers and hepatomas for TAT, SDH, and

other enzymes were carried out using the same animals (87). The
data in the two reports (3, 87) are presented in similar fashion
in relation to time of day, to dietary protein, and following hormone treatment. The data show complex relationships between nutritional and endocrine factors that probably could only be domon-
strated with animals on controlled feeding and lighting protocols.
Data on the distribution ratios for AIB in the hepatomas, and in
control and host liver (3, Chart 3) were presented in relation to
the data on TAT and SDH and other enzymes (67, 87 Charts 6B and 7B)
in a review by Potter (55, Fig 8). There is a clear relationship
between increased AIB distribution ratio and increased TAT or SDH.
Especially striking is the ability of the hepatomas to hold a fixed
level of the enzymes that bears no relation to dietary protein and
instead parallels the AIB distribution ratio. Further modulation
of these parameters involved hormone treatments (see below).

F. Hormonal Inductions

     From the earliest studies on Morris hepatomas the rich back-
ground on the induction of various enzymes by hydrocortisone in rat
liver presented an opportunity to ask whether the enzymes could be
induced in the hepatomas to the same extent by the same means. The
failure of the hepatomas to respond to dietary protein in the mode
followed by control liver raised the question of whether they would
respond to hormones in a way comparable to normal liver. The available data on variations due to diet suggested that the controlled
lighting and feeding protocol be adopted for the hormone studies,
including more than one level of dietary protein and carbohydrate.
The enzyme data were reported by Watanabe et al. (3) and reviewed
by Potter (55). The data are remarkably reinforced by the availability of parallel experiments on the different diets. Thus when hydrocortisone was administered for 1, 3 or 7 days to rats on 12, 30 or
60% dietary protein, the values for TAT in normal liver were still
proportional to dietary protein but had increased by a substantial
amount on all diets after one day, were back to control values by 3
days, and were below controls at 7 days (87, Chart 4). The behavior
of SDH was quite different although all the curves showed a linear
relationship to dietary protein: There was no change after one day
of hydrocortisone, elevation after 3 days, and further elevation at
7 days (87, Chart 5). As in previous reports, glucose-6-phosphate
dehydrogenase (87, Chart 6) behavior was reciprocally altered in
comparison to SDH.
     These experiments were extended to include the effect of glu-
cagon superimposed on the 3 diets and the 4 time periods after hydrocortisone (0, 1, 3 and 7 days). All animals receiving glucagon were
sacrificed 6 hours later. It is especially interesting to compare
the data for TAT (87, Charts 1, 2, and 3) with data on AIB transport
(3, Charts 4, 5, and 6); Both were strongly enhanced by glucagon in
animals treated for 3 or 7 days with hydrocortisone but the effect
on TAT was more pronounced on 12% and 30% dietary protein, while the

effect on AIB transport was more pronounced on 30% and 60% dietary protein. The interaction between hydrocortisone and glucagon was borne out by later studies on liver cell cultures (see below).

The application of similar protocols to animals bearing Morris hepatomas 7800, 5123C, 9633 and 9618A brought out the diversity in these tumors as well as the concordance between TAT data and AIB transport data. For example both parameters were strongly enhanced by glucagon after 7 days hydrocortisone and 30% dietary protein in host liver and both parameters were absolutely unaffected by glucagon in hepatoma 9633 (87, Chart 23, and 3, Chart 10). Again, concordance was seen in both parameters in the case of hepatoma 9618A but in this tumor both parameters responded to glucagon after 7 days of hydrocortisone treatment (87, Chart 27B and 3, Chart 11). The response to glucagon by hepatoma 9618A and the lack of response by 9633 was confirmed in later experiments in which cyclic AMP was shown to accumulate in 9618A after glucagon, but not in 9633 (see below).

The AIB studies (3) involving hydrocortisone and glucagon reported concurrent effects on 4 other enzymes (87) which cannot be detailed here, as well as supporting data from adrenalectomized animals. These reports led directly to studies on another parameter, which will now be referred to.

G.   Cyclic AMP Induced by Glucagon in Vivo (from 1971)

The studies on AIB transport and TAT induction were greatly extended by Dr. D.F. Scott in collaboration with Dr. F.R. Butcher, who brought in the techniques for measuring cyclic AMP (14) and with Mr. R.D. Reynolds. Initial studies involved concurrent measurements of TAT activity and AIB distribution ratios in normal liver by various combinations of glucagon and theophylline, which was known to be an inhibitor of cyclic AMP diesterase (76). Animals trained to an "8+16" protocol showed no increase in TAT or AIB ratio when not given food, but both parameters increased about 5-fold over a period of 5 hours following theophylline at 10 mg per 100 g body weight. Both parameters gave remarkably parallel results over a wide range of values with theophylline at 0, 2.5 and 10 mg per 100 g body weight in all possible combinations with glucagon at 0, 0.24 and 2.0 mg per 100 g body weight, tested at 4 hours after injections. Both parameters were strongly elevated by dibutyryl cyclic AMP at 5 mg/100 g body weight (76).

The studies on normal liver were now extended to include measurements of cyclic AMP, which rises to a maximum and declines long before the other two parameters reach their peaks (18). It was found that the route of administration of glucagon markedly affected the results with subcutaneous glucagon at 0.2 mg per 100 g clearly established as more effective than the same dose given intraperitoneally (17).

With a background based on normal liver, concurrent measurements on AIB ratio and TAT induction by combinations of glucagon, theophylline, food intake, and dexamethasone were carried out on control liver, host liver, neonatal liver and 5 Morris hepatomas of which one was carried in intact and in adrenalectomized rats (70). All of the hepatomas differed from each other and from host and control liver responses, and host liver differed from controls. Neonatal liver gave clearcut inductions of TAT after the 3rd postnatal day. The range of hepatoma values was spanned by the range of values from birth to adulthood including induced values.

The major contributions in this series were reported in 1972, with TAT and AIB ratio reported by Scott et al. (74) and cyclic AMP induced and uninduced levels reported by Butcher et al. on the same animals (19). Eleven Morris hepatomas and their host livers were studied following induction of the 3 parameters by glucagon, epinephrine, isoproterenol, theophylline and dibutyryl cyclic AMP. Different animals had to be used to determine cyclic AMP-induced levels at 15 minutes after stimulant injection, while TAT and AIB were measured concurrently in animals killed at 3.5 hours after injection. Glucagon effects were studied in all animals but no experiments with dexamethasone alone or in combination were carried out. Such experiments were reported by Reynolds et al. (70) but did not include cAMP measurements.

The studies on the co-induction of the 3 parameters in 15 groups of hepatoma bearing rats were most instructive in that the induced levels were more revealing than the basal levels. However even the latter showed a proportionality between TAT and AIB. For the hepatomas the plot of TAT versus AIB ratio simply extended the curve for host liver about 3 fold for both parameters maintaining the same slope. Thus the maximum for the host livers was 1.5 and 10 respectively for TAT and AIB ratio, while the maximum among all the hepatomas was 6 and 30 respectively (74, Charts 1 and 2). The same slope was maintained in host livers stimulated by glucagon but now the values for TAT and AIB ratio moved out to a maximum of 12 and 40 respectively (74, Chart 6). In the case of the hepatomas there were two kinds of responses. Certain hepatomas responded to glucagon by increasing the value for both TAT and AIB ratio along the normal slope (74, Chart 5) a response that coincided with their ability to produce cyclic AMP under the influence of glucagon (19, Chart 1). Other hepatomas showed increases in TAT but not in AIB ratio (74, Chart 5) and this coincided with their absolute failure to produce cyclic AMP under the influence of glucagon (19, Chart 1). Closer inspection of the latter data reveals that the hepatomas responding to glucagon with increases in all 3 parameters resembled normal adult liver in several respects including a low basal level for all three

parameters (AIB ratio under 5) while the hepatomas that made no
glucagon response for either AIB ratio or cyclic AMP all had basal
levels for AIB ratio higher than 10 and up to 30. Yet these same
hepatomas responded to glucagon with respect to the third parameter,
TAT. This latter finding raises the question of whether an increase
in cyclic AMP is obligatory for the induction of TAT and suggests
that it is not if AIB transport is already high. Further experiments showed parallelism between TAT and AIB responses to adrenergic
agents and to dibutyryl cyclic AMP in host liver again maintaining
the "normal" slope, while there was a strong divergence in hepatoma
behaviors. Again those with high AIB ratios responded by increasing
TAT without going to higher AIB ratios, while those with low AIB
ratios responded poorly in the cases tried. As in other connections,
the hepatoma spectrum represented various combinations of neonatal
and adult properties. It was shown that neonatal liver and adult
liver have low cAMP and low AIB ratios, while neonatal liver responds
poorly to glucagon in both these parameters but quickly matures to
the good response in adult liver and in the hepatomas with similar
low AIB ratios. In contrast, the hepatomas that seem "derepressed"
and independent of glucagon for their AIB ratios, resemble neonatal
liver in their lack of response with cyclic AMP. The numerous
studies on TAT, AIB ratio and cyclic AMP in various kinds of normal
liver and in hepatomas under the influence of glucocorticoids, glucagon, and dietary manipulation led to a general concept of each
parameter as the resultant of a non-linear relationship between responses at the transcriptional level and responses at the translational level. The difficulty in carrying out in vivo studies on multiple
parameters influenced by multiple variables became obvious at an
early date and led to studies with cell cultures, first with hepatomas and more recently with adult liver (see below).

H. Hepatomas in Replicating Cell Cultures (From 1964)

     Another area that is a direct consequence of the availability
of the Morris hepatomas is the culture of well differentiated hepatoma cells in which many properties of liver cells still remain (56).
The development occurred first in the case of a single hepatoma, then
others were placed into serial culture, and clones were established.
Next cultures of fetal liver were studied, and finally primary cultures of adult liver cells were prepared. In a comprehensive review
of the role of cyclic AMP (cAMP) in the regulation of protein synthesis Wicks (92) called attention to these developments noting especially the first culture of hepatoma cells that were shown to respond to a hormone by inducing tyrosine aminotransferase (TAT) in our
laboratory in 1964 (46), thanks to the thesis efforts of Paul Morse,
and to the culture of fetal liver with similar properties in organ
culture by Wicks in 1968 (91). Wicks pointed out that these two culture systems "allowed studies of the direct action of hormones and
cyclic nucleotides to be made under conditions where many of the

complications associated with whole-animal studies (multiple hormone excretions, etc.) could be avoided." (92). He remarked that
"Although the physiologic normalcy of these culture systems is
clearly open to question, the results obtained through their use
have been remarkably similar to those ultimately observed in rat
liver". Here it must be noted that the various hepatoma cell cultures and sub-clones deviate from normalcy in much the same way
that E. coli and Neurospora mutants differ from their wild type
parents, so that the hepatoma cell lines seem to retain many normal
regulatory mechanisms and to deviate in interesting ways in a few.
The 1964 report (46) led to the development in 1966 of another hepatoma cell line designated HTC in the laboratory of the late Gordon
Tomkins starting with Morris hepatoma 7288c (79). The many contributions from that laboratory have recently been described by
Baxter et al. (5).

     Potter et al. (66) reported parallel studies on tyrosine amino-
transferase (TAT) and ornithine aminotransferase (OAT) in the H4-II-
E or H35 cell line showing induction of TAT by cortisone and by insulin and additive effects when both were present, but no increase
in OAT under any combination of hormones tested. Krawitt et al. (32)
confirmed the TAT inductions and showed that insulin-free glucagon
obtained from Dr. Ronald Chance failed to induce either TAT or AIB
uptake, while previous lots of glucagon had stimulated both. In this
system, AIB transport was increased by insulin but not by hydrocortisone, while both hormones increased TAT activity. Thus the results
with cultures differed from those in whole animal experiments (see
above). Later experiments with liver cell cultures have resolved
these differences (see below). Butcher et al. (15) demonstrated induction of TAT in the H-35 monolayers by dibutyryl cAMP (DBC) alone
or superimposed on cells maximally induced by hydrocortisone. The
response to DBC was much greater in the presence of hydrocortisone
and the "permissive" effect of hydrocortisone for DBC action was
noted and attributed to the possible production of mRNA for TAT by
the steroid and to "post-transcriptional" events for the action of
DBC and of insulin, a view subsequently reinforced. That the H35
cells respond to DBC while the Tomkins line of HTC cells do not was
also noted. This difference has been subsequently exploited by
Granner et al. (21) who showed that a line of HTC cells demonstrates
an absolute requirement for steroid pretreatment in order to obtain
any stimulation by DBC. Perhaps the only direct comparison of H35
cells and HTC cells in culture was made by Butcher et al. (16) who
showed that the H35 cells have about 30 times more TAT activity than
the HTC cells when both are maximally induced with cortisol. In the
absence of cortisol the H35 cells contained about 730 milliunits/mg.
In both cell lines addition of either cordycepin or actinomycin D
blocked the cortisol effect. It appears that the Granner results (21)
may stem from an extremely low level of mRNA for TAT in the absence of
cortisol and only a small amount of TAT mRNA even when cortisol is

present.

Walker et al. (82) examined a replicating culture of cells derived from adult rat liver and reported a 100% expression of fetal
liver isozymes and 0% expression of adult liver isozymes in the case
of hexokinase (adult form is "glucokinase"), aldolase (A, not B) and
pyruvate kinase (III, not I). Further properties of the pyruvate
kinase were reported by Walker and Potter (84).

Studies by Bushnell et al., using the H-35 cell line showed
that camptothecin blocked the induction of TAT by the steroid hormone (12) supporting the earlier work with cordycepin (16). Both
inhibitors block RNA synthesis but do not cause the "superinduction"
seen with actinomycin D. Ultraviolet light was shown to be an excellent inhibitor of transcription but not translation (13) and its
effects were enhanced by incorporation of bromodeoxyuridine (BrdU)
into DNA (11). The latter study grew out of a comprehensive examination by Gurr et al. (22) of the effects of incorporating BrdU
into the DNA of the H-35 cells. Each of several enzymes responded
differently with respect to increased or decreased basal levels or
levels induced by dexamethasone.

Additional hepatoma cell lines have been derived from known
transplantable Morris hepatomas. Two hepatoma lines known to
secrete large amounts of alphafetoprotein (AFP) into rat serum in
vivo were placed in culture by deNechaud et al. (20) and Becker et
al. (17). Both lines have continued to secrete AFP into the medium
and differ from each other in their response to dexamethasone. The
experience with replicating hepatoma cell lines was helpful in the
development of techniques for the study of cultures of normal adult
rat liver parenchymal cells (see below).

I. Adult Liver Cells in Primary Non-replicating Cell Cultures (From 1974)

With the development of the Berry and Friend collagenase perfusion technique many laboratories began to place rat liver cells
into short-term suspension cultures or into sterile monolayers with
a longer period of usefulness. Bonney et al. (8) chose the latter
course using regenerated liver while subsequent work has employed
normal intact adult rat liver. The first studies demonstrated induction of TAT by hydrocortisone within a few hours when added to
cultures that had been maintained one to several days.

Pariza et al. (36, 39) reported induction of ornithine decarboxylase by insulin but not by dexamethasone and showed that the insulin
effect was strongly dependent on the medium on which the cells were
maintained. Evidence for the repair of initial cell damage with the
passage of time up to 2 or 3 days was presented.

A series of reports followed which seemed to help explain the many previous observations on the role of hydrocortisone, glucagon, insulin and catecholamines on the induction of TAT, AIB transport, and cyclic AMP, although further studies continue. Kletzien et al. (30) began the study of AIB transport in liver cell monolayers in serum-free media, in which the effect of a single hormone could be studied. In contrast to responses in vivo where the effect of single hormones cannot be observed, dexamethasone did not induce AIB transport but it exerted a "permissive" effect on the induction by glucagon. Pariza et al. (37) showed that during the lag period after glucagon was added there was a striking production of cyclic AMP. The AIB transport system required the continued presence of both dexamethasone and glucagon and decayed rapidly in their absence, but either cycloheximide or puromycin could stop the decay. Further experiments showed that epinephrine like glucagon gave a striking increase in cyclic AMP and a subsequent increase in AIB transport but in the presence of propranolol the increase in cyclic AMP was completely blocked but the increase in AIB transport still occurred (38). The synergistic effect of dexamethasone and glucagon or exogenous cyclic AMP has been shown to depend dramatically on the postulated repair process as the monolayers are allowed to stabilize over a period of 48 to 72 hours (Gurr, Becker and Potter, unpublished) and the stabilized monolayers may be useful in the search for nutrients or hormones that will initiate replication, a phenomenon not yet observed for our cultures as a whole, while the replicating cultures obtainable from liver appear to have a whole new set of properties as described earlier (82, 84). It is still not clear whether such cultures derive from a tiny minority among the starting cultures or whether dedifferentiation of adult phenotypes can occur with appropriate culture conditions.

J. Autochthonous Slowly Growing Hepatomas in Vivo (From 1977)

Most autochthonous or primary hepatomas have been obtained under strongly carcinogenic conditions. With the advent of the Morris hepatomas the concept of deliberately using weakly carcinogenic conditions to induce minimally deviated hepatomas came into being. The idea was further advanced by the work of Peranio et al. (107) who used mild initiating conditions followed by a diet containing 0.05% phenobarbital. Kelley and Potter (29) used the Peraino protocol to produce 123 usable hepatomas in 43 rats and showed AIB ratios that were lower than those of normal liver and within a fairly narrow range relative to the ratios seen eralier with a spectrum of Morris hepatomas. However enzyme studies by Gurr et al. (unpublished) revealed a great diversity in several enzyme activities. The Peraino protocol and its modifications should produce in the future a wealth of experimental material which will be easier to interpret on the basis of established facts regarding the Morris hepatomas.

III.   INTERPRETATION

    The Morris hepatomas have now been studied in dozens of labo-
ratories all over the world and probably no one is cognizant of all
the implications that can be deduced from the total literature on
these cells. The present report covers only a partial list of the
contributions from one laboratory. From this admittedly narrow
view it is nevertheless possible to see that the available lines of
transplantable hepatomas form a spectrum of phenotypic diversity
that illustrates the breadth of the possible within the limits permitted by the definition of a cancer cell.

    The studies on AIB transport that have been herein reported
have led to the view that the transport elements in the cell membrane are simply localized enzymes that have the properties of other
enzymes in that their synthesis involves transcription and translation both of which are subject to regulation. In addition the
half-life of the system may be quite short, and is also probably
subject to regulation (37, 38). It appears that the synthesis of
the AIB transport system is responsible for many pleiotropic effects
resulting from alterations in the internal aminoacid pool, since we
have shown that a wide range of enzyme activities is correlated with
the level of AIB transport. The early in vivo studies measured only
the equilibrium value between tissue and blood based on an injection
of labeled AIB the previous day, but the more recent studies on monolayers in cell culture are based on initital rates and are probably
valid measures of the amount of the actual transport system (37, 38).
We have shown in the case of normal liver that there are several
levels of control. The glucocorticoid hormones alone cannot increase
the amount of the transport system but probably act by increasing the
amount of mRNA for the system. This sets the stage for the action of
glucagon, which may act via cyclic AMP (37) while the action of epinephrine appears not to be mediated by cAMP (38). Glucagon alone can
increase the amount of AIB transport slightly but not to the level
made possible by the prior action of dexamethasone. Recent unpublished experiments by Dr. D. Kelley have shown a more primitive type of
control not involving hormones but suggesting a combination of "trans-
inhibition" and direct repression of transcription by free amino acids.
Taken as a whole the data suggest that the Morris hepatomas with the
higher levels of AIB transport have become more and more independent
of hormonal control and have become "locked-in" to a derepressed level
of activity, possibly by internal manipulation of the free amino acid
pool thus using the primitive method of control.

    In terms of cell regulation the concept of multiple critical
nutrients as seen by Holley (23, 24, 25) is certainly supported.
Moreover the focus on the outer cellular membrane viewing cancer as a
membrane disease (85) with emphasis on signal reception and nutrient
transport is certainly justified. Both of these views of cancer are

completely compatible with the views of cancer as altered gene expression and, to be more specific in the case of liver, as a spectrum of different degrees of blocked ontogeny following retrodifferentiation. In this connection the apparent disagreement between
Pierce (41) and Uriel (80) seems unnecessary and probably is a result of focusing on different experimental material. Retrodifferentiation (80) or dedifferentiation seems applicable in liver carcinogenesis with the occurrence of various sites of residual blocked
ontogeny when the cells resume their progress toward the terminal
differentiated state (54, 55, 83).

    The available data are relevant to the question of whether the
widely documented literature on phenotypic diversity support the
concept of cancer as a highly random accumulation of blocks in the
ordered process of differentiation and development. According to
this view cancer is a process of natural selection within a multi-
cellular organism leading to the evolution of any combination of
phenotypic properties that can achieve enough autonomy to continue
to proliferate with no overall control that operates in the interest
of the host organism. This process of natural selection moves
naturally in the direction of faster growth and greater autonomy
leading occasionally to an impression of order and predictability
(89) and certainly to a collection of blocks in the ontogenic development that normally leads to cells whose proliferation is not autonomous but in fact tuned to the needs of the whole organism in a
changing environment.

REFERENCES

1. Ballard, P.L. and Tomkins, G.M. J. Cell Biol. 47 (1970) 222.

2. Baril, E.F. and Potter, V.R. J. Nutr. 95 (1968) 228.

3. Baril, E.F., Potter, V.R. and Morris, H.P. Cancer Res. 29
    (1969) 2101.

4. Baril, E.F., Watanabe, M. and Potter, V.R. In: Regulatory
    Mechanisms for Protein Synthesis in Mammalian Cells. Third
    Kettering Symposium, A. San Pietro, M.R. Lamborg, and F.T.
    Kennedy (eds). Academic Press, New York (1968) 417.

5. Baxter, J.D., Rousseau, G.G., Higgins, S.J. and Tomkins, G.M.
    In: The Biochemistry of Gene Expression in Higher Organisms,
    Pollak and Lee (eds). Australia and New Zealand Book Co, Sidney,
    (1973) 206.

6. Becker, F.F. In: Biology of Tumors: Cellular Biology and Growth,
    Cancer, A Comprehensive Treatise, Plenum Press, New York 3 (1975).

7. Becker, J.E., DeNechaud, B. and Potter, V.R. In: Oncodevelop-
    mental Gene Expression, W.H. Fishman and S. Sell (eds). Academic
    Press, New York (1976) 259.

8. Bonney, R.J., Becker, J.E., Walker, P.R. and Potter, V.R. In
    Vitro 9 (1974) 399.

9. Bottomley, R.H., Pitot, H.C. and Morris, H.P. Cancer Res. 23
    (1963) 392.

10. Bottomley, R.H., Pitot, H.C., Potter, V.R. and Morris, H.P.
    Cancer Res. 23 (1963) 400.

11. Bushnell, D.E. Biochem. Biophys. Res. Comm. 74 (1977) 92.

12. Bushnell, D.E., Becker, J.E. and Potter, V.R. Biochem. Biophys.
    Res. Comm. 56 (1974) 815.

13. Bushnell, D.E., Yager, J.D. Jr., Becker, J.E. and Potter, V.R.
    Biochem. Biophys. Res. Comm. 57 (1974) 949.

14. Butcher, F.R. Horm. Metab. Res. 3 (1971) 336.

15. Butcher, F.R., Becker, J.E. and Potter, V.R. Exp. Cell Res. 66
    (1971) 321.

16. Butcher, F.R., Bushnell, D.E., Becker, J.E. and Potter, V.R.

Exp. Cell Res. 74 (1972) 115.

17. Butcher, F.R., Scott, D.F. and Potter, V.R. Endocrinol. 89 (1971) 130.

18. Butcher, F.R., Scott, D.F. and Potter, V.R. FEBS Letters 13 (1971) 114.

19. Butcher, F.R., Scott, D.F., Potter, V.R. and Morris, H.P. Cancer Res. 32 (1972) 2135.

20. DeNechaud, B., Becker, J.E. and Potter, V.R. Biochem. Biophys. Res. Comm. 68 (1976) 8.

21. Granner, D.K., Lee, A. and Thompson, E.B. J. Biol. Chem. 252 (1977) 2891.

22. Gurr, J.A., Becker, J.E. and Potter, V.R. J. Cell Physiology 91 (1977) 271.

23. Holley, R.W., Baldwin, J.H. and Kiernan, J.A. Proc. Nat. Acad. Sci. U.S.A. 71 (1974) 3976.

25. Holley, R.W. and Kiernan, J.A. Proc. Natl. Acad. Sci. U.S.A 71 (1974) 2908 and 2942.

26. Hopkins, H.A., Bonney, R.J., Walker, P.R., Yager, J.D. Jr., and Potter, V.R. Advan. Enzyme Regul. 11 (1973) 169.

27. Hopkins, H.A., Campbell, H.A., Barbiroli, B. and Potter, V.R. Biochem. J. 136 (1973) 955.

28. Kalckar, H.M. J. Cellular Physiol. 89 (1976) 503.

29. Kelley, D. and Potter, V.R. Biochem. Biophys. Res. Comm. 75 (1977) 219.

30. Kletzien, R.F., Pariza, M.W., Becker, J.E. and Potter, V.R. Nature 256 (1975) 46.

31. Kletzien, R.F., Pariza, M.W., Becker, J.E. and Potter, V.R. J. Cellular Physiol. 89 (1976) 641.

32. Krawitt, E.L., Baril, E.F., Becker, J.E. and Potter, V.R. Science 169 (1970) 294.

33. Nowell, P.C., Morris, H.P. and Potter, V.R. Cancer Res. 27 (1967) 1565.

34. Ono, T., Blair, D.G.R., Potter, V.R. and Morris, H.P. Cancer Res. 23 (1963) 240.

35. Ono, T., Potter, V.R., Pitot, H.C. and Morris, H.P. Cancer Res. 23 (1963) 385.

36. Pariza, M.W., Becker, J.E., Yager, J.D.Jr., Bonney, R.J. and Potter, V.R. In: Differentiation and Control of Malignancy of Tumor Cells, W. Nakahara, T. Ono, T. Sugimura and H. Sugano (eds). U. Tokyo Press, Tokyo (1974) 267.

37. Pariza, M.W., Butcher, F.R., Kletzien, R.F., Becker, J.E. and Potter, V.R. Proc. Nat. Acad. Sci. U.S.A. 73 (1976) 4511.

38. Pariza, M.W., Butcher, F.R., Becker, J.E. and Potter, V.R. Proc. Nat. Acad. Sci. U.S.A. 74 (1977) 234.

39. Pariza, M.W., Yager, J.D.Jr., Goldfarb, S., Gurr, J.A., Grossman, S.H., Becker, J.E., Barber, T.A. and Potter, V.R. In: Gene Expression and Carcinogenesis in Cultured Liver, E.B. Thompson, and L.E. Gerschenson (eds). Academic Press, New York (1975) 137.

40. Peraino, C., Fry, R.J.M., Staffeldt, E. and Kisieleski, W.F. Cancer Res. 33 (1973) 2701.

41. Pierce, G.B. Fed. Proc. 29 (1970) 1248.

42. Pitot, H.C. Bull. Tulane Unive. Med. Fac. 19 (1959) 17.

43. Pitot, H.C. Cancer Res. 20 (1960) 1262.

44. Pitot, H.C. In: Cancer, A Comprehensive Treatise, Plenum Press, New York, 3 (1975) pp. 121-154.

45. Pitot, H.C., Peraino, C., Bottomley, R.H. and Morris, H.P. Cancer Res. 23 (1963) 135.

46. Pitot, H.C., Peraino, C., Morse, P.A. and Potter, V.R. Nat. Cancer Inst. Mono. 13 (1964) 229.

47. Pitot, H.C. and Potter, V.R. Biochim. Biophys. Acta 40 (1960) 537.

48. Pitot, H.C., Potter, V.R. and Morris, H.P. Cancer Res. 21 (1961) 1001.

49. Potter, V.R. Univ. Mich. Med. Bull. 23 (1957) 401.

50. Potter, V.R. Fed. Proc. 17 (1958) 691.

51. Potter, V.R. Cancer Res. 21 (1961) 1331.

52. Potter, V.R. In: The Molecular Basis of Neoplasia, M.D. Anderson Hospital and Tumor Institute (eds). Austin Univ. Texas Press, (1962) 367.

53. Potter, V.R. Adv. Enz. Regul. 1 (1963) 279.

54. Potter, V.R. Canadian Cancer Conf. 8 (1969) 9.

55. Potter, V.R. Miami Winter Symposia 2 (1970) 291.

56. Potter, V.R. Cancer Res. 32 (1972) 1998.

57. Potter, V.R. In: Cancer Medicine, J.F. Holland and E. Frei,III (eds). 2nd Edition in press. Lea and Febiger, Philadelphia (1977).

58. Potter, V.R. and Auerbach, V.H. Lab. Invest. 8 (1959) 495.

59. Potter, V.R., Baril, E.F., Watanabe, M. and Whittle, E.D. Fed. Proc. 27 (1968) 1238.

60. Potter, V.R., Gebert, R.A., Pitot, H.C., Peraino, C., Lamar, C. Jr., Lesher, S. and Morris, H.P. Cancer Res. 26 (1966) 1547.

61. Potter, V.R. and Ono, T. Cold Spring Harbor Sym. on Quant. Biol. 26 (1961) 355.

62. Potter, V.R., Pitot, H.C., Ono, T. and Morris, H.P. Cancer Res. 20 (1960) 1255.

63. Potter, V.R., Reynolds, R.D., Watanabe, M., Pitot, H.C. and Morris, H.P. Advan. Enzyme Regul. 8 (1970) 299.

64. Potter, V.R., Walker, P.R. and Goodman, J.I. Gann Mono. 13 (1972) 121.

65. Potter, V.R. and Watanabe, M. In: Proceeedings of the International Leukemia-Lymphoma Conference, C.J.D. Zarafonetis (ed). Lea and Febiger, Philadelphia (1968) 33.

66. Potter, V.R., Watanabe, M., Becker, J.E. and Pitot, H.C. Adv. Enzyme Regul. 5 (1967) 303.

67. Potter, V.R., Watanabe, M., Pitot, H.C. and Morris, H.P. Cancer Res. 29 (1969) 55.

68. Reynolds, R.D. and Potter, V.R. Life Sci. II 10 (1971) 5.

69. Reynolds, R.D., Scott, D.F., Potter, V.R. and Morris, H.P.
    Adv. Enzyme Resul. 9 (1971) 335.

70. Reynolds, R.D., Scott, D.F., Potter, V.R. and Morris, H.P.
    Cancer Res. 31 (1971) 1580.

71. Risser, W.L. and Gelehrter, T.D. J. Biol. Chem. 248 (1973)
    1248.

72. Schmitz, H., Potter, V.R. and Hurlbert, R.B. Cancer Res. 14
    (1954) 58.

73. Schmitz, H., Potter, V.R., Hurlbert, R.B. and White, D. Cancer
    Res. 14 (1954) 66.

74. Scott, D.F., Butcher, E.R., Potter, V.R. and Morris, H.P. Cancer
    Res. 32 (1972) 2127.

75. Scott, D.F., Butcher, F.R., Reynolds, R.D. and Potter, V.R.
    In: Biochemical Responses to Environmental Stress, I.A.
    Bernstein (ed). Plenum Press, New York (1971) 51.

76. Scott, D.F., Reynolds, R.D., Pitot, H.C. and Potter, V.R. Life
    Sciences II, 9 (1970) 1133.

77. Sell, S. and Morris, H.P. Cancer Res. 34 (1974) 1413.

78. Shatton, J.B., Morris, H.P. and Weinhouse, S. Cancer Res. 29
    (1969) 1161.

79. Thompson, E.B., Tomkins, G.M. and Curran, J.F. Proc. Nat. Acad.
    Sci. U.S.A. 56 (1966) 296.

80. Uriel, J. In: Cancer, A Comprehensive Treatise, Plenum Press,
    New York, 3 (1975 pp. 21-55.

81. Walker, P.R. Life Sciences 15 (1975) 1507.

82. Walker, P.R., Bonney, R.J., Becker, J.E. and Potter, V.R. In
    Vitro 8 (1972) 107.

83. Walker, P.R. and Potter, V.R. Adv. Enzyme Regul. 10 (1972) 339.

84. Walker, P.R. and Potter, V.R. J. Biol. Chem. 248 (1973) 4610.

85. Wallach, D.F.H. In: Membrane Molecular Biology of Neoplastic
    Cells, Elsevier, Amsterdam (1975).

86. Watanabe, M., Potter, V.R. and Pitot, H.C. J. Nutr. 95 (1968) 207.

87. Watanabe, M., Potter, V.R., Pitot, H.C. and Morris, H.P. Cancer
    Res. 29 (1969) 2085.

88. Watanabe, M., Potter, V.R., Reynolds, R.D., Pitot, H.C. and
    Morris, H.P. Cancer Res. 29 (1969) 1691.

89. Weber, G. Adv. Enzyme Regul. 1-14 (1963-1977).

90. Weinhouse, S. Cancer Res. 32 (1972) 2007.

91. Wicks, W.D. J. Biol. Chem. 243 (1968) 900.

92. Wicks, W.D. In: Advances in Cyclic Nucleotide Research, P.
    Greengard and G.A. Robinson (eds). Raven Press, New York,
    4 (1974) pp. 335-438.

93. Yanagi, S., Campbell, H.A. and Potter, V.R. Life Sciences,
    17 (1975) 1411.

THE MOLECULAR CORRELATION CONCEPT OF NEOPLASIA: RECENT ADVANCES

AND NEW CHALLENGES

George Weber[1], Harutoshi Kizaki, Taiichi Shiotani,
Diana Tzeng and Jim C. Williams

Laboratory for Experimental Oncology
Indiana University School of Medicine
Indianapolis, Indiana 46202

SUMMARY

This paper critically evaluates the advances made with the
molecular correlation concept as a conceptual and experimental approach in elucidating the biochemical strategy of the cancer cells.
New advances made in gaining an insight into the behavior of pyrimidine metabolism are also used to illustrate the method and current
status of the molecular correlation concept. Investigation of the
hepatomas of different growth rates and comparison with appropriate
control systems such as the normal, differentiating and regenerating liver has led to the discovery that in neoplastic cells there
is an ordered pattern of enzymatic and metabolic imbalance. We
documented in detail the linking of biochemical discriminants with
neoplastic transformation and progression in carbohydrate, pentose
phosphate, purine, pyrimidine, ornithine and polyamine metabolism
and in membrane cAMP systems. We pointed out the importance of
selecting for such investigations the analysis of the activity, concentration and isozyme pattern of opposing key enzymes in antagonistic pathways of synthesis and degradation. We demonstrated that the
control of gene expression operates through reciprocal regulation of
opposing key enzymes in antagonistic and competing metabolic pathways.

Current investigations on the behavior of the opposing key enzymes, thymidine kinase and dihydrothymine dehydrogenase, support
our earlier reports on the antagonistic behavior of the opposing
pathways of thymidine utilization for synthesis and degradation.
Ongoing investigations on the behavior of enzymes involved in uridylate and CTP biosynthesis show that CTP synthetase is the rate-

limiting enzyme in the overall pathway culminating in CTP production. The activity of UDP kinase was elevated in all the hepatomas, indicating that the behavior of this enzyme was transformation-linked. The activities of uridine kinase, uracil phosphoribosyl-transferase and CTP synthetase were also significantly increased in all tumors and 6- to 11-fold elevated in the rapidly growing neoplasms. These three enzymes are both transformation- and progression-linked in the hepatoma spectrum. Concurrent with this increased capacity for CTP biosynthesis, the capacity of the degradative pathway was decreased.

From this and earlier work and also from results of other laboratories, we have extensive evidence that the cancer cells through a reprogramming of gene expression exhibit a meaningful and ordered biochemical imbalance that confers selective advantages to the cancer cells. Neoplasms may show random fluctuations in some biochemical parameters; this behavior is apparently coincidental and not related to the core of neoplasia. What is essential about neoplastic transformation and progression is ordered and what is not, is the randomness and diversity. The presence of the operation of an ordered pattern is no longer at issue, but rather the challenge is to discover the molecular mechanisms that can account for the highly integrated, purposeful, ordered, poly-enzyme, multi-pathway alterations.

The metabolic imbalance in the hepatomas is specific to neoplasia and no similar pattern has been observed in fetal, differentiating, regenerating or adult normal liver. The applicability of some aspects of the metabolic imbalance discovered in the hepatoma spectrum has also been shown in kidney and mammary cancer in the rat, lymphomas in the mouse, viral-induced hepatoma in the chicken and most importantly in human primary hepatomas and renal cell carcinomas.

With the progress in elucidation of the biochemical strategy of malignancy, a significant challenge is the application of this knowledge to the design of drug treatment. In this laboratory advances were made in achieving a successful design in tissue culture on the basis of enzyme-pattern-targeted chemotherapy. Such applications of the insight into the enzymic and isozymic pattern of tumors and relevant host tissues should permit the design of more selective chemotherapy and biochemical rescue methods to achieve a successful treatment of neoplastic diseases.

INTRODUCTION

The molecular correlation concept has been the steering element in our enquiry in this laboratory into the molecular basis of neoplastic transformation and progression (17, 18). The objective of this enquiry is to elucidate the pattern of reprogramming of gene expression as it is manifested in the information content revealed in the activity and behavior of key enzymes, isozymes and metabolic pathways. As remarked by Medawar and Medawar, in biology the term 'information' "connotes order and orderliness or anything that embodies it - e.g., a message or set of instructions specifying order... 'Noise' connotes the very opposite of information, that is to say randomness and disorderliness. A signal which conveys no information in a context in which it might have been expected to have done so is dismissed as noise" (9). The molecular correlation concept made progress in identifying the order and neoplasia-linked biochemical imbalance as it was first recognized in the spectrum of hepatomas of different growth rates (14). This approach also identified biochemical changes that show no relationship to the core of neoplasia as coincidental alterations - the 'noise' or diversity. Clarification of these issues was made possible by our introduction to cancer research of the key enzyme concept on the basis of our observations that the strategy of gene expression is carried out by regulation of a few antagonistic or competing enzymes in the various metabolic pathways. The amount, activity and isozyme pattern of the key enzymes are stringently controlled as the regulation of gene expression is modulated. Such conditions occur in development, endocrine regulation, regeneration and neoplasia (14, 17-19). The obstacles that litter the road of progress are the unreasonable expectations of researchers that every scrap of metabolic change must make sense and be relevant to neoplasia. We drew attention to the need to concentrate on the behavior of key metabolic components. Our pointing out the presence of coincidental alterations in neoplasia, mostly involving the behavior of enzymes that were present in great excess and our recognition of the noise nature of these findings prevented our being bogged down in a mire of non-cancer-related observations. Once the key enzymes were identified and the relationship of these parameters with transformation and progression was elucidated, then the ordered pattern was discovered. Thus, the molecular correlation concept provided a powerful pattern of explanation from which the observations would become explicable as a matter of course. Our utilization of a number of available hepatocellular carcinomas as a continuous system according to their biological behavior (growth rate) provided a suitable model in which the heuristic value of the molecular correlation concept was first tested.

In summarizing the main achievements of the molecular correlation concept and some of the recent results, we pay respect to Professor Harold P. Morris with whom a harmonious and productive collaboration has been carried out for nearly two decades.

MATERIALS AND METHODS

Biological Systems: Tumors. Aspects of the biology and biochemistry of the hepatoma spectrum have been reviewed previously

(10, 14, 15, 17-19). The rats were kept in separate cages, with water and Purina Laboratory Chow available ad libitum. The tumors were maintained as bilateral subcutaneous transplants in inbred strains of ACI/N or Buffalo male rats. The tumors were harvested at a diameter of about 1.5 cm as described elsewhere (17). It is important that in all experiments rats were killed between 9:00 a.m. and 10 a.m. and normal rats of the same age, sex, strain, and weight were killed at the same time for control tissues.

Studies on the Spectrum of Kidney Tumors of Different Growth Rates. These neoplasms were produced specifically on my suggestion by Dr. Morris and they are discussed elsewhere (7, 11, 31). Investigations on mouse lymphomas were referred to previously.

Studies on Human Primary Liver and Kidney Tumors. Investigations on primary hepatocellular carcinoma and renal cell tumors from human cases were compared with control tissues obtained from the same host at operations as reported elsewhere (21, 23, 26).

Studies on Fetal, Differentiating and Regenerating Liver. Our investigations on the conditions and the respective usefulness of the biochemical information obtained in these control biological systems were outlined elsewhere (14, 15, 17, 18).

Enzyme Assays and Metabolic Techniques. The preparation of homogenates and subcellular fractions, tissue slices and freeze clamp preparations were reported (2, 15, 17, 18, 28).

The methods for determination of protein, DNA and nuclear counts were given in detail earlier (14, 17, 18, 23).

Expression and Evaluation of Results. The biological, histological and biochemical quantitation of tumor malignancy, i.e., growth rate, were evaluated and discussed in detail elsewhere (2, 14, 17, 18). Enzymatic, metabolic and isozymic results were quantitated and compared on the basis of various biochemical variables. For instance, enzyme activities were expressed in micromoles or nanmoles of substrate metabolized per hr at 37°C at a specified pH per wet weight of tissue, per mg protein, per DNA, or per average cell. It has been explained elsewhere that per cell is the preferred basis of expression. Ready comparability with reports of others in the literature is obtained by our providing the data as specific activity (per mg protein). The data were tabulated for comparison as percentages of the relevant normal liver of adult fed rat. The results were statistically evaluated where significance was accepted for p values < 0.05. The correlation coefficient was also calculated when approriate for the growth rate and the biochemical activity.

RESULTS AND DISCUSSION

The Molecular Correlation Concept and the Key Enzyme Concept.
An insight into the ordered pattern of biochemical and enzymatic
imbalance was made possible, in part at least, by the introduction
of the molecular correlation concept and the concept of key enzymes.
The molecular correlation concept was introduced as a theoretical
and experimental method aimed at discovering the pattern of biochemical imbalance and its linking to neoplastic transformation and
progression (14, 15, 17, 18). The concept of key enzymes was proposed to account for observations made in this laboratory that
identified certain enzymes through which regulation of the rate and
direction of opposing synthetic and catabolic pathways was controlled.
The evidence indicated that the control of gene expression was exerted through regulation of certain enzymes that opposed each other or
competed with each other at strategic points in opposing and competing synthetic and degradative pathways (19).

The molecular correlation concept proposed that the biochemical
strategy of the genome in neoplasia can be identified by elucidation
of the pattern of gene expression revealed in the concentration,
activity and isozyme pattern of key enzymes and their linking with
neoplastic transformation and progression, Thus, from determination
of the end product of the expression of the gene program, the concentration of specific enzyme proteins, the strategy of gene expression and its quantitative and qualitative alterations can be measured
(17-19). The advantages of this concept included the following facts.
(1) Precise predictions can be made which can be tested and disproven
or verified, (2) Not only can the molecular correlation concept provide candidates for metabolic alterations in relation to transformation and progression but the extent and direction of alterations can
be predicted and tested, (3) From the relationship of the behavior of
the enzyme activities in the hepatoma spectrum the linking of the
metabolic imbalance with transformation and progression can be discovered, (4) By pointing out the opposing key enzymes as prime candidates in discovering the altered patterns of gene expression, the
logic of gene expression can be analyzed, (5) By identifying the
operation of an isozyme shift in neoplasia the qualitative aspects of
the reprogramming of gene expression can be studied, (6) By determining the linking of the enzymatic alterations to transformation and
progression, the road was opened to use the enzymes in the biochemical
diagnosis and grading of malignancy, (7) In identifying the key enzymes that were stringently linked with transformation and progression,
it was possible to discover the selective advantages the reprogramming
of gene expression confers to cancer cells, (8) By recognizing the
selective advantages, the key enzymes were identified as promising
targets in the design of anti-cancer selective chemotherapy. (9) By
identifying an ordered pattern of enzymatic and biochemical imbalance,
the specificity of this pattern to neoplasia can be established using

a series of control biological systems, (10) By identifying the
specificity to neoplasia of the altered pattern of gene expression,
it became possible to test the applicability of this information to
tumors other than hepatomas in animals and to primary tumors of different types in human.

The linking of the behavior of the activities of enzymes and
metabolic pathways with transformation and progression provides a
classification of these parameters according to their stringent linking with neoplasia or their coincidental alterations in the cancer
cells (Table 1). With the approaches of the molecular correlation
concept the biochemical imbalance in the hepatoma spectrum was
critically evaluated in a number of metabolic areas that were summarized in Table 2. The conclusion that emerged from these studies
is that an ordered pattern is revealed in the progression- and transformation-linked alterations. The apparent diversity that occurs for
some biochemical parameters apparently is due to their less stringent
linking with regulatory events which marked these changes as coincidental to the core of neoplasia. The conclusion was drawn that what
is important about cancer is ordered - what is not, is the random
element and the diversity.

Recently an account was given of the main experimental observations that led us to the formulation of the present integrated concept of the biochemical strategy of the neoplastic cells as achieved
by application of the molecular correlation concept (17, 18). In
Table 3 an overview is provided of the main achievements reached by
application of the molecular correlation concept in the spectrum of
hepatomas of different growth rates.

Some of the current work in this laboratory has been directed to
the elucidation of the enzymology of pyrimidine synthesis in normal
and neoplastic cells. Therefore, this area of investigation will be
used to demonstrate some of the approaches and considerations of the
molecular correlation concept.

Correlation of Opposing Overall Pathways of Thymidine Utiliza-tion and Key Enzyme Activities in the Spectrum of Hepatomas.

Earlier work (2) recently extended and brought up to date (20)
demonstrated that the utilization of thymidine for DNA synthesis
(TdR to DNA) correlated positively, whereas the opposing catabolic
pathway, the degradation of thymidine to CO_2 (TdR to CO_2), correlated
negatively with the increase in growth rate and malignancy of the
various tumor lines in the spectrum of hepatomas. As a result the
ratio of TdR to DNA/TdR to CO_2 correlated with tumor growth rate was
over several orders of magnitude in the log scale. This TdR ratio
provides the best biochemical correlate to tumor malignancy to date.
The results are summarized in Fig 1, which illustrates the antagonis-

Table One
Analysis of Biochemical Strategy of the
Cancer Cell by the Molecular Correlation Concept

Class	Linking of biochemical discriminants[a] with malignancy[b]	Indicators of reprogramming of gene expression; activities of enzymes, isozymes, pathways
1	Progression-linked	Activities correlate with tumor malignancy:
		stringent linking with degrees of expression of neoplastic program
2	Transformation-linked	Activities increase or decrease in all hepatomas:
		stringent linking with malignant transformation per se.
3	Coincidental alterations	Activities do not relate to malignancy:
		random fluctuations not linked with transformation or progression

[a] Biochemical features that quantitatively or qualitatively differentiate pattern of hepatic neoplasia from that of normal, adult, fetal, developing or regenerating lvier.

[b] Measured growth rates of various tumor lines.

Table Two
The Biochemical Imbalance in the Hepatoma
Spectrum was Characterized in the Following Metabolic
Areas

Pyrimidine (de novo and salvage pathways)

Purine (IMP synthesis, degradation and utilization)

Carbohydrate (gluconeogenesis, glycolysis)

Pentose phosphate (oxidative and non-oxidative pathways)

Urea cycle

Ornithine (synthesis, degradation and utilization)

Polyamine biosynthesis

Membrane cAMP (synthesis and degradation)

Protein and amino acid (synthesis and degradation)

Conclusion: An ordered pattern is revealed in:

Progression-linked alterations[a] (Class 1)

Transformation-linked alterations[a] (Classs 2)

---

[a] In activities of key enzymes, isozymes and opposing metabolic
pathways.

Table Three
Conceptual and Experimental Advances Achieved by Application
of the Molecular Correlation Concept

Key enzymes	The role of antagonistic key enzymes and synthetic and catabolic pathways was identified in neoplasia.
Reciprocal Behavior	The opposing behavior of antagonistic key enzymes and pathways was recognized in neoplasia; the ratios of key enzymes and pathways were shown to be the most sensitive discriminants in recognizing transformation and characterizing the different degrees in the expression of neoplasia (progression).
Isozyme Shift	The qualitative alterations of reprogramming of of gene expression were identified in the isozyme shift.
Ordered Pattern	In the biochemical phenotype malignant transformation and progression were expressed as an ordered pattern of quantitative and qualitative imbalance.
Linking with Malignancy	The biochemical imbalance was stringently linked with neoplastic transformation and with the degrees of expression of malignancy (progression).
Specificity	The biochemical pattern of ordered imbalance was specific to neoplasia and no similar pattern has been observed in fetal, differentiating, adult or regenerating liver.
Generalization	The ordered pattern of ordered imbalance was applicable to various chemically-induced tumors in rat and in mouse, to viral-induced hepatoma in chicken and to primary hepatoma and renal cell tumors in human.
Predictive power	The molecular correlation concept was able to provide predictions for quantitative and qualitative biochemical alterations and for the extent and direction of the changes.
Selective Advantages	The molecular correlation concept revealed the selective advantages (replicative advantages) that the reprogramming of gene expression confers to cancer cells.
Diagnosis and Grading	The ordered pattern of quantitative and qualitative biochemical imbalance which was elucidated can be employed in the diagnosis and grading of tumor malignancy.
Chemotherapy	The imbalance in the activities of key enzymes and the recognition of the selective advantages points out the key enzymes as possible sensitive targets for selective anti-cancer chemotherapy.

Table Four

Reciprocal Alterations Linked with Degrees of Expression of Neoplastic Transformation (Progression)

Functions Increased		Functions Decreased	
Pathways	Enzymes	Pathways	Enzymes
RNA and DNA Metabolism			
CTP synthesis	Aspartate carbamoyl-transferase	CTP degradation	Dihydrouracil dehydrogenase
	Dihydro-orotase		
	Uridine kinase		
	CTP synthetase		
De novo pathway	Ribonucleotide reductase		
	dCMP deaminase		
	dTMP synthase		
Salvage pathway (TdR to DNA)	TdR kinase	Thymidine degradation (TdR to CO_2)	Dihydrothymine dehydrogenase
	dTMP kinase		
	DNA polymerase		
Carbohydrate Metabolism			
Glycolysis	Hexokinase	Gluconeogenesis	Glucose-6-phosphatase
	Phosphofructokinase		Fructose 1,6-diphosphatase
	Pyruvate kinase		Phosphoenolpyruvate carboxykinase
			Pyruvate carboxylase
Ornithine Metabolism			
Ornithine to polyamine synthesis	Ornithine decarboxylase	Ornithine to urea cycle	Ornithine carbamoyl-transferase
cAMP Metabolism in Membrane			
cAMP metabolism	cAMP phosphodiesterase	cAMP synthesis	Adenylate cyclase

tic behavior of opposing synthetic and catabolic pathways, the
sensitivity of the ratios to neoplastic transformation (the ratio
is increased 7-fold in the slowest growing hepatoma) and the usefulness of the ratio in characterizing malignancy.

Recently we tested the applicability of the proposition that
the antagonistic enzymes involved in channeling thymidine to DNA
and degradation of thymidine to CO_2 would correlate with the behavior of the overall metabolic pathways. For this study the enzyme in the biosynthetic pathway, thymidine kinase, was selected
because it is involved in the immediate utilization of thymidine,
channeling it to the synthetic pathway. In the catabolic pathway,
the rate-limiting enzyme of degradation, dihydrothymine dehydrogenase, was selected. The behavior of these two opposing enzymes
has never been tested previously in the same tissue preparations.
Such experiments also provided a comparison of the behavior of the
activity of opposing enzymes measured in tissue extracts with the
behavior of overall metabolic pathways that were quantitated in
tissue slices. The outcome of these experiments is shown in Fig
2. The results indicate that the behavior of thymidine kinase
paralleled that of the incorporation of thymidine into DNA, whereas
the dehydrogenase paralleled that of the catabolic pathway. This
good agreement between the activities and reciprocal behavior of
the overall metabolic pathways and key enzymes provides further
support for the usefulness of the molecular correlation concept
and the key enzyme concept as conceptual and experimental tools for
gaining insight into the molecular basis of neoplasia.

Reciprocal Alterations in Key Enzyme Activities Linked with
Degrees of Expression of Neoplastic Transformation (Progression).

The recognition that the antagonistic enzymes show opposing
behavior was first made in this laboratory in studies on the behavior of enzymes of glucogenesis and glycolysis under nutritional
and hormonal regulation and during differentiation (19). The reciprocal regulation manifested under these regulatory conditions
was found to apply to the enzymatic changes in neoplasia. An example of the opposing behavior of key enzymes of thymidine utilization was shown above in Fig. 2. Our investigations elucidated that
reciprocal alterations in gene expression occur in a number of metabolic pathways and some of these expressions of metabolic imbalance
are linked with the degrees of expression of the neoplastic transformation. Thus, the reciprocal alterations are linked with progression in the hepatoma spectrum. Some of these reciprocal alterations are tabulated in Table 4. Such observations were originally
made in carbohydrate metabolism and then reciprocal regulation was
tested and found to apply to RNA, DNA and ornithine metabolism and
to cAMP metabolism in the plasma membrane. Thus, the principle of

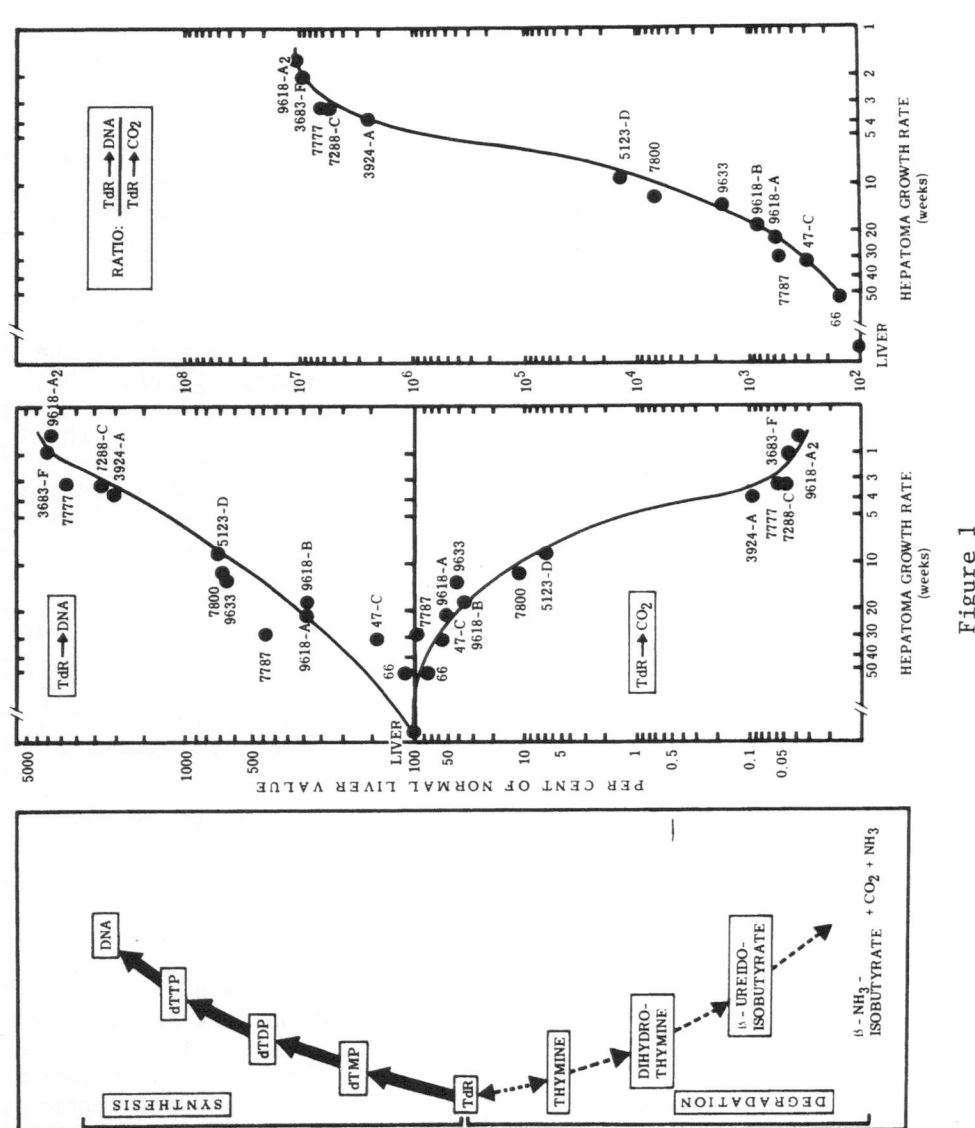

Figure 1

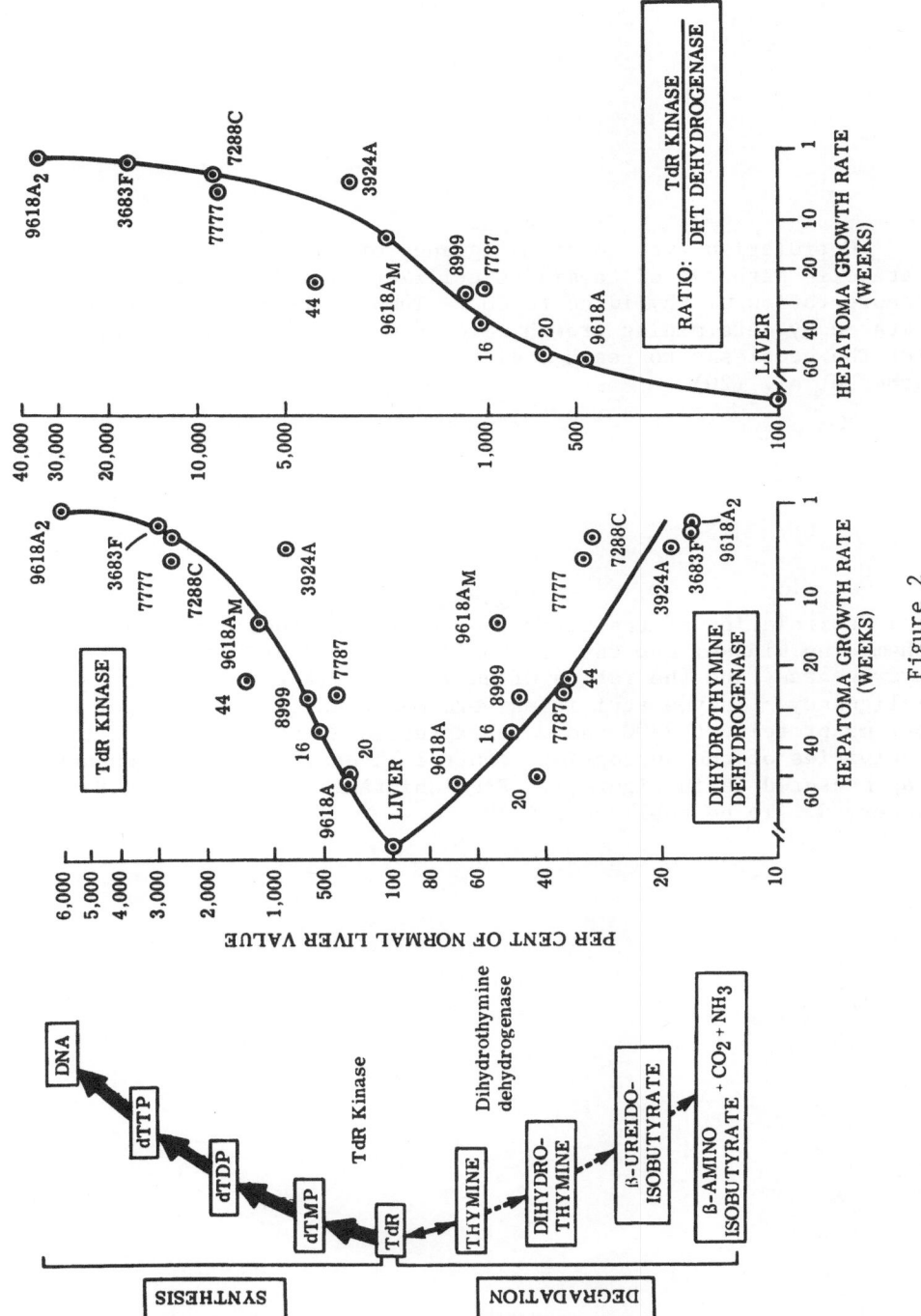

Figure 2

Figure 1
Correlation with tumor malignancy of the synthetic and
catabolic pathways of thymidine utilization and the ratio of
incorporation of thymidine to CO_2. Tumor malignancy was quantitated by determining growth rate as measured in weeks required
for the neoplasms to reach a diameter of 1.5 cm. From data of
Weber et al. (20).

Figure 2
Correlation of the activities of the synthetic enzyme,
thymidine kinase, and the catabolic enzyme, dihydrothymine dehydrogenase, and the ratios of enzyme activities with tumor
malignancy. Enzyme activities were measured in nanmoles per hr
per mg protein at 37°C and were expressed as percentages of the
activities of the appropriate control livers. Tumor malignancy
was measured as in Figure 1. From Shiotani, T., Morris, H.P. and
Weber, G. To be published, 1978.

reciprocal regulation appears to pervade all metabolic areas and
its further testing in other fields should provide more information on the applicability of the strategy of gene expression and
genic logic as an effective method of biological information control. These studies demonstrated the linkage with progression of
the behavior of antagonistic key enzymes in hepatomas of different
growth rates. Thus, any explanation postulating a mechanism at
the molecular level would have to account for this inheritable
linking of the reciprocal control in the different lines of hepatomas (See below). These observations underline the ordered pattern of biochemical imbalance and the usefulness of the molecular
correlation concept in pinpointing the enzymes, the directions of
the alterations and even the extent of rise or decrease as has
been discussed elsewhere (17, 18). It is clear that the reciprocal
changes in the opposing enzymatic activities should amplify the
metabolic imbalance and the reprogramming of gene expression manifested in these alterations should provide selective proliferative
advantages to the cancer cells.

Enzymatic Imbalance in Uridylate and CTP Biosynthesis in Hepatomas.

In what follows I will use current work in my laboratories to
illustrate certain of the approaches of the molecular correlation
concept as applied to a metabolic area of special interest in the
control of RNA and DNA metabolism, drug activation and targeting of
anti-cancer antimetabolites. The metabolic area of the biosynthesis
or uridylates and of CTP is of particular relevance to neoplasia
because these precursors are strategic shared metabolites for both
DNA and RNA production. The biosynthesis of UMP and CTP has proved
to be a sensitive target to inhibition by antimetabolites (8) and
in this laboratory we have made progress in designing an enzyme-
pattern-targeted, organ-specific chemotherapy against this pathway
3, 4). Because of our earlier observations that orotate did not enter in any appreciable quantity to hepatomas (27), it became of interest to consider a rescue by orotate of the bone marrow, intestine
and other organs in presence of high concentrations of anti-metabolites of the biosynthetic pathways of uridylate and CTP. To gain a
deeper insight into the enzymology of UMP and CTP formation, a systematic investigation is currently being carried out in my laboratory
to elucidate the behavior of key enzymes of CTP biosynthesis in a
spectrum of hepatomas of different growth rates and in the meaningful biological systems we use as controls such as differentiating and
regenerating liver and resting liver of adult rats.

The area of uridylate and CTP metabolism also holds an attrac-
tion for the biochemist because it provides an opportunity to examine the display of the informational program triggered by transformation and progression. Our studies demonstrated that in the

formation of uridylates and CTP the final enzyme, CTP synthetase, has the lowest activity and this appears to be rate-limiting in the sequence. Consequently, on strictly arguing for efficiency one may assume that an increase in the activity of CTP synthesis might be sufficient to achieve a rise in the output of this pathway from where the metabolites may be channeled to RNA and DNA biosynthesis. That the activity of this enzyme should be increased in neoplasia also follows from our consideration of the principle of reciprocal regulation because the absolute activity of CTP synthesis is lower than that of the rate-limiting catabolic enzyme, dihydrouracil dehydrogenase.

In attempting to gain a fuller insight into the biochemical aspects of the neoplastic program, attention also has to be paid to the three enzymes involved in the production of the strategic precursor, UMP. (a) OMP decarboxylase is the final enzyme in the de novo biosynthesis of UMP and its behavior was examined by Sweeney et al. (13); we interpret their data as signalling that this enzyme activity was increased in all five examined hepatomas. (b) Uridine kinase is a so-called salvage enzyme that produces AMP from uridine. (c) UMP can also be provided by the salvage of uracil which may be recycled in presence of PRPP through uracil phosphoribosyltransferase activity.

The outcome of our studies on the behavior of enzymes of CTP biosynthesis in the spectrum of hepatomas of different growth rates is reported in Table 5. A comparison shows that the absolute activities of the enzymes of CTP biosynthesis differ widely, with the highest being that of UDP kinase (30). The activity of uridine kinase is orders of magnitude lower than that of uracil phosphoribosyltransferase (22) and CTP synthetase (29) is another order of magnitude lower. UDP kinase activities were elevated in all hepatomas, indicating that this is a transformation-linked enzyme (30). The activities of uridine kinase, uracil phosphoribosyltransferase and CTP synthetase were significantly increased in all tumors and 6- to 11-fold elevated in the rapidly growing neoplasms. These three enzymes are both transformation- and progression-linked. Thus, the information expressed in cancer cells entails not only a step-up in the activity of the rate-limiting enzyme, CTP synthetase, but also an elevation in the activities of the other enzymes involved in the biosynthesis of UMP and CTP.

Earlier studies pointed out a relationship between the absolute activity in resting liver of the adult fed rats and the extent of rise in enzyme activity in the rapidly growing tumors. This principle was shown to apply to enzymes of pyrimidine and DNA synthesis (17, 18), and, in recent work, to enzymes of purine biosynthesis (24). Table 5 suggests the operation of this principle in CTP biosynthesis. UDP kinase, the enzyme with the highest activity, increased the least

Table Five
Behavior of Enzymes of Uridylate and CTP Biosynthesis in
Hepatomas of Different Growth Rates

Tissues	Protein (mg/g)	UDP kinase	Uridine kinase	Uracil phospho-ribosyl-transferase	CTP synthetase
Liver	100.0 ± 0.6	$444,000 \pm 10,000$[a] 100	$156+5$[a] 100	15 ± 0.6[a] 100	$5.5+0.5$[a] 100
Hepatomas					
9618A	93	244	242	263	340
16	84	300	200	293	
28A	78		273	240	359
8999	82	193	220	367	184
7787	82	191	230	300	188
44	88	191	245	350	222
9633F	77		168		277
7800	79	311	193		
7777	63	270			464
3924A	72	183	614	467	702
7288C	80		552	557	999
9618A$_2$	72	203	527	357	911
3683F	74	298	694	760	1122

[a] Specific activities (nmoles/hr/mg protein) were expressed as % of control liver activities. All tumor activities were significantly higher than those in control livers ($p = <0.05$). Details of the techniques of extraction and assay of the various enzymes are given elsewhere (22, 28, 29).

whereas CTP synthetase, the enzyme with the lowest activity, was elevated the highest in the rapidly growing hepatomas. The phenotypic evidence for reprogramming of gene expression in hepatic neoplasia for CTP metabolism is summarized in Table 6.

Specificity to Neoplasia of the Biochemical Imbalance in CTP Biosynthesis

The discriminating power of the biochemical pattern can be judged from the differences between tissues that have similar growth rates, such as the rapidly growing hepatomas and newborn and regenerating liver. Results in Table 7 show that the alterations in the activities of enzymes involved in CTP biosynthesis are specific to neoplasia and that no similar pattern was observed in any of the control tissues, as shown by the quantitative and qualitative discriminants.

Progression-linked Discriminants: Enzymatic Markers of the Degrees of Malignant Transformation

In elucidating the linking of the biochemical strategy with biological malignancy in neoplasia, it was observed that the display of the malignant genic program may be expressed in different degrees that range from mild through advanced to the fullblown pattern. This graded expression of the neoplastic program in the different tumor lines in the spectrum of hepatomas of the same cell type is termed progression. Our studies indicated that the activities and concentration of certain key enzymes increased and those of the opposing enzymes decreased in parallel with the malignancy of the different hepatoma lines. These are the enzymatic markers of malignant progression and a summary of some of these enzymatic changes is provided in Table 8.

Transformation-linked Discriminants: Enzymatic Markers of Malignancy - The Shared Program in Cancer Cells.

It has rightly been stressed by Busch that neoplasia is manifested by transformation that is hereditable and characterizes every tumor cell (1). The molecular correlation concept postulated that since there is a shared program of commitment to proliferation in all cancer cells, certain enzymes should exhibit the same type of alterations in all the tumors in a spectrum of neoplasms. Our observations have provided evidence that such all-or-none alterations that are stringently linked with transformation do indeed occur in neoplasms and an up-to-date summary of these enzymatic markers of malignancy is provided in Table 9. This table indicates that the principle of reciprocal regulation also applies to the transformation-linked enzymatic alterations. The activities of certain key enzymes in pentose phosphate, purine, pyrimidine and DNA

Table Six

CTP Metabolism: Phenotypic Evidence for Reprogramming of Gene Expression in
Hepatic Neoplasia

Synthetic enzymes	Key enzymes of UMP[a], and CTP[b] synthesis	Increased
Degradative enzymes	Key enzymes of degradation[c]	Decreased
Enzymatic imbalance	Ratios of synthetic/catabolic enzymes	Increased
Metabolic imbalance	Ratios of synthetic/catabolic pathways	Increased
Linking to malignancy	Alterations are co-variant with growth rate	Progression-linked imbalance
	Alterations present in all hepatomas	Transformation-linked im-balance
Biological role	Imbalance in anabolic/catabolic enzymes of CTP metabolism provide increased capacity for de novo and salvage CTP production	Confers selective advantages to cancer cells

a Carbamoyl-phosphate synthase (glutamine), aspartate carbamoyltransferase, dihydro-orotase, orotate phosphoribosyltransferase, OMP decarboxylase, uridine phosphorylase, uridine kinase, uridine phos-phoribosyltransferase

b UDP kinase, CTP synthetase

c Dihydrouracil dehydrogenase

Table Seven

Discriminating Power of Biochemical Pattern in CTP Biosynthesis: Key Differences Between Rapidly Growing Neoplastic, Newborn and Regenerating Liver

Enzymes: Pyrimidine markers of substrate gene expression	K_m (mM)	Normal fed adult nmoles/hr/mg protein	Livers		Hepatoma
			Regenerating (24 hr) % of adult liver	Newborn (6-day-old) % of adult liver	Rapidly growing (3683) % of adult liver
		% of adult liver			
UDP kinase	0.5	440,000	100	100[b]	100[b]	298
Uridine kinase	4.0	156	100	120[a]	30[b]	694
Uracil phosphoribo-syltransferase	1.0	15	100	213[a]	56[b]	760
CTP synthetase	0.5	5.5	100	200[a]	31[b]	1,122

[a] Quantitative discriminant from hepatoma.

[b] Qualitative discriminant from hepatoma.

Table Eight

Progression-linked Discriminants: Enzymatic Markers of the Degrees of Malignant Transformation

Nucleic Acid Metabolism	Carbohydrate Metabolism	Protein Metabolism	Other Metabolic Areas
Pyrimidine, RNA & DNA synthesis Increased: Carbamoyl-phosphate synthase (glutamine) Aspartate carbamoyltransferase Dihydro-orotase Uridine phosphorylase Uridine kinase Uridine phosphoribosyltransferase CTP synthetase Ribonucleotide reductase Deoxycytidylate deaminase Thymidylate synthetase Thymidine kinase DNA polymerase DNA nucleotidyltransferases tRNA methylase Pyrimidine catabolism-decreased: Dihydrouracil dehydrogenase Purine synthesis-increased: IMP dehydrogenase AMP aminase Purine catabolism-decreased: Adenylate kinase	Glucose catabolism-increased: Hexokinase Phosphofructokinase Pyruvate kinase Glucose synthesis-decreased: Glucose 6-phosphatase Fructose 1,6-diphosphatase Phosphoenolpyruvate carboxykinase Pyruvate carboxylase Specific phosphorylating enzymes-decreased: Fructokinase Glucokinase Fructose utilization-decreased: Thiokinase Aldolase Isozyme shift-decreased: High K_m isozymes Isozyme shift-decreased: Low-K isozymes R-5-P utilization-increased: PRPP synthetase	Protein synthesis-increased: Amino acid incorporation into protein (alanine, aspartate, glycine, serine, isoleucine, valine) Activity of postmicrosomal protein synthesizing system Enzymes catabolizing amino acids-decreased: Glutamate dehydrogenase Glutamate-oxaloacetate transaminase Tryptophan pyrrolase Serotonin deaminase 5-Hydroxytryptophan decarboxylase Urea cycle-decreased: Ornithine carbamoyltransferase	Polyamine synthesis-increased: Ornithine decarboxylase Polyamine synthesis-decreased: S-Adenosylmethionine synthetase Membrane cAMP metabolism: cAMP phosphodiesterase increased Adenylate cyclase:decreased Ketone-body utilization-increased: Succinyl coA: acetoacetate coA transferase Lipid metabolism-decreased: α-Glycerophosphate dehydrogenase HMG-CoA synthase

Table Nine

Transformation-linked Discriminants: Enzymatic Markers of Malignancy

Metabolic areas	Synthetic pathways: Increased	EC No.	Degradative Pathways Decreased	EC No.
Pentose phosphate	Glucose 6-phosphate dehydrogenase	1.1.1.49		
	Transaldolase	2.2.1.2		
	PRPP synthetase[a]	2.7.6.1		
Purine	Glutamine PRPP aminotransferase	2.4.2.14	Inosine phosphorylase	2.4.2.1
	Adenylosuccinate synthetase	6.3.4.4	Xanthine oxidase	1.2.3.2
	Adenylosuccinase	4.3.2.2	Uricase	1.7.3.3
	AMP deaminase[a]	3.5.4.6		
	IMP dehydrogenase[a]	1.2.1.14		
Pyrimidine & DNA	Thymidine kinase[a]	2.7.1.75	Dihydrothymine dehydrogenase	1.3.1.2
	Orotate phosphoribosyltransferase	2.4.2.10	Thymidine phosphorylase	2.4.2.4
	Orotidine 5'-phosphate decarboxylase[a]	4.1.1.23		
	Uracil phosphoribosyltransferase	2.4.2.9		
	Uridine kinase	2.7.1.48		
	UDP kinase	2.7.4.6		
	CTP synthetase[a]	6.3.4.2		

[a] Also linked with progression.

biosynthesis were increased and opposing enzymes were decreased
in all the examined hepatomas. The applicability of these enzymatic markers of malignant transformation to other tumor types
is of particular interest as they may assist in the biochemical
diagnosis of neoplasia.

Generalization: Applicability of the Biochemical Imbalance Identified in the Spectrum of Rat Hepatomas to Other Types of Tumors in Rat, Mouse, Chicken and in Human Neoplasms

Recent studies carried out in this laboratory demonstrated
that the biochemical imbalance was applicable to mouse lymphomas
(26), and to rat renal cell carcinomas (7, 31) and studies in
other centers indicated that the imbalance also applied to other
rat neoplasms (5). Our work in primary hepatomas in human (23)
and our current investigations on a series of 15 cases of renal
cell carcinomas in human (26), documented the applicability of
the metabolic imbalance to primary human neoplasms (Table 10).

Recent important work in the laboratory of Professor Lapis
(6) and the interesting studies of Prajda et al. (12) demonstrated
that the metabolic imbalance discovered in the chemically-induced
transplantable hepatomas also applies to a viral-induced transplantable hepatoma in the chicken.

These investigations ranging from rodents to avian to human
and from chemically-induced to viral-induced to "spontaneous"
primary neoplasms in man share the information content and program
display indicating that neoplastic transformation and progression
at the biochemical level may entail a similar readout that may
be stringently linked with the core of neoplasia. The utilization
of the various hepatomas produced by Harold P. Morris thus has made
possible the testing of the predictions and principles of molecular
correlation concept in the first biological system available for a
systematic and meaningful study of the biochemistry of neoplasia.
It may not be superflous to emphasize at this point that we do not
consider the elucidation of the biochemical pattern of neoplasia by
any means a completed task, because a very great deal of further insight is needed into the many vital areas of metabolic alterations
in cancer cells.

Criteria to be Fulfilled by an Account of the Molecular Mechanisms that Underlie the Ordered Pattern of Imbalance in Cancer Cells

An important further task is to understand the molecular mechanisms that may account for the highly ordered and meaningful metabolic imbalance that has been discovered. The various metabolic aspects of the transformation- and progression-linked alterations would

Table 10
Generalization: The Biochemical Imbalance Discovered
in Rat Hepatomas is Applicable to Other Types of Tumors in
Different Species

A.   RODENT TUMORS

     Rat kidney tumors (renal cell carcinomas)

     Rat mammary carcinomas

     Mouse lymphomas

B.   AVIAN TUMOR

     Chicken hepatoma

C.   HUMAN TUMORS

     Primary hepatoma

     Kidney tumors (renal cell carcinoma)

require an explanation at the molecular level that would account
for a number of aspects of the ordered biochemical pattern revealed in the strategy of the cancer cells.

Thus, any mechanism proposed should account for the well-
known observation that the biochemical pattern is hereditable and
that the gene pool is remarkably stable as manifested in the constancy of the biological malignancy (17, 18) and the extent of the
metabolic imbalance of the different tumor lines in the spectrum.
Any proposed mechanisms must account for the observation that the
enzymatic imbalance appears to be irreversible and that it entails
a highly integrated multi-enzyme imbalance involving enzymes the
production of which is specified on different genes in separate
chromosomes. Any proposed molecular mechanism should account for
the observations that many of the stringently linked biochemical
alterations that are progression-linked and that other alterations
occur in all tumors and thus are transformation-linked. An explanation should account for the emergence of qualitative alterations which are expressed in the isozyme shift and in the altered
responsiveness to regulate the activity and the amount of the
various enzymes in the tumor lines. In any final analysis the
mechanisms proposed should account for the specificity to neoplasia
of the biochemical imbalance as no similar pattern has been observed in fetal, differentiating, regenerating or normal liver. I
have discussed the main possibilities in terms of genetic or epi-
genetic mechanisms and work is in progress in my laboratory to throw
more light on this important problem (16, 25).

Phenotypic Markers of Neoplasia and Targets of Chemotherapy: Key Enzymes

In this paper, as in an earlier review (17, 18), an attempt was
made to integrate some of the most relevant quantitative and qualitative differences in the biochemistry of the cancer cell, discriminating it from that of normal cells. We discovered that in
cancer cells there operates an ordered pattern of enzymatic imbalance that is linked stringently with the malignant transformation
and the gradations in the expression of the neoplastic properties
(progression). We also identified the biological advantages that
the metabolic imbalance confers on the cancer cells. This insight
into the molecular biology of neoplasia points out the key enzymes
as sensitive targets of selective anti-cancer drugs. It is recognized that the selective advantages observed in the cancer cells,
short-term as they are, are expressed in the net proliferative advantage of the neoplastic gene pool and information content in the
host. The integrated enzymic imbalance in cancer cells suggests
that the genes participating in the control of opposing key enzymes
of pyrimidine, purine, carbohydrate, pentose phosphate, polyamine
and ornithine utilization and other strategic metabolic pathways are

closely coadapted during evolution, so as to represent one, or a
complex, or integrative or master genes (16-18, 25). In the
design of selective chemotherapy there should be a particular advantage in targeting the combination chemotherapy against several
of the key enzymes. For this purpose we tested experimental approach in which the specialized enzymatic pattern characteristic
of the tissue of origin of a tumor might be exploited to target
and enhance drug selectivity (3, 4). In some of our studies D-
galactosamine-induced depletion of UTP, primarily a hepatic event,
was employed to enhance the growth inhibition caused by 3-deaza-
uridine. In cultured cells the drug effect was most pronounced in
the slower growing, well-differentiated hepatoma lines (e.g., hepatoma 8999) where the activities of certain liver metabolic pathways and key enzymes, though decreased, were still efficiently
operative. In such cell lines the effects of galactosamine and
deazauridine were strongly synergistic. In contrast, in non-
hepatic cell lines these drugs were merely additive. Similar enzyme-pattern-targeted drug selectivity was also succefully tested
with the other anti-metabolites of pyrimidine biosynthesis (3, 4).
With current experiments employing orotate that is not taken up by
neoplastic cells and with 5-deazauracil, an irreversible inhibitor
of the rate-limiting catabolic enzyme, dihydrouracil dehydrogenase,
which can increase the circulating level of thymidine, powerful approaches can be brought to bear upon attempts to increase the organ-
and cell-specificity of combined anti-cancer modalities.

[1] Recipient of USPHS Grants CA-13526 and CA-05034, to whom requests
for reprints should be addressed at the Laboratory for Experimental Oncology, Indiana University School of Medicine, Indianapolis,
Indiana 46202.

REFERENCES

1. Busch, H. In: <u>The Molecular Biology of Cancer</u>, Academic Press, New York (1974).

2. Ferdinandus, J.A., Morris, H.P. and Weber, G. Cancer Res. 31 (1971) 550.

3. Jackson, R.C. and Weber, G. Biochem. Pharmacol. 25 (1976) 2613.

4. Jackson, R.C., Williams, J.C. and Weber, G. Cancer Treat. Reports 60 (1976) 835.

5. Knox, W.E., Linder, M. and Friedell, G.H. Cancer Res. 30 (1970) 283.

6. Kovalszky, I., Jeney, A., Asbot, R. and Lapis, K. Cancer Res. 36 (1976) 2140.

7. Lea, M.A., Morris, H.P. and Weber, G. Cancer Res. 28 (1968) 71.

8. McPartland, R.P., Wang, M.C., Bloch, A. and Weinfeld, H. Cancer Res. 34 (1974) 3107.

9. Medawar, P.B. and Medawar, J.S. The Life Science. Current Ideas of Biology, Harper & Row, New York (1977)

10. Morris, H.P. and Meranze, D.R. Recent Res. in Cancer Res. 44 (1974) 103.

11. Morris, H.P., Wagner, B.P. and Meranze, D.R. Cancer Res. 30 (1970) 1362.

12. Prajda, N., Lapis, K. and Eckhardt, S. In: <u>New Approaches to the Study of Environmental Hepatocarcinogenesis</u>,K. Lapis (ed) In press, Hungarian Academy of Sciences, Budapest (1978).

13. Sweeney, M.J., Parton, J.W. and Hoffman, D.H. Adv. in Enzyme Reg. 12 (1974) 385.

14. Weber, G. Adv. in Cancer Res. 6 (1961) 403.

15. Weber, G. In: <u>The Molecular Biology of Cancer</u>, H. Busch (ed). (1974) 487.

16. Weber, G. In: <u>Cancer Enzymology</u>, Miami Winter Symposia J. Schultz and F. Ahmad (eds). Academic Press, New York 9 (1976) 63.

17. Weber, G. New Eng. J. Medicine 296 (1977) 486.

18. Weber, G. New Eng. J. Medicine 296 (1977) 541.

19. Weber, G. In: Search and Discovery. Symposium dedicated to Dr. Albert Szent-Gyorgyi, B. Kaminer (ed). Academic Press, New York, in press (1977).

20. Weber, G., Ferdinandus, J.A., Queener, S.F., Dunaway, G.A., Jr. and Trahan, L.J.P. Adv. in Enzyme Reg. 10 (1972) 39.

21. Weber, G., Goulding, F.J., Jackson, R.C. and Eble, J.N. In: Biological Characterization of Human Tumors, W. Davis and C. Maltoni (eds). Excerpta Medica, American Elsevier, in press (1977)

22. Weber, G., Kizaki, H., Shiotani, T., Tzeng, D. and Williams, J.C. In: New Approaches to the Study of Environmental Hepato-carcinogenesis, K. Lapis (ed). In press, Hungarian Academy of Sciences, Budapest (1978).

23. Weber, G., Malt, R.A., Glover, J.L., Williams, J.C., Prajda, N. and Waggoner, C.D. In: Biological Characterization of Human Tumors, W. Davis and C. Maltoni (eds). Excerpta Medica, American Elsevier (1976) 60.

24. Weber, G., Prajda, N. and Jackson, R.C. Adv. in Enzyme Reg. 14 (1976) 3.

25. Weber, G., Prajda, N. and Williams, J.C. Adv. in Enzyme Red. 13 (1975) 3.

26. Weber, G., Jackson, R.C., Williams, J.C., Goulding, F.J. and Eberts, T.J. Adv. in Enzyme Reg. 15 (1977) 53.

27. Weber, G., Singhal, R.L. and Srivastava, S.K. Adv. in Enzyme Reg. 3 (1965) 396.

28. Weber, G., Stubbs, M. and Morris, H.P. Cancer Res. 31 (1971) 2177.

29. Williams, J.C., Kizaki, H., Morris, H.P. and Weber, G. Submitted for Publication (1978).

30. Williams, J.C., Morris, H.P. and Weber, G. Nature 253 (1975) 567.

31. Williamson, D.H., Krebs, H.A., Stubbs, M., Page, M.A., Morris, H.P. and Weber, G. Cancer Res. 30 (1970) 2049.

EXPRESSION MECHANISM OF ABNORMALITY OF ORNITHINE AMINOTRANSFERASE LEVEL IN MORRIS HEPATOMAS

Nobuhiko Katunuma and Keiko Kobayashi

Department of Enzyme Chemistry, Institute for Enzyme Research, School of Medicine, Tokushima University Tokushima 770, Japan

INTRODUCTION

Ornithine aminotransferase (OTA) plays a role in both the production of glutamate or proline from ornithine via glutamic δ-semialdehyde and in the production of ornithine from proline. Therefore, the activity of OTA might regulate the ornithine level in liver. The ornithine concentration in liver controls the urea cycle activity and is also important as a source to make putrescine by ornithine decarboxylase. On the other hand, although the OTA proteins from liver and kidney are identical, the inducibilities of the liver enzyme and that from kidney to individual hormones or dietary condition are different. Since the different hormonal responsiveness in different organs were elucidated from aspects of the synthesis and degradation of the enzyme, it is interesting to know OTA levels in the spectrum of Morris hepatomas which differ in the degree of deviation from normal liver (11) and to elucidate the expression mechanisms of the abnormalities of OTA levels.

BEHAVIOR OF OTA IN INDIVIDUAL ORGANS TOWARD VARIOUS HORMONES

Studies on changes in OTA activity in liver and kidney under various biological conditions, hormones and diet protein, have been reported (1-5). OTA in the liver was induced by a high protein diet or by glucagon administration and the treatment of rats with estrogen increased the OTA activity in the kidney, but not in the liver. In our laboratory, OTA in liver and kidney was crystallized and these enzyme proteins from liver and kidney were identical (3, 6). Furthermore, it was shown by immunochemical analysis that these increased activities were due to an increase in the amount of these enzyme pro-

teins (3). The half-life of OTA in liver was about 4 times as
rapid as that in kidney. Morris et al. reported that the induction
of OTA activity in liver by a high protein diet was due to an increase in the rate of enzyme synthesis (7). As shown in Table 1
(8), the increased amount of kidney OTA in estrogen treated rats is
due to an increase in the rate of the biosynthesis, not to a decrease in the rate of degradation. However, no changes in the rates
of biosynthesis and degradation of liver OTA were observed after
administration of estrogen. It is interesting to consider the abnormal expression of OTA levels in the spectrum of hepatomas and
furthermore if there are abnormal hormonal responses in some hepatomas.

Table One
Rate Constants of Degradation and Synthesis of Liver and Kidney Ornithine Amino-transferase

	Content (units/g wet weight)	t1/2 (days)	Kd (day $^{-1}$)	Ks (units/g wet weight/day)
Liver				
Control	2.80 + 59*	0.95	0.73	2.04
Estrogen-treated	3.0 + 30*	0.92	0.75	2.31
Kidney				
Control	3.04 + 59*	4.0	0.17	0.52
Estrogen-treated	15.10 + 81*	4.7	0.15	2.27

Values are means + standard deviations of values in fifteen animals.

BEHAVIOR OF OTA ACTIVITY IN HEPATOMAS OF DIFFERENT GROWTH RATES

The results in Fig 1 (9) show that the level of OTA per mitochondria in the rapidly growing hepatomas was markedly decreased and
in the slowly growing hepatomas showed about the same level as that
of normal liver (9). However, we found an exception in this connection, that is, hepatomas 21, 47C and 44 showed unexpectedly high
levels of OTA. OTA activity in the regenerating liver was in the
normal range exhibited by the liver of the sham-operated controls.
The completely purified OTA from slowly growing hepatoma 44 and from
rapidly growing hepatoma 7777 were identical proteins with that of
normal liver as judged by kinetic parameters, acrylamide gel electrophoresis and immunochemical methods. To examine whether the alterations in activity represented changes in concentration, the OTA amount

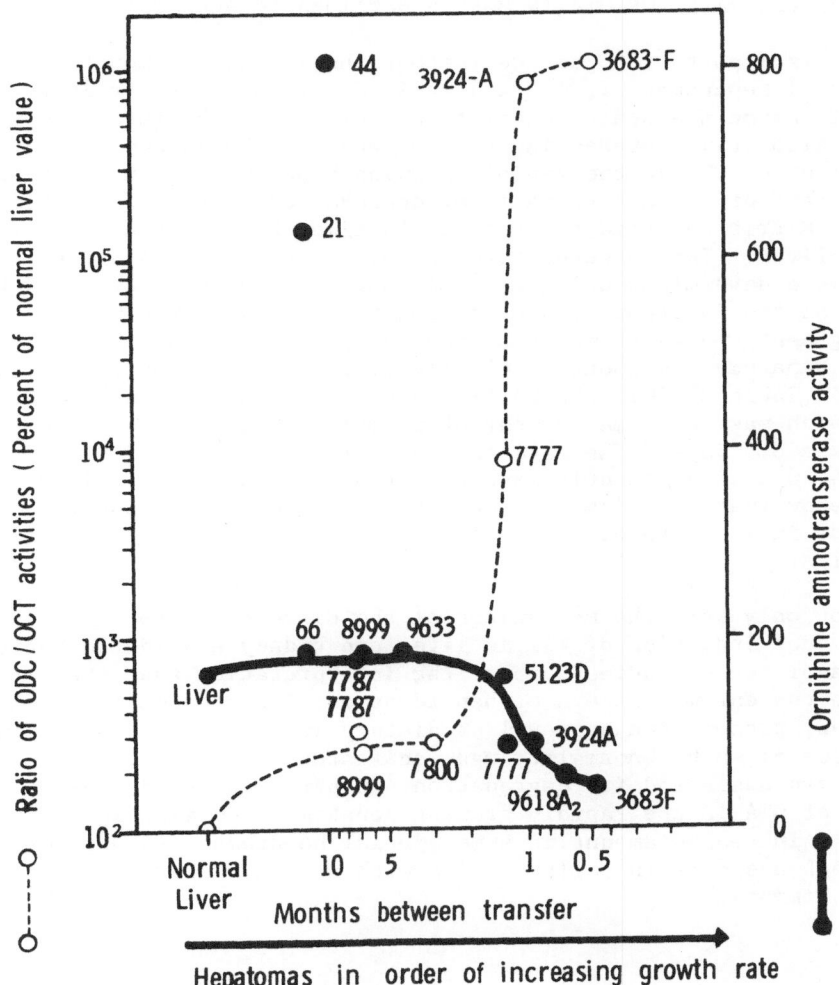

Figure 1
Correlation of the ornithine aminotransferase activity with hepatoma
growth rate.

was measured by by the immunochemical technique. The OTA amount of liver and hepatomas (44, 8999, 9633, 7777 and 3924A) showed a parallel with these enzyme activities.

TURNOVER RATES OF OTA IN MORRIS HEPATOMA 44 AND HOST LIVER

It is important to decide whether the increased amount of OTA in special hepatomas 21, 47C and 44 is due to an increase in the rate of enzyme synthesis and/or to a decrease in the rate of degradation. Also it is interesting to know whether the marked decrease in the amount of OTA in the rapidly growing hepatomas is due to a change in the rate of enzyme synthesis or degradation or both. The OTA content of Morris hepatoma 44 is about 15 times higher than that of normal liver. The turnover rates of OTA in hepatoma 44 and host liver were determined using L-[^{14}C]leucine. Studies shown in Table 2 (10) on the incorporation of radioactive leucine into OTA in rats bearing hepatoma 44 showed that the rate of synthesis of this enzyme in the hepatoma was about 5-fold higher than that of host liver. As shown in Table 3 (10), the half-life of OTA in host liver was 0.98 day, which was the same as that of normal liver, whereas in hepatoma 44 it was 3.5 days. The rate constant of degradation of OTA in hepatoma 44 was significantly less than that of host liver. These results show that the high OTA content of hepatoma 44 is due to both an increase in its rate of synthesis and a decrease in its rate of degradation.

Not only were the mechanisms of the different responsiveness to hormonal induction of OTA in liver and kidney elucidated but the results of these studies support the interpretation that the alteration in the enzyme pattern of hepatomas entails abnormal gene expression, rather than hormonal or dietary influences. Expression mechanism of such abnormality was manifested from the viewpoint of enzyme synthesis and its degradation, in part, in the decreased amount of OTA in the rapidly growing hepatomas and also in the abnormally increased amount in some special hepatomas. (A part of this work was done in collaboration with Drs. G. Weber, H.P. Morris and I. Tomino).

Editor's Note:

Studies such as the above reflect the complexity of regulation in cancer tissues. Not only is the synthesis of specific proteins under rigid control, but so also their degradation. Therefore, it should never be unexpected to learn that both synthetic and degratory mechanisms are modified in cancers.

Table Two
Relative Rates of Synthesis of Ornithine
Aminotransferase in Hepatoma 44 and Host Liver

	Content of OTA (units/g wet weight)	TCA soluble (cpm/g wet weight)	L-[^{14}C]Leucine incorporation		
			A	B	Ax10^4/B
			OTA (cpm/g wet weight)	Total soluble protein (cpm/g wet weight)	Relative rate of synthesis
Host liver	1.86	1.36 x 10^4	303	18.19 x 10^4	16.66
	2.18	1.63 x 10^4	433	24.20 x 10^4	17.90
	1.15	1.56 x 10^4	186	21.75 x 10^4	8.59
Hepatoma 44	26.07	1.52 x 10^4	1,189	13.69 x 10^4	86.83
	25.52	1.71 x 10^4	1,454	16.42 x 10^4	88.58
	25.68	2.02 x 10^4	1,972	22.36 x 10^4	88.21

Rats bearing hepatoma 44 were given a single intraperitoneal injection of L-[^{14}C]leucine (10 μCi per 100 g body weight). Two hours later they were killed and the radioactivities incorporated into ornithine aminotransferase (OTA), total soluble protein and the trichloroacetic acid-soluble fraction (TCA-soluble) were determined.

Table Three
Rate Constants of Degradation and Synthesis
of Ornithine Aminotransferase in Hepatoma 44 and
Host Liver

	Content (units /g wet weigt)	t1/2 (days)	Kd (day $^{-1}$)	Ks (units/g wet weight/day)
Host Liver	1.47 ± 0.32*	0.98	0.71	1.04
Hepatoma 44	25.15 ± 1.99*	3.50	0.20	5.03

* Values are means ± standard deviations of values in fourteen animals.

REFERENCES

1. Katunuma, N., Matsuda, Y. and Tomino, I. J. Biochem. 56 (1964) 499.

2. Katunuma, N., Okada, M., Matsuzawa, T. and Otuka, Y. J. Biochem. 57 (1965) 445.

3. Sanada, Y., Suemori, I. and Katunuma, N. Biochim. Biophys. Acta 220 (1970) 42.

4. Herzfeld, A. and Greengard, O. J. Biol. Chem. 244 (1969) 4894.

5. Herzfeld, A. and Knox, W.E. J. Biol. Chem. 243 (1968) 3327.

6. Matsuzawa, T., Katsunuma, T. and Katunuma, N. Biochem. Biophys. Res. Comm. 32 (1968) 161.

7. Morris, H.P., Chee, R.Y. and Swick, R.W. Biochem. Biophys. Acta 354 (1974) 29.

8. Kobayashi, K., Kito, K. and Katunuma, N. J. Biochem. 79 (1976) 787.

9. Tomino, I., Katunuma, N., Morris, H.P. and Weber, G. Cancer
    Res. 34 (1974) 627.

10. Kobayashi, K., Morris, H.P. and Katunuma, N. J. Biochem. 80
    (1976) 1085.

11. Weber, G. In: The Molecular Biology of Cancer, Academic Press,
    New York (1974) pp. 487-521.

CONTROLS OF NUCLEOLAR FUNCTION IN CANCER CELLS*

H. Busch, N.R. Ballal, R.K. Busch, Y.C. Choi, F. Davis,
I.L. Goldknopf, S.I. Matsui, M.S. Rao, and L.I. Rothblum

Department of Pharmacology
Baylor College of Medicine
Houston, Texas 77030

The protein synthesizing machinery of the cell in which the ribosomes play a key role is of great importance to its rate of growth (1). The availability of ribosomes is dependent upon the activity of the nucleolus (Fig 1), which is the sole site of synthesis of preribosomal RNA and of assembly of preribosomal particles. The high rate of protein synthesis is one reason why the attention of oncologists has been directed to analysis of nucleolar structure and function (2). Another interesting feature of the nucleolus of cancer cells is that its size and shape vary markedly in relationship to the degree of malignancy and in the most actively growing tumors, the nucleoli are almost completely aneuploid (2, 3).

Our understanding of the many components of actively synthesizing ribosomes has increased enormously in the last decade. In addition to four RNA species, ribosomes contain almost 100 proteins that have been shown to be parts of the protein synthesizing systems which include GTP, initiation factors, elongation factors and termination factors.

Behind the mystery of the continued and unresponsive growth of cancer cells are basic mechanisms that lack the sensitivity of feedback controls of nontumor cells. Whether these mechanisms constitute factors that are positive gene derepressors or factors that interfere with gene repression is still the subject of intense investigation. Both types of possibilities have been suggested. Possible repressors such as protein A24 and protein A11 (possibly a phosphorylated H1 histone) are markedly reduced in nucleoli of cells undergoing rapid growth and division. On the other hand, possible derepressors include nucleolar antigens of tumor cells that are not present in nontumor cells. Interestingly, other nucleolar antigens have been found

CARCINOGENESIS

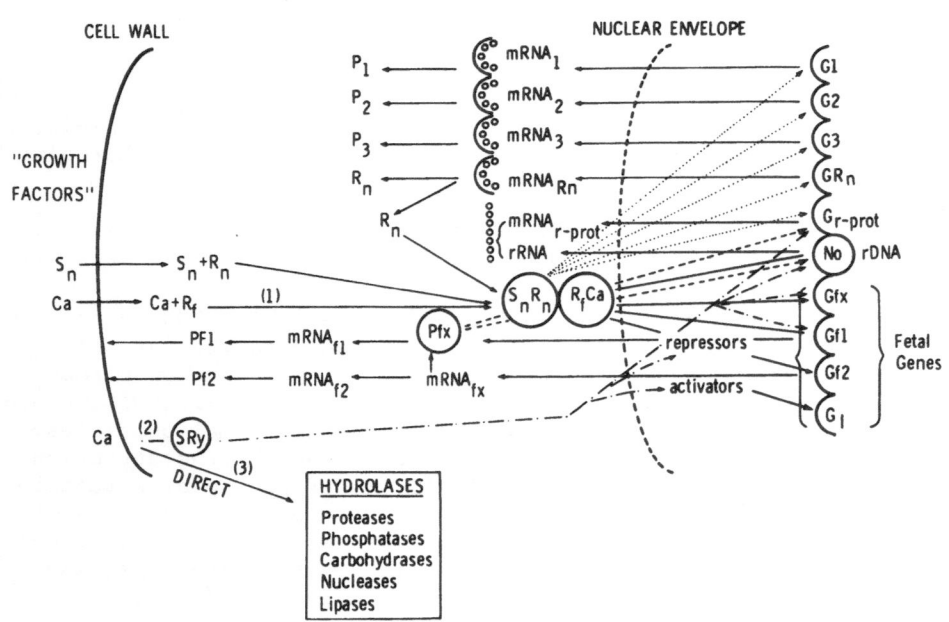

Figure 1A
Effects of carcinogenic agents on cellular responses. It is
envisioned that carcinogens permit structural genes to function in
production of normal products but that, through several mechanisms,
fetal genes are activated to produce a variety of fetal products,
including Pf1 and Pf2, which are important to invasiveness and
metastasis. The carcinogen may act with a fetal receptor to directly interact with the genome or may cause a new stimulus within the
cell to interact with a receptor that will interact with the genome.
Alternatively, the carcinogen may interfere with degradative reactions that are involved in normal growth controls. Ca, carcinogen;
R_1-Rn, cytoplasmic receptor proteins; G1-GR_1, structural genes including genes for receptor proteins (GR_1); Gf1-Gfn, fetal genes
with functions indicated; G_1, inhibitor genes; No, rDNA genes; and
G_r-prot, genes for ribosomal proteins (1).

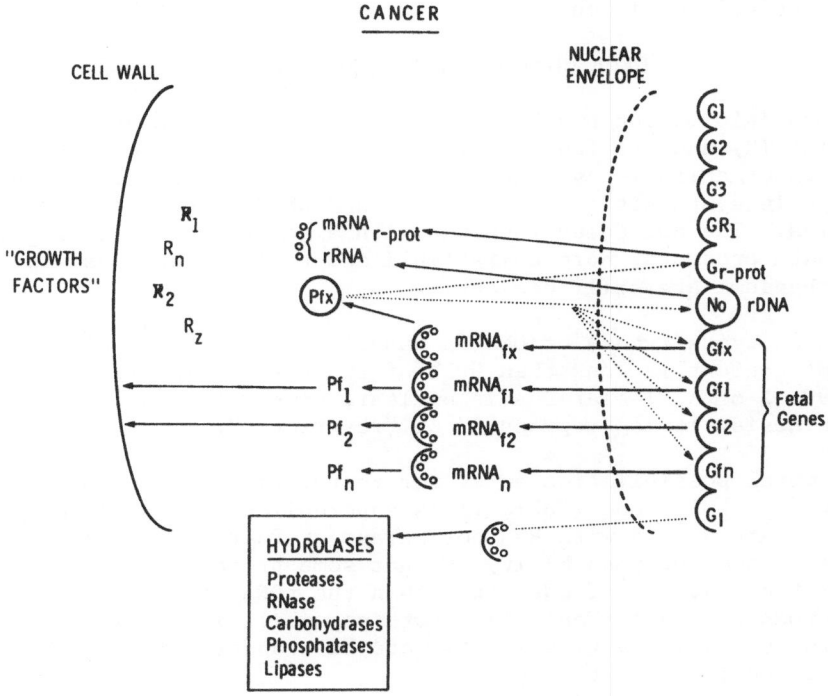

Figure 1B

    This diagram indicates the expression of cancer as a con-
tinuous production of gene products involved in growth, invasiveness and metastasis. Such cells no longer produce R1, R2 (blocked,
R_1, R_2) or others that may have phenotypic specificity. It is
envisioned that these gene products and their derepressors are
produced or maintained in high concentration through mitosis and
keep these genes activated during new cell formation. Moreover,
the lack of fetal extracellular regulatory mechanisms do not permit
these genes to be inactivated as they would be during fetal growth
and development (1).

in nontumor cells that are not present in tumors.

There are multiple elements in the various feedback arms that may control activity of specific chromatin elements. The task of sorting out these factors continues to be a complex one that is of importance in comprehension of the cancer problem as well as normal growth and cell division.

GENE CONTROL IN THE NUCLEOLUS

Much information has been developed on the structure of the nucleolus (2) and its function in synthesis of ribosomes. However, little information is available on the controls of the many genes involved in synthesis of the proteins and RNA of nucleolar rRNP particles. The nucleolus responds with alacrity to cellular demands for growth products, hormonal stimuli and toxic substances. However, the mechanisms are still unclear.

An enormous excess of DNA is associated with the nucleolus; its rDNA content is less than 0.5% of the total. The role of the other 99.5% of nucleolar DNA is unclear; since it is not read during RNA synthesis, it is "repressed" or "restricted".

Several possibilities exist for restriction of nucleolar gene readouts to rDNA. One (Table 1) is supercoiling which prevents physical interaction with RNA polymerase or factors for nucleolar readouts. Another possibility is that some proteins specifically inhibit the readouts of DNA other than the rDNA or specifically activate rDNA readouts (Table 1). Both possibilities could also be true fro rDNA which varies in its rate of transcription in varying states of nucleolar activity.

Restriction of transcription of the nucleolus-associated DNA is due to special proteins. When the nucleolus is deproteinized the oligonucleotide fingerprints of its transcriptional products markedly changed and the specific oligonucleotides of the fingerprint of the nucleolar readout were totally lost and replaced by random readouts. Uncharacteristic fingerprints of other RNA products appeared. Thus, one role of the nuclear proteins is to specifically "restrict" transcription of nucleolar DNA other than rDNA.

What other mechanisms operate on expression of nucleolar function? Hildebrandt and Suaer (4) reported a polyphosphate that inhibits nucleolar initiation of rRNA in Physarum. This inhibitor is selective and reversibly binds to RNA polymerase 1. It is released during differentiation but not during growth. During starvation this inhibitor increases in amount and after refeeding, it decreases in amount. Accordingly, control mechanisms in Physarum might involve transient changes in concentration of this inhibitor.

Table One
Nucleolar Control Factors

I. Chromatin Structure

    A. Supercoiling

    B. Restriction Proteins

II. rDNA Activators

    A. Proteins

        1. Preribosomal

        2. S-R Complexes

        3. RNA POL I-Activation (rapid, slow)

    B. Soluble Factors - polyamines, O.D.C.

III. Inhibitors

    A. Gene Repressors (macromolecular)

    B. Polyphosphates (PPXPP analogs)

Table Two
Compositions of Nucleoli and Nucleolar
Chromatin[a]

| | DNA | RNA | Protein | |
			Acid Soluble[b]	Acid Insoluble[c]
Nucleoli	1.00	1.51	5.60	2.60
Nucleolar chromatin	1.00	0.30	2.65	0.79

[a]
 Values are relative to DNA and averages of three different
 preparations.
[b]
 Soluble in 0.25 N HCl.
[c]
 Insoluble in 0.25 N HCl.

DNA was determined by a modified diphenylamine reaction and RNA by
alkaline hydrolysis.

Positive controls of nucleolar function have been suggested by electron microscopic observations and labeling analyses of 45S RNA synthesis in lectin-activated lymphoctytes and other growing cells. The "triggering" events that result in the 15-50 fold increases in nucleolar rDNA readouts may include:

(a) Polyamines and ornithine decarboxylase (ODC) which have been reported to enhance RNA polymerase I activity (5);

(b) ribosomal proteins which produced a marked shift in the activity of nuclei to the synthesis of preribosomal products (6) and tissue specific proteins (7).

A number of cautions must be exercised in evalution of these results. Matsui et al. (8) and Ballal et al. (9) showed a huge increase in "nucleolar synthesis" when whole nucleolar DNA or E. coli RNA polymerase were added to nucleoli. Unfortunately, a corresponding increase in the characteristic T_1 RNase oligonucleotides was not demonstrated by homochromatography. Accordingly, it is important to demonstrate fidelity of the product as well as increased labeling.

Nuclear Gene Expression

Although in eukaryotes less than 10% of the total genome is expressed at a given time in any type of cell (10), the large variety of types of mRNA and other RNA species transcribed complicates the evaluation of expression of specific genes. For studies of specific gene expression nucleoli and nucleolar chromatin have the advantage that rDNA is virtually the only active gene set in nucleoli and, thus, rRNA is the major product in vivo and in vitro (2, 11-15). An advantage of this system is that rRNA is distinguishable from many other RNA species by its high GC content. RNA polymerase I which synthesizes rRNA is readily isolated in high purity (11, 16-23).

Nucleolar preribosomal 45S RNA (pre-rRNA) is the initial rDNA transcript (2), and improvements in homochromatography-fingerprinting have simplified its characterization (16). This technique permits evaluation of the fidelity of transcription in vitro and analysis of the specific sequences of rRNA and nonconserved spacer regions. Also, the unique oligonucleotides resulting from complete or partial T_1 RNase digestion have been identified (9, 16, 24-28) and are absent from other RNA species (29). Isolated nucleoli synthesize RNA in vitro that resembles pre-rRNA in base composition, marker oligonucleotides, and hybridization (8, 15-20). Recently, Grummt (15) demonstrated by DNA-RNA dehybridization experiments that nucleolar transcripts can be competed by 45S pre-rRNA; these experiments provide evidence that the major product of isolated nuclei is rRNA.

Fractionation of Nucleolar Proteins

Over 200 different species of nucleolar proteins could be found

by 2-dimensional gel electrophoresis (7). Even in the highly purified nucleolar RNP particles almost 100 proteins were present including a large number of high molecular weight proteins which were
clearly not ribosomal proteins. To further fractionate the nucleolar
proteins into groups that were chemically functional, a study was
undertaken of products extractable in various salt and EDTA buffers.
These studies demonstrated that the usual NaCl-EDTA wash and the Tris
wash(II) for preparation of chromatin (I) extracted more than 50% of
all the nucleolar proteins including the vast bulk of RNA polymerase
I and nucleolar protein kinase. In addition, the Tris wash extracted
more of the nucleolar RNP particles. Interestingly, the residue fraction ("nucleolar chromatin") retained its transcriptional specificity
(8, 9). Thus, the "restriction proteins" for rDNA remain in this
fraction. The locus of the proteins that affect rates of readouts of
RNA in nucleoli is not yet defined.

Antibodies to Nucleolar Proteins

     Antibodies to nucleoli in this laboratory were prepared by
immunization of rabbits with whole nucleoli of Novikoff hepatoma and
normal rat liver (2, 30). Immunoflourescence analysis studies showed
specificity of localization of the antibodies to the nucleolus (30).

     Immunological studies on chromatin proteins of tumors and other
tissues demonstrated the presence of an antigen, NAg-1 (31) in tumors
and fetal liver. These results are consistent with the presence in
tumor nuclei of fetal proteins that were not detected in normal growing or nongrowing tissues (1, 31-34).

     With the techniques developed in studies on NAg-1 (31), a re-
investigation was made of the antigens in nucleoli and nucleolar
chromatin. In addition to NAg-1, tumor nucleoli contain another antigen, noAg-1 which is different from NAg-1 and appears to be more limited in localization. noAg-1 was not found in normal liver nucleoli.
Three antigens were found in normal liver that were not present in
tumor nucleoli or nuclei.

PROPERTIES OF THE NUCLEOLAR TRANSCRIPTIONAL SYSTEMS

RNA Synthesis by Isolated Nucleoli and Nucleolar Chromatin

     The chemical compositions of isolated nucleoli and nucleolar
chromatin (Table 2) indicated that the preliminary extractions for
chromatin preparation removed substantial amounts of RNA and protein
from the nucleoli. Also, nucleolar chromatin is richer in RNA and
acid-soluble proteins than whole nuclear chromatin (10).

     The kinetics of RNA synthesis by isolated nucleoli, nucleolar

chromatin and nucleolar DNA (Fig 2) showed that after extensive
washing with 0.075 M NaCl-0.025 M EDTA and 10 mM Tris-HCl, nucleolar
chromatin retained sufficient RNA polymerase I activity to synthesize
RNA at approximately 1/5-1/10 the rate of whole nucleoli (Table 3
and Fig 2). Transcription was linear up to 10 minutes, the standard
incubation time. The sedimentation peaks of incorporation were at
19, 20 and 25S for chromatin, DNA and molecular transcripts, respectively (Fig 3).

Fidelity of in vitro rRNA Synthesis by Isolated Nucleoli and Nucleolar Chromatin

Nucleotide compositions determined by incorporation of each
labeled nucleotide showed that RNA synthesized by the nucleoli and
nucleolar chromatin was rich in GMP and CMP; its composition was
very similar to that of rRNA or preribosomal RNA (Table 4). When
RNA polymerase I was added to the nucleolar chromatin the rate of
synthesis was increased; the purine content of the RNA product was
essentially the same with whole nucleoli or chromatin as template.
The pyrimidine content differed; less CMP and more UMP was incorporated. With DNA as the template (Table 4), much more AMP and UMP
were incorporated than with whole nucleoli or nucleolar chromatin.

RNA treated with DNase I to eliminate trace amounts of contaminating DNA was hybridized to nucleolar DNA fractionated on CsCl
gradients. The nucleolar transcripts hybridized mainly to DNA of
density 1.715 g/cm^3; little hybridized to the main band DNA (1.692
g/cm^3).

The base composition and hybridization of the RNA products
(Table 4, Fig 4) showed that they contained ribosomal products and
products of main band DNA (Fig 4).

To more specifically determine the fidelity of transcription of
rRNA, homochromatography-fingerprinting of T$_1$ RNase digestion products was used. Figure 5A shows the pattern obtained from Novikoff
hepatoma nucleolar 45S pre-rRNA labeled in vivo with ^{32}P orthophos-
phate (16). Structural studies have established identity of many
fragments (Fig 5B) with fragments of the 45S pre-rRNA (8, 16, 27-29).

Figure 6 shows a similar pattern for RNA transcribed in vitro
(28-35S) with isolated nucleoli using α-^{32}P-labeled nucleotides.
Four spots that contain five oligonucleotides of the in vivo product
were not found (Fig 5B). Oligonucleotides Y$_1$-3 (C$_6$A$_6$U$_4$,ψ,GmA,UmC,
G-18S; C$_3$,A$_7$,U$_5$,AmGmCmA,G-28S) and Y$_1$-4 (C$_5$,A$_5$,U$_6$,GmU,G-28S) each
contain a Gm residue. Three spots (Fig 6, pointers) were found in
the in vitro transcripts and not in the 45S pre-rRNA. It is possible
that the missing fragments were undermethylated (35) and cleaved by
T$_1$ RNase. Specificity of the expression of rDNA genes was retained

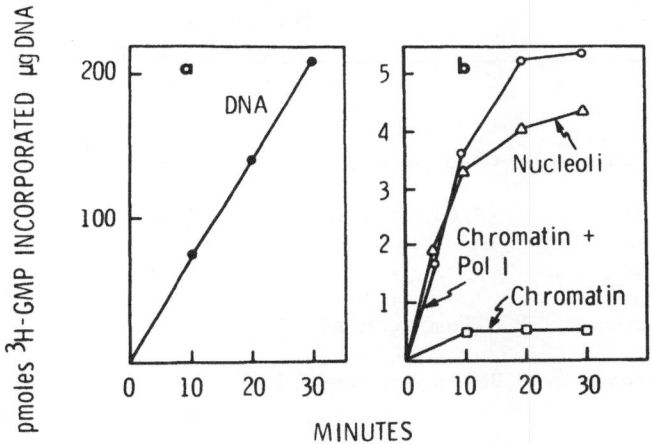

Figure 2
Kinetics of RNA synthesis in vitro. (a) RNA synthesis by
nucleolar DNA + RNA polymerase I. (b) RNA synthesis by isolated
nucleoli($\triangle$), chromatin ($\square$), and chromatin + RNA polymerase I (o).
When RNA polymerase I was added, the assay was performed under
conditions where only the template was rate limiting. The values
are in pmol of [^{3}H]GMP incorporated/µg of DNA (8).

Table Three
Transcriptional Activity of Nucleoli and Nucleolar
Chromatin

Components	pmol of GMP incorporated/µg of DNA per 10 min	%
Nucleoli	5.74	100
Nucleoli + α-amanitin (0.5 µg/ml)	6.79	118
Nucleoli + rifampicin AF/013 (60 µg/ml)	7.10	124
Nucleolar chromatin	0.46	8
Nucleolar chromatin + rifampicin AF/013	0.69	12
Nucleolar chromatin + RNA polymerase I (28 units)	0.72	12.5
Nucleolar chromatin + RNA polymerase I (28 units) + rifampicin AF/013	0.79	13.8
Nucleolar chromatin + E. coli RNA polymerase (25 units)	3.22	56.0

Incorporation of [^{3}H]GTP by isolated nucleoli or nucleolar chromatin was determined. Nucleolar RNA polymerase was purified through a DEAE-Sephadex column. (9).

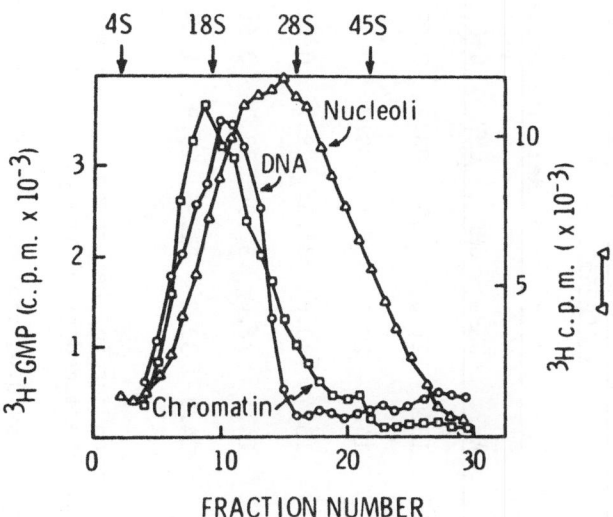

Figure 3
Sucrose gradient centrifugation pattern of RNA synthesized
in vitro. Samples were run on 30-ml gradients of 5 to 45% sucrose-
0.1 M NaCl-0.02 M acetate buffer (pH 5.1)-0.01 M EDTA for 18 hrs
at 85,000 g; (Δ) nucleolar transcripts; (□) chromatin transcripts;
(o) DNA transcripts (8).

Table Four

Nucleotide Composition Analysis by Relative Nucleotide Incorporation

Condition	No. of Determinations	AMP	UMP	GMP	CMP	Relative Nucleotide Incorporation[a] A+U/G+C
Nucleoli	3	13.0	21.0	35.5	30.5	0.52
Nucleolar 45S RNA[b]		14.6	20.5	35.1	29.7	0.54
Chromatin	2[c]	13.4	20.6	37.3	29.7	0.52
Chromatin + polymerase I	4[c]	14.5	24.4	37.9	23.2	0.66
DNA + polymerase I	2	24.9	32.3	21.9	20.9	1.34

[a] Values based on 10 min transcription carried out in the presence of α-amanitin (10 μg/ml).

[b] Nucleotide composition of nucleolar 45S RNA determined by ultraviolet spectra analyses.

[c] The endogenous incorporation by chromatin was 0.46 pmol of [^{3}H]GMP per μg of DNA per 10 min. With exogenous enzymes, the incorporation was 3.52 pmol of [^{3}H]GMP per μg of DNA per 10 min.

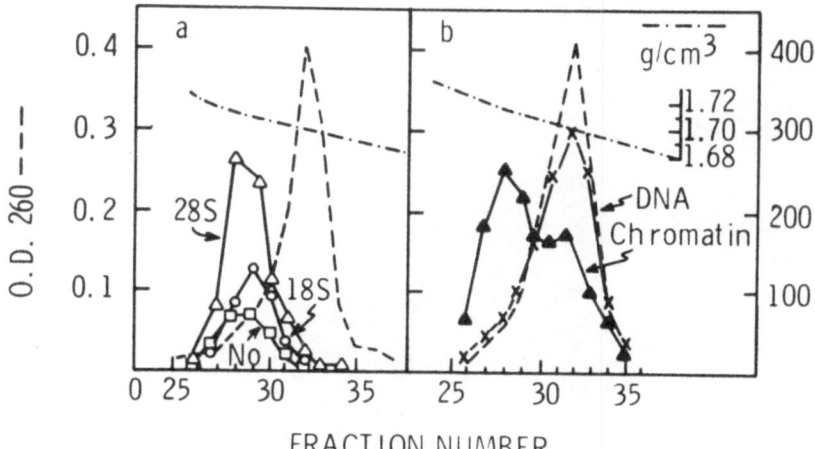

Figure 4

    Hybridization of rRNA and <u>in vitro</u> transcripts to nucleolar
DNA fractionated on CsCl gradients. Samples containing 50 μg of
nucleolar DNA (mol. wt. 10 x 10^6) were centrifuged in a neutral
CsCl gradients (5 ml) at 68,700 g for 72 hr. The DNA in each
fraction was denatured with 0.1 N NaOH, adsorbed to a Millipore
filter, and hybridized with the appropriate RNA in 2 x SSC-30%
formamide-25 mM Hepes-0.1% sodium dodecyl sulfate at 45° for 48
hr.   (a) Hybridization with ^{3}H-labeled 28S rRNA (△), ^{3}H-labeled
18S rRNA (o), and ^{3}H- labeled nucleolar transcripts (□). In this
particular experiment, the incorporation rate was 0.41 pmol of
GMP incorporated per μg of DNA per 10 min for endogenous activity
and 4.0 pmol of GMP incorporated per μg of DNA per 10 min with
exogenous enzyme. Specific activities of rRNA and nucleolar
transcripts were 2.06 x 10^5 and 3.0 x 10^3 cpm/μg, respectively.
Input: 1 μg/ml for rRNA and 15 μg/ml for nucleolar transcripts.
(b) Hybridization with ^{3}H-labeled chromatin transcripts with
exogenous RNA polymerase I (▲) and ^{3}H-labeled DNA transcripts
with exogenous RNA polymerase I (X). Specific activities of
chromatin and DNA transcripts were 1.25 x 10^4 and 1.74 x 10^6 cpm/
μg, respectively. Input: about 0.3 μg/ml (8).

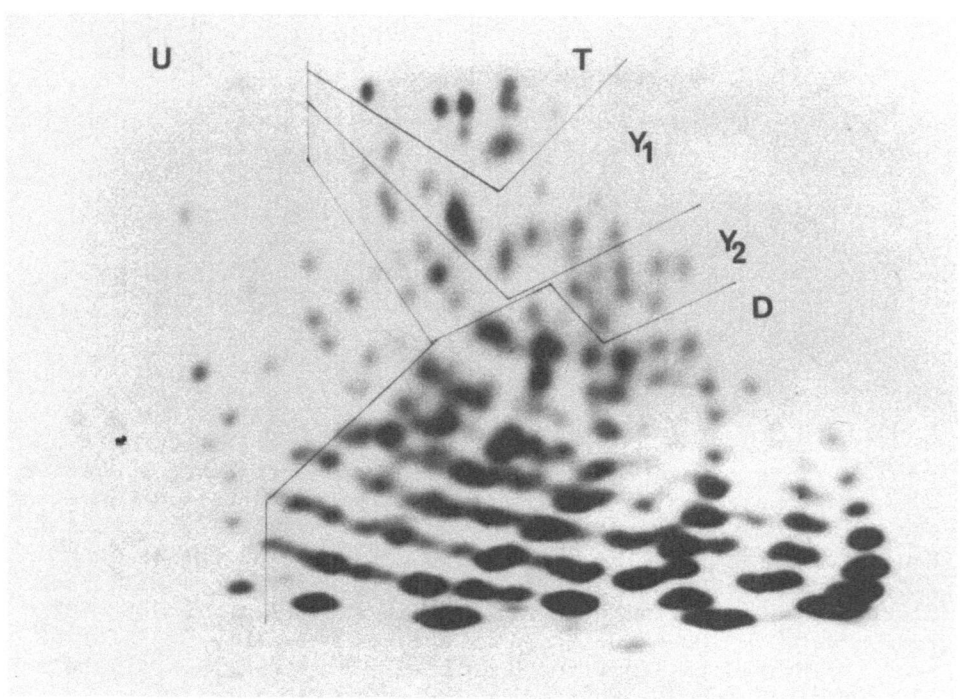

Figure 5A
Homochromatography of T_1 RNase digests of 45S pre-rRNA
labeled in vivo. For convenience, the pattern was divided into
regions; U (uridylate-rich), T (top triangle), Y_1 (Y-shaped),
Y_2 (below Y_1) and D (approximately decanucleotides) (9).

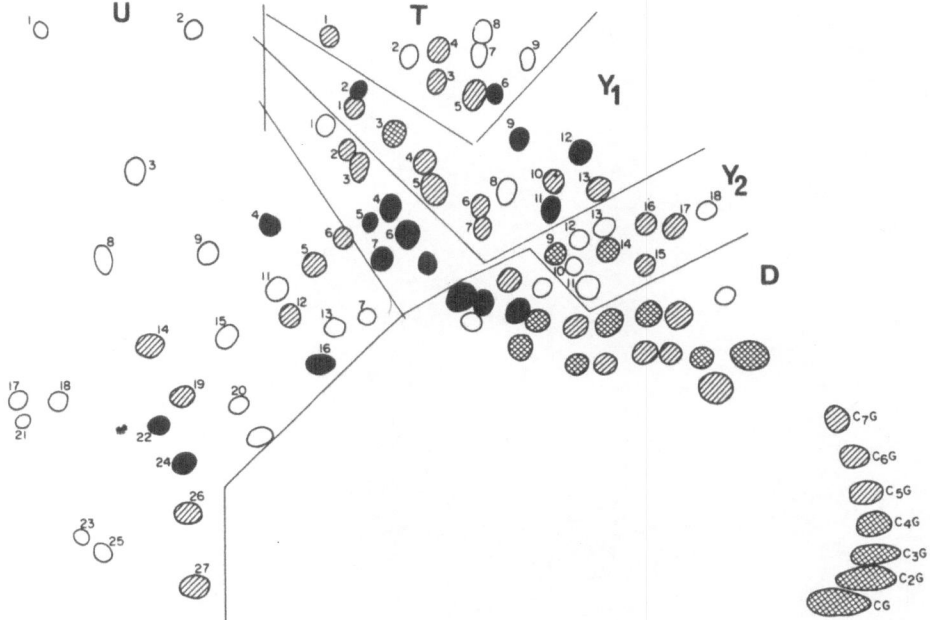

Figure 5B
Diagrammatic map of the oligonucleotide homochromatogram in
Fig 5A. Closed circles represent oligonucleotide spots found in
18S rRNA; hatched circles represent fragments found in 28S rRNA;
crosshatched circles represent fragments present in both 18 and
28S rRNA; open circles represent oligonucleotide fragments present
in the spacer segments of pre-RNA. Spot T-9 was a variable spot
which was occasionally missing from the digests (9).

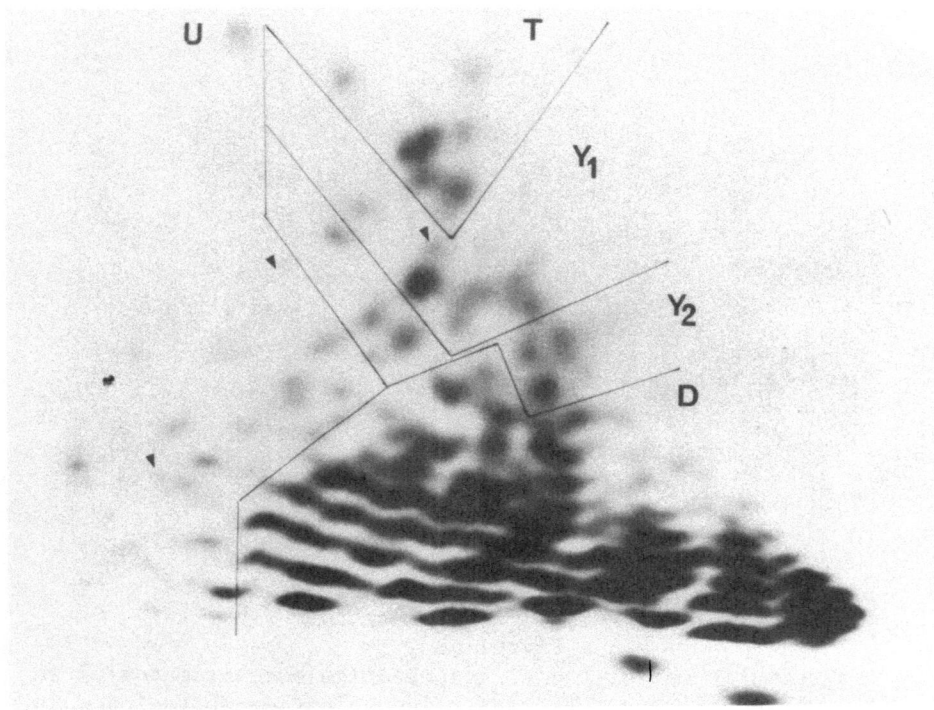

Figure 6A
Homochromatography of the T_1 RNase digestion products of RNA
products synthesized _in vitro_ in isolated Novikoff hepatoma nucleoli. Pointers indicate spots that are absent in 45S pre-rRNA
(9).

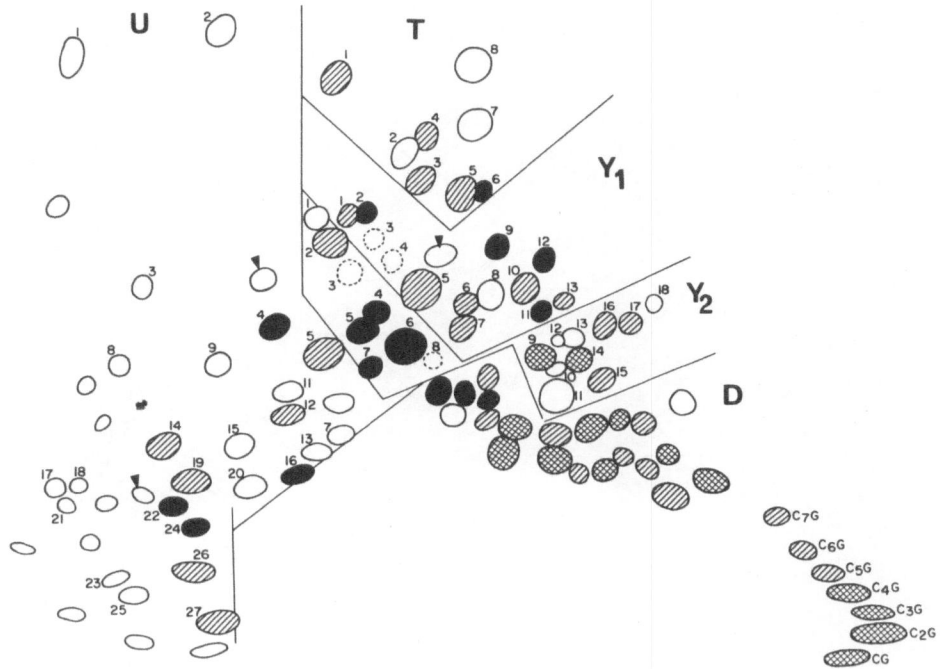

Figure 6B
Diagrammatic map of the oligonucleotide homochromatogram in
Fig 6A. Broken circles represent spots of 45S RNA that are absent
from this RNA. See legend for Fig 5B (9).

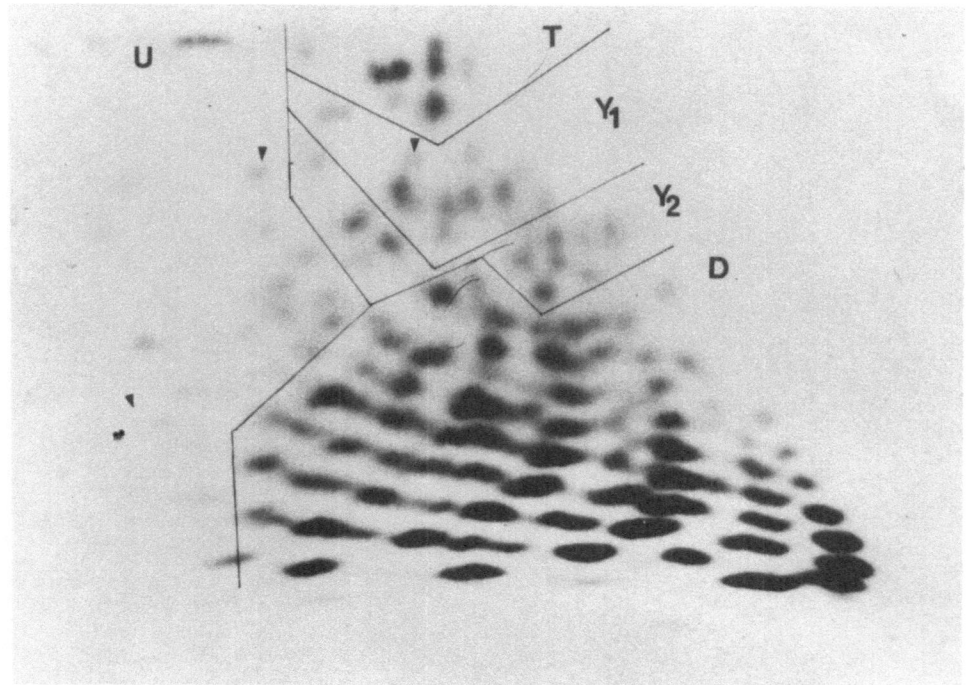

Figure 7A
Homochromatography of the T_1 RNase digestion products of RNA
products synthesized _in vitro_ in nucleolar chromatin with RNA polymerase I.   The sedimentation coefficient of this RNA was approximately 18S-28S.   Pointers respresent spots that are absent in 45S pre-
rRNA (9).

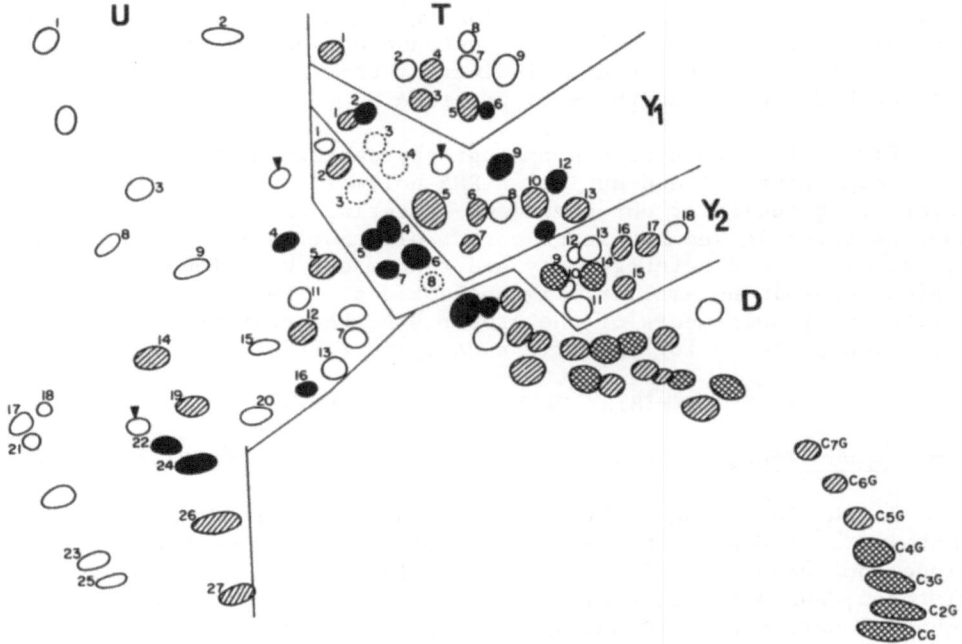

Figure 7B
Diagrammatic map of the oligonucleotide homochromatogram in
Fig 7A. See legends for Figure 5B and 6B (9).

in the nucleoli and nucleolar chromatin (Fig 7).

Since the system containing nucleolar RNA polymerase I was not as efficient in transcription of nucleolar chromatin as whole nucleoli, the efficiency and fidelity of transcription were tested with E. coli RNA polymerase. Even though the rate of transcription of nucleolar chromatin was 4-5 times greater with E. coli polymerase than with RNA polymerase I (Table 3), it was still less than that of the whole nucleoli. When the labeled RNA was subjected to homochromatography-fingerprinting, the spot pattern (Fig 8) indicated that all of the larger oligonucleotide markers of preribosomal RNA and oligonucleotides C_5G through C_7G were absent from these transcripts. Even in the lower chain length region of the map, instead of discrete spots in the tetra- and pentanucleotide region, only continuous stripes were visible, indicating that many sequences were transcribed other than those of pre-rRNA.

Figure 9 shows a homochromatography pattern of RNA transcribed using nucleolar DNA and nucleolar RNA polymerase I. As with transcripts from nucleolar chromatin and bacterial RNA polymerase, these spot patterns lacked any large marker oligonucleotide spots of preribosomal RNA and heterogeneity and randomness were found in the regions containing smaller oligonucleotides. These results demonstrate the requirements of the proper DNA, RNA polymerase and restriction proteins for specific rDNA transcription.

CHEMISTRY OF NUCLEOLAR PROTEINS

Numbers and Types of Nucleolar Proteins

In the nucleolus a ratio of protein to RNA or DNA is approximately 8. The proteins in the nucleolus are of many types and include the precursors of ribosomal proteins as well as enzymes, histones, and nonhistone proteins. The histones are present in an equal amount to DNA and account for 1/8 of the total nucleolar proteins (10).

Until the first demonstration by Orrick et al. (7), it was generally assumed that there were relatively few species of nucleolar acid soluble proteins; however, the current evidence shows that there are approximately 200. Included in this group of proteins are approximately 40 phosphorylated proteins of which proteins C23-25 and C26 and C27 have been most intensively studied (10). They are typical nonhistone proteins with large quantities of glutamic and aspartic acid and, in addition, they are the first proteins in which clusters of acidic residues have been found associated with the phosphorylated sites (36).

During the nucleolar hypertrophy produced by thioacetamide

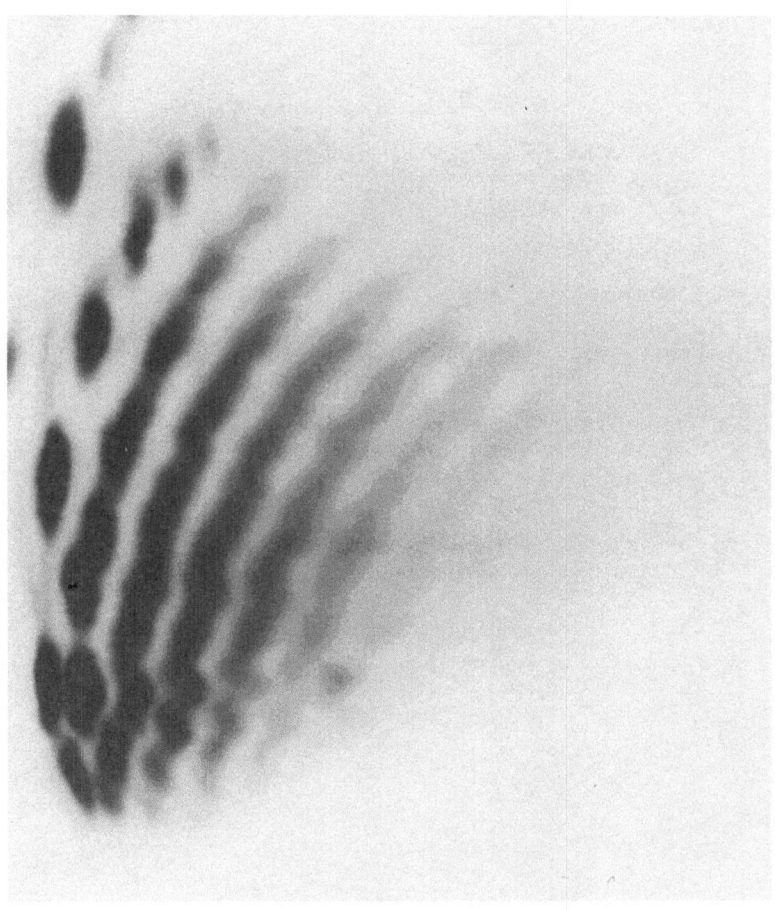

Figure 8
Homochromatography of the T_1 RNase digestion products of RNA
transcribed _in vitro_ with nucleolar chromatin and _E. coli_ RNA
polymerase (9).

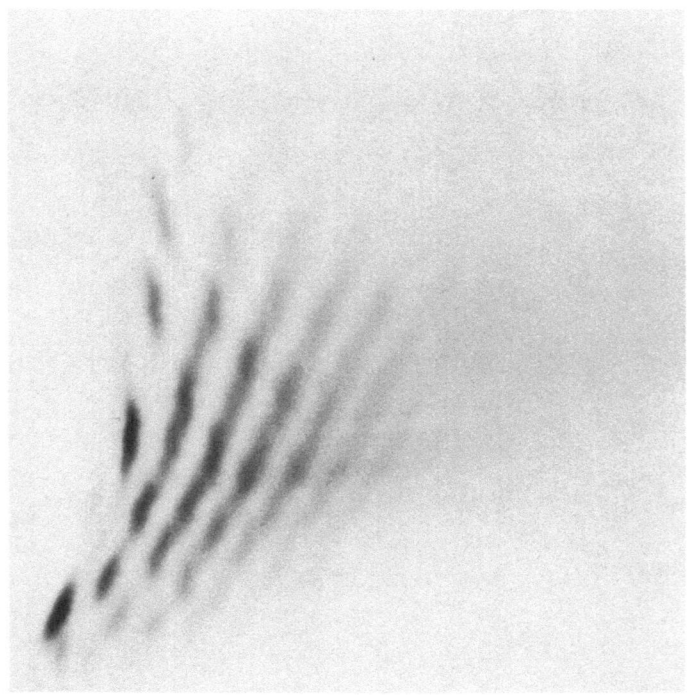

Figure 9
Homochromatography of the T_1 RNase digestion products of RNA
transcribed in vitro with nucleolar DNA and RNA polymerase I (9).

treatment, a series of rapid changes occur in nucleolar proteins, some of which are markedly decreased and others, associated with synthesis of preribosomal ribonucleoprotein particles, are markedly increased in amount (37, 38). These changes were studied by one- and two-dimensional polyacrylamide gel electrophoresis of the 0.4 N H_2SO_4 soluble nucleolar proteins, which showed an overall increase in the ratio of nonhistone proteins to histones following thioacetamide treatment. Most spots that increased in size and density had electrophoretic mobilities of proteins of the preribosomal ribonucleoprotein particles. One spot (A25) remained constant in size and density during the course of the treatment. Interestingly, marked decreases were found very early in two protein spots (A11 and A24) while two other protein spots (C13 and C14) decreased slowly with time. These results indicate that the nucleolus rapidly exhibits multifaceted changes during alterations in cell function.

Protein A24 -   Isolation and initial chemical characterization indicated that protein A24 was a nonhistone chromosomal protein with approximately equal amounts of acidic and basic amino acids; it constituted approximately 1.9% of the sum of histones 2A, 2B, 3, and 4 (39). Protein A24 was found to contain the tryptic and chymotryptic peptides of histone 2A as well as additional peptides and, accordingly, it was suggested that protein A24 contained a "nonhistone-like" polypeptide linked to a histone 2A molecule (39-44). More recently (40, 41), protein A24 was found to contain as one amino-terminal sequence:

```
1               5                    10
Met-Gln-Ile-Phe-Val-Lys-Thr-Leu-Thr-Gly-
11              15                   20
Lys-Thr-Ile-Thr-Leu-Glu-Val-Glu-Pro-Ser-
21              25                   30
Asp-Thr-Ile-Glu-Asn-Val-Lys-Ala-Lye-Ile-
31              35
Gln-Asp-Lys-Glu-Gly-Ile-Pro
```

The identity of this structure to that of ubiquitin (42)

```
                              10
NH2-Met-Gln-Ile-Phe-Val-Lys-Thr-Leu-Thr-Gly-
                              20
    -Lys-Thr-Ile-Thr-Leu-Glu-Val-Glu-Pro-Ser-
                              30
    -Asp-Thr-Ile-Glu-Asn-Val-Lys-Ala-Lys-Ile-
                              40
    -Gln-Asp-Lys-Glu-Gly-Ile-Pro-Pro-Asp-Gln-
                              50
    -Gln-Arg-Leu-Ile-Phe-Ala-Gly-Lys-Gln-Leu-
                              60
    -Glu-Asp-Gly-Arg-Thr-Leu-Ser-Asp-Tyr-Asn-
                              70
```

-Ile-Gln-Lys-Glu-Ser-Thr-Leu-His-Leu-Val-

-Leu-Arg-Leu-Arg-COOH

was very quickly noted by Hunt and Dayhoff (43). This sequence is
not homologous to histone sequences.

The Second Amino Terminus of Protein A24

Comparison of tryptic peptide maps of histone 2A and protein
A24 revealed remarkable similarities (44). A peptide designated
16 was not previously detected in protein A24 because it did not
stain with the ninhydrin-cadmium or fluorescamine procedure, which
require the presence of a primary amino group. This peptide contained the blocked amino terminus of histone 2A (44, 45):
                    N-Acetylserine-Gly-Arg.

The Single Carboxyl Terminus of Protein A24

Carboxypeptidase A and B digestion indicated that protein A24 contains the carboxyl-terminal sequence (40, 41) identical to that of
histone 2A (45):
                -His-His-Lys-Ala-Lys-Gly-Lys
                123 124 125 126 127 128 129
                (histone 2A residue number)

Quantitative hydrazinolysis released molar yields of carboxyl-
terminal lysine of 1.01 and 0.88 for protein A24 and histone 2A,
respectively; not other carboxyl-terminal amino acids were detected
in protein A24.

The Branched Tryptic Peptide of Protein A24

The detection of two amino termini and one carboxyl terminus
suggested that the protein A24 molecule was branched and that the
nonhistone polypeptide was linked to histone 2A in a manner that
prevented detection of its carboxyl terminus. The amino acid composition and carboxyl terminus of peptide 17 of histone 2A (Table
5) were the same as that reported for a peptide containing amino
acid residue 119-125 of the histone 2A sequence (45). Edman degradation (Table 6) confirmed the identity and amino acid sequence
of this peptide (Fig 9). The amino acid sequence analysis of tryptic
peptide 17' of protein A24 (Fig 10A) showed that it contains tryptic
peptide 17 of histone 2A, Lys-Thr-Glu-Ser-His-His-Lys. Lysine 119,
the amino terminus of this peptide, which is derived from the histone
2A portion of protein A24, is linked by an isopeptide bond to the
carboxyl group of a glycine residue. Accordingly, the branched
structure of protein A24 is proposed in Fig 10B.

Table Five
Amino Acid Ratios and Carboxyl Termini of
Peptides 17 of Histone 2A and 17' of Protein A24

	17	17'
Gly	–	1.64
Lys	1.67	1.68
His	1.71	1.61
Thr	0.91	0.93
Ser (=1.00)	1.00	1.00
Glu	0.95	0.94
COOH terminus*	Lys (0.57)[+]	Lys (0.64)[+]
Molar yield[‡]	0.67	0.74

* Data obtained by hydrazinolysis; only lysine was found.

+ Data in parantheses are molar yield of carboxyl-terminal lysine.

‡ Nanmoles of peptide recovered from tryptic peptide maps per
nanmole of protein digested.

Table Six
Sequential Edman Degradation of Peptides
17 and 17' (nmol of amino acids per nmol of
peptide released from thiazolinones after
hydrolysis with HI)

Amino Acid	Edman cycle			
	1	2	3	4
Peptide 17 of histone 2A				
Gly				
Lys	0.5			
Thr		1.0		
Glu			0.9	
Ser				0.3
Peptide 17' of protein A24				
Gly	1.6	0.5		
Lys	0.4	0.1		
Thr		1.1		
Glu			0.8	
Ser				0.3

(Ref. 41).

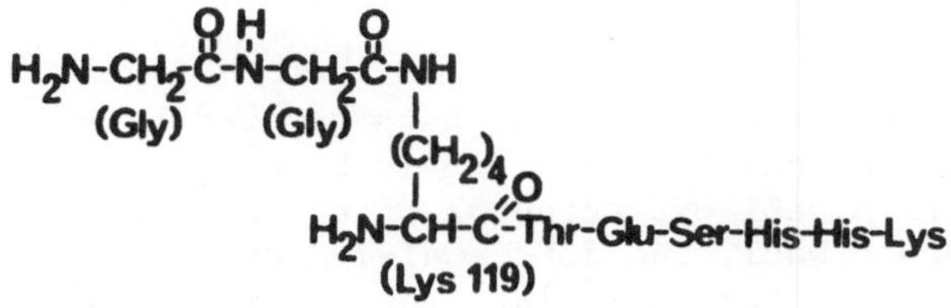

Figure 10A
Amino acid sequence of the branched peptide of protein A24
(41).

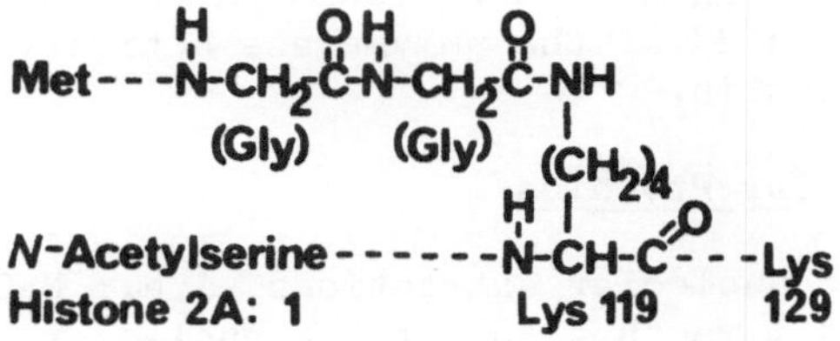

Figure 10B
Idealized sequence of protein A24 (41).

FRACTIONATION OF NUCLEOLAR PROTEINS

Distribution of Nucleolar Proteins in Salt Fractions

When nucleoli were extracted with 0.075 M NaCl-0.024 M EDTA, 19% of the nucleolar proteins were removed (Table 7). Subsequent washes with 10 mM Tris extracted another 35% of the nucleolar proteins (47). These two buffers extracted 54% of the nucleolar proteins (Fig 11A,B, Table 7).

The remainder of the proteins were removed by extraction with salt solutions, and may be more tightly bound to the DNA or chromatin. 0.15 M NaCl extracted 5% of the nucleolar proteins and 0.35 M NaCl, 0.6 M NaCl, and 3 M NaCal-7 M urea each extracted approximately 14% of the nucleolar proteins (Table 7).

Distribution of RNA polymerase and Protein Kinase

Both RNA polymerase I and protein kinase (46) activities were assayed in whole nucleoli and the various fractions (47). The 0.075 M NaCl-0.025 M EDTA and 10 mM Tris washes contained 40% and 60% of the extracted nucleolar protein kinase activity, respectively. Only 13% of the extracted RNA polymerase I was in the NaCl-EDTA extracts; 87% of the RNA polymerase I was in the 10 mM Tris extracts (Table 8).

The nucleolar chromatin residue (after the NaCl-EDTA and 10 mM Tris extractions) contained only 22% of the nucleolar RNA polymerase I activity, and 25% of the nucleolar protein kinase (Table 9). 0.15 M NaCl extracted 17% of polymerase I and 15% of the protein kinase from the chromatin residue. After two 0.35 M NaCl extractions, less than 3% of the polymerase activity remained associated with the chromatin.

Analysis of Nucleolar Proteins

The first two nucleolar extractions, i.e., NaCl-EDTA and 10 mM Tris, extracted more than 50% of the nucleolar proteins. The proteins in the NaCl-EDTA extract of nucleoli were heterogeneous; it contained a minimum of 25 polypeptides (Fig 11A). In the C region, the most prevalent proteins were C23-25, C6, C14, CI and CG. In contrast, the 10 mM Tris extract consisted predominantly of proteins B18, B23-25, and C23-25 (Fig 11B).

The initial RNA:DNA ratio of nucleoli was 1:1; following the NaCl-EDTA and 10mM Tris extracts, the RNA:DNA ratio of the residue was 0.2:1. Accordingly, a significant amount of the nucleolar ribonucleoproteins had been extracted. 10 mM Tris extracts were sedimented at 105,000 x g for 18 hours over a 1 M sucrose cushion.

Table Seven

Distribution of Nucleolar Proteins[a]

Fraction	% Total Nucleolar Protein	% Total Dissociated Nucleolar Chromatin Protein
NaCl-EDTA	19 ± 3	
10 mM Tris	35 ± 5	
Chromatin	46 ± 5	100%
0.15 M NaCl	5 ± 1	14 ± 1.4
0.35 M NaCl	13 ± 4	27 ± 4.0
0.6 M NaCl	14 ± 4	30 ± 4.8
3 M NaCl/7 M urea	14 ± 6	28 ± 7.6

[a] Nucleoli were extracted as indicated above, and the amount of protein extracted determined and represented here as the % of the total amount extracted. Data presented is the mean ± the standard error of the mean.

Table Eight
Distribution of RNA Polymerase I and Protein
Kinase in the NaCl-EDTA and Tris Extracts of Nu-
cleoli[a]

Protein Kinase[b] (CPMx10^{-5})   RNA Polymerase[b] (Unitsx10^{-3})

NaCl-EDTA   11.2 (40)   10.4 (12.5)

10 mM Tris   18.4 (60)   67.9 (87.5)

a
 Enzyme activities are expressed as CPM of ^{32}P incorporated into
casein for protein kinase and as units for RNA polymerase.
Numbers in parentheses are the percent of the total extracted.

b
 Protein kinase represents 77% of the total nucleolar activity;
RNA polymerase represents 73% of the total nucleolar activity.
(47).

Table Nine
Distribution of RNA Polymerase I and Protein
Kinase in Subnucleolar Fractions[a]

	RNA Polymerase I			Protein Kinase
	I	II	III	
Nucleoli	20.8	106.6	170.6	38.4
Chromatin	4.8 (23)	22.5 (21)	38.6 (23)	8.8 (23)

a
 RNA polymerase activity determined as described in "Methods"
using: I. Endogenous template, II. Endogenous template and
added nucleolar DNA, and III. Extracted nucleoli or chromatin
Protein kinase activity is expressed as CPM of ^{32}P incorporated
into casein. Numbers in parentheses are the percentage of the
total nucleolar activity.(47).

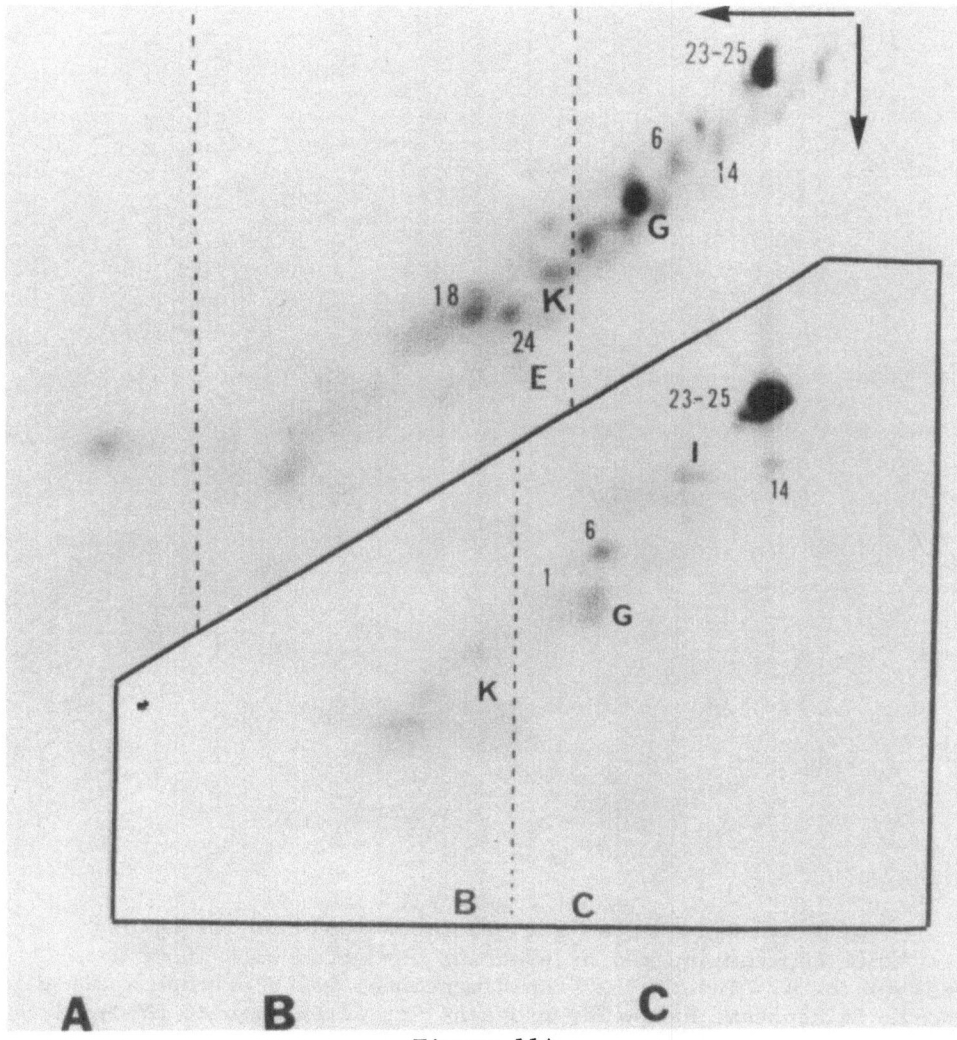

Figure 11A
Two-dimensional polyacrylamide gel electrophoresis of 200
μg Novikoff hepatoma nucleolar proteins extracted with NaCl-EDTA.
Samples were run in the first dimension on disc gels of 10%
acrylamide, 6 M urea, 0.9 N acetic acid. For the second dimension
electrophoresis, a 12% acrylamide, 0.1% SDS slab gel was run (referred to below as 10/12 two-dimensional polyacrylamide gel electrophoresis). Inset. Two-dimensional polyacrylamide gel electrophoresis of Novikoff hepatoma nucleolar proteins extracted with NaCl-
EDTA. Samples were run in the first dimension on the disc gels of
6% acrylamide, 6 M urea, 0.9 N acetic acid. For the second
dimension an 8% acrylamide, 0.1% SDS slab gel was run (referred to
below as 6/8 two-dimensional gel electrophoresis) (47).

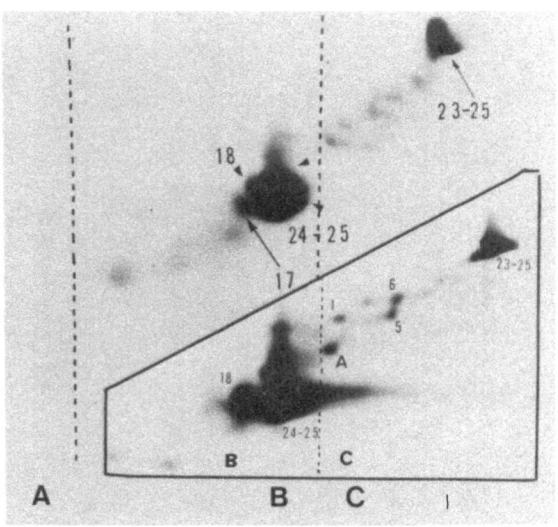

Figure 11B
10/12 two-dimensional gel electrophoresis of 110 μg of
Novikoff hepatoma nucleolar proteins extracted with 10 mM Tris-
HCl (pH 8.0).   Inset.   6/8 two-dimensional gel electrophoresis of
Novikoff hepatoma nucleolar proteins extracted with 10 mM Tris-
HCl (pH 8.0) (47).

10% of the extracted proteins were in the pelleted particles; they were extracted from the pellet with 3 M NaCl-7 M urea, 20 mM Tris HCl, pH 8.0. The two-dimensional electrophoretogram (Fig 12) of these proteins was essentially identical to those of the nucleolar ribonucleoprotein particles (48, 49).

The 0.15 M NaCl extract of chromatin consisted almost entirely of proteins with molecular weights greater than 30,000 (Fig 13). The sample was of limited heterogeneity; proteins B17, B18 and C24 were the densest spots present. The 0.35 M NaCl (Fig 14) extract of chromatin contained many proteins not extracted by 1.15 M NaCl. For example, proteins B24, B25, C14, C17 and C27 which were dense spots in the 0.35 M NaCl extract (Fig 14) were not found in the 0.15 M NaCl extract (Fig 13). On the other hand, proteins B35 and B17 were not present in the 0.35 M NaCl extract; they were in the 0.15 M NaCl extracted group of proteins.

The H1 histone spots were dense and large in the 0.6 M NaCl extract (Fig 15); proteins C17 and C24 also were dense spots. When the post 0.6 M NaCl chromatin residue was extracted with 3 M NaCl-7M urea, the histones, other than the H1 histones, were the major polypeptides present (Fig 16).

In addition, several low molecular weight proteins including A7, A15, A24, and A25 were also found in the 3 M NaCl-7M urea extract. Additional dense spots in this fraction were B7, B9, B13, BJ, and CA, C6, CM, CM', CI, CP, and CQ which were previously found by Yeoman et al. (50) in chromatin fraction II, and by Olson et al. (51) in nucleolar chromatin fraction II.

Translational Factors in Nucleoli

Recent studies in our laboratory have established the presence of elongation factors in nucleoli (52). The data shown in Table 10 show that the specific activity of EF-1α in nucleoli is higher than that of the whole homogenate. Inasmuch as the rDNA is a very small percentage of active nucleolar DNA, the concentration of the translational factors at rDNA loci may be much higher than indicated by the overall specific activity in terms of units/mg DNA. Preliminary studies indicate that both EF-2 and initiation factors may be concentrated in nucleoli. Whether they have a role in the assembly of preribosomal particles or as control elements in nucleolar function remains to be established by future studies.

IMMUNOLOGY OF NUCLEOLAR PROTEINS

noAg-1 - In previous studies (31), a chromatin antigen (NAg-1) was found in Novikoff hepatoma nuclei and fetal liver that was not found in normal liver cells. This antigen was purified and found to be a

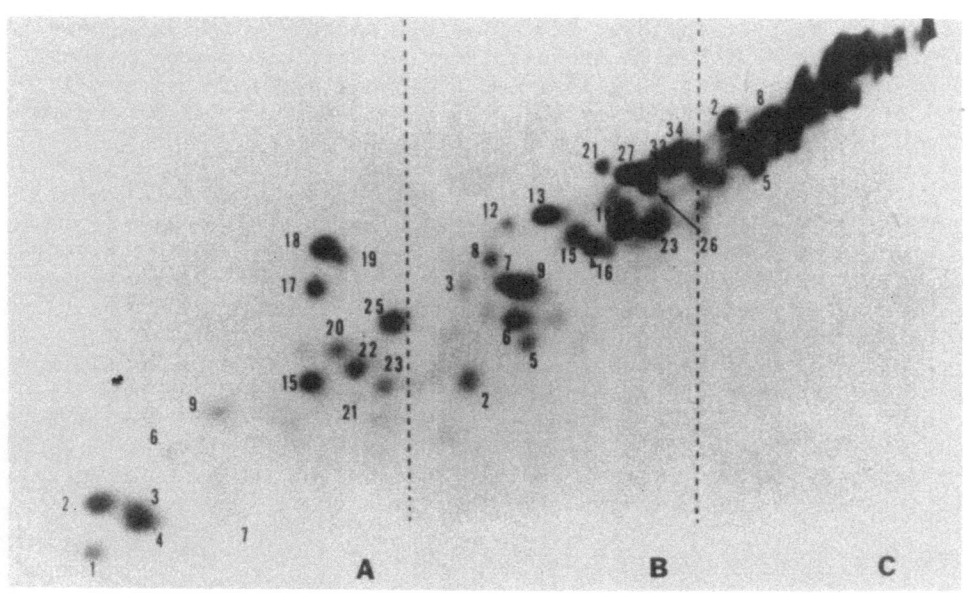

Figure 12
10/12 two-dimensional gel electrophoresis of 300 µg of
Novikoff hepatoma nucleolar preribosomal particle proteins extracted with 10 mM Tris-HCl (pH 8.0) (47).

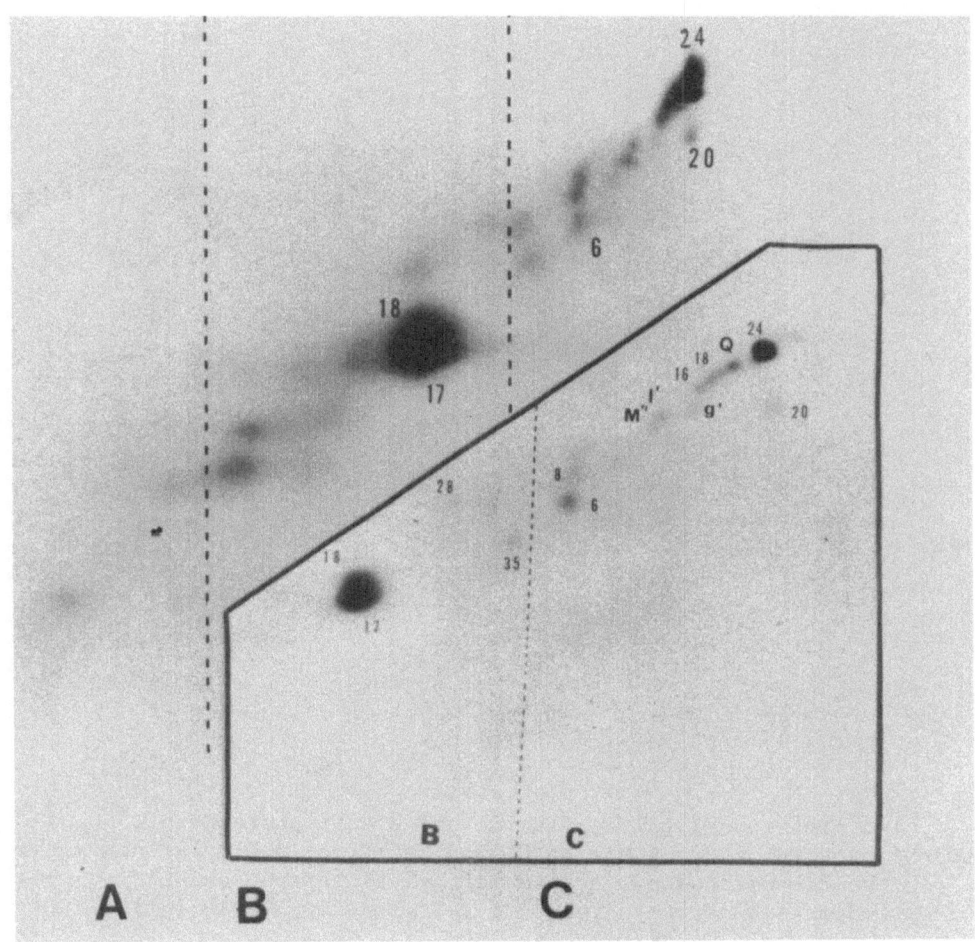

Figure 13
Two-dimensional polyacrylamide gel electrophoresis of 200 μg
of the proteins extracts with 0.15 M NaCl from nucleolar chromatin.
10/12 two-dimensional polyacrylamide gel electrophoresis. Inset.
6/8 two-dimensional polyacrylamide gel electrophoresis (47).

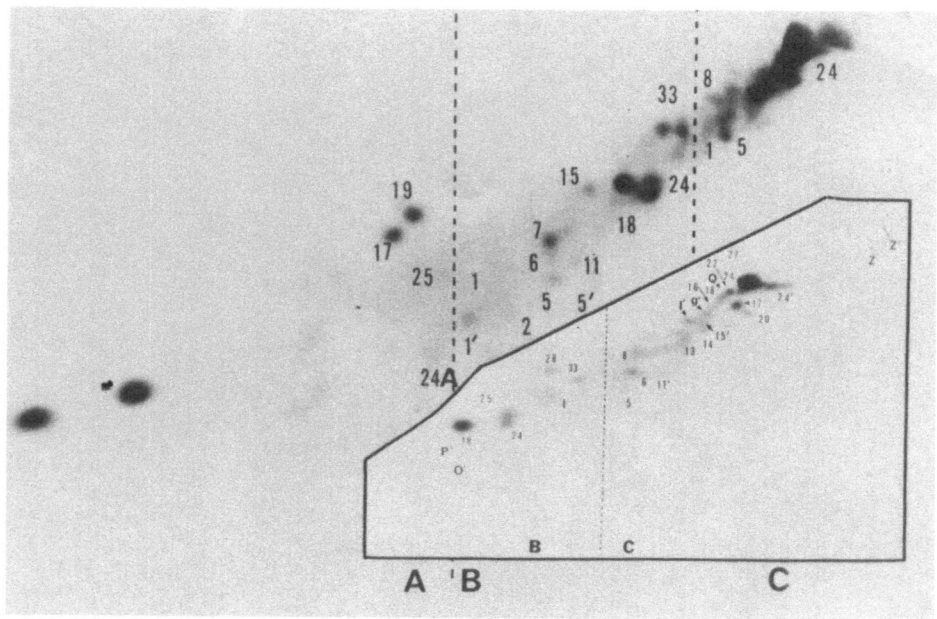

Figure 14
Two-dimensional polyacrylamide gel electrophoresis of 550 μg
of the proteins extracted with 0.35 M NaCl from nucleolar chromatin.
10/12 two-dimensional polyacrylamide gel electrophoresis. Inset.
6/9 two-dimensional polyacrylamide gel electrophoresis (47).

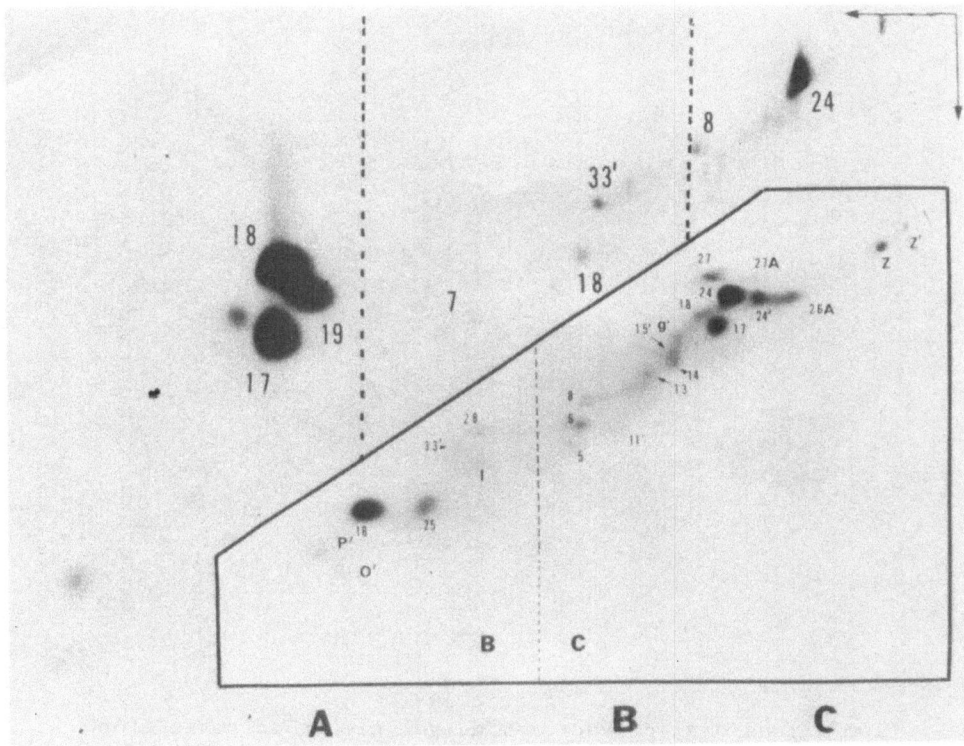

Figure 15
Two-dimensional polyacrylamide gel electrophoresis of 575 µg
of the proteins extracted with 0.6 M NaCl from nucleolar chromatin.
10/12 two-dimensional polyacrylamide gel electrophoresis.   Inset.
6/8 two-dimensional electrophoresis run (47).

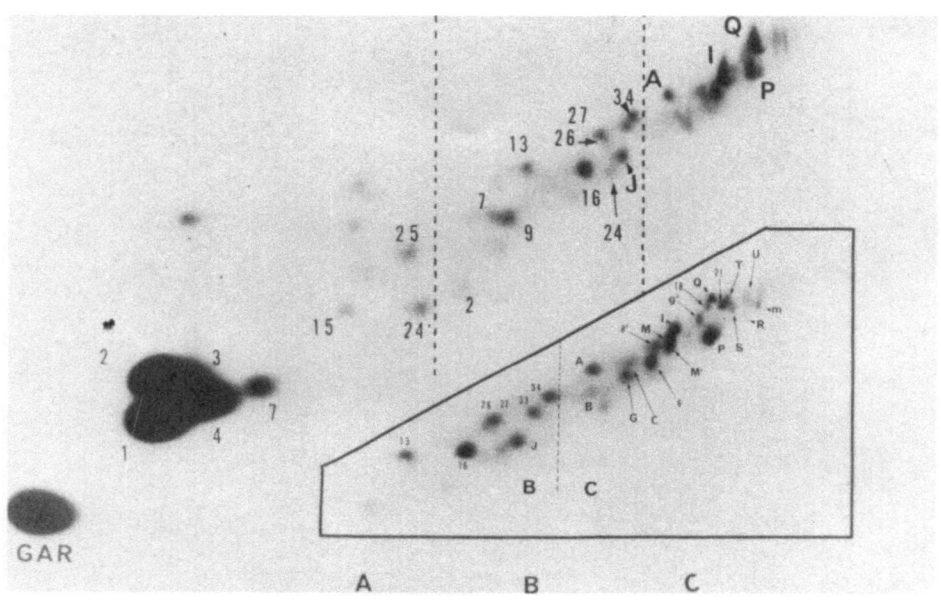

Figure 16
Two-dimensional polyacrylamide gel electrophoresis of 600
μg of the residual chromatin proteins extracted by 3 M NaCl-7 M
urea. 10/12 two-dimensional polyacrylamide gel electrophoresis.
Inset. 6/8 two-dimensional gel electrophoresis (47).

Table Ten
Elongation Factor 1 in Cellular Fractions

Fractions	Percent Distribution of EF-1	Specific activity of EF-1α (units/ mg protein x 10^{-2})	Specific activity of EF-1α (units/ mg DNA x 10^{-3})
Whole Homogenate	100	2.2	23
Nuclei	14	6.2	3.1
Nucleoplasm	9.5	5.7	3.0
Nucleoli	0.9	6.4	3.5

* One unit is the equivalent of one pmole of phenylalanyl-tRNA bound to ribosomes in 10 minutes at 37°C. Each value is an average of three independent experiments.

Elongation factor 1α assay incubation mixture included the following in a total volume of 100 µl: Tris-HCl, pH 7.5, 40 mM; MgAc, 7 mM; NH$_4$Cl, 50 mM; KCl, 50 mM; GTP, 50 µM; DTT, 2 mM; creatine perosphate, 1.25 mM; creatine phosphokinase, 2.5 ug, poly U, 40 µg; salt washed ribosomes, 0.8 A$_{260}$ units; and ^{3}H-phenylalanine-tRNA, 30 pmoles. The reaction is carried out at 37° for 5 minutes with all the constituents except ^{3}H-phenyl-alanine tRNA and enzyme. After preincubation, enzyme and tRNA were added and incubation was continued for 10 minutes. 80 µl of the assay mixture were filtered through Millipore filters and washed with 3 ml of ice-cold buffer containing 0.05 M Tris-HCl, pH 7.5; 0.05 M KCl; and 0.001 M DTT.(52).

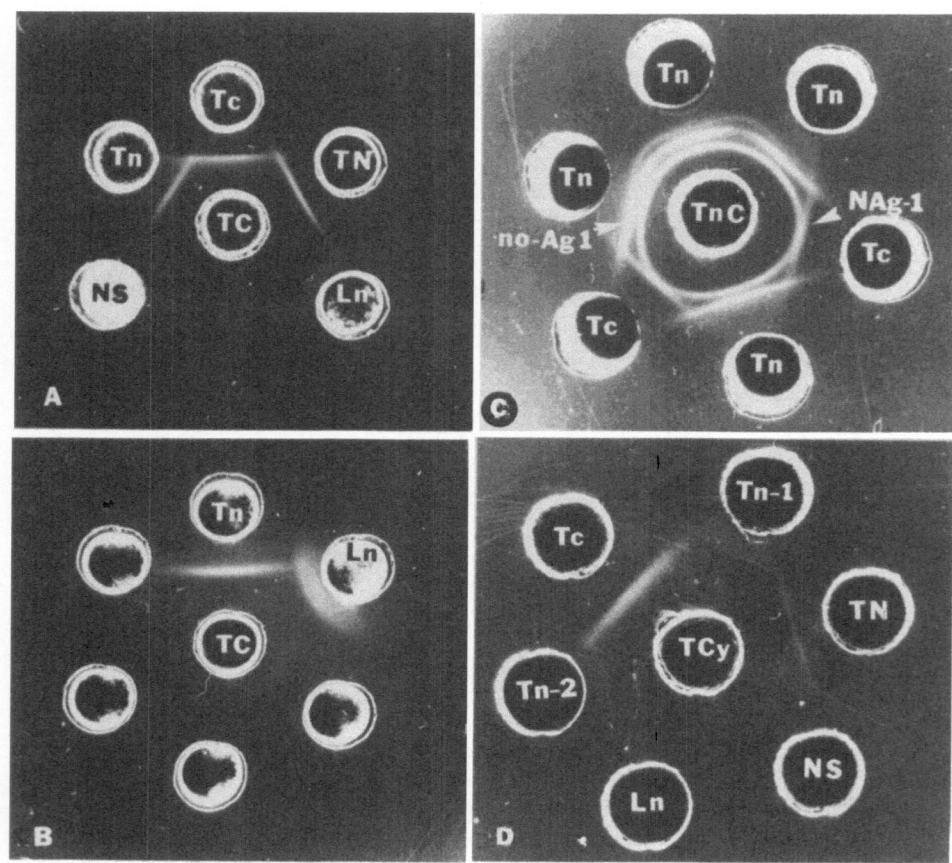

Figure 17A
Immunodiffusion plate which contains a 0.6 M NaCl extract of
tumor nuclear chromatin (TCAg) as the antigen in the center well
(300-400 μg). The antigen formed precipitin bands with 33 μl of
the following antisera in the side wells: TnAb - tumor nucleolar,
TcAb - tumor chromatin, TNAb - tumor nucleolar and LnAb - liver
nucleolar. A normal serum control (NS) is negative (53).

Figure 17B
Immunodiffusion plate which contains a 0.6 M NaCl extract
of tumor nucleolar chromatin TCAg as the antigen in the center
well (300-400 μg). The antigen formed different precipitin bands
with tumor-TnAb and liver-LnAb nucleolar antisera (33μl) in the
side wells.

Figure 17C
Immunodiffusion plate which contains a 0.6 M NaCl extract
of tumor nucleolar chromatin TnCAg as the antigen in the center
well (280-300 μg). The antigen formed three bands with the tumor
nucleolar antibodies (TnAb) which was added to three side wells
(33 μl per well). The antigen also formed two bands with TcAb,
the tumor chromatin antiserum which was added to two side wells
(33 μl per well). The specific bands for noAg-1 and NAg-1 are
shown with arrows (53).

Figure 17D
Immunodiffusion plate which contains a fraction of tumor
cytosol TCyAg (prepared from Novikoff Nonidet nuclei) in the center
well as the the antigen (300-400 μg). The antigen formed a dense
precipitin band with antibodies to tumor chromatin TcAb and faint
bands with antibodies to tumor nucleoli TnAb-1 and TnAb-2, and
tumor nuclei TNAb (33μl contained in each side well). There were
no visible bands with normal serum NS or liver nucleolar antiserum
(53).

glycoprotein (31). Initial evidence (53) suggested that tumor nucleolar chromatin contained a different antigen (noAg-1). Figure
17A shows the immunoprecipitin bands formed with tumor chromatin
antigens (TCAg) and antibodies to tumor nuclei (TNAb), tumor chromatin (TCAb), tumor nucleoli (TnAb) and liver nucleoli (LnAb). The
lack of antigenic identity of the bands (TCAg-TnAb) with the tumor
nucleolar antibodies and tumor chromatin antibodies (TCAg-TcAb) is
apparent. Antibodies to liver nucleoli did not form the same bands
with antigens from tumor chromatin as did antibodies to tumor nucleoli (Fig 17A, B).

Is noAg-1 distinct from NAg-1? - To compare noAg-1 and NAg-1, tumor
nucleolar chromatin antigens (TnCAg) were tested for immunoprecipitation with tumor nucleolar antibodies (TnAb) and tumor chromatin antibodies (TcAb). As shown in Figure 17C, three bands formed with TnAb
and two with TcAb. The inner band is common to both types of antibodies. The dense band between TcAb and TnCAg shows tumor nucleolar
chromatin contains NAg-1 as well as noAg-1 which is the middle of the
three bands between TnCAg and TnAb.

Does NAg-1 form immunoprecipitin complexes with nucleolar antibodies?
Figure 17D provides an analysis of the interaction of a purified
preparation of NAg-1 in a concentrated preparation of tumor cytoplasmic proteins (TCyAg) with a variety of antibody preparations.
TCyAg was shown earlier to contain NAg-1 (31). Figure 17D shows
that this preparation formed a dense band with TcAb. However, with
TNAb and TnAb only faint bands were present. Since TnAb formed dense
bands with noAg-1 (Fig 17C), these results show that antibodies that
reacted strongly with noAg-1 did not react strongly with NAg-1.
Accordingly, noAg-1 differs from NAg-1. Thus, NAg-1 is present in
the nucleus and cytoplasm bu noAg-1 is localized to the nucleolus
and nucleolar chromatin.

Evidence that noAg-1 is tightly bound to tumor chromatin - noAg-1
was not extracted from tumor nucleoli with 0.075 M NaCl-0.025 M
EDTA, pH 8.0 since tumor nucleolar antibodies did not react with proteins in this extract. Tumor nuclear antibodies (TNAb), however,
formed a dense band with antigens of tumor nucleolar chromatin (TnCAg),
but formed only a faint band with these soluble antigens (NaEAg, Fig
18A, B). The band for NAg-1 was readily observed when tumor chromatin
antibodies (TcAb) were reacted with either TnCAg or EaEAg. Thus, the
saline-EDTA extraction (NaEAg) solubilized NAg-1 but not noAg-1.

Is antigen noAg-1 in normal liver? - Evidence provided earlier indicated that NAg-1 was not present in a variety of normal adult growing
and nongrowing tissues. Although antibodies to liver nucleoli (LnAb)
and liver chromatin antigens formed bands with the tumor nucleolar
antigens they were diffuse and close to the antibody well. Adsorption
with tumor nucleoli of the antiserum for liver nucleoli eliminated

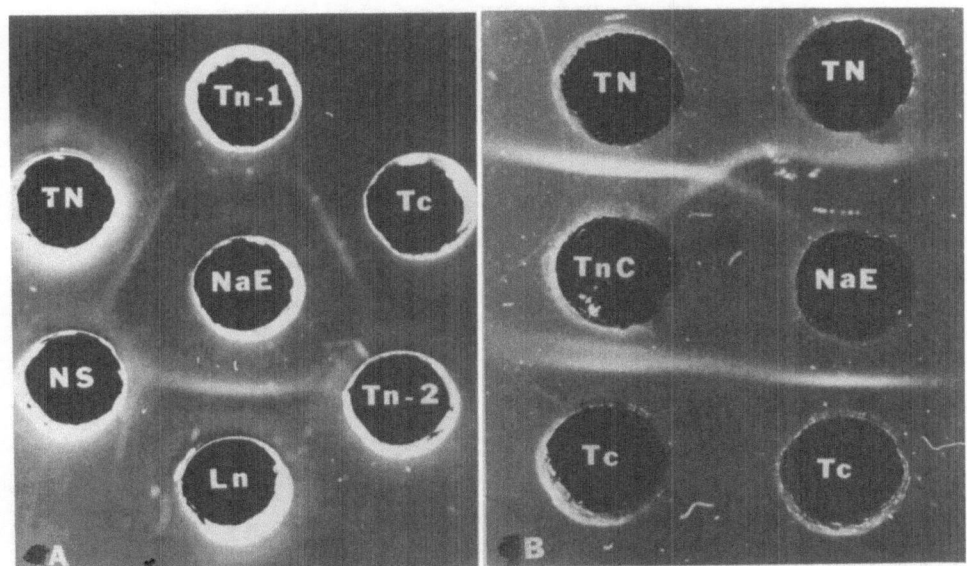

Figure 18A
Immunodiffusion plate which contains a NaCl-EDTA (NaEAg) chromatin extract in the center well (300–400 µg/33 µl). This antigen formed precipitin bands with antibodies (33µl/well) to tumor nuclei (TNAb), to tumor chromatin (TcAb) and to liver nucleoli (LnAb). There were no precipitin bands formed with this antigen and the tumor nucleolar antiserum (TnAb) and normal serum (NS).

Figure 18B
Immunodiffusion plate which contains a 0.6 M NaCl extract of tumor nucleolar chromatin (TnC) as the antigen in the left center well and NaCl EDTA nucleolar chromatin extract (NaEAg) as the antigen in the center right well (300–400 µg). Antigen TnCAg formed precipitin bands with antibodies to tumor nuclei (TNAb) and tumor chromatin, TcAb (33 µl per well) and antigen NaEAg formed bands with antibodies to tumor nuclei (TNAb) and tumor chromatin (TcAb).

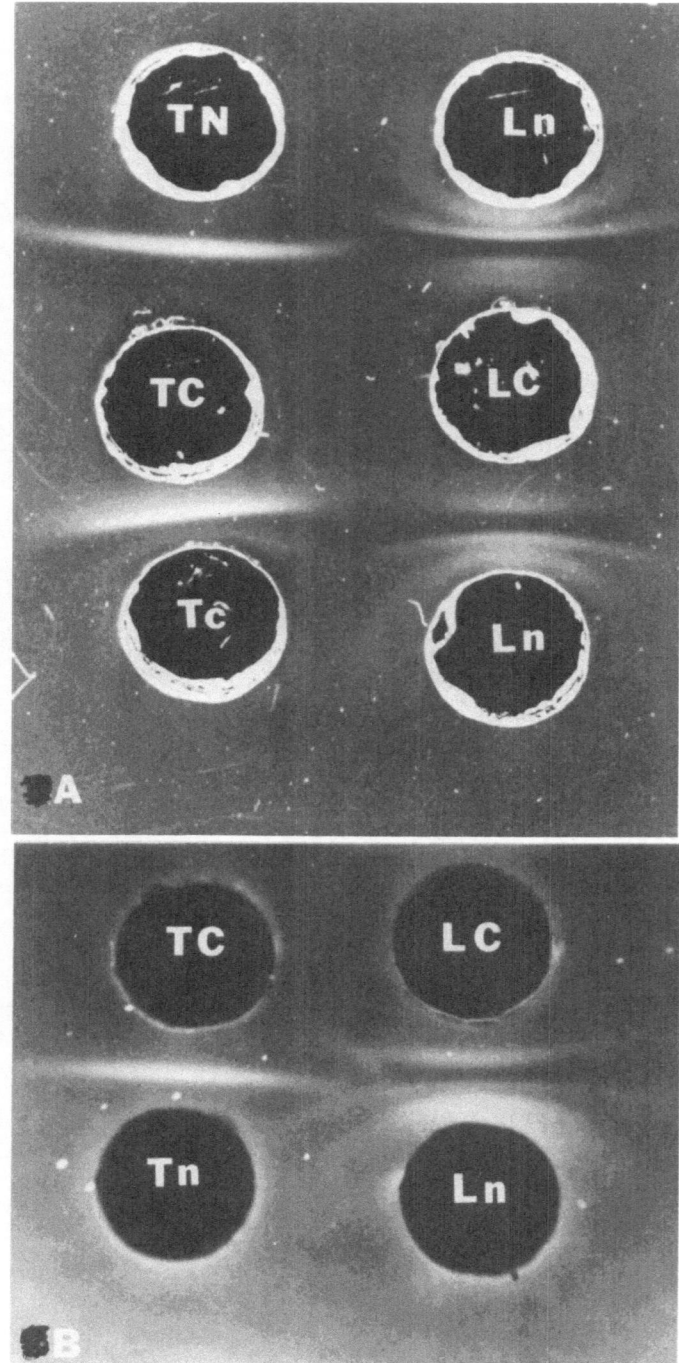

Figure 19A
    Immunodiffusion plate which contains a 0.6 M NaCl extract
of tumor nuclear chromatin TCAg in the left center well and liver
chromatin LCag in the right center well (300-400 µg) as antigens.
The TCAg formed precipitin bands with tumor nuclear (TNAb) and
tumor chromatin (TcAb) antibodies. The LCAg antigen formed at
least three precipitin bands with the liver nucleolar (LnAb)
antibodies. The antibody wells contain 33$_\mu$l (53).

Figure 19B
    Immunodiffusion plate which contains 0.6 M NaCl extracts of
tumor nuclear chromatin TCAg in the top left well and liver nuclear
chromatin LNAg in the top right well (300-400 µg). The tumor
chromatin antigen formed a precipitin band with the tumor nucleolar antiserum (TnAb). The LCAg antigen formed at least three
precipitin bands with the liver nucleolar antibodies (LnAb). The
antibody wells contain 33 $_\mu$l (53).

the formation of these immune complexes.

Liver nucleolar antibodies (LnAb) formed several bands with the liver chromatin antigens. Evidence that these immunoprecipitin bands are not the same as those found in the corresponding tumor samples is shown in Figure 19. The single dense bands formed between the nucleolar (TnAb), chromatin (TcAb), nuclear (TNAb) antibodies, and the chromatin antigens of the tumor (TCAg) did not show identity with the bands formed between LnAb and LCAg.

These results indicate that the antigen recognized by the antinucleolar antibodies to the tumor was not demonstrable in normal liver nucleoli. Conversely, several liver nucleolar chromatin antigens were not found in the Novikoff hepatoma nucleoli.

Immunoelectrophoretic analysis in which the samples shown in Figure 20 were placed in the wells and a new antitumor nucleolar antisera was placed in the trough showed multiple arcs formed with tumor and liver nucleolar proteins extracted with 0.075 M NaCl-0.025 M EDTA. Of these arcs the one marked by the arrow was uniquely found in the tumor nucleolar extract. This result supports the results shown above which indicate the presence of unique antigens in tumor nucleoli. It is noteworthy that these were not demonstrated in the fetal liver nuclei.

DISCUSSION

This brief review of analytical and isolation studies in our laboratory reflects the overall progress in our knowledge of the various elements of nucleolar activity and nucleolar gene control. Nevertheless, there are many more important questions fundamental to future understanding of nucleolar function, gene control and tumor growth.

1) "Restriction proteins": Structure and function - Current studies in our and other laboratories (8, 9, 14) show that specificity of readout of rDNA genes persists in nucleolar residues after extraction of nucleoli with the Zubay-Doty buffer (0.075 M NaCl-0.025 M EDTA, pH 7.4) and with 0.01 M Tris (pH 8.0). Under these circumstances more than 50% of the nucleolar proteins were extracted including most of the RNA polymerase I, protein kinase and most of the RNP particles (47). The less soluble proteins that remain can be fractionated into two groups: (a) those that are referred to as the TBP (tight binding proteins, 10) and (b) those soluble in 3 M NaCl-7 M urea. The latter contain the "restriction proteins" inasmuch as the DNA residue containing the TBP is read for genes other than rDNA. Further studies on the nature and specificity of the "restriction proteins" are in progress. They must be isolated and reconstituted with the chromatin to determine which proteins specifically "restrict"

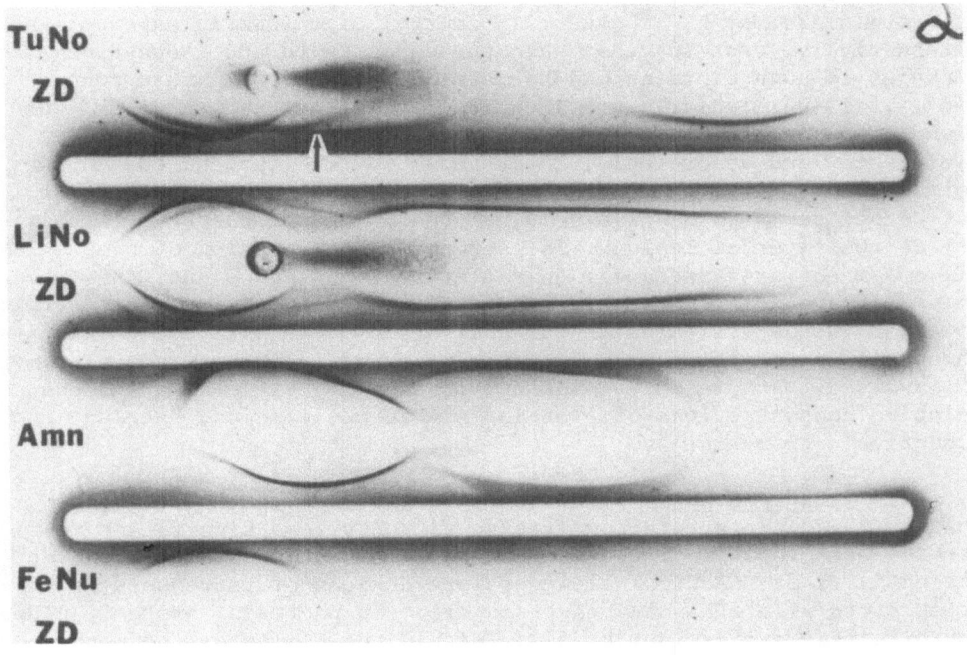

Figure 20
      Immunoelectrophoretic profile of nucleolar antigens. Zubay-
Doty extracts (0.075 M NaCl, 0.025 M EDTA, pH 8.0, containing 1
mM PMSF) were made from nucleoli isolated by the calcium sucrose
procedure from Novikoff hepatoma nucleoli (TuNoZD) and from rat
liver nucleoli (LiNoZD) and from nuclei prepared by the NP40
sucrose procedure from livers of 19-day fetal rats (FeNuZD).   20
μg of each of these extracts and of the amniotic fluid of the fetal
rats was analyzed by electrophoresis for 35 min at 75 V in 1%
agarose (Immunoagaroslides, Millipore Biomedica, Acton, Mass.).
50 μl of an immunoglubulin fraction at 80 mg.ml, which was prepared from the serum of a rabbit immunized against whole Novikoff
nucleoli, was placed in each trough and precipitin arcs were
allowed to develop for 24 hr. Precipitin arcs were stained with
Coomassie blue. Note the presence of a precipitin arc in the extract from Novikoff nucleoli which is not detected in the other
fractions (arrow).

and how they function. Clearly, both the restriction proteins and
the RNA polymerase affect the type of readout obtained (9, 54, 55).

   2) Chromatin supercoiling - At present methods are improving
for separation of "active" and "inactive" chromatin. Proteins such
as protein A24 may be important in control of chromatin supercoiling.
Alternatively, proteins that have the capacity to add isopeptide
linkages to such proteins may be rate-determining. In this connection, it is particularly pertinent to recall that as nucleolar function increased, the concentrations of protein A24 and A11 rapidly
diminished, and accordingly, their possible role in gene control was
anticipated. Protein A24 does not seem to be a specific repressor,
but rather seems to be inversely related in amount to the total activity of the liver nucleolus. The structure and function of protein
A11 are much less adequately characterized. In any event, the mechanisms of nucleolar chromatin supercoiling and uncoiling are of great
interest and necessitate careful analysis of both active and inactive
chromatin to determine what specific roles of individual proteins may
be involved. At present, Goldknopf et al. (56) are evaluating the
relative concentrations of proteins A24 in nucleosomes, "active" and
"inactive" chromatin.

   3) Derepression - Nucleolar synthesis is subject to rapid
change (2, 57), e.g., in specific in vitro systems significant increases were found in 1 hour in RNA Pol I. Such changes may reflect
the activity of RNA Pol I alone or interactions of repressors or
stimulators with rDNA and its promoters. In bacterial systems, ppGpp
inhibits rRNA synthesis (58, 59). Within the limits of the methods
available, neither ppGpp, cAMP, cGMP or their analogs exert effects
on eukaryotic nucleolar activities. The polyphosphate of Hildebrandt
and Suaer (4) reduced rates of rRNA synthesis; in growing or dividing
cells, the rates may be increased by removal of such inhibitory cellular elements.

   An event of relative rapidity is the phosphorylation of dephosphorylation of nuclear proteins, such as RNA polymerase. Much
effort has been dovoted to the study of phosphorylated proteins C23-
25 and C26, 27 (35). However, variation in their phosphorylation
parallels rather than precedes changes in nucleolar activity. Phosphorylation of RNA polymerase I has been reported but like changes
in nucleolar protein kinases, it is an associated rather than a
primary event in nucleolar function.

   4) Moment-to-moment controls. What then are the driving
factors that influence the rate rather than the specificity of nucleolar functions? Both the supercoiling of nucleolar chromatin and
its specificity of readout are probably long-acting rather than
moment-to-moment control mechanisms.

5) Systems for analysis of controls of nucleolar function -
A key problem in studies on mechanisms has been the lack of satisfactory systems for rDNA activation and inhibition. Recently,
Andersen et al. (60) have been analyzing rates of activation of
nucleoli in thioacetamide treated livers. A 10-fold increase in
nucleolar RNA synthesis occurred in the 7-hour period following
administration of the drug. At 48-72 hours, there was a return to
the normal level. This system offers a simple tool for analysis
of nucleolar function with opportunity to determine correlates
between the reduction of ribosome levels in the cytoplasm (2),
activation of cytoplasmic RNases and "feedback" circuitry of the
nucleolus.

Other systems that may be useful include the "refeeding"
system recently described by Mauck (57) in which rapid stimulation
of RNA polymerase has been found. In this system, a rapid increase
in rRNA synthesis occurs in cells that were stationary and grow
after refeeding.

6) Feedback systems - It has been postulated that ribosomes
or ribosomal products could be important feedback factors in nucleolar function (2). Studies in our laboratory (61) and those of
Warner (62) directed attention to the close correlation of the relationship of ribosomal protein synthesis and that of rRNA. In
addition, both Highashi's group (63) and Muramatsu's group (64)
have shown that inhibition of protein synthesis by cycloheximide
produced cessation of nucleolar function.

Recently, Bolla et al. (6) have done the interesting experiment of adding ribosomal proteins to nuclei of liver cells. They reported that these proteins caused a shift in synthesis from mRNA
to pre-rRNA suggesting that r-proteins redirect nuclear to nucleolar
synthetic activity.

At the same time, our group, which demonstrated that the nucleoli contain many ribosomal proteins (49), has been evaluating
elongation and initiation factors in nucleoli. Recently, Rao et al.
(52) have found both initiation and elongation factors (both EF-1
and EF-2) in rat liver nucleoli in concentrations higher (activity/
mg protein) than those of the nucleoplasm or cytoplasm. Since the
nucleolus contains high concentrations of the preribosomal proteins
and other preribosomal elements, the higher concentration of the
initiation and elongation factors may be important to the overall
biosynthetic and/or assembly reactions of the nucleolus.

In our earlier studies (49), the nucleolar RNP particles were
shown to contain a number of high molecular weight proteins in
addition to ribosomal proteins. These particles are easily extractable from the nucleoli (2); they are identical in size and ultra-

structure to the large ribosomal subunit and are precursors of the
ribosomes. These early findings have now been confirmed (47);
2-D electrophoresis also showed that the RNP particles contain
higher molecular weight proteins corresponding in migration to the
initiation and elongation factors (52) purified by Merrick's group
(65) and others (66). Studies are now in progress to determine
whether the 0.5 M KCl extract of nucleoli contains all the initiation and elongation factors of the cytoplasmic ribosomes (52).

  7) Reconstitution systems - Reconstitution techniques may
provide the types of answers required for analysis of the rate-
limiting factors involved in nucleolar function (26, 32, 67-74).
Further analysis of this technique is in progress in this and other
laboratories.

  8) Tumor nucleolar antigens (noAg-1) - There have been many
reports of unusual antigens in tumor cells including carcinoembryonic antigens (75), α-fetoproteins (76), "pre-neoplastic antigens"
(77) as well as viral antigens, including T antigen (78) and the
Epstein-Barr nuclear antigen (79). An extractable nuclear antigen
has also been described (80). Chromatin extracted from tumor nuclei contains an antigen (noAg-1) which appears to be limited in
location to nucleoli (53). This antigen was not found in normal
liver nuclear or nucleolar chromatin, in cytoplasmic fractions of
tumor or in the 0.075 M NaCl-0.025 M EDTA and 0.01 M Tris-HCl extracts of nucleoli.

  Although immunoprecipitation analysis showed the presence of
noAg-1 in tumor nucleoli, the fact that it was not detected in
liver may reflect (a) its absence from liver, (b) a very small
amount of the antigen in the liver, (c) masking of the antigen, and
(d) association with other macromolecules altering its extractability.

  Evidence that antigen noAg-1 differs from NAg-1 (53) was obtained in studies showing that antibodies to tumor chromatin proteins
soluble in 0.15 M NaCl-0.35 M urea did not form an immunoprecipitin
band with this antigen. While antibodies to whole nucleoli formed
a dense immunoprecipitin band with this antigen, the two immunoprecipitin lines crossed over one another. The antinucleolar antibodies
did not react with a more purified preparation of NAg-1 obtained from
tumor cytosol, while the anti-chromatin antibodies produced a dense
band with this preparation.

  Interestingly, the antibodies raised against liver nucleoli
reacted with different proteins than those of the Novikoff hepatoma
nucleoli or nuclei. The immunoprecipitin bands formed did not exhibit identity with those formed with antigens of the Novikoff hepatoma nuclei, chromatin, nucleoli or nucleolar chromatin. This result is interesting because the normal liver nucleolus operates in

a highly repressed state, i.e., the rDNA is transcribed at only one-tenth to one-fifteenth the rate of transcription in Novikoff hepatoma (2), and possibly these repressors are in the liver antigens. Also, some nucleolar enzymes, including RNA methylases (81) and protein kinases (82) have been reported to differ in tumors and other tissues and may be among the antigens detected in these studies.

The possibility also exists that noAg-1 may serve as a derepressor protein which may increase readouts of rDNA (1). Feedback stimulation of nucleolar function was suggested by studies on estrogen-stimulated systems (83-85). It may be that protein All is a phosphoprotein (such as phosphorylated lysine-rich histone F10) that serves a similar function as ppGpp (58, 59) or the polyphosphate of Hildebrandt and Suaer (4). If noAg-1 were a phosphotase that reduced its content, nucleolar activity might well reach the large levels that characterize these tumors.

Tests of the effects of various proteins which are currently being isolated in sufficient quantities for further studies are now being rapidly improved. The key development has been the evidence that the nucleolus in vivo and in vitro synthesizes unique gene products which can be simply assayed for by homochromatography fingerprinting of T_1 RNase digests. This development permits demonstration of fidelity and offers the opportunity to correct the lack of fidelity. The methods for reconstitution of nucleolar activity require further development and standardization. With this system, and the vastly improved techniques for separating and isolating proteins, the next decade should bring rapid advances in our understanding of nucleolar gene control.

*   These studies were supported by the Cancer Research Center Grant
    CA-10893 awarded by the National Cancer Institute, DHEW, the
    Davidson Fund, the Wolff Memorial Foundation and a generous gift
    from Mrs. Jack Hutchins.

REFERENCES

1. Busch, H. Cancer Res. 36 (1976) 4291.

2. Busch, H. and Smetana, K. The Nucleolus, Academic Press, New York (1970).

3. Caspersson, T.O. Cell Growth and Cell Function. A Cytochemical Study, Norton, New York (1950).

4. Hildebrandt, A. and Suaer, H.W. Biochem. Biophys. Res. Comm. 74 (1977) 466.

5. Manen, C.A. and Russell, D.H. Science, 1965 (1977) 505.

6. Bolla, R., Roth, H.E., Weissbach, H. and Brot, N. J. Biol. Chem. 252 (1977) 721.

7. Orrick, L.I., Olson, M.O.J. and Busch, H. Proc. Natl. Acad. Sci. U.S.A. 70 (1973) 1316.

8. Matsui, S., Fuke, M. and Busch, H. Bichemistry 16 (1977) 39.

9. Ballal, N.R., Choi, Y.C., Mouche, R. and Busch, H. Proc. Natl. Acad. Sci. U.S.A. 74 (1977) June.

10. Busch, H., Ballal, N.R., Olson, M.O.J. and Yeoman, L.C., In: Methods in Cancer Reserach, H. Busch (ed). Academic Press, New York 11 (1975) 43.

11. Blatti, S.P., Ingles, C.J., Lindell, T.J., Morris, P.W., Weaver, R.F., Weinberg, F. and Rutter, W.J. Cold Spring Harbor Synp. Quant. Biol. Med. 35 (1970) 649.

12. Zylber, E.A. and Penman, S. Proc. Natl. Acad. Sci. U.S.A. 68 (1971) 2861.

13. Grummt, I. and Lindigkeit, R. Eur. J. Biochem. 36 (1973) 244.

14. Beebee, T.J.C. and Butterworth, P.H.W. Eur. J. Biochem. 51 (1975) 537.

15. Grummt, I. Eur. J. Bicohem. 57 (1975) 159.

16. Choi, Y.C., Ballal, N.R., Busch, R.K. and Busch, H. Cancer Res. 36 (1976) 4301.

17. Yu, F.L. and Feigelson, P. Proc. Natl. Acad. Sci. U.S.A. 69 (1972) 2833.

18. Liau, M.C., Hunt, J.B., Smith, D.W. and Hurlbert, R.B. Cancer Res. 33 (1973) 323.

19. Ferencz, A. and Seifart, K.H. Eur. J. Biochem. 53 (1975) 605.

20. Ballal, N.R. and Rogachevsky, L. Proc. Amer. Assoc. Cancer Res. 17 (1976) 162.

21. Roeder, R.G. and Rutter, W.J. Nature 224 (1969) 234.

22. Roeder, R.G. and Rutter, W.J. Proc. Natl. Acad. Sci. U.S.A. 65 (1970) 675.

23. Chambon, P., Gissinger, F., Kedinger, C., Mandel, J.L. and Meilhac, M. In: The Cell Nucleus, H. Bushc (ed). Academic Press, New York, 3 (1974) 269.

24. Inagaki, A. and Busch, H. Biochem. Biophys. Res. Comm. 49 (1972) 1398.

25. Eladari, M.E. and Galibert, F. Eur. J. Biochem. 55 (1975) 247.

26. Matsui, S., Fuke, M. and Busch, H. J. Cell Biol. 67 (1975) 266a.

27. Fuke, M. and Busch, H. J. Mol. Biol. 99 (1975) 277.

28. Fuke, M. and Busch, H. Nucleic Acids Res. 4 (1977) 339.

29. Woo, S.L.C., Rosen, J.M., Liakaros, C.D., Choi, Y.C., Busch, H., Means, A.R. and O'Malley, B.W. J. Biol. Chem. 250 (1975) 7027.

30. Busch, R.K., Daskal, I., Spohn, W.H., Kellermayer, M., and Busch, H. Cancer Res. 34 (1974) 2362.

31. Yeoman, L.C., Jordan, J.J., Busch, R.K., Taylor, C.W., Savage, H.E. and Busch, H. Proc. Natl. Acad. Sci. U.S.A. 73 (1976) 3258.

32. Chytil, F. and Spelsberg, T.C. Nature New Biol. 233 (1971) 215.

33. Wakabayashi, K. and Hnilica, L.S. J. Cell Biol. 55 (1972) 271a.

34. Zardi, L., Lin, J. and Baserga, R. Nature New Biol. 245 (1973) 211.

35. Nazar, R.N., Sitz, T.O. and Busch, H. FEBS Lett. 59 (1975) 83.

36. Mamrack, M.D., Olson, M.O.J. and Busch, H. Biochem. Biophys. Res. Comm. 76 (1977) 150.

37. Balla, N.R., Goldknopf, I.L., Goldberg, D.A. and Busch, H.
    Life Sci. 14 (1974) 1835.

38. Ballal, N.R., Kang, Y.J., Olson, M.O.J. and Busch, H. J. Biol.
    Chem. 250 (1975) 5921.

39. Goldknopf, I.L. and Busch, H. Biochem. Biophys. Res. Comm.
    65 (1975) 951.

40. Olson, M.O.J., Goldknopf, I.L., Guetzow, K.A., James, G.T.,
    Hawkins, T.C., Mays-Rothberg, C.J. and Busch, H. J. Biol. Chem.
    251 (1976) 5901.

41. Goldknopf, I.L. and Busch, H. Proc. Natl. Acad. Sci. U.S.A.
    74 (1977) 864.

42. Schlesinger, D.H., Goldstein, G. and Niall, H.D. Biochemistry
    14 (1975) 2214.

43. Hunt, L.T. and Dayhoff, M.O. Biochem. Biophys. Res. Comm.
    74 (1977) 650.

44. Sugano, N., Olson, M.O.J., Yeoman, L.C., Johnson, B.R., Taylor,
    C.W., Starbuck, W.C. and Busch, H. J. Biol. Chem. 247 (1972)
    3589.

45. Yeoman, L.C., Olson, M.O.J., Sugano, N., Jordan, J.J., Taylor,
    C.W., Starbuck, W.C. and Busch, H. J. Biol. Chem. 247 (1972)
    6018.

46. Kang, Y.J., Olson, M.O.J. and Busch, H. J. Biol. Chem. 249 (1974)
    5580.

47. Rothblum, L.I., Mamrack, P.M., Olson, M.O.J. and Busch, H. In
    manuscript.

48. Daskal, Y., Prestayko, A.W. and Busch, H. Exptl. Cell Res. 88
    (1974) 1.

49. Prestayko, A.W., Klomp, G.R., Schmoll, D.J. and Busch, H.
    Biochemistry 13 (1974) 1945.

50. Yeoman, L.C., Taylor, C.W., Jordan, J.J. and Busch, H. Exptl.
    Cell Res. 91 (1975) 207.

51. Olson, M.O.J., Ezrailson, E.G., Guetzow, K. and Busch, H. J.
    Mol. Biol. 97 (1975) 611.

52. Rao, M.S., Rothblum, L.I. and Busch, H. In manuscript.

53. Busch, R.K.and Busch, H. In manuscript.

54. Honjo, T. and Reeder, R.H. Biochemistry 13 (1974) 1896.

55. Reeder, R.H. J. Mol. Biol. 80 (1973) 229.

56. Goldknopf, I.L., French, M.F., Musso, R. and Busch, H. In manuscript.

57. Mauck, J.C. Biochemistry 16 (1977) 793.

58. Travers, A. Nature 244 (1973) 15.

59. Travers, A. Nature 263 (1976) 641.

60. Andersen, A., Ballal, N.R. and Busch, H. In manuscript.

61. Wu, B.C., Rao, M.S., Gupta, K.K., Rothblum, L.I., Mamrack, P. C. and Busch, H. Cell Biol. Internatl. Rpts. 1 (1977) 31.

62. Warner, J.R. In: Ribosomes, M. Nomura, A. Tiessieres and P. Lengyel (eds). Cold Spring Harbor Laboratories (1974) 461.

63. Hisgashi, K., Matsushita, T., Kitao, A. and Sakamoto, Y. Biochim. Biophys. Acta 166 (1968) 388.

64. Muramatsu, M., Shimade, N. and Higashinakagawa, T. J. Mol. Biol. 53 (1970) 91.

65. Kemper, W.M., Berry, K.W.and Merrick, W.C. J. Biol. Chem. 251 (1976) 5551.

66. Weissbach, H. and Ochoa, S. Ann. Rev. Biochem. 45 (1976) 191.

67. Paul, J. and Gilmour, R.S. J. Mol. Biol. 34 (1968) 305.

68. Bekhor, I., Kung, G.M. and Bonner, J. J. Mol. Biol. 39 (1969) 351.

69. Spelsberg, T.C., Hnilica, L.S. and Ansevin, A.T. Biochim. Biophys. Acta 228 (1971) 550.

70. Stein, G.S. and Farber, J. Proc. Natl. Acad. Sci. U.S.A. 69 (1972) 2918.

71. Axel, R., Cedar, H. and Felsenfeld, G. Biochemistry 14 (1975) 2489.

72. Bluthmann, H., Mrozek, S. and Gierer, A. Eur. J. Biochem. 58

(1975) 315.

73. Stein, G.S., Mans, R.T., Gabbay, E.J., Stein, J.L., Davis, J. and Adawakar, P.D. Biochemistry 14 (1975) 1859.

74. Daubert, S., Peters, D. and Dahmus, M.E. Arch. Biochem. Biophys. 178 (1977) 381.

75. Gold, P. and Freedman, S.O. J. Exptl. Med. 122 (1965) 467.

76. Abelev, G.I., Avenirova, Z.A., Engel-gardt, N.V., Baidakova, Z.L. and Stephanchenok-Rudnik, G.I. Proc. Acad. Sci. U.S.S.R. Engl. Transl. 124 (1959) 51.

77. Okita, K., Kligman, L.H. and Farber, S. J. Natl. Cancer Inst. 54 (1975) 199.

78. Suzuki, M. and Himuna, Y. Intl. J. Cancer 14 (1974) 753.

79. Todaro, G.J., Habel, K. and Green, H. Virology 27 (1965) 179.

80. Morris, A.D., Littleton, C., Corman, L.C., Esterly, J. and Sharp, C.G. J. Clin. Invest. 55 (1975) 903.

81. Liau, M.C., Hunt, M.E. and Hurlbert, R.B. Biochemistry 15 (1976) 3158.

82. Thomson, J.A., Chiu, J.F. and Hnilica, L.S. Biochim. Biophys. Acta 407 (1975) 114.

83. Arnaud, M., Beziat, Y., Borgna, J.L., Guilleux, J.C. and Mourrseron-Canet, M. Biochim. Biophys. Acta 254 (1971) 241.

84. Dierks-Ventling, C. and Bieri-Bonniot, F. Nucleic Acids Res. 4 (1977) 381.

85. Cohen, M.E. and Hamilton, T.H. Proc. Natl. Acad. Sci. U.S.A. 72 (1975) 4346.

NUCLEAR MACROMOLECULAR CHANGES IN HEPATOMAS

Jen-Fu Chiu, Lubomir S. Hnilica, Luc Belanger and
H.P. Morris*

Department of Biochemistry, Vanderbilt University
School of Medicine, Nashville, Tennessee 37232
*Department of Biochemistry, Howard University
School of Medicine, Washington, D.C. 20001

SUMMARY

A new DNA polymerase (6-8S) was detected and isolated from nuclei of several experimental hepatomas. This new polymerase activity could not be found in normal adult rat tissues. However, it
appeared in liver nuclei about 2 weeks after dietary introduction
of 3'-methyl-4-dimethylaminobenzene (3'-MDAB), increased considerably with time, and reached a prominent maximum between 30-40 days on
the diet. The activity of 6-8S nuclear DNA polymerase of the Morris
hepatomas could be directly correlated with their degree of differentiation and growth rates.

Dehistonized chromatin was found to be antigenic, capable of
producing tissue-specific antibodies. The changes of immunospecificity of dehistonized chromatin in experimental hepatomas were studied.
Administration of 3'-MDBA to Fischer rats produced an early change of
the immunospecificity of liver chromatin to a new type, common to
many experimental malignancies. The affinity of various hepatoma dehistonized chromatin preparations for the Novikoff hepatoma antiserum
approximately paralleled the degree of their differentiation as well
as their individual growth rates. The fast growing and poorly differentiated 7777 and 3942A hepatomas were more reactive than the slow
growing and better differentiated 7800 and 7787 tumors.

Nuclear phosphoprotein kinase activities and nuclear nonhistone
protein phosphorylation patterns were studied in the experimental hepatomas. The kinase activities were several times higher in hepatoma
than in normal rat liver. The enzyme activities both in hepatomas and
normal liver had similar optimal requirements for pH and Mg concentra-

tion. Selective changes in the phosphorylation pattern of chromosomal proteins were observed between the normal liver and experimental
hepatomas. Most affected was the area of high molecular weight of
nonhistone proteins. Supported by U.S. Public Health Service Grants
CA-18668 and by National Cancer Institute Contract NO1-CP-65730.

INTRODUCTION

Cell proliferation and differentiation are related, often inversely (3), e.g. during normal growth, as differentiation proceeds,
cells mature and decrease their rate of division. Malignant cells
may be induced to undergo differentiation to benign cells (28).
Weiler (41) has suggested that the expression of the neoplastic
phenotype is possibly coupled with the loss of some differentiated
traits of the normal stem cells. Potter (30) in his study of the
"minimal deviation hepatomas" also comes to the conclusion that the
key to malignant transformation may be in altered responses to the
factors that normally program cell maturation.

Since nuclear function is necessary for both differentiation and
proliferation, the molecules that regulate DNA replication and transcription must play a most important regulatory function in the cell.
In this communication, we discuss the activities of DNA polymerases,
immunospecificities of nuclear antigens, as well as some properties
of phosphoproteins and phosphoprotein kinases in the nuclei of normal
rat liver and hepatomas.

Materials and Methods

DNA polymerases were extracted from nuclear fractions of different tissues with 0.2 M sodium phosphate buffer pH 7.4 containing 2 mM
β-mercaptoethanol (14). The extract was then centrifuged at 15,000
rpm at 0°C in an International Refrigerated Centrifuge Model B-20 for
60 min. The supernatant was dialyzed against 0.01 M sodium phosphate
pH 7.4, 2mM mercaptoethanol and used for sucrose gradient studies or
for further purification.

Sucrose density gradient sedimentation patterns were obtained by
assaying the DNA polymerase activities in each fraction after sucrose
density gradient centrifugation of the enzymatic extarcts (13). The
sample was layered over a sucrose gradient from 5-20% w/v and centrifuged in a Spinco SW 39 L rotor at 37,000 rpm for 16 hours. The DNA
polymerase activities were assayed as described previously (12).

For hepatocarcinogenesis experiments, male Fischer rats (120-150
gm initial weight) were maintained on Wayne laboratory meal pellets
(Allied Mills) soaked with 10% corn oil containing either 0.06% 3'-
methyl-4-dimethylaminoazobenzene (3'-MDAB) or 0.05% α-naphtyl-isothio-
cyanate (αNIT). Each experimental point represents an average of 4

or 5 rats. All experimental points were repeated at least twice.

Morris hepatomas 7777, 7787, 7800 and 3924A were transplanted by Dr. H.P. Morris at the Biochemistry Department, Howard University, Washington, D.C. and shipped to our laboratory.

The isolation of nuclei and chromatin was described previously (33). Briefly, the livers or hepatomas of rats were homogenized in 10 vol of 0.32 M sucrose containing 3 mM $MgCl_2$, and centrifuged at 1,000 x g for 10 min. The supernatant, after recentrifugation at 105,000 x g for 1 hr, was used to determine the activity of cytoplasmic phosphokinase. The sediment was rehomogenized in 10 vol of 2.2 M sucrose containing 5 mM $MgCl_2$ and centrifuged at 100,000 x g for 1 hr. The pelleted nuclei were used either for further preparation of chromatin or for isolation of phosphoproteins and phosphoprotein kinases.

Phosphoproteins and phosphosprotein kinases were isolated by the method described by Kish and Kleinsmith (22). Isolated nuclei were homogenized in 0.14 M NaCl to remove cytoplasmic contaminants and nuclear sap. The nonhistone proteins were extracted by homogenizing the nuclear pellets in equal vol. of 2 M NaCl, 0.05 M Tris, pH 7.5. The resulting solution was mixed with 1.5 vol. of 0.02 M Tris, pH 7.5, and the precipitated nucleo-histone and nuclear debris were removed by centrifugation at 81,500 x g for 1 hr. The nuclear phosphoproteins and kinases were further purified by Bio-Rex 70 chromatography and calcium phosphate gel absorption as described by Kish and Kleinsmith (22).

The protein phosphokinase activities were asssayed (36) in a reaction mixture which contained 30 µl of 0.43 M Tris (pH 7.5), 10 µl of 0.75 M $MgCl_2$, and specified amounts of enzyme preparations. 10 µl of [γ-^{32}P] ATP (0.6 ^{um}/ml, 0.5 ^{Ci}/mM ATP) was added to each assay to start the reaction and the tubes were incubated at 30° C for 10 min. The reaction was terminated by addition of 10% trichloroacetic acid. The precipitate was collected and washed on Millipore membrane filters. The radioactivities were determined in the Packard scintillation spectrometer.

The nonhistone protein-DNA complexes (dehistonized chromatin) were obtained by dehistonization of chromatin in 2.0 M NaCl, 5.0 M urea, sodium phosphate buffer, pH 6.0. Ultracentrifugation of this mixture at 110,000 x g for 36 hr produced a pellet of DNA and nonhistone proteins leaving histones and about 20% of the nonhistone proteins in the supernatant. The dehistonized chromatins were used for immunization of rabbits according to the schedule described by Chytil and Spelsberg (18). The antisera were decomplemented by heating at 56°C for 30 min and the γ-globulin fraction of rabbit serum was obtained by ammonium sulfate precipitation and DEAE cellulose chromatography (31).

The immunospecificity of the nonhistone proteins-DNA complexes was determined by the modified microcomplement fixation method of Wasserman and Levine (40).

RESULTS

Nuclear DNA Polymerases

One of the most outstanding features of malignant cells is their capability of perpetual division, out of control by the host. Among the principal macromolecular events obligatory to growth and cellular proliferation is the replication of nuclear DNA. The loss of control of DNA synthesis is a basic element for the transformation of cells from normal to the malignant state. The elucidation of regulatory mechanisms concerning the DNA synthesis in living cells, both normal and abnormal, may be essential for the understanding and control of neoplastic growth. Therefore, studies on nuclear DNA polymerase may help to the understanding of the process of neoplasia.

It was suggested (5, 14) that a DNA polymerase which has a molecular weight of 3-4 S, is principally associated with the nucleus. A second DNA polymerase activity, 6-8 S, was detected in proliferating tissues, such as developing rat brain (15), regenerating rat liver (2, 9, 25, 27), and cancerous tissues (2, 7, 19, 27). In this work we have studied the nuclear DNA polymerases in the Morris hepatomas and in rat livers during the course of 3-MDAB hepatocarcinogenesis.

In contrast to the normal and αNIT animals, the activities of DNA polymerase in the 3'-MDAB rats began to increase in about 8 days and reached a prominent peak between 30-40 days of the exposure to this carcinogen (Fig 1). After 40 days, the DNA polymerase activities decreased gradually. The sucrose density gradient patterns of DNA polymerase activities are shown in Fig 2. As can be seen, only the 3-4S DNA polymerase activity could be detected in the control and αNIT rats, and during the early periods on the carcinogenic diet. The high molecular weight 6-8S DNA polymerase activity appeared prominently in rats exposed to 3'-MDAB diet for 24 days. It reached a peak around 40 days and then decreased rapidly, disappearing altogether after 104 days of exposure to this carcinogen.

Figure 3 compares the nuclear bound form of the DNA polymerase activity in rapidly and intermediately growing Morris hepatomas with that of normal adult rat liver. Poorly differentiated, rapidly growing Morris hepatomas 7777 and 3924A contained highly active 6-8S nuclear DNA polymerase enzyme. On the other hand, well differentiated, hepato-cellular carcinomas with an intermediate growth rate contained only low DNA polymerase activity in the 6-8S DNA polymerase regions.

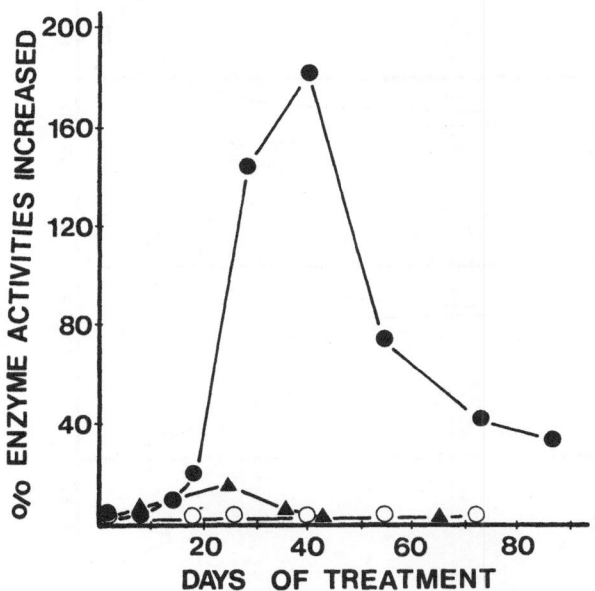

Figure 1
DNA polymerase activities of rat liver during hepato-carcinogenesis. ● = rats fed with diet containing 3'-MDAB; ▲ = rats fed
with diet containing NIT; O =rats fed with control diet.

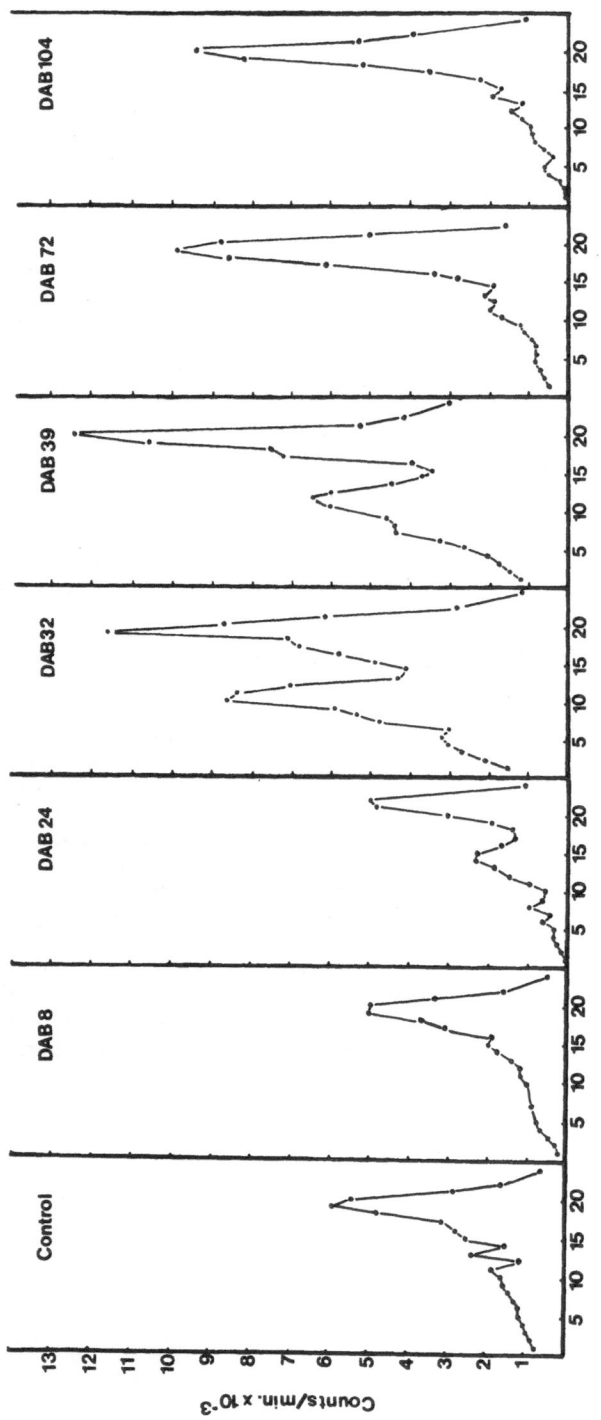

Figure 2

Sucrose density gradeint centrifugation of DNA polymerases in control and 3'-MDAB treated rat livers. The bottom of the gradient is to the left. DAB-8 (etc): Days on 3'-MDAB diet.

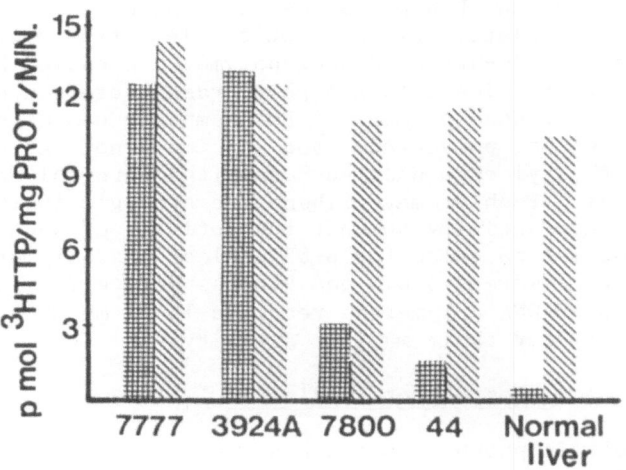

Figure 3
The activities of nuclear DNA polymerase in Morris hepatoma
7777, 3924A, 7800 and 44. (▦▦▦): 6-8S nuclear DNA ploymerase;
(/////////): DNA ploymerase β.

Because of the many similarities between the biochemical and metabolic properties of embryonic and neoplastic cells, the distribution of 6-8S nuclear DNA polymerase in developing rat livers was also investigated. As can be seen in Fig 4, only the low molecular weight DNA polymerase is present in the adult and one month old rat liver nuclei, while both the low and high molecular weight DNA polymerase activities are present in fetal and neonatal rat livers.

The 6-8S and 3-4S nuclear DNA polymerases were further purified by ammonium sulfate fractionation and DEAE-cellulose column chromatography (7). Their characteristics were also studied. The 3-4S DNA polymerase exhibited a high preference for native DNA; very little incorporation occurred with heated DNA as template. On the other hand, 6-8S nuclear DNA polymerase used both native and heat-denatured DNA as template. By addition complementary oligoribonucleotides, the single-stranded deoxypolymer was copied by 6-8S nuclear DNA polymerase. The 3-4S DNA polymerase preferred deoxyribose template with deoxyribose primer. A DNA template was essential for the activity of either polymerase, and RNA could not satisfy this requirement. Sulfhydryl compounds such as dithiothreitol enhanced both enzyme activities. P-chloromercuribenzoate strongly inhibited the 6-8S DNA polymerase activity but not the activity of 3-4S DNA polymerase. The optimal pH value for 6-8S nuclear DNA polymerase and 3-4S DNA polymerase were 7.5-8.0 and 9.0 respectively. The 6-8S DNA polymerase and 3-4S DNA polymerase required 15-25 mM $MgCl_2$ and 10 mM $MgCl_2$ respectively for their maximal activity.

Phosphoproteins and phosphoprotein kinases

Our interest in phosphoprotein kinases and nuclear phosphoproteins was stimulated by evidence suggesting that the phosphorylation and dephosphorylation of ceratin nuclear proteins may play a key role in the specific regualtion of gene activities in eukaryotes (23, 24). These phosphorylated nuclear nonhistone proteins are heterogenous and tissue specific (29, 35), bind specifically to homologous DNA (32, 25), and can stimulate the transcription of specific genes (24, 37).

The activities of phosphoprotein kinase enzymes which are responsible for the phosphorylation of nuclear proteins dramatically increased in the rat liver cytoplasm and chromatin after the administration of an azo dye carcinogen as shown in Fig 5. The increases of phosphoprotein kinase activities were accompanied by a similar increase in the capacity of chromatin to template for RNA synthesis (110% increase at 36-days of treatment).

To determine which proteins are phosphorylated by the increased phosphoprotein kinase activities, ^{32}P incorporation into electrophoretically separated chromatin proteins (histones and nonhistone proteins) was compared. The exposure of rats to the carcinogenic diet

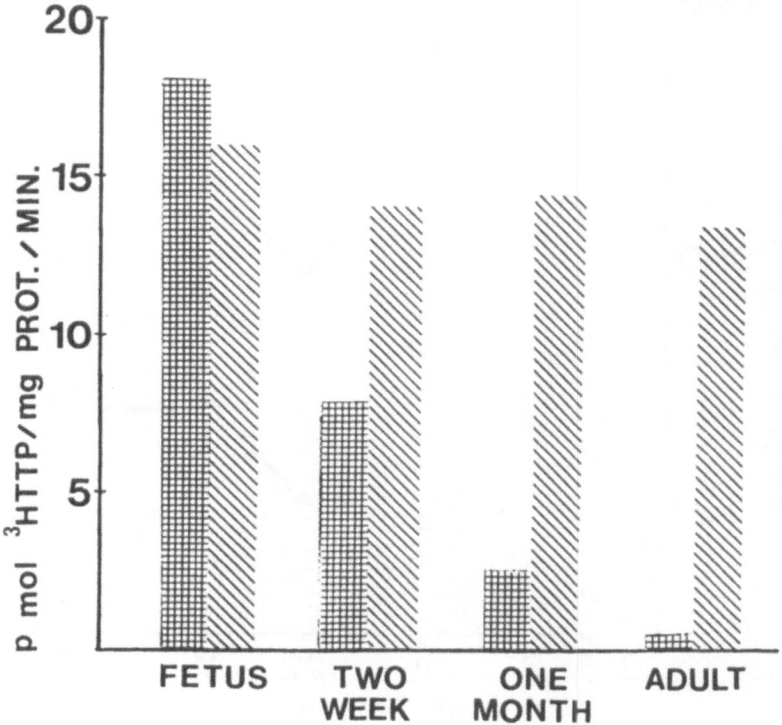

Figure 4
The activities of nuclear DNA polymerase in developing rat liver.
(//////): 6-8S nuclear DNA polymerase; (///////): DNA polymerase β.

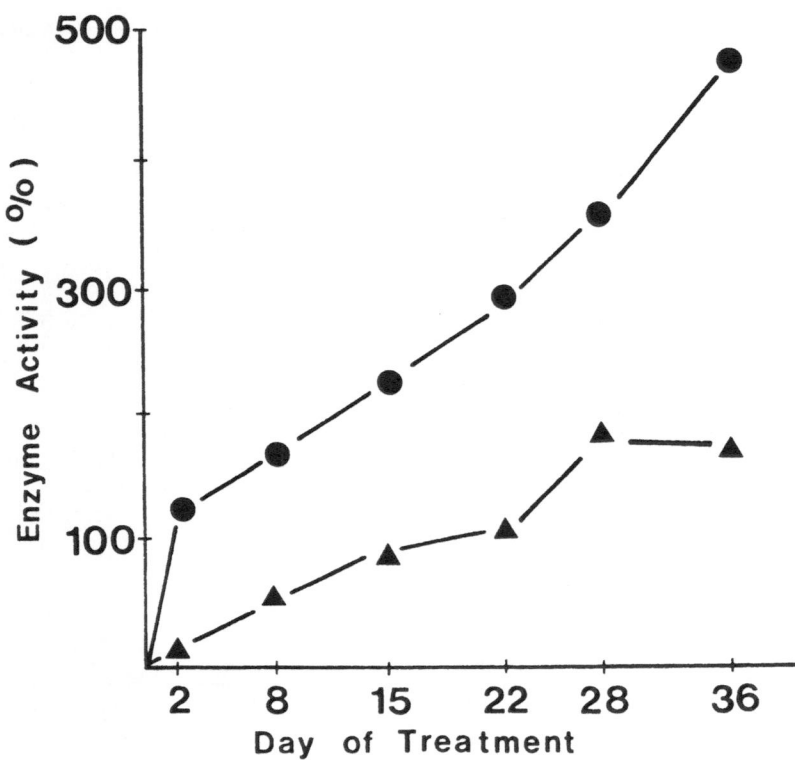

Figure 5
The phosphoprotein kinase activities in control and 3'-MDAB fed rat
livers.   0 = cytoplasmic phosphoprotein kinases; Δ = chromatin bound
phophoprotein kinases.

for 28 days produced a selective change in the phosphorylation
pattern of chromosomal proteins in liver.

Histones, although present in large quantities (Fig 6) were,
with the exception of the H1 fraction, only marginally phosphorylated. Indeed, all the histone phosphorylation accounted for less than
10% of the ^{32}P incorporated into chromatin proteins. The phosphorylation of H1 histone can be correlated with cell proliferation.
It is of interest that only few nonhistone protein bands exhibited
increased phosphorylation during the first 28 days of 3'-MDAB diet.

Phosphoproteins and their kinase activities were also studied
in spontaneous human hepatoma. Phosphoprotein kinases were isolated
from hepatoma nuclei by the method of Kish and Kleinsmith (22). As
shown in Fig 7, nuclear phosphoprotein kinases in human hepatoma were
at least four times more active than those of non tumor liver (adjacent to the hepatoma).

Optimal conditions for phosphoprotein kinase activity were
further characterized by studying the effects of varying the Mg^{2+}
or Mn^{2+} concentration and the pH of the incubation medium. A dual
optimal pH (7.6 and 8.4) was found both in hepatoma and normal liver.
The optimal concentration of Mg^{++} was 30 mM. The amount of radioactivity incorporated in the presence of Mn^{++} was compared to the
amount of radioactivity incorporated in the presence of Mg^{2+}. Mn^{2+}
ion could not replace Mg^{2+}ion for maximal activity of phosphoprotein
kinase. However, the phosphoprotein kinases isolated from hepatoma
were stimulated much more than those from non tumor liver when assayed in the presence of Mn^{2+} as compared with the presence of Mg^{2+} ions.
These results are consistent with the reports of Thomson et al. (36)
and Kang et al. (20) who showed that a tumor-specific phosphoprotein
kinase fraction is activated by Mn^{2+} and that specific substrates can
be found in neoplasms. Such substrate specificity of the Mn^{2+} responsive nuclear protein phosphokinase(s) is confirmed in Fig 8. In this
experiment, the phosphorylation of endogenous non histone proteins by
kinases in the presence of Mn^{2+} was analyzed by polyacrylamide gel
electrophoresis. The non tumor liver proteins were not phosphorylated
as much as the hepatoma proteins. Further, the profiles show the
phosphorylation of one major protein band (approximate molecular
eight 70,000). This suggests the presence of specific nuclear protein
phosphokinase(s) and their substrate(s) in human hepatoma and other
malignant neoplasms (20, 36).

Immunospecificities of Nuclear Antigens

Cancerous growth can be regarded as an error in maintenance of
normal differentiated state brought about by specific modifications
of cellular genetic information and its phenotypic expression. A key
factor in the cellular differentiation is the composition and function-

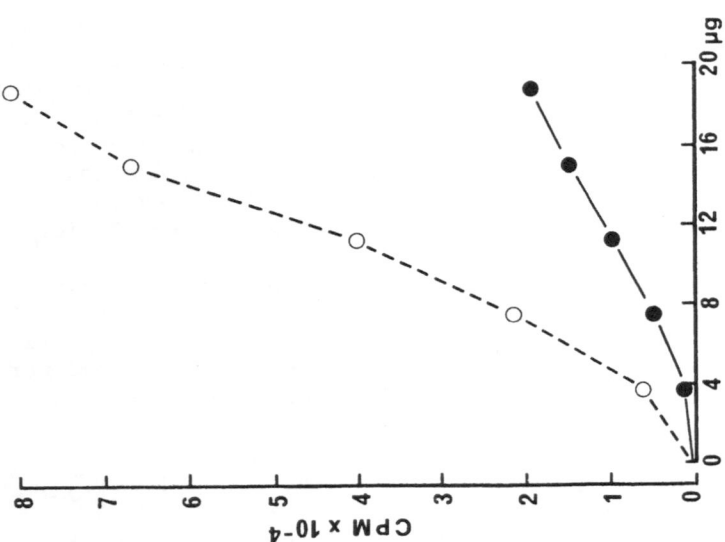

Figure 7
Incorporation of label from γ32P-ATP into phosphoprotein, as a function of protein concentration, in a case of human hepato-carcinoma. 0———0 non tumor liver; 0————0 hepatoma.

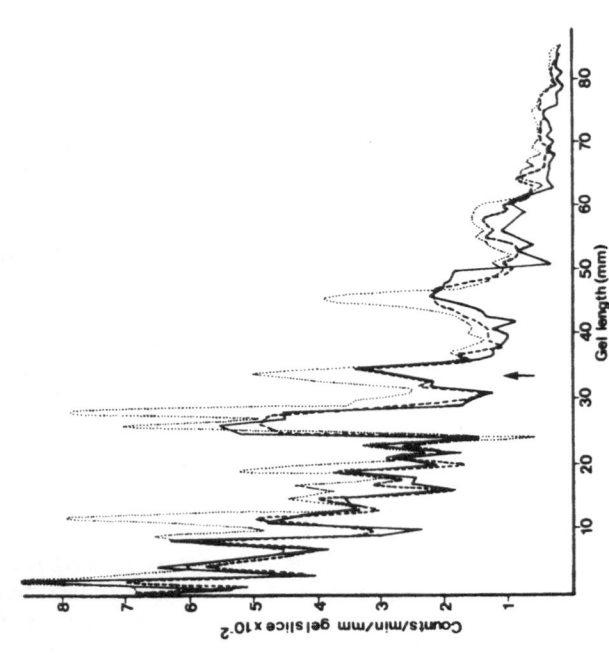

Figure 6
Radioactivity (32P) distribution of liver chromatin proteins on polyacrilamide gels. •••••: control rats; ————: Rats on 3'-MDAB diet for 15 days; ———: Rats on 3'-MDAB diet for 28 days.

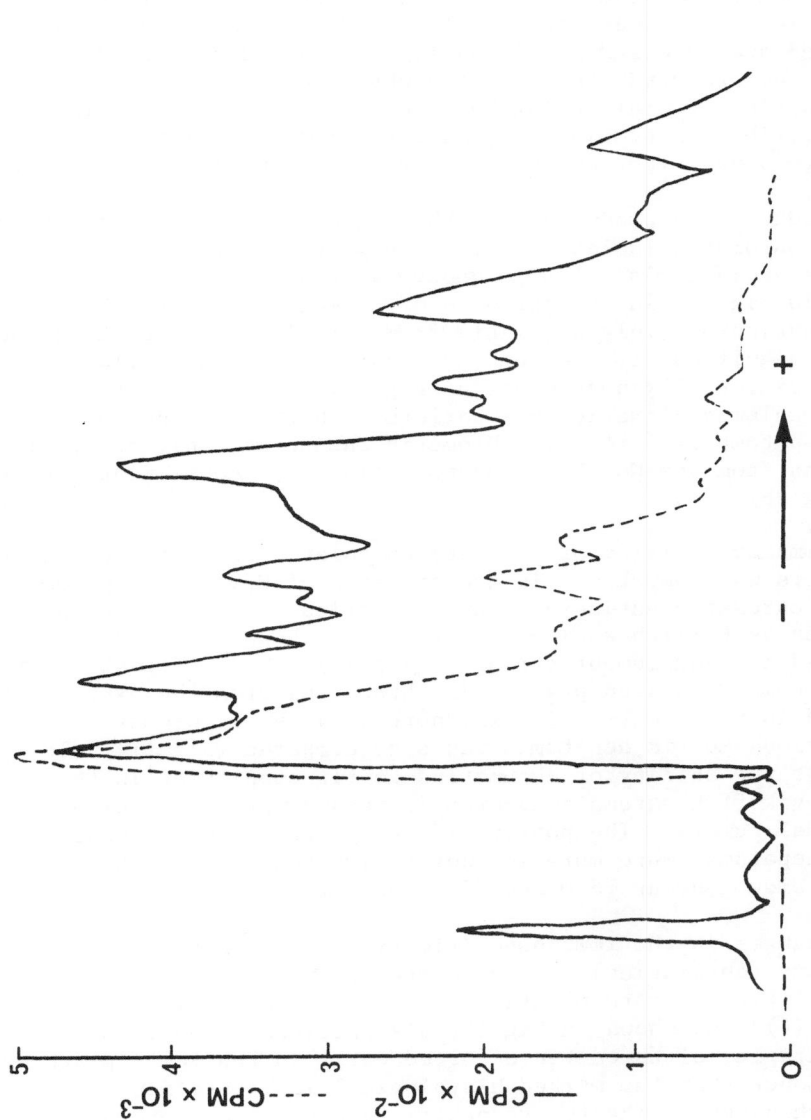

Figure 8

Phosphorylation pattern of nonhistone proteins (kinase activation by Mn^{++}), in a case of human hepatocarcinoma, 0——0 non tumor liver; ---- hepatoma.

al status of its genetic material, most of which is located in the
nucleus in the form of chromosomes. Several investigators (18, 32,
42) have shown that tissue-specific antibodies can be elicited in
rabbits by injecting them with complexes of chromosomal non histone
proteins and homologous DNA. Immunological methods can be used as
a powerful tool to study the specific change of composition or structure of genetic material during hepatocarcinogenesis. In this section we describe how neoplasia changes the immunospecificity of
chromatin to a new type, common to many experimental malignancies.

Antibodies were produced in rabbits against preparations of dehistonized chromatin isolated from either normal rat liver or rat
Novikoff hepatoma cells. The immunospecificities of these antibodies
are shown in Fig 9. In the presence of normal rat liver dehistonized
chromatin antiserum, only chromatin from normal rat liver fixed the
complement significantly. Chromatin preparations from Novikoff hepatoma were essentially non-reactive (Fig 9a). On the other hand,
when the complement fixation was performed in the presence of
Novikoff hepatoma dehistonized chromatin antiserum, only chromatin
preparations from the Novikoff hepatoma fixed the complement extensively (Fig 9b).

The immunoreactivity of chromatins isolated from various experimental tumors was compared. In the presence of Novikoff hepatoma dehistonized chromatin antiserum, the chromatins prepared from various
tumors, such as Ehrlich ascites tumor, Morris hepatomas and Walker
tumor, fixed the complement strongly (Fig 10). This suggests that
there is a common antigen present in chromatins from the experimental
tumors used in the assays. The immunoreactivity of chromatins isolated from various Morris hepatomas was also compared (Fig 11). It
appears that the ability of chromatins to fix complement in the presence of Novikoff hepatoma antiserum increased with the growth rates
of individual tumors. The poorly differentiated, fast growing 7777
and 3924A hepatomas were more immunoreactive than the better differentiated and slow growing 7800 and 7787 tumors.

The changes in the immunospecificity of the non histone protein
DNA complexes (chromatins) during hepatocarcinogenesis were studied
in livers of Fischer rats maintained on a diet containing 3'-MDAB
carcinogen (4). As shown in Fig 12, a significant change in the
immunospecificity of chromatin occurred early in the feeding schedule.
This was sooner than the marked histological manifestation of the
cancerous phenotype. The tumor-specific non histone proteins-DNA
complexes did not appear in liver chromatin of rats fed with γNIT
as determined by immunoassay (Fig 12).

According to our previous findings, the immunospecificity of
chromatins depends on their specific non histone proteins association
with homologous DNA (38, 39). Non histone proteins separated from

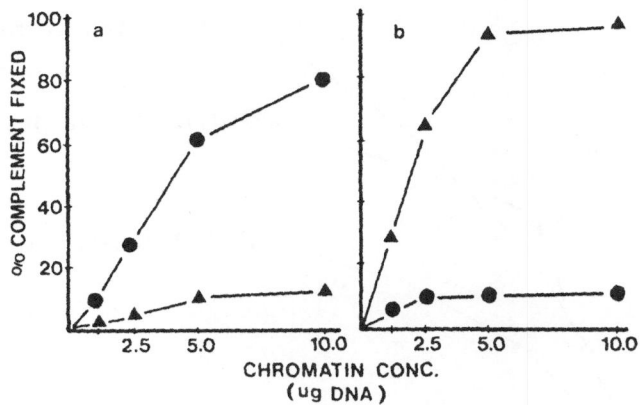

Figure 9
The immunospecificity of chromatin. A complement fixation
assay was performed in the presence of antisera against dehistonized
chromatin from rat liver (a) or Novikoff hepatoma (b) all assays were
corrected for anticomplementarity. ● = Normal rat liver chromatin;
▲ = Novikoff hepatoma chromatin.

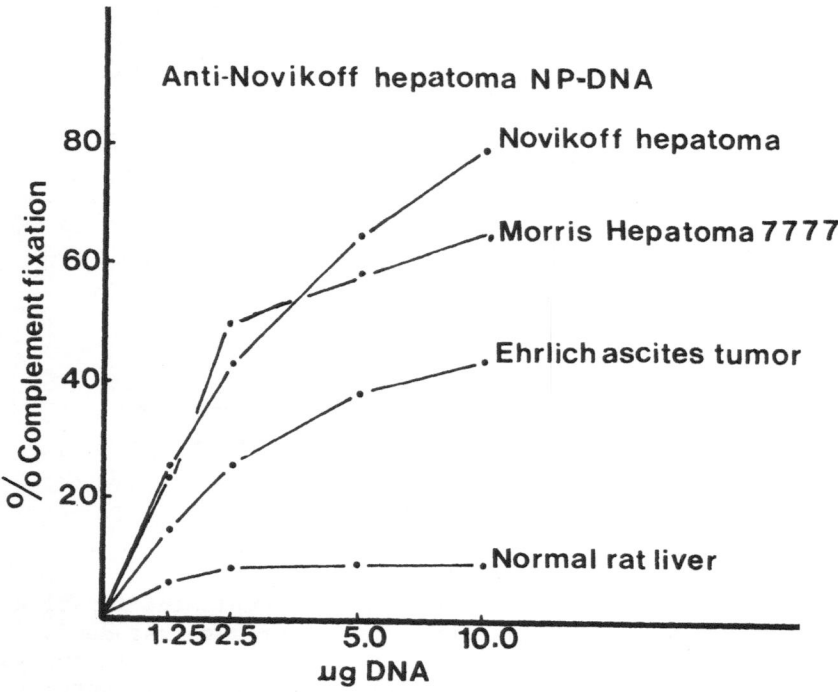

Figure 10
Complement fixation of chromatins isolated from various experimental
tumors in the presence of antiserum against Novikoff hepatoma dehistonized chromatin. All experimental points were corrected for anticomplementarity.

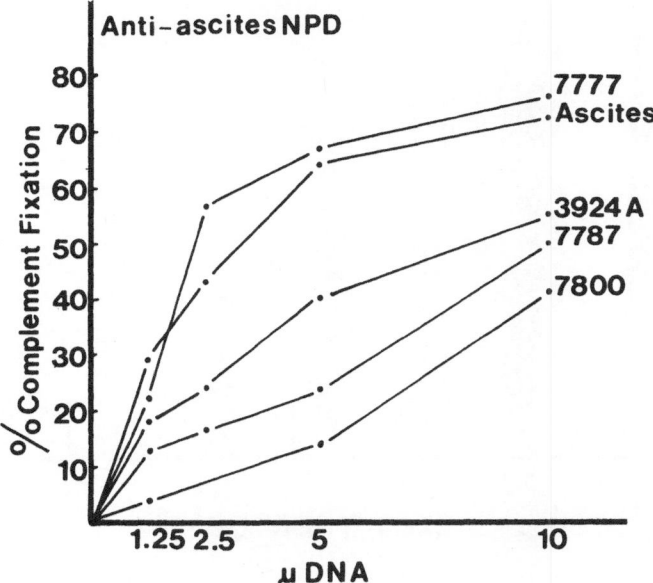

Figure 11
Complement fixation of chromatins isolated from Novikoff hepatoma and various Morris hepatomas in the presence of antiserum against Novikoff hepatoma dehistonized chromatin. All experimental points were corrected for anticomplementarity.

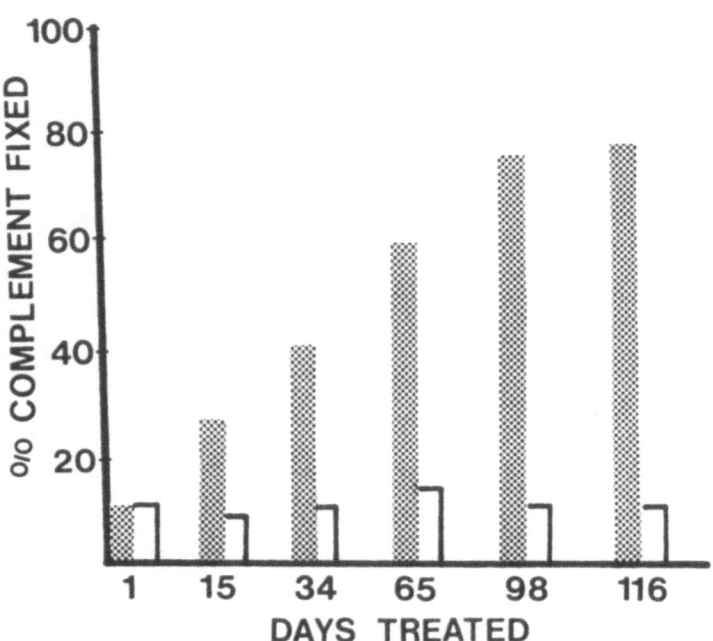

Figure 12
Time course of increasing complement fixation of chromatins
isolated from liver of rats maintained on 3'-MDAB containing diet.
The complement fixation assay was performed in the presence of antisera against Novikoff hepatoma dehistonized chromatin. ▨▨▨▨ : Rats
maintained on 3'-MDAB,   ▭▭▭ : Rats maintained on γNIT.

their DNA were antigenic but the antibodies were not tissue speficic
(39). Using the fractionation schedule for chromatin proteins as
described in previous paper (10), a small fraction of immunospecific
non histone proteins could be isolated. The immunochemical tissue
specificity can be transferred by reconstituting immunospecific non
histone proteins from one tissue to the DNA from another tissue of
the same species (8). It is noteworthy that this fraction of non
histone proteins also contains proteins which selectively associate
with homologous DNA (10, 39). These complexes are immunologically
tissue-specific and change qualitatively during differentiation
(8, 17).

DISCUSSION

Experiments presented here show that nuclear macromolecules
change significanly during carcinogenesis. The administration of
a carcinogen, 3'-MDAB to Fischer rats changed the immunological
specificity of chromatin from the type characteristic of normal
tissue (liver) to a new type, common to several experimental tumors.
The immunospecificity of chromatin depends on the complexes of immunospecific non histone proteins with homologous DNA which interact in
a highly specific manner. This interaction specificity changes with
cellular differentiation (8, 17), chemical (10) or viral (42) carcinogenesis and phase of the cell cycle (our unpublished data). It
appears that alterations in the composition and perhaps the structure
of nuclear non histone proteins are closely associated with the process of cytodifferentiation and carcinogenesis. Recently we (11)
have shown that tissue specific antisera will inhibit the in vitro
transcription of chromatin. This phenomenon is tissue specific in
that individual chromatins will be inhibited only by their homologous
antisera. This points to the possible presence of gene regulatory
proteins in the imminospecific protein fraction. We have also employed the chicken reticulocyte chromatin system to analyze the
effects of chromosomal proteins on the in vitro transcription of
globin genes. The immunospecific protein fraction was found to be
essential for the in vitro transcription of globin mRNA by chromatins
reconstituted from DNA and isolated chromosomal protein components
(16). All these results indicate that modifications of gene regulation occur in cancerous tissues.

The evidence of abnormal gene expression in neoplastic disease
also provided by studies on phosphoprotein and their kinases in neoplastic tissues. As described in this communication, we have found
that the phosphoprotein kinase activities were several times higher
in hepatomas than in the normal liver. Selective difference in the
phosphorylation pattern of chromosomal proteins were observed between
the normal liver and experimental hepatomas. Apparently the phosphoproteins in the nucleus play an important role in the regulation of
gene expression (23, 24, 29, 32, 24, 25, 27). Evidence from many

laboratories supports the view that the specific array of nuclear
non histone proteins in chromatin determines the overall potential
of gene expression at any given steady state of differentiation of
a particular cell. The degree of protein phosphorylation may determine to what extent specific genetic loci are transcribed at any
given time in response to specific stimuli (23, 34). Evidence has
been recently presented by Thomson et al. (37) that phosphoproteins
activate the transcription of histone specific gene. Our data
(Figs 6, 7 and 8) are in accord with this report. The observed
functional modification of chromatin accompanied by changes in the
phosphorylation of its proteins and by the increased activity of the
phosphokinase enzymes may represent one of the early steps neccessary
for the establishment of neoplastic phenotype.

Neoplastic transformation results in unbalanced DNA biosynthesis.
A 6-8S nuclear DNA polymerase which is not presented in adult normal
tissue, appears in the liver during carcinogenesis. This 6-8S nuclear DNA polymerase increases in hepatomas and regenerating rat
liver. Indeed, the activity of 6-8S nuclear DNA polymerase in nuclei parallels the rate of DNA synthesis throughout liver regeneration and hepatocarcinogenesis (7). It seems likely that the 6-8S
nuclear DNA polymerase functions as a replicative enzyme. Recently,
the evidence for direct participation of RNA synthesis in DNA replication has been reported (26). According to Chang and Bollum, oligoribonucleotides are effective initiators of DNA synthesis catalyzed
by DNA polymeraseα (6) and Keller (21) reported that DNA synthesis
by KB cell polymerases is stimulated by the coupled reaction with RNA
polymerase (21). These results indicate that DNA synthesis in vitro
can be initiated by RNA primer. The 6-8S nuclear DNA polymerase described in this paper can use oligoribonucleotides as primer. This
observation lends additional support for a role for the 6-8S nuclear
DNA polymerase in the replication of nuclear DNA. Further correlation of the activity of this enzyme with DNA replication in normal
and malignant tissues is under investigation.

REFERENCES

1. Balhorn, R., Chalkley, R. and Granner, D. Biochemistry 11 (1972)
    1094.

2. Baril, E.F., Jenkins, M.D., Brown, O.E., Laszlo, J. and Morris,
    H.P. Cancer Res. 33 (1973) 1187.

3. Bruni, C. and Rust, J.H. J. Natl. Cancer Inst. 54 (1975) 687.

4. Capizzo, F. and Roberts, R.J. Toxicol. Appl. Pharmacol. 19
    (1971) 176.

5. Chang, L.S. and Bollum, F.J. Biochemistry 11 (1972) 1264.

6. Chang, L.M.S. and Bollum, F.J. Biochem. Biophys. Res. Comm.
    46 (1972) 1354.

7. Chiu, J.F., Craddock, C., Morris, H.P. and Hnilica, L.S.
    Cancer Biochem. Biophys. 1 (1974) 13.

8. Chiu, J.F., Craddock, C., Morris, H.P. and Hnilica, L.S. FEBS
    Lett. 42 (1974) 94.

9. Chiu, J.F. and Hnilica, L.S. FEBS Lett. 36 (1973) 235.

10. Chiu, J.F., Hunt, M. and Hnilica, L.S. Cancer Res. 35 (1975) 913.

11. Chiu, J.F., Chytil, F. and Hnilica, L.S. In: Onco-Developmental
    Gene Expression W.H. Fishman and S. Sell (eds). Academic Press,
    New York (1976) p. 271.

12. Chiu, J.F. and Sung, S.C. Biochim. Biophys. Acta 269 (1972) 364.

13. Chiu, J.F. and Sung, S.C. Biochim. Biophys. Acta 209 (1970) 34.

14. Chiu, J.F. and Sung, S.C. Biochem. Biophys. Res. Comm. 46 (1972)
    1830.

15. Chiu, J.F. and Sung, S.C. J. Neurochem. 20 (1973) 617.

16. Chiu, J.F., Tsai, Y.H., Sakuma, K. and Hnilica, L.S. J. Biol.
    Chem. 250 (1975) 9431.

17. Chytil, F., Glasser, S.R. and Spelsberg, T.C. Developmental
    Biol. 37 (1974) 295.

18. Chytil, F. and Spelsberg, T.C. Nature New Biol. 233 (1971) 215.

19. DePhilip, R.M., Lynch, W.E. and Lieberman, I. Cancer Res. 37 (1977) 702.

20. Kang, Y.J., Olson, M.O.J. and Busch, H. J. Biol. Chem. 249 (1974) 5580.

21. Keller, W. Proc. Natl. Acad. Sci. U.S.A. 69 (1972) 1560.

22. Kish, V.M. and Kleinsmith, L.J. J. Biol. Chem. 249 (1974) 250.

23. Kleinsmith, L.J. J. Cell Physiol. 85 (1975) 459.

24. Kleinsmith, L.J., Stein, J.S., and Stein, G.S. Proc. Natl. Acad. Sci. U.S.A. 73 (1976) 1174.

25. Lynch, W.E., Short, J. and Lieberman, I. Cancer Res. 36 (1976) 901.

26. Okazaki, R., Suzino, A., Hirose, S., Okazaki, T., Imae, Y., Karinumakuroda, R., Ogawa, T., Arisawa, M. and Kurusawa, Y. In: DNA Synthesis In Vitro, R.D. Wells, and R.B. Inman (eds). University Park Press, Baltimore (1973) p. 83.

27. Ove, P., Coetzee, M.L. and Morris, H.P. Cancer Res. 29 (1973) 1557.

28. Pierce, G.B. and Wallace, C. Cancer Res. 31 (1971) 127.

29. Platz, R.D., Kish, V.M. and Kleinsmith, L.J. FEBS Lett. 12 (1970) 38.

30. Potter, R. V. Cancer Res. 28 (1968) 1901.

31. Rapp, H.J. In: Immunochemical Methods, J.F. Ackbayed (ed). F.A. Davis Co., Philadelphia, Penn. (1964).

32. Shea, M. and Kleinsmith, L.J. Biochem. Biophys. Res. Comm. 50 (1973) 473.

33. Spelsberg, T.C. and Hnilica, L.S. Biochim. Biophys. Acta 228 (1971) 202.

34. Stein, G.S., Spelsberg, T.C. and Kleinsmith, L.J. Science 183 (1974) 817.

35. Teng, C.S., Teng, C.T. and Allfrey, V.G. J. Biol. Chem. 246 (1971) 3597.

36. Thomson, J.A., Chiu, J.F. and Hnilica, L.S. Biochim. Biophys.

Acta 407 (1975) 114.

37. Thomson, J.A., Stein, J.L., Kleinsmith, L.J. and Stein, G.S. Science 194 (1976) 428.

38. Wakabayashi, K. and Hnilica, L.S. Nature New Biol. 242 (1973) 153.

39. Wakabayashi, K., Wang, S. and Hnilica, L.S. Biochemistry 13 (1972) 1027.

40. Wasserman, E. and Levine, L. J. Immuno. 87 (1961) 290.

41. Weiler, E., In: Carcinogenesis Ciba Foundation Symposium,"Loss of Specific Antigens in Relation to Carcinogenesis", Little, Brown and Co., Boston (1959).

42. Zardi, L., Lin, J.C. and Baserga, R. Nature New Biol. 245 (1973) 211.

ENZYMATIC MODIFICATION OF NUCLEAR PROTEINS DURING NEOPLASTIC GROWTH

Woon Ki Paik, Samuel Nochumson and Sangduk Kim

Fels Research Institute
Department of Biochemistry
Temple University School of Medicine
Philadelphia, Pa. 19140

SUMMARY

Post-synthetic modifications of nuclear proteins, especially histones, are frequently investigated enigmatic reactions. The biological significance of these particular modification reactions is not thoroughly understood. The relatively high degree of evolutionary stability of the histone's primary structure and to a large extent its modification sites suggests that proper chromatin organization depends a great deal on precise post-synthetic modification reactions. This idea is substantiated by a number of reports indicating that these reactions occur predominantly around the time that cells, in preparation for division, are replicating their chromosomes and processing newly synthesized histones.

A description of histone modification sites and the enzymes that catalyze these reactions are discussed. In addition, the relationship of these modification reactions to the cell cycle is presented.

INTRODUCTION

Post-translational modification of protein amino acid residues is a well known metabolic phenomenon. These modification reactions include methylation, acetylation, phosphorylation, thiolation, hydroxylation, ADP-ribosylation, adenylation, carboxylation and glycosylation of numerous classes of proteins. One such class of proteins is the nuclear proteins which includes histones, "acidic" proteins and non-histone chromosomal proteins. These proteins are found complexed with DNA and RNA to form the chromatin within the nucleus.

205

Modification of chromosomal proteins has been strongly implicated
as a means for gene activation in the cases of phosphorylation and
acetylation; however, methylation is believed to play more of a
structural role in the formation of chromatin.

Histones have been studied extensively since their discovery
in 1884 (1). These basic proteins are grouped into distinct classes in higher animals and some plants. These include the (a) lysine-
rich: H1, (b) slightly lysine-rich: H2A and H2B, (c) arginine-rich:
H3 and H4, and (d) a last class which is unique to nucleated erythrocytes, the lysine-rich H5*. Histones are synthesized in the
cytoplasm and are generally found in the nuclei associated with the
chromatin of most eukaryotes (2). A remarkable feature of histones
is the fact that throughout evolution there has remained a high
degree of conservation of the primary amino acid sequence, especially in histone H4, which is the most evolutionarily conserved protein
known today. Thus, there are very similar but not identical chemical
and physical properties among each histone class isolated from different species and tissues. It is this quality which makes it difficult to reconcile with the hypothesis that histones play a major
role in gene expression and are consequently responsible for phenotypic differences between cells. However, histones undergo a number
of post-translational modifications which could conceivably play a
major role in cellular differentiation.

Neither the "acidic" proteins nor the non-histone chromosomal
proteins are as clearly defined or characterized as the histones,
although considerable progress has been made in recent years towards
resolution of this problem. The non-histone chromosomal proteins
have been described as "those proteins (excluding the histones) that
isolate together with DNA in purified chromatin or chromosome" (3).
Therefore this class of proteins by definition is clearly distinguishable from other non-histone nuclear proteins, which have been
derived from whole nuclei (4). There appears to be a greater diversity among the non-histone chromosomal proteins which has attracted much attention towards a regulatory function in the chromatin as
well as structural and enzymic roles (3). Like histones, non-histone
chromosomal proteins are also modified post-translationally with
phosphorylation being the most prevalent modification reaction, resulting in a subclass of phosphoproteins (5). Methylation has also
been reported and, in particular, the modification of arginine residues by protein methylase I [S-Adenosylmethionine:protein-arginine
methyltransferase; EC 2.1.1.23] may be highly significant for the
functioning of some of the non-histone nuclear proteins (6-8). Thus,
it is the purpose of this article to provide some insight into the

---

* Histone nomenclature is that adopted by the Ciba Foundation
Symposium 28 (see reference 16).

nature of the post-synthetic modifications of nuclear proteins and to suggest the consequences that may result from these reactions.

SITES OF PROTEIN MODIFICATION

Histone Methylation

The first identification of ε-N-methyllysine in histones was reported by Murray in 1964 (9). Since then, two other ε-N-methyl-lysine derivatives have been found in histones: ε-N-Dimethyllysine by Paik and Kim (10), and ε-N-trimethyllsine by Hempel et al. (11). It has subsequently been established that these methylated amino acids occur mainly in the arginine-rich histones H3 and H4. Sequence studies have revealed that H3 histone contains a mixture of ε-N-monomethyl, ε-N-dimethyl, and ε-N-trimethyllysine at positions 9 and 27 (12, 13). It has recently been found that a minor site at lysine residue 4 in H3 histone is also methylated in developing trout testis (14). Histone H4 from animals also contains either ε-N-monomethyl or ε-N-dimethyl-lysine, however, this occurs only at position 20 (15-18). The fact that histone H4 from plants does not contain any methylated lysine residues has led to speculation that there is a specific enzyme responsible for its methylation. Although methylated arginine residues have been found in histones using radioactive S-adenosyl-L-[methyl-^{14}C] methionine as a methyl donor, the exact locations of these compounds have not been identi-fied (19).

Histone fractions, from Chinese hamster ovary (CHO) cells grown in the presence of [methyl-^{14}C]methionine, were found to have a measurable portion of the radioactivity incorporated into a labile form which became volatile following either acid or alkali hydrolysis (20). The volatile component was identified as methanol and is most likely derived from the formation of carboxyl-methyl ester of either aspartyl or glutamyl residues or possibly from the free carboxyl-terminal end of the histone molecules. Protein carboxyl-methyl esters are notoriously unstable (21) and have been difficult to isolate and identify in vivo. Recently the γ-carboxyl-methyl ester of glutamic acid has been shown to be present in a bacterial protein (22, 23).

The presence of 3-methylhistidine in histone H1 and H5 from duck erythroid cells has also been reported (24). However, the exact position of this modified histidyl residue has not been determined.

Histone Phosphorylation

The primary acceptor of phosphate groups among the histone fractions is the very lysine-rich histone H1, although all of the other histone fractions have also been reported to accept phosphate groups (2, 25-29). Serine residues have been shown to be the major acceptors of phosphate groups, involving an ester linkage (25, 29). Unlike the consistency of the metabolically stable ε-N lysine methylation sites, there is a wide variation in the pattern of phosphorylation which is dependent on whether or not the cell is in a dividing or nondividing situation (18, 30).

Potential histone H1 phosphorylation sites which have been identified include serine 38, 106, 157, 172 and 196 (18). All others have one identifiable site: H2A - serine 1, H2B - serine 6, H3 - serine 10, H4 - serine 1, and a lysine-rich histone found in trout testis H6 at serine 5. It has been observed that histones H2A, H2B, H3, H4 and H5 phosphorylation occurs at the N-terminal region which contains a cluster of basic residues (18). Thus, the introduction of a negative phosphate group in this region would tend to reduce the basicity of the molecule. In histone H1, the phosphate groups are at the C-terminal region which contains a predominant basic region and this would also produce a neutralizing effect, tending to lessen the interaction between histone H1 and DNA.

Histone Acetylation

Histones were first reported to be acetylated at the amino terminal in 1963 by Phillips (31). He demonstrated that histones H1, H2A and H4 had their N-terminal serine residues acetylated. Therefore, the N-terminal serine of histone H2A and H4 appear to be rather unique in that these residues are subjected to two different post-translational modification reactions, namely, phosphorylation and acetylation. The N-terminal acetyl groups are apparently metabolically stable (32), while the acetylation of interior ε-amino groups of lysine residues are metabolically unstable (33, 34). It has been shown by numerous investigators that the arginine-rich histones H3 and H4 are the best acceptors of labile acetyl groups; H3 contains at least three ε-N-acetyllysine residues and H4 has at least two labile acetyl sites (2).

Calf thymus arginine-rich histones, H4, was found to be partially acetylated at lysyl residue 16 (35), whereas the same histone from pea seedlings was found to be acetylated at lysyl residues 5 and 16 (36). Two out of 14 possible lysyl residues of calf thymus histones (H3) have been found to be acetylated (37). In trout testis during spermatogenesis, at least four lysyl residues of histone H4 are modified by acetylation at lysyl residues 5, 8, 12 and 16 (38). In addition, trout testis histones H2A and H4 are identical in the first six N-terminal amino acids in which lysine residue 5 is acetylated. This may indicate that both molecules are acetylated by the same enzyme. Lysine residue 5 in histone H2B is also acetylated and is followed by a phosphorylated serine residue.

Having so many variations in modifications raises the question of whether or not modification reactions are arranged in some sort of hierarchy in which one reaction must occur before an enzyme catalyzing another type of reaction on the same protein can function. More work on the substrate specificity of protein-modifying enzymes is required to determine the effects which different protein modification reactions that occur on the same protein may have on each other. In any case, the precise data on acetylation sites in histones is probably not complete largely due to the metabolic lability of these groups.

Modifications of Non-Histone Nuclear Proteins

Identifications of the modification sites in non-histone nuclear proteins have not progressed nearly as much as for the histones. At this time, it is apparent that these proteins undergo the same types of modification reactions as to the histones (3). In particular, modification of non-histone nuclear proteins by methylation of arginine residues seems to be most significant as opposed to lysine methylation is histones (6-8). A nuclear protein complexed with HnRNA which was isolated from the lower eukaryote Physarium polycephalum has been shown to contain a substantial amount of N^G, N^G-dimethylarginine (7). The significance of this modified residue is not known but its presence in both higher and lower organisms indicates an important functional role in the HnRNP protein. This observation has been confirmed by Boffa et al. (8) who reported that histone chromosomal proteins isolated from rat liver while N^G-monomethylarginine is present in trace amounts. Also, the proteins associated with rapidly labeled HnRNA contain over half of the N^G, N^G-dimethylarginine found in the cell nucleus.

ENZYMOLOGY OF THE PROTEIN MODIFICATION REACTION

Protein Methyltransferase

Three enzymes have been characterized, each responsible for methylating a specific protein amino acid residue. The methylation of the guanidino portion of arginyl residues is catalyzed by protein methylase I [S-Adenosylmethionine:protein-arginine-methyltransferase; EC 2.1.1.23], protein methylase II [S-Adenosylmethionine:protein-carboxyl methyltransferase; EC 2.1.1.24] catalyzes the formation of carboxyl-methyl esters of glutamyl and aspartyl residues and the methylation of the ε-amino group of lysyl residues is catalyzed by protein methylase III [S-Adenosylmethionine:protein-lysine methyltransferase; EC 2.1.1.43]. Protein methylase I has bee purified approximately 120-fold from calf brain (39).

It is mainly a cytosolic enzyme, which has

been shown to catalyze the formation of N^G-monomethylarginine, N^G, N^G-dimethylarginine and N^G,N'^G-dimethylarginine. The enzyme favors histones as its protein substrate and appears to be different from another protein methylase I which is responsible for methylating a myelin basic protein (AI protein) at arginine residue 107 (40). Whether or not histones are the in vivo substrate remains to be demonstrated, however, in view of the fact that non-histone nuclear proteins contain a large amount of N^G,N^G-dimethylarginine (6-8), it would be worthwhile to try these proteins as substrates. At any rate, the location of this enzyme primarily in the cytosol would suggest that methylation of some nuclear proteins might occur outside the nucleus.

Protein methylase II has been purified to apparent homogeneity from calf thymus. It is a soluble enzyme found mainly in the cytosol of various tissues (41). Since its endogenous substrate has yet to be identified, the role it plays in modification of carboxyl residues of nuclear proteins is entirely speculative and will not be discussed.

Protein methylase III's have been found to be associated with chromatin in isolated nuclei from rat liver (42, 43). Thus, they are examples of non-histone chromosomal proteins which have enzymatic properties. Since the enzyme is associated with chromatin, its isolation following solubilization has been difficult due to its extreme instability (44). Following incubation of rat liver chromatin in the presence of S-adenosyl-L-[methyl-^{14}C]methionine, it was shown that the amino acid residue that accepted the [methyl-^{14}C] group was lysine (19, 43). Solubilized protein methylase III from rat liver nuclei was also shown to methylate predominantly arginine-rich histones from calf thymus (44). In vivo experiments involving synchronized HeLa cells also confirmed that histones H3 and H4 are the only histones which are methylated (45).

As mentioned previously, there may be a different enzyme involved in the methylation of histones H3 and H4, since histone H4 is not methylated in plants presumably because plants are lacking a specific histone H4-methylating enzyme. Thus, protein-lysine methyltransferases may have strict substrate requirements. Recent studies with a protein methylase III from Neurospora crassa showed that this enzyme was responsible solely for the methylation of cytochrome c and could not catalyze a methyl transfer to a number of different protein substrates, including histones (46). This example emphasizes the importance of having the proper substrate in identifying a specific protein methylase III activity: Purification of this enzyme revealed that it is a single enzyme which catalyzes the formation of ε-N-trimethyllysine at lysine residue 72 of cytochrome c (47) whereas the products of histone methylation involves a mixture of ε-N-monomethyllysine, ε-N-dimethyllysine, and ε-N-trimethyllysine also at specific sites as discussed previously.

The presence of a DNA-dependent protein methylase activity has been reported in bull seminal plasma (48). Endogenous basic seminal plasma proteins were able to accept methyl groups from S-adenosyl-L-[methyl-^{14}C]methionine when DNA was present, with heterologous DNA being the most effective. Approximately 70% of the enzymatically modified amino acid residues in the methylated proteins were tentatively identified as 0-methylated amino acid ethers. Apparently no methylated lysyl, arginyl, histidyl, or carboxyl residues were formed. The functions of this unusual enzyme activity is not known.

Protein Phosphotransferase

Phosphorylation of histones can be catalyzed by either a cAMP-dependent histone kinase or a less specific cAMP-independent phosphoprotein kinase, both enzymes have been located in liver cytoplasm (49). It has since been established that histones are good substrates in general for protein kinases and that histone kinase is identical to the phosphorylase kinase kinase (50). Although histone kinase preferentially phosphorylates histones, it has been observed that a significant cAMP-activated phosphorylation of non-histone chromosomal protein is also catalyzed by this enzyme (51). Recently, Moll and Kaiser (52) have purified a cAMP-dependent histone kinase from bovine brain using a new assay procedure involving [^{14}C] adenosine triphosphate. The enzyme is capable of hydrolyzing ATP in the absence of histone substrate and it is suggested that there is competition between water and histones as the acceptors for the phosphate group.

Lake (53) has identified and separated two major histone Hl kinases from M-arrested Chinese hamster ovary (CHO) cells by gel filtration. One activity was cAMP-dependent and specific for a major phosphorylation site in the N-terminal portion of histone Hl. The other activity was cAMP-independent and specific for seven major sites in the histone Hl molecule, corresponding to the metaphasic cell-specific phosphorylation sites observed in vivo. Thus it was suggested that the cAMP-independent histone Hl kinase activity predominates during the G_2 - M transition. Hashimoto et al. (54) have shown that both a cAMP-dependent and a cGMP-dependent protein kinase from silkworm pupae are specific for seryl residue 38 of histone Hl. Thus the cAMP-dependent histone kinase appears to have a single site specificity for histone Hl, while the cAMP-independent histone kinase is responsible for multiple-site phosphorylation.

Langan (50) has suggested that protein kinases do not recognize primary structure in their protein substrates, but rather that recognition is based on a specific three-dimensional configuration. Thus, he proposed that this may account for the lack of specificity

in vitro. More investigation is needed in understanding the factors
which govern the substrate specificity of protein kinases in the
cell in order to clarify the function of histone phosphorylation.

The phosphorylation of the non-histone nuclear proteins appears
to be a much more complex situation. Kish and Kleinsmith (51) have
separated twelve distinct enzyme fractions containing protein kinase
activity from the non-histone chromatin phosphoprotein fraction of
beef liver nuclei. These fractions exhibit varying specifications
for casein, histone and non-histone protein substrates. In addition,
the effect of cAMP on these protein kinase fractions was found to be
either inhibitory or stimulatory, depending on the fraction and substrate used. Other investigators have reported from two to four
protein kinases (55-58). This discrepancy in the number of enzymes
involved may be due to the problem of not employing the proper substrate, a case which is similar to that emphasized for the cytochrome
c-dependent protein methyltransferase in N. crassa (46).

Protein Acetyltransferase

Enzymatic acetylation occurs mainly in the arginine-rich histones H3 and H4 (2). Three different histone acetyltransferases
have been partially purified from rat thymus nuclei (59). None of
the three enzymes exhibits any absolute specificity towards any one
histone fraction, although histones are the only proteins which act
as acetyl group acceptors. Two forms of histone acetyltransferases
have been found to occur in rat liver nuclei having a specificity
toward the arginine-rich histones (60). Histone acetyl-transferases
have also been partially purified from the nuclei of rat brain (61),
pigeon (62) and rat liver (63). In addition, Racey and Byvoet have
found histone acetyltransferases to be associated with chromatin (64).

Dixon et al. (18) have characterized the acetylation of internal
lysine residues into two major categories: Type A includes ε-N-acetyllysine bordered on either side by a neutral amino acid, which is most
often glycine but can also be alanine, serine or threonine and type B
in which ε-N-acetyllysine is present as a member of a Lys-Arg, Arg-
Lys or Lys-Lys pair. Thus, these two separate classes may indicate
at least two different histone acetyltransferases with distinct specificities.

Non-enzymatic Modification of Proteins

Aside from the enzymatic reactions in which nuclear proteins are
modified, both the acetyl donor, acetyl CoA and the methyl donor, S-
adenosyl-L-methionine can react in the absence of enzyme to produce a
modified protein. The non-enzymatic acetylation reaction has a pH
optimum between 9 and 10 with poly-L-lysine being the most efficient
acceptor, followed by histones (65, 66). The product of the reaction

was solely ε-N-acetyllysine.

Non-enzymatic methylation of proteins was first described by Paik et al. (67). This reaction had two pH optima, one at 6.3 and the other at 12.5. Egg white globulin was the best acceptor at pH 6.3, while polyarginine reacted to the greatest degree at pH 12.5. Histones reacted only at pH 12.5. The major amino acid residues to be modified are these carboxyl groups forming alkali-labile methyl esters. Whether or not these non-enzymatic reactions have a biological significance has not yet been resolved.

PROTEIN MODIFICATION REACTIONS AND THEIR BIOLOGICAL IMPLICATIONS

Trying to ascribe a functional role to post-translational nuclear protein modification reactions, investigators have primarily used two different approaches: An in vitro approach in which much evidence has been gathered to document that histones can effectively block the template activity of DNA for both DNA or RNA synthesis and that the effectiveness of the blockage is reduced when the histone is phosphorylated (68); and, the second approach, which uses in vivo studies designed to determine the temporal relationship between protein modification, DNA, RNA and protein synthesis, Inferences drawn from these kinds of studies have been criticized on the basis of whether or not these correlations are directly related or merely a coincidence of indirectly related events (69).

It is generally accepted that DNA replication and histone synthesis are tightly coupled in somatic cells of higher eukaryotes. Exceptions to this have been implicated in the lower organisms of yeast (70, 71) and Physarum polycephalum (72) in which histone synthesis is unaffected when DNA replication is partially inhibited. In higher eukaryotes, male gametes during meiosis do not seem to conform to the general rule of DNA replication coupled to histone synthesis (73-75). Also, in non-dividing avian reticulocytes, the synthesis of histone H5 continues in the absence of DNA replication (76).

Where and when nuclear protein modification reactions occur in the sequence of events in dividing and differentiating cells is what we shall now discuss.

Methylation: Modification of histones by methylation has also been studied in various in vivo systems in an attempt to understand its biological significance. Histone methylation was investigated in regenerating adult rat liver by Tidwell et al. (77, 78) and it was found that maximum methylation of lysine residues occurred approximately six hours after DNA and histone synthesis, but prior to mitosis. These findings substantiate the suggestion (19) that histone methylation may result in structural alteration of chromatin prior to mitosis.

Paik and his coworkers (45, 79) found that lysine methylation of histones H2B, H3 and H4 occurred throughout the entire HeLa S-3 cell cycle and increased in G_2 phase and mitosis. In addition, histone H3 contained significant amounts of methylated arginine and histidine residues, which were formed at a maximum rate during S-phase. Turnover of the methyl groups were found to be quite low in contrast to phosphate and acetyl groups. The fact that the major portion of histone-lysine methylation occurred prior to mitosis has again led to speculation that the reaction may be necessary for chromatin condensation (45). It has also been found that the increase in histone-lysine methylation parallels the increase in protein methylase III activity in synchronized HeLa S-3 cells (79). If DNA and histone synthesis are inhibited, the increase in protein methylase III activity still occurs, but results in an "over-methylation" of previously synthesized histones toward more di- and tri-methyllysine rather than mono- and di-methylation. In studying the kinetics of histone methylation in Erlich ascites tumor cells, Thomas et al. (80) found that methylation of histones commences immediately after their biosynthesis, which would place this event in S-phase; however, since the rate of methylation is slower than that for histone synthesis, the peak of histone methylation occurs at a later time in late S or at G_2 phase. Both the rate and the mechanism of histone H3 and H4 methylation were found to be different, suggesting that two different enzymes are responsible for methylating each of these histones.

In cells from trout testis, it was found that both the larger, diploid spermatocytes and stem cells, which are still active in DNA and histone synthesis, were actively undergoing histone methylation (81). The investigators suggested a possible role for the methylation of histones H3 and H4 in chromatin condensation prior to mitosis. They ruled out the possibility of methylation being involved in the mechanism of histone replacement by protamines, since this occurs in spermatids and is primarily thought to require histone acetylase (18). The histone methyl groups, once attached to the lysyl residue, were relatively stable. A temporal sequence of modification was suggested for histone H4 in which, following its synthesis, it was acetylated, deacetylated and then phosphorylated, either coincidently with or shortly after methylation. According to this scheme, acetylation is not a prerequisite for methylation to occur.

During in vivo studies of histone turnover in the rat brain, Duerre and Lee (82) were not able to incorporate either radioactive lysine or methionine into the brain histones of adult rats since cell division is a rare occurrence at this late stage of development. Thus, using newborn rats, they showed that histones and their methyl groups turned over quite rapidly for the first 40-50 days following the administration of precursor isotopes. Afterwards, the histones and the incorporated methyl groups had a much greater stability.

These results correlate well with rat brain development, in which, during the first two months, there is considerable cellular proliferation and thereafter, the brain is essentially mature with limited cellular proliferation. They also found that the N-methyl groups on the histone H3 and H4 lysyl residues do not turn over independently from the backbone polypeptide chain. Byvoet et al. (20) have also shown in Chinese hamster ovary cells that there is no turnover of methyl groups relative to the histone polypeptide backbone. This was subsequently confirmed in vivo in a number of rat tissues (83). Although a mitochrondrial enzyme has been found which can demethylate histones as well as ε-N-methyllysine, its role in methylated histone metabolism remains obscure (84, 85).

Since histone methylation appears to be a metabolically irreversible modification reaction, Byvoet and Baxter (86) argue against the speculation that it is involved in the preparation of chromatin for mitosis. Rather, they envision histone methylation as a finalization process, in which the methylated histones are firmly bound to other macromolecules, in the actual formation of a stable chromatin complex. In support of this hypothesis, they found that increased methyl substitution of the ε-amino group of lysine results in a progressive decrease in charge density which would increase the affinity of these residues for anionic species such as the DNA in chromatin (87). In addition, it was shown that histones which were methylated to the greatest extent, were the most difficult to remove from chromatin by various displacing agents (86). Furthermore, those highly methylated portions of histones were not released from chromatin following trypsin treatment, indicating that these regions are protected from this protease by being firmly bound to DNA. In view of the fact that the degree of methylation of histones contributes to the affinity of their binding to DNA, it seems worthwhile to examine whether or not the ratio of various methylated amino acid residues (primarily those of lysine) change during different times of the cell cycle. Duerre and Chakrabarty (83) have examined the distribution of methylated lysine residue in histone isolated from various adult rat organs. They found that histones H3 and H4 contained methylated amino acid residues that were only in the form of various N-methyl substituted lysyl derivatives. Thus, histone H4 contained mostly ε-N-dimethyllysine and trace amount of ε-N-monomethyllysine at approximately 1.0 mol/mol of polypeptide in all organs examined. On the other hand, histone H3 contained ε-N-monomethyllysine, ε-N-dimethyllysine and ε-N-trimethyllysine in an approximate molar ratio of 0.55:1.0:0.35. This ratio did not vary significantly from organ to organ and the total methylated lysine content was between 1.8 - 1.9 mol/mol of polypeptide. As already mentioned, histone H3 is found methylated at lysyl residues 9 and 27, while H4 is methylated at lysyl residue 20.

In a study comparing the amino acid composition and peptide

maps of histone H4 from human leukemic, embryonic and other neoplastic cells, Desai and Foley (88) found them to be remarkably
similar except for the ratio of ε-N-monomethyllysine to ε-N-dimethyllysine at lysyl residue 20. In the case of H4 from leukemic lypho-
blasts, Novikoff hepatoma and fetal thymus ε-N-monomethyllysine was
present in twice the amount as ε-N-dimethyllysine, whereas in calf
thymus histone H4, the ratio is reversed to give four times as much
ε-N-dimethyllysine as ε-N-monomethyllysine. Thus, according to
previous findings (86), histone H4 in these rapidly proliferating
cells would have less of an affinity for DNA than normal and may
possibly result in a loosely organized chromatin structure. A
shift towards a decrease in the ε-N-dimethyllysine to ε-N-monomethyllysine ratio of the arginine-rich histones has also been observed
in continuously dividing HeLa S-3 cell culture (45). However,
Shephard et al.(89) have observed a majority of ε-N-dimethyllysine
in the more normal Chinese hamster ovary tissue culture cells.
Whether or not a change in the ratio of the methylated lysine derivatives in arginine-rich histones is a characteristic difference
between neoplastic and normal tissues requires more information.
This possibility is well worth investigating in light of the previous
mentioned work and may implicate histone methylation as an improtant
factor in the malignant process. In support of this notion is the
interesting finding by Kass (90) in which he found methylated arginines in histones isolated from bone marrow erythroid precursors of
patients with chronic erythremic myelosis (DiGuglielmo's syndrome).
These methylated arginines were not found in the bone marrows of
patients with nonmalignant disorders of erythropoiesis. The arginine-
rich histones in most cases contained both N^G,N^G-dimethylarginine and
N^G, N'^G-dimethylarginine. Based on these findings, Kass (91) developed a procedure for the metachromatic staining of basic nucleoprotein
in chronic erythremic myelosis.

  Investigations of the levels of protein-histone methyltransferase activities in neoplastic tissues have been conducted in an attempt
to determine which methylating enzymes are elevated in these rapidly
proliferating cells. Initially, in studies performed on whole homogenates of Morris and Novikoff hepatomas, Paik and his coworkers (92)
found that the level of protein methylase I activity paralleled the
growth rate of these slow to fast growing tumors. Protein methylase
II activity remained essentially the same in tumors, host livers and
normal rat livers. Protein methylase III showed no significant
change between the tumors and host livers except in the Novikoff hepatoma in which the enzyme activity was increased two to three fold.
Later, upon reinvestigation of these enzymes, in which protein methylase I and III were assayed from the cytosol and nuclear fractions respectively, a much more significant difference in these enzyme levels
between the tumors of different growth rates was observed. Protein
methylase I activity was found to be about seven-fold higher in the
fast-growing tumors than that of the slower growing tumors. Whereas

previously there was no significant difference seen for protein
methylase III activity assayed from whole homogenates (92), the
activity from the nuclear fraction showed a two to three fold increase in the fast- and moderately fast-growing tumors than for
the slow-growing tumors (6). This may indicate that some inhibitory
factor is present in the cytosol which previously masked these differences. In the same study, it was found that a significant qualitative difference in the methylated amino acids could be distinguished between the histone and non-histone nuclear proteins. Histones
contained their usual complement of methylated lysines while the non-
histone proteins contained mainly methylated arginine derivatives,
as well as a large amount of as yet unidentified compounds.

Turner and Hancock (93) have also found an elevation of two to
nine fold of cytosolic histone methyltransferase in embryonic liver
and mouse hepatomas. However, the elevated levels of protein methylase III in these fast-growing hepatomas may not be directly related
to histone and DNA synthesis since in synchronized HeLa S-3 cells,
the induction of this enzyme was not dependent upon new synthesis of
its histone substrate nor of DNA (79). Whether or not there is a
causal relationship between histone methylation and rapid cell proliferation requires much more investigation.

Effect of Carcinogens on Histone Methylation

Some carcinogens are potent alkylating agents and, as such,
have been shown to modify certain amino acid residues in vivo. Dimethylnitrosamine, which is oxidized by a microsomal enzyme system
to formaldehyde and an active methylating intermediate, has been
shown to modify lysyl, histidyl, cysteinyl and possibly methionyl
residues in histones (94). However, in assessing the role of chemical
alkylation of histones, there is no apparent correlation between the
extent of alkylation and the ultimate carcinogenic effect. For
example, a certain dosage of dimethyl-nitrosamine used was sufficient
to cause kidney tumors but not liver tumors;however, the liver histones were found to be alkylated to a greater extent than those of
the kidney (94). Methyl methanesulphonate was also found to alkylate
rat liver histones to form S-methylcysteine, N-methyllysine, 1-N-
methylhistidine and 3-N-methylhistidine (94). This compound has not
been shown to be a rat liver carcinogen, thus again there is no correlation between histone alkylation and the carcinogenic effect. This
does not rule out that the alkylation of histones over a longer time
may have a cumulative effect since methylation of histone-lysine residues is an irreversible process.

Baxter and Byvoet studied the direct effect of a number of carcinogens of protein methylases I and III (95, 96). They found that
when the carcinogen L-ethionine is in its biologically active form,
as S-adenosyl-L-ethionine, it is able to be utilized by protein

methylase I to form ethylated histones and when in the presence of
the methyl donor S-adenosyl-L-methionine, it inhibits the enzyme
non-competitively. N-Hydroxy-2-aminofluorene was the most potent
inhibitor tested while dimethylnitrosamine showed no inhibitory
effect. In the case of protein methylase III, S-adenosyl-L-ethionine
was a competitive inhibitor of the enzyme in the presence of S-
adenosyl-L-methionine, while in its absence, there was a minimal
amount of histone ethylation detected, in contrast to what was found
for protein methylase I. Like protein methylase I, N-hydroxy-2-
aminofluorene was the most potent inhibitor tested on protein methylase III, while dimethylnitrosamine had no effect. Since these studies
were done in vitro, and many carcinogens are metabolized in vivo
either to active or inactive forms, it would be of interest to look
at the effects of the metabolites on the protein methylases. Also,
some carcinogens are specific for different organs, thus it may be
of interest to isolate the enzymes from these organs and to see how
the carcinogen affects the histone methylating activity. It may also
be possible that carcinogens may react with the enzyme to cause a
change in its specificity with respect to a specific amino acid residue in the histone. Another possibility is that the carcinogen may
react directly with the histone, as seen for the metabolite of dimethylnitrosamine, and form a potent inhibitor of the enzyme.

Phosphorylation: In a situation where cells are dividing, such as
regenerating liver, hepatoma and hepatoma tumor cells (HTC) in
culture, synchronized HeLa and Chinese hamster cells, and trout
testis spermatogonia and spermatocytes, there is considerable agreement that up to 85% of histone H1 molecules are phosphorylated at 1
to 4 sites (18). This situation is completely different in non-
dividing liver cells treated with hormones known to increase the
levels of cAMP. In this case, phosphorylation of histone H1 occurs
at serine 38 alone and is limited to approximately 1% of all the histone H1 molecules (97099). Based on these observations, Langan suggested that this phosphorylation represented an activation of those
liver genes whose expression is influenced by hormones which raise
the cAMP levels.

    Bradbury et al. (100), studying histone phosphorylation in
Physarum polycephalum, proposed that phosphorylation of histone H1
is the initiation step for mitosis. Thus, it was implied that phosphorylation of the middle region of histone H1 (seryl residues 38 and
106) could possibly control the condensation of chromatin. However,
the studies of Dixon and his coworkers (18), using the developing
testis of the rainbow trout for studying protein modification reactions, have shown that phosphorylation in these rapidly dividing cells
occurs at up to four sites located in the highly basic carboxyl-
terminal quarter of the molecule and does not take place significantly
at seryl residues 38 and 106. Three of the sites which contain phosphorylated serine have been characterized in the trout histone H1 and

all three have the same amino acid sequence: Lys-Ser-Pro-Lys-Lys-
at residues 155-159, 171-175, and 195-199. The location of a fourth
phosphorylation site at the carboxyl-terminal end is not yet clear.
Interestingly, Sherod et al. (101) have made identical observations
regarding the pattern of phosphorylation in histone H1 in dividing
mammalian cells. The authors used Ehrlich ascites tumor cells and
hepatoma tissue culture cells to show that the increase of histone
H1 phosphorylation during S-phase occurs at the carboxyl-terminal
half of the molecule and serine-38 phosphorylation is not associated
with cell replication.

Identification of carboxyl-terminal phosphorylation sites for
comparative purposes of histone H1 from various species and tissues
would be of value in determining the conservation of these sites
throughout evolution. This type of analysis will help interpret
the molecular function of histone H1 phosphorylation.

Two distinct kinds of histone phosphorylation have been described in synchronized HeLa S-3 cells (102). In the first type,
histone H2B (and/or H2A) molecules are phosphorylated throughout
the cell cycle and are independent of DNA replication. This is in
contrast to Shephard et al. (103) who reported that histone H2B was
phosphorylated only in G_1 and S-phase of synchronized Chinese hamster
ovary cells. The second type of phosphorylation involves histone H1
and is dependent on the phase of the cell cycle (102). Pulse-label-
ing studies showed that the rate of phosphorylation of histone H1 is
low during G_1-phase, but does follow the increase in the rate of DNA
replication during S-phase. During this time, over 90% of all H1
molecules are converted into one of two phosphorylated forms, thus
both the "old" and newly synthesized forms must be phosphorylated.
After mitosis histone H1 molecules are extensively dephosphorylated
during G_1-phase until DNA replication begins, at which time the phosphorylation cycle commences once again. Unfortunately, the sites of
phosphorylation with regard to amino- or carboxyl-terminal locations
were not determined. If DNA replication and histone synthesis are
inhibited, only about 50% of histone H1 phosphorylation is inhibited,
indicating that this reaction is only partially coupled to DNA synthesis. This observation has also been seen in x-irradiated Chinese
hamster ovary cells, where the turnover of histone H1 was completely
arrested but phosphorylation decreased by 50%, however the phosphorylation of histone H2A was unaffected (104). This result suggests that
the phosphorylation of histone H1 and H2A may serve different biological functions.

A comparison of the histone phosphorylation pattern of metaphase
and interphase Chinese hamster ovary cells, HeLa S-3 cells and rat
nephroma cells was made by Lake et al. (105)by locating the phosphorylated histones on polyacrylamide gels before and after treatment
with alkaline phosphatase to remove protein-bound phosphate. The

authors found that during metaphase there was a pronounced phosphorylation of histone H1 and a rapid dephosphorylation as the cells
enter G_1-phase. It has been suggested that histone H1 phosphorylation has an influence on chromatin condensation (106-108). However,
if histone phsophorylation is intimately involved with transcription
and replication by decreasing the binding to DNA (109), then during
mitosis when transcription is arrested and the chromatin is condensed,
histone H1 should appear in a dephosphorylated form. This is contrary to the previously mentioned data of Lake et al. (105) and as a
result they caution against misinterpretation of in vitro studies
on the interaction of protein and DNA. They suggest that histone H1
phosphorylation during metaphase may be a general case of the more
specific process of gene repression in differentiated tissues.

Three discrete phosphorylations of histone H1 have been described throughout the cell cycle of Chinese hamster ovary cells,
occurring at late G_1-, S- and M-phases (110). Based on these findings, the investigators suggested a model of the relationship of
histone phosphorylation to the cell cycle- (a) phosphorylation of H1
two hours prior to DNA synthesis in G_1-phase is involved with chromatin structural changes necessary for cell proliferation, (b) phosphorylation of H1 during S-phase is involved with DNA replication and
(c) phosphorylation of H1 and H3 during mitosis are involved in
chromosome condensation.

Investigating phosphorylation of histone H1 during the cell
cycle of Chinese hamster ovary cells, Hohmann et al. (111) have
looked at phosphorylation in specific regions of the molecule. They
have found that interphase phosphorylation of H1 began in late G_1-
phase, at a serine in the carboxyl-terminal portion of the molecule
and continued throughout S-phase and mitosis. However, in mitosis,
an additional threonine as well as serine residues are phosphorylated
at the carboxyl-terminal region of the H1 molecule and the amino-
terminal portion of H1 as well became phosphorylated on both of these
residues. The exact positions are not known since the molecule has
not yet been sequenced, but at least four possible phosphorylation
sites exist in mitotic cells. Lake (112) found that histone H1 during
interphase in Chinese hamster V-79 cells was phosphorylated at both
the amino-terminal and carboxyl-terminal regions of the molecule.
This difference may be due to a nonconserved phosphorylation site in
the amino-terminal region of H1 reported by Langan et al. (99).

The amino-terminal phosphorylation of H1 observed during mitosis
in Chinese hamster ovary cells is different from that which has been
observed in dividing cells of trout testis (18) and Erlich ascites
cells (101) as mentioned previously and requires further investigation
of the primary structure to determine which phosphorylation site in
the molecule is highly conserved. In effect, more information on the
position of phosphorylation sites of H1 and their relationship during

DNA interaction is needed to ascribe a function to this modification reaction in mitotic cells.

Acetylation: Much experimental evidence has accumulated which shows that an increase in histone acetylation precedes an increase in RNA synthesis (113-116). This has led to the speculation that histone acetylation may function in the process of gene activation be lessening its interaction with DNA and allowing for the transcription of previously masked nucleotide sequences (2). Involved in this hypothesis would be the enzymatic acetylation of the internal lysyl residues of histone H2A, H2B, H3 and H4, but not H1, which is not usually subjected to this type of modification reaction in vivo, although its amino-terminal serine is acetylated. However, Shepherd et al. (117) have observed a significant amount of metabolically unstable acetylations of histone H4 in synchronized Chinese hamster ovary cells. Since histone acetylation has also been observed in nondividing cells such as mature erythrocytes, it does not always have to be related to the general phenomena of gene activation (76). It also occurs quite extensively in the non-dividing spermatid cells of trout testis and may be related to the replacement process of histones by protamines (18). Aside from the correlations of gene activation with histone acetylation, there are also correlations between gene deactivation and histone deacetylation (32), which lend further evidence for a role in controlling transcription.

The acetylation of the amino-terminal serine residues of histone occurs in the cytoplasm and in the case of histone H4 this reaction takes place when the nascent chains are still attached to the cytoplasmic polysomes (32, 118). This reaction is irreversible and, unlike the acetylation of lysyl residues, N-acetylserine is a permanent modification.

Once synthesized, histones rapidly enter the nucleus where acetylation of particular lysyl residues within the polypeptide chain occurs. As mentioned previously, this process is metabolically reversible and, as a result a deacetylating enzyme has been described (119-121). It should be pointed out that modification reactions such as histone acetylation result in a heterogeneity of the different classes of histones. Therefore, despite the evolutionary stability of amino acid sequence of histone structure, the variability resulting from post-synthetic reactions can be large. Dixon et al. (18) were able to resolve nine modified species of trout testis histone H4 on starch gels and follow the kinetics of the modification reactions of newly synthesized H4 polypeptides, They found that from the time histone H4 is synthesized and finally appears as a "mature" histone H4, the molecule undergoes an obligatory series of acetylation and deacetylations and that no appreciable H4 phosphorylation occurs until after the acetylation cycle is completed. This finding of acetylation and deacetylation preceding other post-synthetic modification reactions

is consistent with Shephard et al. (117) who found that acetylation
of histones began in the middle of S-phase or shortly thereafter,
followed by a loss of acetyl groups after cessation of DNA synthesis,
whereas phosphorylation and methylation occurs later in the cell
cycle.

In dividing duck erythroid cells, newly synthesized histone H4
is pictured as undergoing amino-terminal serine and internal ε-N-
lysine acetylation reactions as well as amino-terminal serine phosphorylation in the cytoplasm (32). After entrance into the nucleus,
the ε-N-acetyl groups and the amino-terminal serine phosphate groups
are removed. Later modifications of nuclear histone H4 include a
stepwise acetylation of the polypeptide chain at specific sites in
preparation for its organization into the chromosome. These results
are basically consistent with Jackson et al. (122) who found that
newly synthesized histone H4 molecules in HTC cells are immediately
modified, primarily by acetylation either prior to or at the time of
their entrance into the nucleus or shortly thereafter. Newly synthesized histone H3 was about 50% acetylated, while histone H2A and
H2B showed only a small degree of modification. The fate of these
newly synthesized histone molecules progressed as follows: (1) a
large degree of modification of histone H4 rapidly shifted toward the
lesser modified parental form, (2) histones H3, H2A and H2B which
were modified to varying degrees initially, remained mainly in their
present form, and (3) histone H1 showed a continuous progression from
its initial unmodified form to the phosphorylated modified form. The
investigators suggested that the extensive modifications of the newly
synthesized histones may be associated in some way with deposition of
these molecules in the organization of the chromosomes.

Since histone acetylation appears to be the most extensive of the
post-synthetic modification reactions, it seems likely that it may
have a multiplicity of functions, which do not only include gene activation, but also deposition and chromatin organization.

FREE METHYLATED AMINO ACIDS AND THEIR EFFECT OF CELLULAR PROLIFERATION

Once formed, N-methylated arginyl and lysyl residues of histones
appear to be metabolically stable. Therefore it has been possible to
detect these free methylated amino acids in the urine (123, 124).
Since many other tissue proteins are also found to be methylated (19),
the presence of these free methylated amino acids cannot be indicative
of the state of histone catabolism. Indeed, very little is probably
contributed by histones, since the turnover has the same constancy as
that of DNA (86). An interesting question has recently been developed
regarding the possible growth-promoting effects of ε-N-trimethyllysine
and that of growth inhibition by N^G-monomethylarginine and N^G,N'^G-
dimethylarginine (125). A growth-promoting effect for three transplantable tumors in mice has been reported for ε-N-trimethyllysine

(126), as well as stimulatory effect of this compound for the transformation of human lymphocytes (127). On the other hand, N^G-methyl-
ated arginine derivatives have been found to have a growth-retarding
effect on tobacco tissue cultures (128, 129). Thus the antagonist action of these two different methylated amino acids is similar to the
findings for both L-arginine and L-lysine (125). Although the potential use of these findings as a method for controlling neoplastic
growth is indeed interesting, more investigation is needed to assess
what effect these compounds have on tissue growth in a variety of
situations (130).

INTERPRETATION

     To date, there is no conclusive evidence which will allow a
specific function to be ascribed to post-synthetic modification
reactions of nuclear proteins. For histones, it is clear that there
has been a remarkable conservation of structure throughout evolution
with the possible exception of histone H1. One would expect that the
structures of histone phosphorylating, acetylating and methylating
enzymes would also exhibit a similar evolutionary conservation as do
their macromolecular substrates. If so, then it would seem that,
rather than playing a role in differentiation or gene activation, a
more likely function, as has been suggested by a number of investigators, would be in the area of precise chromatin organization.
Indeed, the consistence of many of the in vivo sites of phosphorylation, acetylation and methylation of histones from a variety of cell
types lends strong support to this idea. On the other hand, the
modification of the non-histone chromosomal proteins appears to offer
much more diversity which would lend itself to more of a role in the
differentiation process. What is lacking however in this area, as
in the case with histone modifying enzymes, is an extensive characterization of these proteins.

     Phosphorylation and acetylation of internal histone-lysyl resi-
dues can be rapidly reversed and as suggested by Dixon et al. (18),
they may function in allowing histones to achieve the correct conforma-
tion for DNA binding. Once bound, deacetylation will again expose the
positive charge of the lysyl side chains and "lock" the histone into
place by tight ionic linkage. Modification by N-methylation is an
irreversible reaction and may be needed as a "fine" control in fitting
the arginine-rich histones in their precise binding sites. The fact
that carboxyl-methylation of histones is an easily reversible reaction
and results in the neutralization of a negative charge suggests that
it may be important in allowing the proper deposition of histones in
the chromatin. Thus, a likely role for histone modification reactions
would be to serve as a kind of modulator for guiding the molecules
into their designated positions during chromatin formation.

     As far as the role of post-synthetic modification reactions in neoplasia, it is obviously difficult to understand, since their function in general is not really clear. It seems likely that the neoplastic tissues are unable to control these reactions as precisely as normal tissues, however, whether or not there is a cause and effect relationship between aberrant protein modification reactions and neoplasia has never been shown. If highly specific inhibitors of protein-modifying enzymes were available, then one would have a powerful tool for evaluating the significance of a reaction by observing the consequence of blocking its occurrence. Thus far, no such inhibitors are available, although work in this area has been attempted (131).

Like most biosynthetic reactions, protein modification reactions are energy-requiring processes. For phosphorylation and methylation, ATP is the principle energy source, while for acetylation, cleavage of acetyl CoA provides the driving force. In a neoplastic tissue which would presumably be rapidly utilizing its "high energy" compounds for numerous functions, a situation may arise in which the nuclear proteins become "under-modified". This speculation serves to point out the fact that all of the protein modification reactions are energy-dependent and as a result are very much linked to the energy state of the cell. Thus, a deficiency in the level of protein modification may reflect the energy state of the cell and not necessarily a defect in the modification machinery.

Post-synthetic modification reactions of nuclear proteins are still a speculative area which require more definitive investigations to conclusively establish their biological significances.

ACKNOWLEDGEMENTS

This work was supported by research grants AM09602 from National Institute of Arthritis, Metabolism and Digestive Diseases, CA10439 and CA12226 from the National Cancer Institute, and GM20594 from National Institute of General Medical Sciences.

REFERENCES

1. Kossel, AL.K.M.L. Zeitschrift Physiol. Che., 8 (1884) 511.

2. Hnilica, L.S. The Structure and Biological Functions of Histones, The Chemical Rubber Co. (1972).

3. Elgin, S.C.R. and Weintraub, H. Ann. Rev. Biochem. 44 (1975) 725.

4. Gronow, M. and Griffiths, G. FEBS Letters, 15 (1971) 340.

5. Kleinsmith, L.J. and Allfrey, V.G. Biochim. Biophys. Acta 175 (1969) 123.

6. Paik, W.K., Kim, S., Ezirike, J. and Morris, H.P. Cancer Res. 35 (1975) 1159.

7. Christensen, M.E., Beyer, A.L., Walker, B. and LeStourgeon, W.M. Biochem. Biophys. Res. Comm. 74 (1977) 621.

8. Boffa, L.C., Karn, J., Vidali, G. and Allfrey, V.G. Biochem. Biophys. Res. Comm. 74 (1977) 969.

9. Murray, K. Biochemistry 3 (1964) 10.

10. Paik, W.K. and Kim, S. Biochem. Biophys. Res. Comm. 27 (1967) 479.

11. Hempel, V.K., Lange, H.W. and Birkofer, L. Z. Naturforsch, 1 (1968) 37.

12. DeLange, R.J., Hooper, J.A. and Smith, E.L. J. Biol. Chem. 248 (1973) 3261.

13. Hooper, J.A., Smith, E.L., Sommer, K.R. and Chalkley, R. J. Biol. Chem. 248 (1973) 3275.

14. Honda, B.M., Dixon, G.H. and Candido, E.P.M. J. Biol. Chem. 250 (1975) 8681.

15. DeLange, R.J., Fambrough, D.M., Smith, E.L. and Bonner, J. J. Biol. Chem. 244 (1969) 319.

16. Bradbury, E.M. In: The Structure and Function of Chromatin, Ciba Foundation Symposium, Elsevier-Excerpta Medica-North Holland 28 (1975) 1.

17. DeLange, R.J. and Smith, E.L. In: The Structure and Function of Chromatin, Ciba Foundation Symposium, Elsevier-Excerpta Medica-

North-Holland, 28 (1975) 59.

18. Dixon, G.H., Candido, E.P.M., Honda, B.M., Louie, A.J., MacLeod, A.R. and Sung, M.T. In: The Structure and Function of Chromatin, Ciba Foundation Symposium, Elsevier-Excerpta Medica-North-Holland, 28 (1975) 229.

19. Paik, W.K. and Kim, S. In: Advances in Enzymology, A. Meister (ed). John Wiley & Sons, New York 42 (1975) 227.

20. Byvoet, P., Shepherd, G.R., Hardin, J.M. and Noland, B.J. Arch. Biochem. Biophys. 148 (1972) 558.

21. Kim, S. and Paik, W.K. Experientia, 32 (1976) 982.

22. Kleene, S.J., Toews, M.L. and Adler, J. J. Biol. Chem. 252 (1977).

23. Van Der Werf, P. and Hoshland, D.E. J. Biol. Chem. 252 (1977) 2793.

24. Gershey, E.L., Haslett, G.W., Vidali, G. and Allfrey, V.G. J. Biol. Chem. 244 (1969) 4871.

25. Ord, M.G. and Stocken, L.A. Biochem. J. 98 (1966) 888.

26. Sung, M.T., Dixon, G.H. and Smithies, O. J. Biol. Chem. 246 (1971) 1358.

27. Hayashi, T. and Iwai, K. J. Biochem. (Tokyo), 68 (1970) 415.

28. Gutierrez, R.M. and Hnilica, L.S. Science 157 (1967) 1324.

29. Kleinsmith, L.J., Allfrey, V.G. and Mirsky, A.E. Proc. Natl. Acad. Sci. U.S.A. 55 (1966) 1182.

30. Balhorn, R., Chalkley, R. and Granner, D. Biochemistry, 11 (1972) 1094.

31. Phillips, D.M.P. Biochem. J. 87 (1963) 258.

32. Ruiz-Carillo, A., Wangh, L.J. and Allfrey, V.G. Science, 190 (1975) 117.

33. Gershey, E.L., Vidali, G. and Allfrey, V.G. J. Biol. Chem. 243 (1968) 5018.

34. Vidali, G., Gershey, E.L. and Allfrey, V.G. J. Biol. Chem. 243 (1968) 6361.

35. DeLange, R.J., Smith, E.L. Fambrough, D.M. and Bonner, J.

Proc. Natl. Acad. Sci. U.S.A. 61 (1968) 1145.

36. DeLange, R.J. Fambrough, D.M., Smith, E.L. and Bonner, J. J. Biol. Chem. 244 (1969) 5669.

37. DeLange, R.J., Smith, E.L. and Bonner, J. Biochem. Biophys. Res. Comm. 40 (1970) 989.

38. Sung, M.T. and Dixon, G.H. Proc. Natl. Acad. Sci. U.S.A. 67 (1970) 1616.

39. Lee, H.W., Kim, S. and Paik, W.K. Biochemistry, 16 (1977) 78.

40. Miyake, M. J. Neurochem. 24 (1975) 909.

41. Kim, S. Arch. Biochem. Biophys. 157 (1973) 476.

42. Comb, D.G., Sarkar, N. and Pinzino, C.J. J. Biol. Chem. 241 (1966) 1857.

43. Benjamin, W.B. Nature, 234 (1971) 18.

44. Paik, W.K. and Kim, S. J. Biol. Chem. 245 (1970) 6010.

45. Borun, T.W., Pearson, D.B. and Paik, W.K. J. Biol. Chem. 247 (1972) 4288.

46. Nochumson, S., Durban, E., Kim, S. and Paik, W.K. Biochem. J., in press, (1977).

47. Durban, E., Nochumson, S., Kim, S. and Paik, W.K. Manuscript in preparation.

48. Sheid, B. and Pedrinan, L. Biochemistry 14 (1975) 4357.

49. Langan, T.A. In: Some Regulatory Mechanisms for Protein Synthesis in Mammalian Cells, S. Pietro, M. Lamborg and F.T. Kennedy (eds). Academic Press, New York, (1968) p.101

50. Langan, T.A. Adv. in Cyc. Nuc. Res. 3 (1973) 99.

51. Kish, V.M. and Kleinsmith, L.J. J. Biol. Chem. 249 (1974) 750.

52. Moll, G.W. and Kaiser, E.T. J. Biol. Chem. 251 (1976) 3993.

53. Lake, R.S. J. Cell Biol. 58 (1973) 317.

54. Hashimoto, E., Takeda, M., Nishizuka, Y., Hamano, K. and Iwai, K. J. Biol. Chem. 251 (1976) 6287.

55. Takeda, M., Yamamura, H. and Ohga, Y. Biochem. Biophys. Res. Comm. 42 (1971) 103.

56. Ruddon, R.W. and Anderson, S. Biochem. Biophys. Res. Comm. 46 (1972) 1499.

57. Kamiyama, M., Dastugue, B. and Kruh, J. Biochem. Biophys, Res. Comm. 44 (1971) 1345.

58. Desjardins, P.R., Luie, P.F., Liew, C.C. and Cornall, A.G. Can. J. Biochem. 50 (1972) 1249.

59. Gallwitz, D. and Sures, I. Biochim. Biophys. Acta 263 (1972) 315.

60. Luie, P.F., Cornall, A.G. and Liew, C.C. Can. J. Biochem. 51 (1973) 1177.

61. Bondy, S.C., Roberts, S. and Morelos, B.S. Biochem. J. 119 (1970) 665.

62. Nohara, H., Takahashi, T. and Ogata, K. Biochim. Biophys. Acta 127 (1966) 282.

63. Gallwitz, D. Biochem. Biophys. Res. Comm. 32 (1968) 117.

64. Racey, L.A. and Byvoet, P. Exp. Cell Res. 64 (1971) 366.

65. Gallwitz, D. and Sekeris, C.E. Hoppe-Seyler, A. Physiol. Chem. 350 (1969) 150.

66. Paik, W.K., Pearson, D.B., Lee, H.W. and Kim, S. Biochim. Biophys. Acta 213 (1970) 513.

67. Paik, W.K., Lee, H.W. and Kim, S. FEBS Letrs. 58 (1975) 39.

68. Elgin, S.C.R., Froehner, S.C., Smart, J.E. and Bonner, J. Adv. Cell Mol. Biol. 1 (1971) 1.

69. Taborsky, G. Adv. in Prot. Chem. 28 (1974) 1.

70. Hereford, L.M. and Hartwell, L.H. Nature 244 (1973) 129.

71. Williamson, D.H. Biochem. Biophys. Res. Comm. 52 (1973) 731.

72. Mohberg, J. and Rusch, H.P. Arch, Biochem. Biophys. 138 (1970) 418.

73. Bogawov, Y.F., Liapunova, N.A., Sherudilo, A.I. and Antropova,E.N.

Exp.Cell Res. 52 (1968) 59.

74. Bloch, D.P. and Teng, C. J. Cell Sci. 5 (1969) 321.

75. Antopova, E.N. and Bogdanov, Y.F. Exp. Cell Res. 60 (1970) 40.

76. Sung, M.T., Hartford, J., Bundman, M. and Vidakalas, G. Biochemistry, 16 (1977) 279.

77. Tidwell, T., Allfrey, V.G. and Mirsky, A.E., J. Biol. Chem. 243 (1968) 707.

78. Lee, H.W. and Paik, W.K. and Borun, T.W. J. Biol. Chem. 248 (1973) 4194.

79. Lee, H.W. and Paik, W.K. Biochim. Biophys. Acta 277 (1972) 107.

80. Thomas, G., Lange, H.W. and Hempel, K. Eur. J. Biochem. 51 (1975) 609.

81. Honda, B.M., Candido, P.M. and Dixon, G. J. Biol. Chem. 250 (1975) 8686.

82. Duerre, J.A. and Lee, C.T. J. Neurochem. 23 (1974) 541.

83. Duerre, J.A. and Chakrabarty, S. J. Biol. Chem. 250 (1975) 8457.

84. Paik, W.K. and Kim, S. Biochem. Biophys. Res. Comm. 51 (1973) 781.

85. Paik, W.K. and Kim, S. Arch. Biochem. Biophys. 165 (1974) 369.

86. Byvoet, P. and Baxter, C.S. In: Chromosomal Proteins and Their Role in the Regulation of Gene Expression, G.S. Stein and L.J. Kleinsmith (eds). Academic Press, New York (1975) p. 127.

87. Baxter, C.S. and Byvoet, P. Biochem. Biophys. Res. Comm. 64 (1975) 514.

88. Desai, L.S. and Foley, G.E. Biochem. J. 119 (1970) 165.

89. Shepherd, G.R., Hardin, J.M. and Noland, B.J. Arch. Biochem. Biophys. 143 (1971) 1.

90. Kass, L. Proc. Soc. Exp. Biol. Med. 145 (1974) 944.

91. Kass, L. Am. J. Clin. Pathol. 62 (1974) 21.

92. Paik, W.K., Lee, H.W. and Morris, H.P. Cancer Res. 32 (1972) 37.

93. Turner, G. and Hancock, R.L. Life Sci. 9 (1970) 917.

94. Turberville, C. and Craddock, V.M. Biochem. J. 124 (1971) 725.

95. Baxter, C.S. and Byvoet, P. Cancer Res. 34 (1974) 1418.

96. Baxter, C.S. and Byvoet, P. Cancer Res. 34 (1974) 1424.

97. Langan, T.A. Proc. Natl. Acad. Sci. U.S.A. 64 (1969) 1276.

98. Langan, T.A. J. Biol. Chem. 244 (1969) 5763.

99. Langan, T.A., Rall, S.C. and Cole, R.D. J. Biol. Chem. 246
    (1971) 1942.

100. Bradbury, E.M., Inglis, R.J. and Matthews, H.R. Nature 247
     (1974) 257.

101. Sherod, D., Johnson, G., Balhorn, R., Jackson, V., Chalkley, R.
     and Granner, D. Biochom. Biophys. Acta 381 (1975) 337.

102. Marks, D.B., Paik, W.K. and Borun, T.W. J. Biol. Chem. 248
     (1973) 5660.

103. Shepherd, G.R., Noland, B.J. and Hardin, J.M. Arch. Biochem.
     Biophys. 142 (1971) 299.

104. Gurley, L.R. and Walters, R.A. Biochemistry, 10 (1971) 1588.

105. Lake, R.S., Goidl, J.A. and Salzman, N.P. Exp. Cell Res. 73
     (1972) 113.

106. Littau, V.C., Burdick, C.J., Allfrey, V.G. and Mirsky, A.E.,
     Proc. Natl. Acad. Sci. U.S.A. 54 (1965) 1204.

107. Johns, E.W. and Forrester, S. Biochem. J. 111 (1969) 371.

108. Jensen, R.H. and Chalkley, R. Biochemistry, 7 (1968) 4388.

109. DeLange, R.J. and Smith, E.L. Ann. Rev. Biochem. 40 (1971) 279.

110. Gurley, L.R., Walters, R.A. and Tobey, R.A. J. Biol. Chem. 250
     (1975) 3936.

111. Hohmann, P., Tobey, R.A. and Gurley, L.R. J. Biol. Chem. 251
     (1976) 3685.

112. Lake, R.S. L. Cell Biol. 58 (1973) 317.

113. Pogo, B.G.T., Allfrey, V.G. and Mirsky, A.E. Proc. Natl. Acad. Sci. U.S.A. 55 (1966) 805.

114. Takaku, F., Nakao, K., Ono, T. and Terayama, H. Biochim. Biophys. Acta 179 (1969) 396.

115. Pogo, B.G.T., Pogo, A.O., Allfrey, V.G., and Mirsky, A.E. Proc. Natl. Acad. Sci. U.S.A. 59 (1968) 1337.

116. Pogo, B.G.T., Pogo, A.O. and Allfrey, V.G. Genetics, 61 (1969) Suppl. 1, 373.

117. Shepherd, G.R., Noland, B.J. and Hardin, J.M., Biochim. Biophys. Acta 228 (1971) 544.

118. Liew, C.C., Haslett, G.W. and Allfrey, V.G. Nature (London) 226 (1970) 414.

119. Inoue, A. and Fujimoto, D. Biochem. Biophys. Res. Comm. 36 (1969) 146.

120. Inoue, A. and Fujimoto, D. Biochim. Biophys, Acta 220 (1970) 307.

121. Libby, P.L. Biochim. Biophys. Acta 213 (1970) 234.

122. Jackson, V., Shires, A., Tanphaichitir, N. and Chalkley, R. J. Mol. Biol. 104 (1976) 471.

123. Kakimoto, Y. and Akazawa, S. J. Biol. Chem. 245 (1970) 5751.

124. Lange, H.W., Loewer, R. and Hempel, K. Hoppe-Seyler's Z. Physiol. Chem. 354 (1973) 117.

125. Tyihak, E., Szende, B. and Lapis, K. Life Sci. 20 (1977) 385.

126. Szende, B., Tyihak, E., Kopper, L. and Lapis, K. Neoplasma, 17 (1970) 433.

127. Stotz, G., Szende, B., Lapis, K. and Tyihak, E. Expl. Pathol. 9 (1974) 317.

128. Tyihak E., Marot, M., Vagujfalvi, D., Bajusz, S. and Patthy, A. Experientia, 31 (1975) 818.

129. Tyihak, E., Marot, M., Vagujfalvi, D., Bajusz, S. and Patthy A., Acta Agronomica Acad. Scient. Hungar. 24 (1975) 315.

130. Szent-Györgyi, A. Acata Agronomica Acad. Scient. Hungar.

23 (1974) 215.

131.Cory, M., Hewry, D.W., Taylor, D.L. and Koskela, K.J. Chem-
    Biol. Interactions, 9 (1974) 253.

REGULATION OF DNA SYNTHESIS IN ISOLATED MORRIS HEPATOMA NUCLEI

Peter Ove and Mona L. Coetzee

Department of Anatomy and Cell Biology
University of Pittsburgh School of Medicine
Pittsburgh, Pennsylvania 15261

SUMMARY

The preparation of nuclei from rat liver and from Morris hepatoma is discussed. Isolated nuclei incorporate labeled [^{3}H]TTP in an in vitro incubation system and can be used to compare DNA synthesis in normal and malignant tissues. The isolated nuclei, especially nuclei denuded of their membranes by Triton X-100 treatment, can be considered as a DNA replicating complex. It is suggested that a further separation of the nuclear components and reconstitution of such isolated components may lead to the identification of the minimal replicating complex. Such nuclear fractionations are described and it is suggested that investigations of this kind may lead to the identification of alterations that are responsible for the loss of control of growth in hepatoma tissue. It is indicated that an increase in DNA polymerase activity cannot be solely responsible for increased DNA synthesis in hepatomas. Some biochemical characteristics of host liver and hepatoma nuclei are described as are results with some antitumor agents added to the nuclear incorporating system. The possibility to use the system for the screening of potential chemotherapeutic agents and to study their mode of action is discussed.

INTRODUCTION

There might be many different agents responsible for cancer, but the end result is loss of control of growth of the affected cells. This does not imply a rapid growth for all malignant cells, but a deviation from the regular steady state growth pattern of a particular cell population. Lack of control of growth therefore is one of the key problems in malignancy. Since cells do not generally divide with-

233

out replicating their DNA, it seems appropriate to study DNA replication to gain some insight to the loss of control of growth. The
lasting event in neoplastic transformation is most likely a genetic
change. It may be a RNA or DNA virus or a segment of RNA or DNA
functioning either incorporated in the cellular genome or as
episomes. A genetic change may also occur spontaneously or may be
induced by environmental agents. Affected segments of the genetic
material must code for proteins that play a fundamental role in
directing cellular metabolism, especially as related to growth and
DNA replication. It is well recognized that the DNA polymerases
can account for only part of the mechanics required for DNA replication in vivo. Proteins involved in initiation and termination
of nuclear DNA synthesis, proteins associated with the unwinding
of the DNA double helix, enzymes involved with RNA initiation and
possibly structural components of the nucleus must all be part of
a replication complex. The present state of mammalian DNA polymerases has been discussed in several excellent reviews (7, 20,
49, 93).

     To compare control of DNA replication in malignant and healthy
tissues, the Morris hepatomas on the one hand and host or normal
liver on the other represent a well studied system. The Morris hepatomas and the host liver represent normal and malignant tissues
growing in the same animal which can easily be removed without fear
of cross-contamination. An additional advantage of the Morris hepatomas is that they are available in a variety of growth ranges.

     Comparisons of DNA polymerase activities in several Morris hep-
atomas have been reported by a number of investigators (3, 12, 40,
63, 66, 68, 70). Despite reported variations in subcellular localization of several DNA polymerase activities there is general agreement that DNA polymerase activities increase in the hepatomas as
compared to normal or host liver. This increase in activity appears
to be roughly correlated with the growth rate of hepatomas as first
reported in Cancer Research (70). Since mammalian DNA ploymerases,
including those in malignant tissues, have been extensively reviewed, this article will deal with aspects of control of DNA replication in nuclei isolated from Morris hepatomas.

                         PREPARATION OF NUCLEI

     A variety of methods for the isolation of nuclei have been re-
ported. They include citric acid (83), high sucrose density with
acetic acid (33), detergents (1, 15, 36, 82, 87), organic solvents
(4, 71, 81), and glycerol (21, 46). It has been pointed out by
Dounce (18) that the isolation of nuclei from tumor cells is generally more difficult than isolation from cells of control tissue. We
have found this to be true for hepatoma nuclei as opposed to the
liver nuclei.

Nuclear systems for DNA replication have also been reported for HeLa cells (23, 24, 34), rat liver (32, 51), mouse fibroblasts (39), and a variety of other tissues. In our investigation we have used both sucrose nuclei and Triton X-100 extracted nuclei. Host and normal sucrose nuclei were isolated essentially according to Lynch et al, (51). All steps were carried out as rapidly as possible at 0°. Liver samples of 1-2 g were suspended in 20 ml 0.3 M sucrose-4 mM $CaCl_2$ in a loose Dounce homogenizer with 2-3 strokes, followed by 80 strokes using a loose fitting rubber pestle. The homogenate was filtered through 110 mesh nylon screen, and the filtrate centrifuged at 1500 xg for 7 min. The pellet was resuspended in 18 ml 2.0 M sucrose-1 mM $CaCl_2$, homogenized with 8-10 strokes in a loose Dounce homogenizer, layered over 13 ml 2.2 M sucrose, and centrifuged in a Spinco SW 27 rotor for 20 min at 40,000 xg.

In order to obtain an equivalent yield of hepatoma nuclei of comparable purity the method was modified. The bulk of the hepatoma nuclei settles at the 2.2 - 2.0 M sucrose interface during the centrifugation in the Spinco at 40,000 xg. This nuclear layer was removed and rehomogenized in 28 ml 2.0 M sucrose - 1 mM $CaCl_2$ and centrifuged for 30 min in a Spinco SW 27 rotor at 40,000 xg. All nuclear pellets were washed twice with 10 ml 1 M sucrose and once with 10 ml 0.25 M sucrose both in TKMM (50 mM Tris-HCl pH 7.5, 25 mM KCl, 5 mM $MgCl_2$ and 1 mM 2-mercaptoethanol) and were centrifuged for 10 min at 3500 xg, 3500 xg and 1000 xg, respectively. The washes did not extract any measurable DNA polymerase activity. The recovery of nuclei from host or normal liver, hepatoma 7800 and hepatoma 7777 was 0.84 mg DNA per g host liver (38%), 1.02 mg DNA per g hepatoma 7800 (36%), and 1.58 mg DNA per g hepatoma 7777 (34%). Since hepatomas contain more DNA per g tissue than liver does, the recovery is comparable.

As first reported by Aaronson and Blobel (1) liver nuclei can be denuded of their membranes without losing physical integrity by treatment with 2% Triton X-100. The concentration of the Triton X-100 treatment is important. Treatment with 1% Triton X-100 results in the removal of only the outer nuclear envelope. We prepared sucrose nuclei as described above, suspended them in 0.25 M sucrose-TKMM at an optical density of 25 A_{260} and added Triton X-100 to a final concentration of 2%. After 2 min at 0°, 0.5 vol of 1.3 M sucrose-TKMM was underlaid and the samples were centrifuged for 20 min at 1000 xg. The resulting pellet from normal or host liver sucrose nuclei consisted of membrane-denuded nuclei with 95% of the phospholipid removed as compared to sucrose nuclei. Hepatoma nuclei had lost only 90% of their phospholipids. Therefore, the Triton X-100 extraction was repeated with both preparations. After the second extraction 95% of the phospholipids were removed from hepatoma nuclei but no further phospholipids were lost from the liver nuclei. The Triton X-100 treatment removed 15 to 20% of the protein from both liver and hepatoma nuclei. Following this treatment, the nuclear pellets were washed twice with 0.25 M sucrose-TKMM, suspended in 0.25 M sucrose and used immediately for assay or chemical determinations. That the physical integrity of such nuclei is maintained can be seen in Figures 1 and 2.

In order to make valid comparisons of the properties and chemical composition of nuclei from different sources, stringent purity criteria have to be established. In addition to microscopic observations as shown in Figure 3, RNA (55), DNA (9), and protein (50) were determined on the nuclear preparations. The determinations are shown in Table 1. Since the specific activities of such marker enzymes might vary considerably in different tissues it is not sufficient to compare the specific activities of the nuclei from the different tissues but the comparison has to be made with the specific activity of the nuclei as a percentage of the specific activity in the original homogenate. It can be seen in Table 2 that there is less cytochrome c oxidase activity in hepatoma 7800 which is equal to or higher than liver activity. On the other hand both hepatoma tissues showed higher 5'-nucleotidase activity than did host liver. The activities of those marker enzymes in total liver homogenates are in good agreement with other values reported for cytochrome c oxidase (28), glucose-6-phosphatase (27) and 5'-nucleotidase (94, 95). A decreased activity of glucose-6-phosphatase in hepatoma tissue has been reported (92).

It should be pointed out, that these enzyme determinations and the determinations of protein, RNA and DNA are no indication that the nuclear preparations are absolutely free of cytoplasmic contamination, but rather that the preparations from different tissues are comparable with respect to purity.

IN VITRO NUCLEAR INCORPORATING SYSTEMS

A. Sucrose Nuclei

A nuclear system for DNA replication from synchronized HeLa cells has been reported by Friedman and Mueller (23, 24). Since then, numerous papers have appeared dealing with DNA synthesis in nuclear systems (23, 24, 32, 34, 35, 44, 47, 51, 52, 65, 80, 86, 89, 90).

We have compared nuclei prepared from host liver and Morris hepatomas 7800 and 7777 in such an incorporating system. The regular reaction mixture contained 50 µmoles Tris-HCl, pH 7.5; 2 µmoles MgCl$_2$; 4 µmoles 2-mercapto-ethanol; 80 µmoles KCl; 1 µmole ATP; 0.04 µmole each dATP, dCTP, and dGTP; and 0.02 µmole [^{3}H]TTP (50µCi/µmole). Nuclei (50 to 100 ug DNA) were added after a 5 min preincubation of the reaction mixture. The results of such an assay

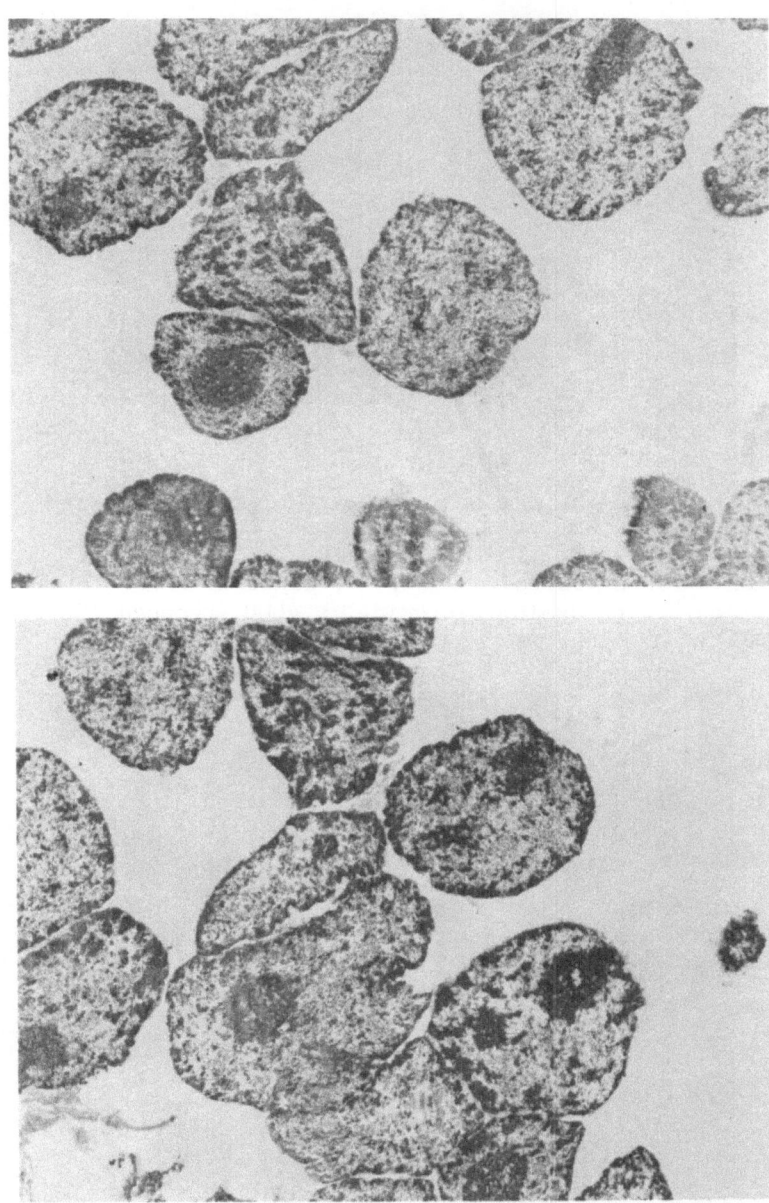

Figures 1A and 1B
Triton X-100 extracted nuclei. A, host liver; B, hepatoma 7800.
Fixed with glutaraldehyde and osmium tetroxide. x 4000

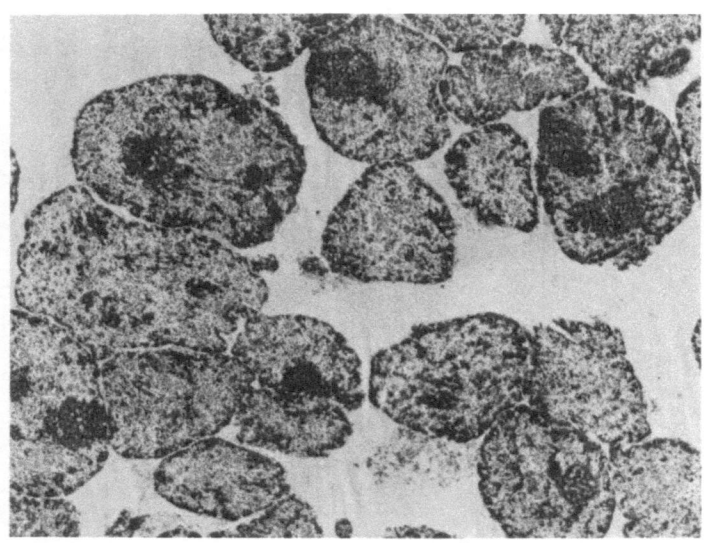

Figure 1C
Triton X-100 extracted nuclei. C, hepatoma 7777. Fixed with
glutaraldehyde and osmium tetroxide. x 4000 (reduced 19% for reproduction).

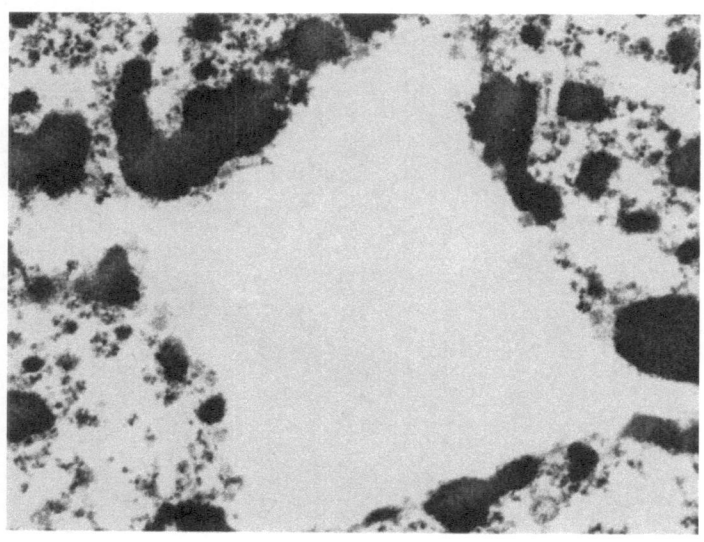

Figure 2A
Triton X-100 extracted nuclei. A, host liver. Fixed with
glutaraldehyde and osmium tetroxide. x 62000 (reduced 19% for reproduction).

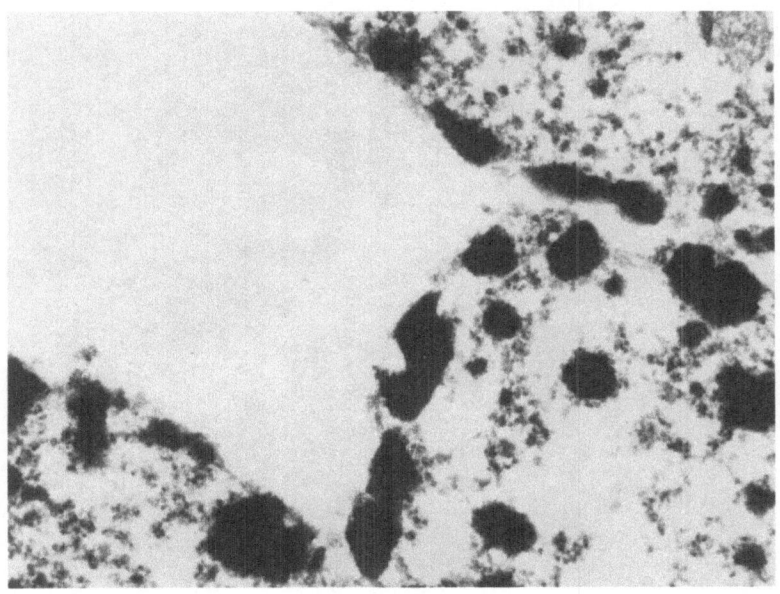

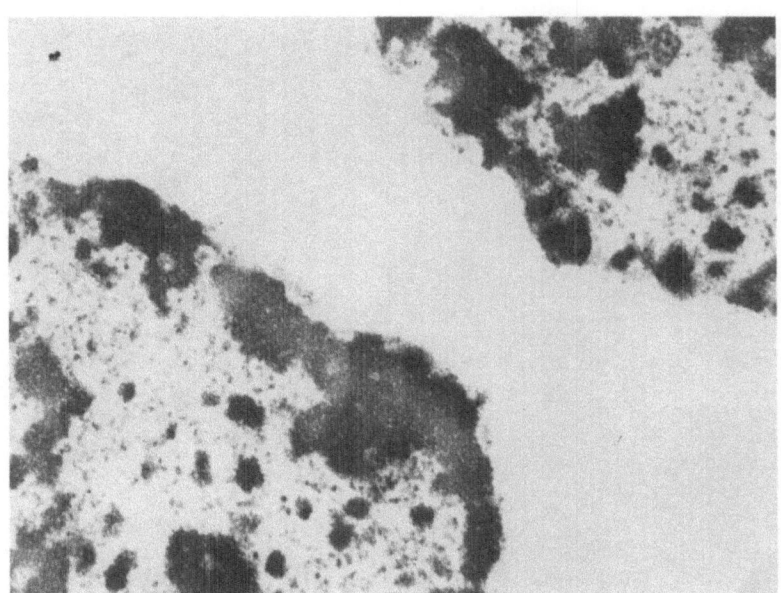

Figures 2B and 2C
Triton X-100 extracted nuclei. B, hepatoma 7800; C, hepatoma
7777. Fixed with gluraraldehyde and osmium tetroxide. x 62,000.

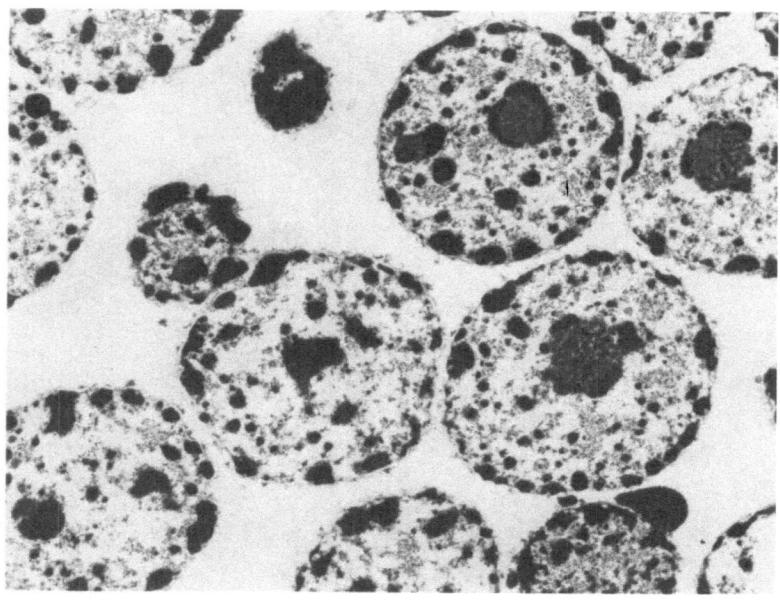

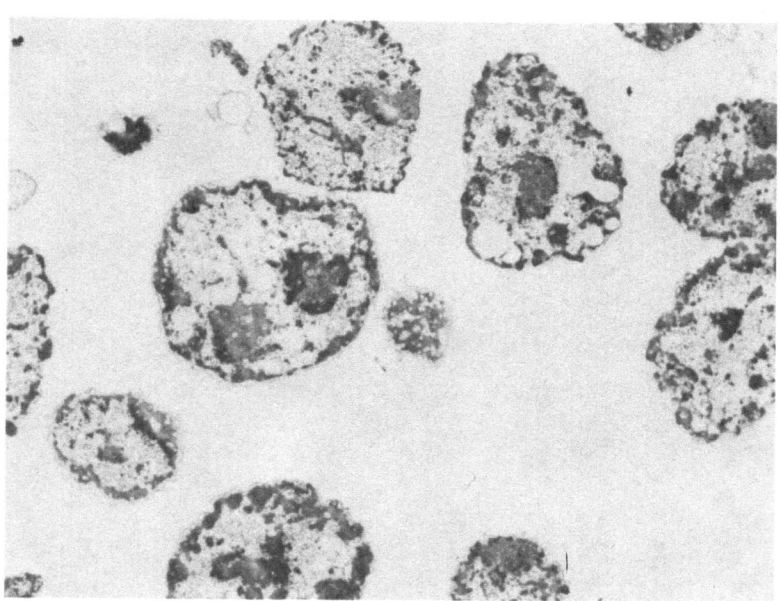

Figures 3A and 3B
Sucrose nuclei from host liver and hepatoma. A, host liver;
B, hepatoma 7800. Fixed with glutaraldehyde and osmium tetroxide.
x 6000.

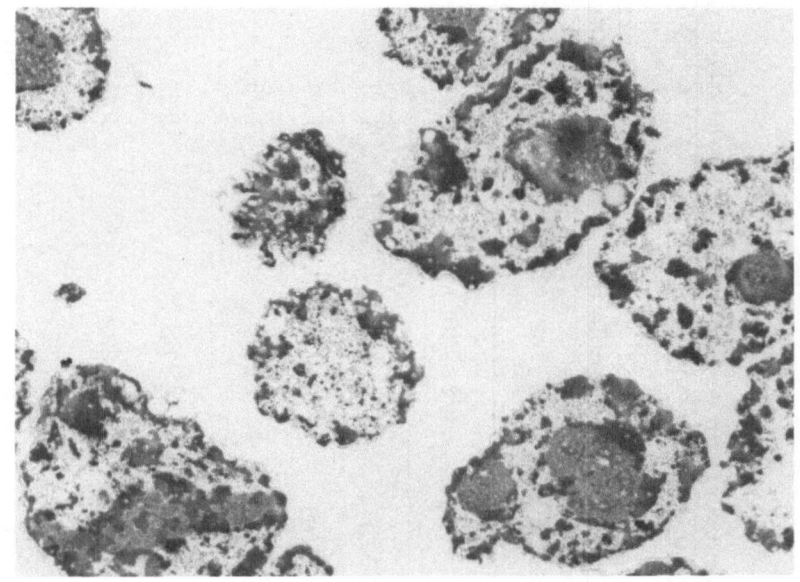

Figure 3C
Sucrose nuclei from host liver and hepatoma. C, hepatoma
7777. Fixed with glutaraldehyde and osmium tetroxide. x 6000.

Table One

Comparison of Sucrose and Triton X-100 Extracted Nuclei with respect
to DNA, RNA and Protein

The ratios given are the averages of the number of determinations indicated
in paranthesis. Individual determinations did not vary by more than 15%. Recovery after Triton X-100 treatment was 95% for DNA, 71% for RNA, and 80% for
protein. The recoveries were the same for the 3 nuclear preparations.

Nuclei	Source	RNA/DNA	Protein/DNA	Protein/RNA
Sucrose	Host liver (15)	0.32	1.8	5.6
	Hepatoma 7800(9)	0.32	1.9	5.8
	Hepatoma 7777(12)	0.30	1.8	6.0
Triton	Host liver (12)	0.24	1.5	6.0
	Hepatoma 7800(5)	0.22	1.4	6.3
	Hepatoma 7777(9)	0.24	1.5	6.3

Table Two

Enzyme Activity Ratios as a Criterion for
Comparable Purity of Host Liver and Hepatoma Nuclei

Enzyme activities were measured in cell homogenates and in suspensions of purified nuclei prepared from the same homogenates. The numbers represent determinations from 4 different experiments. Individual values did not vary by more than 10% from the average.

Source of tissue	Cytochrome c oxidase (µmoles product formed in 1 minute/mg protein)			Glucose-6-phosphatase (µmoles Pi released in 20 minutes/mg protein)			5' nucleotidase (µmoles Pi released in 20 minutes/mg protein)		
	Homogenate	Nuclei	% in nuclei	Homogenate	Nuclei	% in nuclei	Homogenate	Nuclei	% in nuclei
Host liver	0.163	0.39	24	0.755	0.580	77	0.303	0.095	31
Hepatoma 7800	0.179	0.050	28	0.260	0.203	78	0.970	0.390	40
Hepatoma 7777	0.040	0.010	25	0.062	0.044	72	1.380	0.515	27

using sucrose nuclei are shown in Table 3 and Figure 4. The system is proportional with an amount of nuclei used between 20 and 200 μg of nuclear DNA. Addition of DNA or DNase to such a system increases [^{3}H]TTP incorporation considerably. DNase most likely introduces breaks into the nuclear DNA thus making additional initiation sites available.

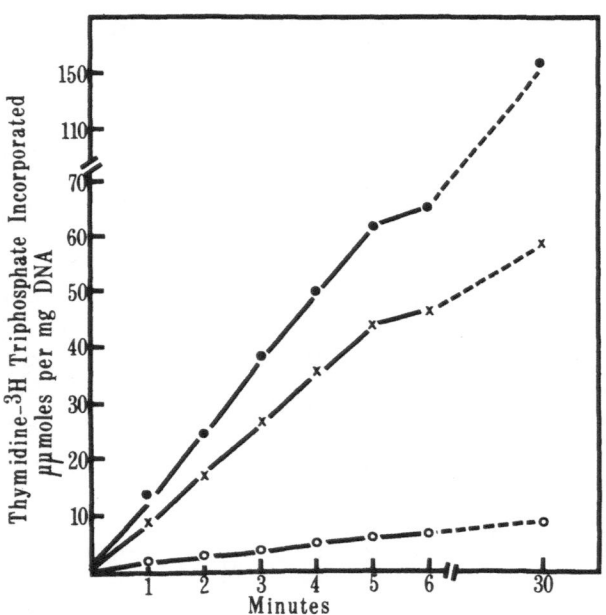

Figure 4
[^{3}H]TTP incorporation in a nuclear system with time. Incorporation with the incomplete incorporating system (dCTP, dGTP, and dATP omitted) has been subtracted from all time points. 0, host liver; X, hepatoma 7800; 0, hepatoma 7777.

Table Three

Incorporation of [^{3}H]TTP into DNA of Whole Nuclei

The complete system contains: 50 µmoles Tris-HCl, pH-7.5; 2 µmoles MgCl2; 4 µmoles 2-mercaptoethanol; 80 µmoles KCl; 1 µmole ATP; 0.04 µmole each dATP, dCTP, and dGTP; 0.02 µmole [^{3}H]TTP (50 µCi/µmole). The reaction mixture was preincubated for 5 min before the addition of nuclei (50-100 µg DNA), in a final volume of 0.5 ml. In the incomplete system, the 3 unlabeled deoxynucleoside triphosphates have been omitted. The numbers are the averages from at least 3 different determinations. Individual numbers did not vary by more than 20%.

| | [3H]TTP incorporated (pmoles/mg DNA in 5 min) | | | | | | | | |
| | Host liver | | | Hepatoma 7800 | | | Hepatoma 7777 | | |
Additions(+) and deletions(-)	Complete system	Incomplete system	Δ	Complete system	Incomplete system	Δ	Complete system	Incomplete system	Δ
None	9.7	3.5	6.2	65.0	20.8	44.2	87.0	25.0	62.0
(-)Mg^{++}	1.1	0.8	0.3	0.9	0.8	0.1	1.2	1.0	0.2
(-)ATP	6.5	2.5	4.0	27.0	15.4	11.6	44.0	12.0	23.0
(+)100 µg native DNA	78.5	26.2	52.3	89.5	38.6	50.9	107.0	42.0	65.0
(+)100 µg denatured DNA	68.0	31.2	36.8	86.5	32.6	53.9	135.0	58.2	76.8
(+)0.2 µg DNase	70.0	42.1	27.9	116.1	56.1	60.0	143.0	61.2	81.8

That the normal system measures a continuation of the in vivo process and uses available intitation sites is indicated by several pieces of evidence. In vitro incorporation is linear for only a short period of time, from 5 to 10 min, presumably finishing incorporation at sites available in vivo. A comparison of in vivo incorporation with in vitro incorporation shows a similar relationship with host liver, hepatoma 7800, and hepatoma 7777, indicating that the in vitro system measures the same difference in DNA synthesis between hepatoma and control tissues that are apparent in vivo. In addition, when rats bearing hepatoma 7777 were injected with hydro-cortisone (5 ug/100 g) at 4 and 2 hours before preparation of nuclei or before animals were pulsed for in vivo [^{3}H] thymidine incorporation, inhibition of incorporation was similar at 42.5% for the nuclear system and at 44.5% for in vivo incorporation in hepatoma 7777.

Further evidence that the nuclear incorporating system measures a continuation of the in vivo process is provided by density gradient analysis (51, 67) of DNA formed in vitro in the nuclear system shown in Figure 5. Rats bearing hepatoma 7777 were given injections of 5-bromodeoxyuridine (10 µmoles/200 g), and 10 min later nuclei were isolated from the hepatomas and used in a nuclear incorporating system. Nuclei were reisolated from the incubation mixture and DNA was extracted (67). The label associated with the nuclei sedimented with the fragments whereas the label found in the supernatant when incorporation had been stimulated with exogenous DNA, was associated with the bulk DNA as was label when there was no BudR in the nuclear DNA. That the stimulation due to exogenous DNA added to the system is incorporation that occurs outside the nucleus is indicated by results shown in Table 4. That this incorporation appears due primarily to a loosely bound DNA polymerase that can be extracted by low salt and may diffuse out during incubation is indicated by results obtained with nuclei that were extracted with 0.2 M potassium phosphate before they were used in the assay system. This treatment extracts a similar amount of DNA polymerase from host liver and hepatoma nuclei, but a tightly bound activity that can be extracted with 2 M NaCl remains (68). When such nuclei are used, they incorporate label as well as untreated nuclei and the greater incorporation with hepatoma nuclei persists. These nuclei, however, are no longer stimulated by exogenous DNA (68). These partially extracted nuclei showed a preference for pH 9.0 whereas untreated nuclei worked just as well at pH 7.5.

Part of the reason for the short period of linear incorporation found in this system might be due to swelling of the nuclei during incubation. This might conceivably lead to the disruption of a possible replicating complex. It was observed that hepatoma nuclei maintained linear incorporation slightly longer (10 min) than host liver nuclei (5 min). By measuring absorbance at 600 nm it was

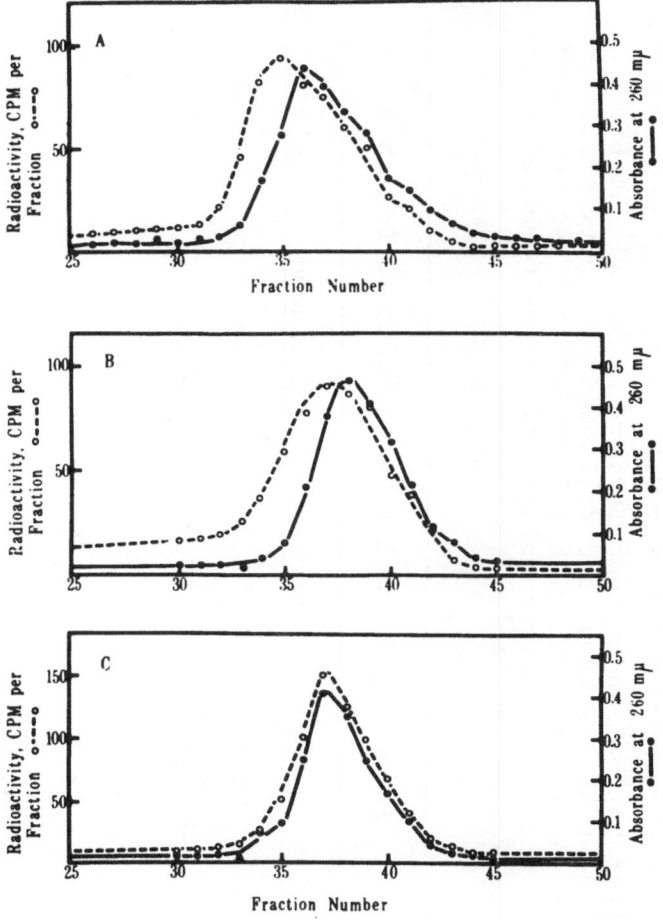

Figure 5
Density gradient analysis of DNA formed <u>in vitro</u> in the nuclear
system. The top of the gradient is to the right. A, nuclei from
incubation without exogenous DNA; B, reisolated nuclei from incubation with exogenous DNA; C, supernatant from incubation with exogenous DNA.

found that the absorbance for host liver nuclei decreased but remained the same for heptoma nuclei after 5 min of incubation (67).
When the density of the incubation medium was changed by the addition of sucrose to a final concentration of 0.8 M, host liver nuclei incorporated more label and linearity of incorporation was
maintained for 10 min. Sucrose had no effect on incorporation with

Table Four

Distribution of Labeled DNA after the
Reisolation of Nuclei

Nuclei were reisolated after incubation by underlaying the 0.5 ml reaction mixture, cooled in ice, with 5 ml 0.34 M sucrose and collected by centrifugation at 1000 xg. The nuclear pellet was washed once with 0.15 M NaCl and recentrifuged. Incorporation was determined in the final nuclear pellet and in the combined supernatants. The incubation mixture was as for Table 3.

Nuclear preparation	Additions	Recovery of labeled DNA (pmoles/mg DNA in 5 min)			
		Nuclei	Supernatant	Total calculated	Total determined
Host liver	None	9.4	1.2	9.6	9.8
Host liver	100 µg denatured DNA	7.9	55.2	63.1	65.0
Host liver	Sucrose	13.3	2.1	15.3	15.4
Hepatoma 7800	None	4.6	2.8	48.1	62.3
Hepatoma 7800	100 µg denatured DNA	44.0	32.2	76.2	84.2
Hepatoma 7777	None	71.0	3.4	74.4	86.2
Hepatoma 7777	100 µg denatured DNA	69.0	41.2	110.2	116.8

hepatoma nuclei as shown in Table 5. The addition of sucrose also prevented a decrease in the absorbance of host liver nuclei after 5 min of incubation.

B.   Triton X-100 Extracted Nuclei

Controversy over a possible regulatory role of the nuclear membrane in DNA synthesis has existed for quite some time and is by no means resolved (16, 17, 19, 25, 38, 39, 42, 48, 56, 57). The preparation of physically intact nuclei with their membrane removed by 2% Triton X-100 treatment was first reported by Aaronson and Blobel (1). Such nuclei, prepared from host liver and from hepatomas, incorporated label in a nuclear incorporating system as shown in Table 6. Despite removal of the membrane, hepatoma nuclei maintain the ability to incorporate more label than liver nuclei. It is also evident that the addition of sucrose does not enhance incorporation in membrane-denuded liver nuclei. This stimulation is the same for host liver and hepatoma nuclei and the difference in incorporation, observed with no exogenous DNA present in the incubation system, is no longer apparent as indicated in Figure 6. That these nuclei can respond to exogenous DNA indicates that the Triton X-100 extraction does not extract all of the loosely bound DNA polymerase from the nuclei and that the loosely bound polymerase activity is not exclusively associated with the nuclear membrane. Reisolation of the membrane-denuded nuclei after [^{3}H]TTP incorporation is completed indicates that the amount of label incorporated due to the exogenous DNA is recovered in the supernatant and is not tightly associated with the nuclei. From these findings it might be concluded that the nuclear membrane does not play an important role in the regulation of DNA synthesis with respect to the observed differences in incorporation with liver and hepatoma nuclei. The possibility that the nuclear pore complexes play an important role cannot be excluded. These nuclei retain 5% of the phospholipid determined for sucrose nuclei. According to Aaronson and Blobel (1) nuclear pore complexes remain tightly bound to the peripheral chromatin after treatment with 2% Triton X-100. We were not able to identify such complexes in our electron micrographs of Triton X-100 extracted nuclei.

CHEMICAL COMPOSITION OF NUCLEI

The biochemical composition of nuclei in general and specifically liver nuclei has been reviewed (10, 11, 22). Considerable work is being done on histones and on non-histone proteins (8, 41, 62, 64). We have been interested in some possible differences in the chemical composition of host liver and hepatoma nuclei. One of our first observations was that hepatoma nuclei contain much more phospholipid than do host liver nuclei (67). This difference in

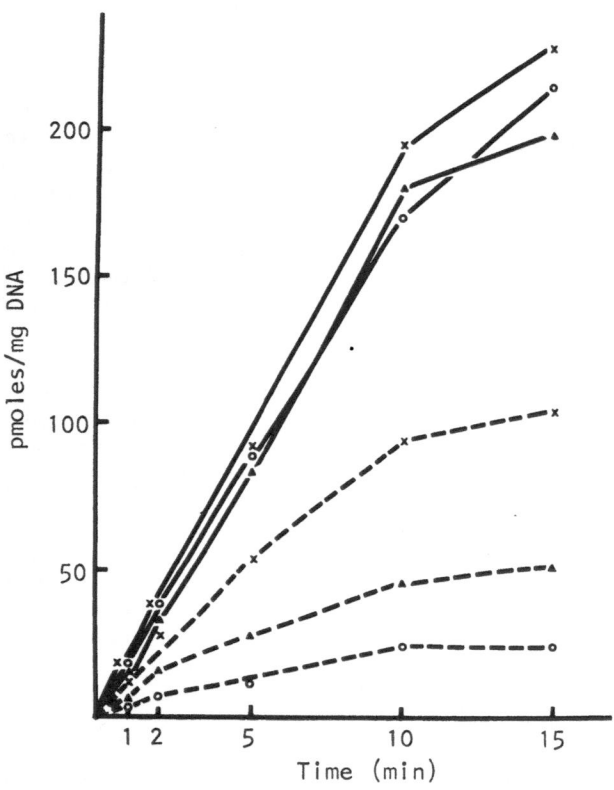

Figure 6
[^{3}H]TTP incorporation into Triton X-100 extracted nuclei with
time. -----, incorporation without the addition of exogenous DNA;
_____, incorporation with 100 μg of calf thymus DNA added per tube.
O, host liver; △, hepatoma 7800, X, hepatoma 7777.

phospholipid content between liver and hepatoma nuclei persists
even when the membranes are removed by Triton X-100 treatment and
only 5% of the total phospholipids found in sucrose nuclei remains.
Some of those phospholipids might of course be associated with nuclear pore complexes that possibly remain attached to the membrane-
denuded nuclei. A considerable amount, however, is found to be
associated with chromatin as indicated when either sucrose or
Triton X-100 extracted nuclei were fractionated (15). A comparison

Table Five

Effect of Sucrose on [³H]TTP Incorporation

The numbers are the averages of 3 different determinations and have been corrected for incorporation with the incomplete system. The complete system is as for Table 3. The final concentration of sucrose was 0.8 M. Individual results did not vary by more than 20%; and incorporation with the incomplete system was about 20% of that of the complete system.

[³H]TTP incorporated (pmoles/mg DNA)

Time of incubation(min)	Host liver		Hepatoma 7800		Hepatoma 7777	
	− sucrose	+ sucrose	− sucrose	+ sucrose	− sucrose	+ sucrose
1	1.5	3.5	9.1	8.7	12.4	11.4
2	2.8	5.5	17.4	16.4	23.8	24.2
4	5.4	12.1	33.4	32.8	51.2	49.6
5	6.4	15.4	40.3	41.1	62.0	58.3
10	7.8	28.3	51.1	49.6	91.0	87.4
15	8.1	28.2	60.0	56.4	110.2	94.3
20	7.9	38.8	59.1	59.5	114.3	107.8

Table Six

Incorporation of [³H]TTP into DNA of Triton X-100 Extracted Nuclei

The complete system is the same as for Table 3. The numbers are the averages from at least 3 different determinations ± S.D. The numbers for hepatoma 16 are from one experiment only.

Complete system	[³H]TTP incorporated (pmoles/mg DNA in 5 min)				
	Host liver	Hepatoma 16	Hepatoma 7800	Hepatoma 7777	
No addition	10.2 ± 1.4	16.4	29.2 ± 3.1	58.4 ± 2.7	
(−) dTP's[a]	4.0 ± 0.8	5.8	10.2 ± 0.6	20.4 ± 4.1	
(−) ATP	8.0 ± 1.0	12.1	18.6 ± 2.6	41.8 ± 3.7	
(+) sucrose (0.8 M final conc)	11.9 ± 1.2	17.2	28.4 ± 2.1	57.6 ± 1.0	
(+) 100 μg native DNA	65.3 ± 3.4	71.3	69.9 ± 4.8	76.2 ± 8.7	
(+) 100 μg "activated" DNA	89.1 ± 8.1	80.4	97.9 ± 2.1	122.9 ± 6.8	

[a]Refers to deoxyadenosine-, deoxycytosine-, and deoxyguanosine triphosphate.

of the phospholipid content in different nuclear preparations from
liver and hepatoma nuclei is shown in Table 7. When the total
phospholipids extracted were separated by thin layer chromatography,
the most dramatic difference was found in sphingomyelin as shown
in Table 8. The fractionation of the nuclei had been described
(15, 83). Fraction 1 seems to represent the inner nuclear envelope, Fraction 2 the outer nuclear envelope, and Fractions 3 and
4 chromatin. The difference in sphingomyelin is primarily found
in the chromatin-associated phospholipids as shown in Table 8.
Histone and acidic nuclear proteins might of course play a major
role in control of DNA synthesis. There are in the literature
some suggestions and there is some evidence that phospholipids
play a role in nuclear events as well. Friedman and Mueller (25)
have reported that a material is associated with replicating DNA
which appears to be a lipopolysaccharide. Mizuno et al, (57)
suggest that newly synthesized DNA at the inner nuclear envelope
is associated with a complex that involves lipoproteins. Others
have shown that the rate of DNA polymerization was depressed when
the DNA template contained phospholipids with a large proportion
of linoleic acid and the enzyme was a DNA ploymerase partially
purified from regenerating rat liver. In the same system, the
rate of polymerization was increased when the template contained
phospholipids with a low distribution of polyunsaturated fatty acids
(29, 30). The association of sphingomyelin with chromatin, specifically with nucleo-histones, has been reported (72, 76, 96). There
is also evidence that sphingomyelin influences the stability of the
DNA double helix (53, 54). Low concentrations of sphingomyelin increase the stability of the double helix and a high concentration
increases the lability. It is possible that high concentrations
of sphingomyelin found associated with chromatin in hepatoma nuclei might make the DNA more accessible to polymerases.

Sialic acid content of sucrose nuclei, fractions of sucrose
nuclei, and of Triton X-100 extracted nuclei has also been determined. Sialic acid was found to be increased in hepatoma nuclei and
the distribution was different in the hepatoma nuclear fractions
from that of host liver nuclear fractions (15, 83). There was a 5-
to 6-fold difference in the amount of sialic acid detectable, depending on whether determinations were made on whole sucrose nuclei
on nuclear fractions. Most likely not all the bound sialic acid
is released when whole nuclei are used. The time of hydrolysis has
to be kept short to prevent extensive hydrolysis of DNA, which inter-
feres with the determination of sialic acid. The values obtained
with nuclear fractions appear to be closer to the true values. An
increase in sialic acid in nuclear membranes of hepatoma 7800 has
been reported (74). At present it is not known what the function of
the sialic acid might be or whether increased levels in hepatoma nuclei are in any way related to a loss of control of growth.

Table Seven

Phospholipid Content of Host Liver and Hepatoma
Nuclei

The procedures for the isolation of citric acid nuclei (83), and chromatin (30) have been described. The Triton extract was precipitated with trichloracetic acid. This precipitate was extracted with chloroform-ethanol as were nuclei. The DNA value for the calculation of the Triton X-100 extract was determined from the extracted nuclei. The values are the averages of the number of determinations indicated in paranthesis ± S.D.

Material extracted	Phospholipid phosphorus (μmoles/mg DNA)			
	Host liver	Hepatoma 7800	Hepatoma 7777	
Sucrose nuclei	0.187 ± 0.02(12)	0.318 ± 0.04(6)	0.507 ± 0.07(12)	
Citric acid nuclei	0.078 ± 0.01(3)	0.124 ± 0.02(3)	0.193 ± 0.02(3)	
Triton X-100 treated nuclei	0.010 ± 0.002(8)	0.016 ± 0.001(3)	0.025 ± 0.003(7)	
Triton X-100 extract	0.133 ± 0.02(4)	0.281 ± 0.03(3)	0.447 ± 0.06(4)	
Chromatin	0.011 ± 0.001(3)	0.017 ± 0.002(3)	0.024 ± 0.003(3)	

Table Eight

Comparison of the Relative Amounts of Different Phospholipids in Host Liver and Hepatoma Nuclear Fractions

Nuclear fractions were prepared from sucrose nuclei as previously described (58). Phospholipid extraction and thinlayer chromatography have been described (83). The numbers represent the results from one determination. Three other determinations for sucrose and Triton X-100 extracted nuclei and a duplicate determination on the nuclear fractions gave similar results.

Fraction	Source	Percent of total extracted phospholipids						
		Origin	LPC[a]	SP	PC	PS+Pi	PE	PGP+PA
Sucrose nuclei	Host liver	0.3	1.9	3.4	51.2	13.9	24.7	4.6
	Hepatoma 7800	0.3	1.7	5.6	48.2	17.1	20.6	6.5
	Hepatoma 7777	0.2	1.9	9.5	48.4	15.6	21.5	2.9
Triton extracted nuclei	Host liver	0	1.2	17.6	34.3	19.1	24.7	3.1
	Hepatoma 7800	0	1.3	22.4	31.9	17.8	23.9	2.7
	Hepatoma 7777	0	1.0	35.7	32.8	13.2	15.1	2.2
Fraction 1	Host liver	0.8	15.5	3.2	48.2	13.5	16.5	2.3
	Hepatoma 7800	0.6	13.8	3.0	46.0	15.6	18.2	2.8
	Hepatoma 7777	0.5	14.7	3.7	47.6	12.6	18.8	2.1
Fraction 2	Host liver	1.0	15.9	2.4	50.9	12.8	15.5	1.5
	Hepatoma 7800	1.5	17.6	4.1	47.1	10.9	17.2	1.6
	Hepatoma 7777	1.0	19.1	7.4	41.8	13.2	15.4	2.1

Table Eight (continued)

Fraction	Source	Origin	Percent of total extracted phospholipids					
			LPC[a]	SP	PC	PS+Pi	PE	PGP+PA
Fraction 3	Host liver	2.7	13.5	2.7	51.7	4.4	21.3	3.7
	Hepatoma 7800	1.9	12.2	6.2	49.4	5.0	22.5	2.8
	Hepatoma 7777	1.3	14.5	8.9	41.1	6.8	23.7	3.7
Fraction 4	Host liver	3.3	15.6	3.6	48.9	5.1	10.2	13.3
	Hepatoma 7800	3.0	16.2	5.2	45.6	4.3	10.8	14.9
	Hepatoma 7777	4.2	14.6	7.1	41.6	6.4	8.1	18.0

[a] LPC, lysophosphatidyl choline; SP, spingomyelin; PC, phosphatidyl choline; PS, phosphatidyl serine; PI, phosphatidyl inositol; PE, phosphatidyl ethanolamine; PGP, poly-glycero phosphatide; PA, phosphatidic acid.

The distribution of labeled DNA in nuclear fractions after a
10 min pulse of an animal with [^{3}H] thymidine and DNA polymerase
activity in the nuclear fractions from host liver and hepatoma 7777
are shown in Table 9. It can be calculated that 82% of the counts
in host liver nuclear fractions and 77% of the counts in the hepatoma 7777 nuclear fractions were found in Fractions 3 and 4. After
a 5 min pulse no counts were found in Fractions 1 and 2. Evidence
obtained with Triton X-100 extracted nuclei in a nuclear-incorporat-
ing system, with the distribution of in vivo labeled DNA in nuclear
fractions, and with the DNA polymerase activity in these fractions
suggests that the difference in DNA synthesis found between host
liver and hepatomas depends at least in part on the physical or
chemical architecture within the nucleus. Some recent reports
suggest that a protein matrix or lamina does exist in the nucleus.

Berezney and Coffey (5, 6) have isolated a nuclear protein
matrix, 98% protein and essentially free of nucleic acids and
phsopholipid. This structure, 12% of the total nuclear protein, is
associated with newly synthesized DNA and regenerating rat liver.
After a 1 minute pulse, more than 90% of the label in nuclear DNA
is associated with the matrix DNA which comprises only 25% of the
total nuclear DNA. This protein matrix is composed primarily of
3 acidic polypeptide fractions with a molecular weight range of
60-70,000 daltons.

Hodge et al. (36) have isolated a subnuclear fraction from
HeLa cells, similar to the nuclear protein matrix of rat liver nuclei with some membraneous components, possibly portions of the
inner nuclear membrane. The phospholipid content was higher in
these structures, but with nucleic acid content only slightly higher
than rat liver nuclear matrices. Gel electrophoresis of the proteins
showed 6 polypeptide bands with 3 being very prominent in the above
mentioned molecular weight range. The polypeptide composition appears to vary with the life cycle of the cell and after infection
with adenovirus.

Nonmembraneous nuclear ghosts isolated from interphase HeLa
cells (43, 47) have been shown to contain annular and rodlike structures interconnected by strands that are sensitive to deoxyribonu-
clease. The isolated nuclear ghost proteins are also composed of
3 major polypeptide bands in the 65-68,000 molecular weight range,
a low molecular weight band and a few of intermediate molecular
weight.

Another nuclear subfraction, the nuclear pore-lamina complex
has been isolated from rat liver nuclei (2) and contains little or
no DNA, RNA or phospholipid. Gel electrophoretic patterns of the
proteins show 3 major and several minor polypeptide bands consistent
with gel patterns reported above (5, 6, 36, 43, 77).

Table Nine

Incorporation of [³H]thymidine and [³H]TTP into Nuclear Fractions

For [³H]thymidine incorporation, a tumor-bearing animal was given an injection of 100 μCi[³H]thymidine per 100 g and tissues were removed 10 min later for preparation of nuclei and nuclear fractions. Nuclear fractions were prepared as described in Table 8. For [³H]TTP incorporation nuclear fractions were prepared and assayed without any additional DNA. The reaction mixture contained 50 μmoles buffer (tris-HCl, pH 7.5 or glycine-NaOH, pH 9.0); 2 μmoles $MgCl_2$; 4 μmoles 2-mercaptoethanol; 0.04 μmole each dATP, dCTP, and dGTP; 0.02 μmole [³H]TTP (50 μCi/μmole), and 20-100 μg protein from nuclear fractions. Counting efficiency was 25%. The numbers are the averages of 3 determinations ± S.D.

Nuclear fraction	Incorporation of [³H]thymidine in vivo cpm/mg protein	Incorporation of [³H]TTP into nuclear fractions pH 7.5 cpm/mg protein	pH 9.0
Host liver			
F 1	17 ± 5	2160 ± 300	650 ± 43
F 2	32 ± 4	1850 ± 95	630 ± 38
F 3	145 ± 21	1260 ± 131	2110 ± 96
F 4	77 ± 15	850 ± 72	4880 ± 318
Hepatoma 7777			
F 1	122 ± 11	2240 ± 191	880 ± 104
F 2	178 ± 32	2370 ± 152	720 ± 81
F 3	480 ± 19	1130 ± 210	2500 ± 196

The presence of such a residual protein structure after various methods of isolation, the likelihood that it is a basic structural component of the nucleus and its association with newly synthesized DNA suggests that it may play a role in DNA replication. Precisely what role remains to be established.

OTHER APPLICATIONS FOR THE NUCLEAR INCORPORATING SYSTEM

Using nuclei from host liver or normal liver and from hepatomas we have applied the nuclear incorporating system to investigate the action of some antitumor agents. The systems might be useful to screen potential antitumor drugs in the future. So far we have looked specifically at the effect of bleomycin on [3H]TTP incorporation into host liver and hepatoma nuclei. It has been reported that liver nuclei were stimulated to take up [3H]TTP in the presence of bleomycin. This incorporation appears to be different from the regular incorporation into nuclei which is linear for a short time. Bleomycin-induced incorporation continued linearly for at least 30 min and was not inhibited by cytosine arabinoside. It was suggested that bleomycin might stimulate repair activity in the nuclei (80).

We found that hepatoma nuclei were also stimulated by the addition of bleomycin but to a far lesser extent than host liver nuclei. The increase in [3H]TTP incorporation during a 20 min incubation due to bleomycin was 12-fold for host liver nuclei, 7.5-fold for hepatoma 7800 nuclei, but only 3.3-fold for hepatoma 7777 nuclei. The possibility that differences in the nuclear membrane might be responsible for the different response of host liver and hepatoma nuclei to stimulation by bleomycin led us to investigate the effect of bleomycin on membrane-denuded nuclei. The results in Table 10 indicate that removal of the nuclear membrane did not affect the level of bleomycin-induced stimulation of [3H]TTP incorporation. By using [111In] bleomycin it was further shown that binding of bleomycin occurred equally well to the chromatin of host liver and hepatoma nuclei. The relatively smaller response of hepatoma nuclei as compared to liver nuclei, to stimulation of [3H]TTP incorporation into newly isolated nuclei. Reaction mixtures from either nuclear preparation supported incorporation similarly. Extraction of DNA from host liver or hepatoma nuclei exposed to bleomycin and analysis of this DNA on alkaline sucrose density gradients showed that bleomycin had caused breaks in the DNA and those breaks were about the same for host liver or hepatoma nuclear DNA as shown in Figures 7 and 8. DNA from bleomycin-treated nuclei was also analyzed on neutral sucrose density gradients. This analysis also indicated that bleomycin induced scissions in the DNA. When bleomycin was removed after a short period of incubation by reisolating the nuclei, and the nuclei were resuspended in bleomycin-free reaction mixtures, repair of DNA scissions could be demonstrated (84). This repair activity was more prominent in host liver nuclei than in hepatoma nuclei. Evidence

Table Ten

Effect of Bleomycin on [³H]TTP Incorporation into Triton X-100–Extracted Nuclei

Conditions for incubation were the same as in Table 3 except for indicated times of incubation. Where indicated the concentration of bleomycin was 1 mg/ml. The numbers are the averages from 2 experiments. Individual numbers did not vary by more than 15% from the average.

Incubation time (min)	Host liver			Hepatoma 7800			Hepatoma 7777		
	Control	Bleomycin	B:C	Control	Bleomycin	B:C	Control	Bleomycin	B:C
2.5	4.9	27.4	5.6	15.2	47.1	3.1	28.7	34.4	1.2
5	9.5	62.1	6.5	28.3	130.2	4.6	58.5	73.1	1.2
10	12.1	142.8	11.8	36.1	223.8	6.2	71.9	144.0	2.0
20	11.9	182.0	15.3	37.2	275.3	7.4	74.8	269.3	3.6

[3H]TTP incorporation (pmoles/mg DNA)

suggesting that the relatively modest response of hepatoma nuclei to bleomycin stimulation might be due to lower levels or activities of repair enzymes in hepatoma nuclei was obtained by using bleomycin-treated template DNA and extracted crude DNA polymerase preparations from host liver and hepatoma tissue (84).

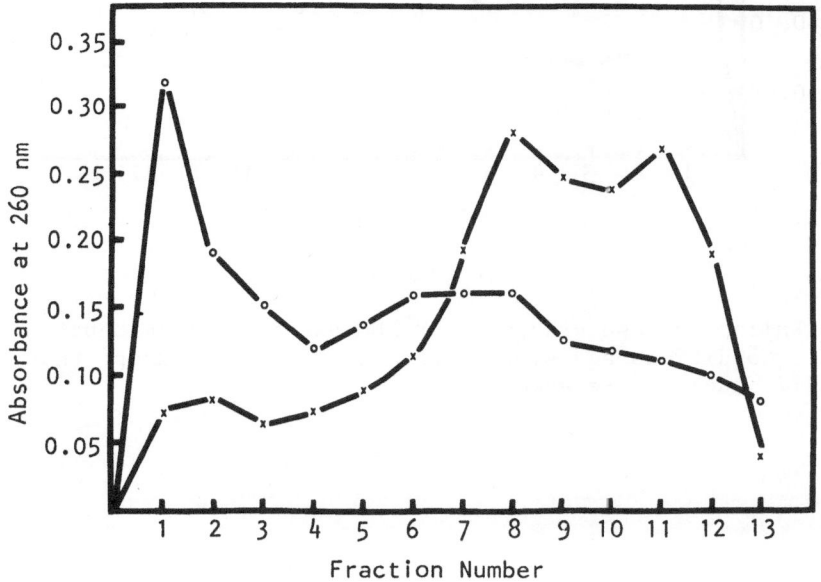

Figure 7

Alkaline sucrose gradients of DNA extracted from liver nuclei. Three to 4 absorbance units of DNA were layered on 5-20% sucrose gradients. Gradients were centrifuged in a SW50L rotor at 25,000 rpm for 18.5 hours. The bottom of the tube is to the left. O, in-cubated without bleomycin in 1.0 ml reaction mixture for 10 min.

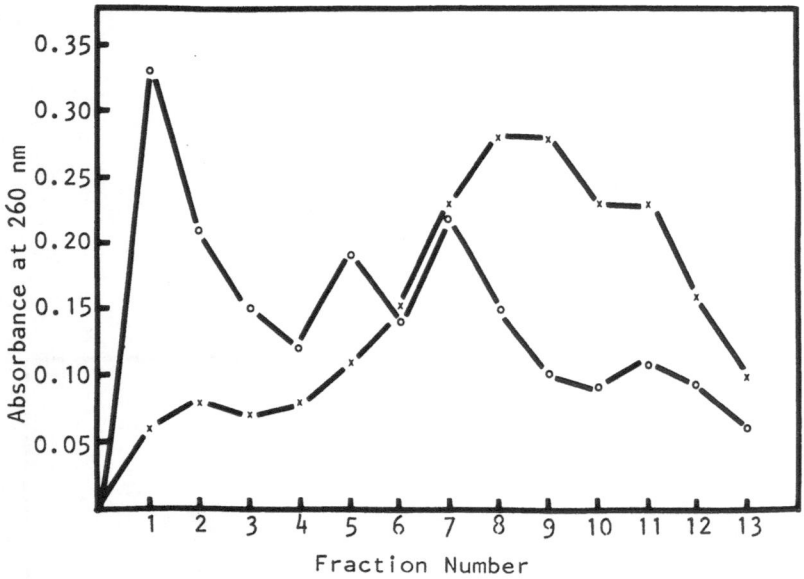

Figure 8

Alkaline sucrose gradients of DNA extracted from hepatoma 7777 nuclei. Conditions and symbols were as for Fig 7 except that hepatoma 7777 nuclei were used.

The action of bleomycin is dependent on the presence of sulfhydryl agents in the incubation mixture (14, 60, 61, 91). Two compounds, N-ethyl maleimide and daunomycin, inhibit the bleomycin-induced incorporation of [3H]TTP preferentially. N-ethyl maleimide inhibits bleomycin-induced activity in liver and hepatoma 7777 nuclei equally. Lower levels of daunomycin inhibit the bleomycin-induced activity in hepatoma 7777 nuclei than are required to inhibit the activity in the liver nuclei. The two compounds inhibit the bleomycin effect by different mechanisms. The addition of N-ethyl maleimide acts by binding to the DNA and by competing with a sulfhydryl agent for bleomycin-sensitive sites on the DNA. Daunomycin apparently inhibits a repair enzyme that is responsible for increased incorporation following bleomycin treatment. Another compound used as an antitumor agent, camptothecin, stimulates bleomycin-induced [^{3}H]TTP incorporation even further. Sucrose density gradients indicated that camptothecin caused additional DNA strand scissions to those produced by bleomycin. Camptothecin alone produced some single strand but no double strand scissions. It was found that camptothecin could partially substitute for sulfhydryl reducing agents. A combination of camptothecin and bleomycin with a sulfhydryl reducing agent absent from the incubation mixture did cause some DNA strand scissions.

The effect of a compound related to bleomycin, phleomycin, on [^{3}H]TTP incorporation into nuclei from a number of mammalian cell lines was investigated by Friedman et al. (26). They also found a stimulation of [^{3}H]TTP incorporation. There was a small response in nuclei from normal diploid cells and a large response in some tumor cell lines. These findings are opposite from those made with host liver and hepatoma nuclei. At present there is no good explanation for this discrepancy. Cells in culture, however, whatever their origin, must make certain adaptive changes to survive in a cell culture environment. Induction of certain enzymes might be one of those changes. Should the postulate be correct, that increased incorporation of [^{3}H]TTP following exposure to bleomycin is due to repair, the system might be useful in chemotherapy. The effect of bleomycin might be enhanced by the addition of daunomycin or adriamycin, which acts identically to daunomycin. It has been shown by several investigators that bleomycin-caused breaks in DNA are repaired in mammalian cells (78, 79, 84, 88). The addition of daunomycin or adriamycin would prevent such repair. Since hepatoma nuclei are more sensitive to repair inhibition by those drugs, it should be possible to use levels that might not inhibit repair in the host cells, thus causing a more selective effect of bleomycin on hepatoma cells.

INTERPRETATION

At present much needs to be learned about regulation of DNA synthesis in mammalian cells. The enzymes involved in DNA replication in eukaryotic cells have not been fully identified and characterized. Initiation sites and their availability at certain periods of the cell cycle have not been characterized. Are there humoral or

cytoplasmic factors involved in some regulatory steps? Is there a
skeletal framework or a matrix on which chromosomes are organized?
How is the double helix separated to allow for copying of the
individual strands? These and many more are questions that await
further elucidation.

The nuclear incorporating system might be useful in obtaining
answers to some of these questions concerned with the basic mechanism
of regulation of DNA replication. By comparing host liver and hepatoma nuclei in such a system it might be possible to identify one
or more steps of the regulatory mechanism that are responsible for
uncontrolled replication and growth of malignant cells.

To provide reasonably good evidence for the involvement of
components in a replicating complex, it will be necessary to separate
some of these components and show by reconstitution which are necessary and at what stage of DNA replication. The nucleus can be
considered such a replicating complex. By comparing sucrose nuclei
with membrane-denuded nuclei, the role of one of the components, the
nuclear envelope has been shown to be of minor importance in regulation of nuclear DNA synthesis. By extracting chromatin, histones
and acidic nuclear proteins under different conditions, and by analyzing any remaining components it should be possible to identify further
components and their role in control of DNA synthesis.

Neoplastic transformation might bring about the production or
alteration of components which reside in the cytoplasm or circulate
in the blood. Neoplastic transformation might also cause changes in
the cell which remove it from control of humoral or cytoplasmic factors that control proliferation in normal cells. The concept that
extranuclear components, cytoplasmic or extracellular, may play a
role in the control of DNA synthesis is based on a variety of observations. A system for DNA replication using HeLa cell nuclei has
been shown to require a cytoplasmic factor (24). In amphibian em-
bryos, nuclei from late embryonic stages which do not show appreciable DNA synthesis, incorporate labeled thymidine within 90 minutes
after transplantation into enucleated egg cytoplasm (31). A similar
effect has been shown in Amoeba (75). The presence and possible importance of humoral factors in the control of DNA synthesis with cross-
circulation of potentially hepatectomized rats is suggested (59). It
is suggested that virally transformed mouse fibroblasts need a serum
factor for growth that is distinct from the factor used by non-transformed cells (37, 73). A serum protein decreases in tumor-bearing
animals as the tumor increases in size (69). This serum protein
stimulates DNA synthesis in isolated membrane-denuded nuclei from
Morris hepatoma 7777 (13). An ammonium sulfate fraction from Novikoff
hepatoma cells has been reported to stimulate DNA polymerase activity
(85). The nuclear incorporating system might be used to investigate
the effect of cytoplasmic or humoral factors from host liver or normal

animals on the nuclear incorporating system derived from hepatomas. The reverse situation, cytoplasmic or humoral factors from hepatoma or hepatoma-bearing animals on the nuclear incorporating system derived from rat liver can also be investigated.

Isolated nuclei appear to continue certain activities with respect to DNA synthesis that were operative in vivo. These events can be studied in an environment removed from the physioloical influences of the organism and from the cytoplasmic influences of the whole cell. At the same time physical or chemical disruptions can be kept to a minimum. It seems reasonable to expect that further studies of this system will result in some answers to the important events in regulation of DNA synthesis and neoplastic transformation.

REFERENCES

1. Aaronson, R.P., and Blobel, G., J. Cell Biol., 62 (1974) 746.

2. Aaronson, R.P., and Blobel, G., Proc. Nat. Acad. Sci. USA, 72 (1975) 1007.

3. Baril, E.F., Jenkins, M.D., Brown, O.E., Laszlo, J., and Morris, H.P., Cancer Res., 33 (1973) 1187.

4. Behrens, M., Hoppe Syler's Z. Physiol. Chem., 209 (1932) 59.

5. Berezney, R., and Coffey, D.S., Science, 189 (1975) 291.

7. Bollum, F.J., Prog. Nuc. Acid Res. Mol. Biol., 15 (1975) 109.

8. Bradbury, E.M., Curr. Top. Dev. Biol., 9 (1975) 1.

9. Burtin, K., Methods Enzymol., 12B (1968) 163.

10. Busch, H. (ed.), The Cell Nucleus, Vol I (1974) Academic Press, N.Y., 1.

11. Busch, H. (ed.), The Cell Nucleus, Vol III (1974) Academic Press, N.Y., 1.

12. Chiu, J-F., Craddock, C., Morris, H.P., and Hnilica, L.S., Cancer Biochem. Biophys., 1 (1974) 13.

13. Coetzee, M.L., Dolan, M.L., and Ove, P., Oncology, 32 (1975) 38.

14. Coetzee, M.L., Sartiano, G.P., Klein, K., and Ove, P., J. Antibiotics, in press (1977).

15. Coetzee, M.L., Spnagler, M., Morris, H.P., and Ove, P., Cancer Res., 35 (1975) 2752.

16. Comings, D., and Kakefuda, T., J. Mol. Biol. 33 (1968) 225.

17. Deumling, B., and Franke, W.W., Hoppe Seyler's Z. Physiol. Chem., 353 (1972) 287.

18. Dounce, A.L., Exptl. Cell Res., Suppl. 9 (1963) 126.

19. Fakan, S., Turner, G.N., Pagano, J.S., and Hancock, R., Proc. Nat. Acad. Sci. USA, 69 (1972) 2300.

20. Fansler, B.S., Int. Rev. Cytol., Suppl.4 (1974) 363.

21. Foster, D.N., and Gurney, T.J., Biol. Chem., 251 (1976) 7893.

22. Franke, W.W., Int. Rev. Cytol., Suppl. 4 (1974) 72.

23. Friedman, D.L., Biochim. Biophys. Acta, 353 (1974) 447.

24. Friedman, D.L., and Mueller, G.C., Biochim. Biophys. Acta, 161 (1968) 455.

25. Friedman, D.L., and Mueller, G.C., Biochim. Biophys. Acta, 174 (1969) 253.

26. Friedman, R.M., Stern, R., and Rose, J.A., J. Natl. Cancer Inst., 52 (1974) 693.

27. Garland, R.C., and Cori, C.F., Biochem., 11 (1972) 4712.

28. Glew, R.H., Kayman, S.C., and Kuhlenschmidt, M.S., J. Biol. Chem., 248 (1973) 3137.

29. Goureau, M.F., and Raulin, J., Bull. Soc. Chim. Biol., 52 (1970) 941.

30. Goureau, M.F., Fichot, O., Raulin, J., and DeRecondo, A.M., Physiol. Chem. Physics, 6 (1974) 379.

31. Graham, C.F., Arms, K., and Gurdon, J.B., Devel. Biol., 14 (1966) 349.

32. Grisham, J.W., Kaufman, D.G., and Stenstrom, M.L., Biochem. Biophys. Res. Commun., 49 (1972) 420.

33. Gurr, M.L., Finean, J.B., and Hawthorne, J.N., Biochim. Biophys. Acta, 70 (1963) 406.

34. Hershey, H.V., Stieber, J.F., and Mueller, G.C., Eur. J. Biochem., 34 (1973) 383.

35. Hershey, H.W., and Taylor, J.H., Exper. Cell Res., 94 (1975) 339.

36. Hodge, L.D., Mancini, P., Davis, F.M., and Heywood, P.J. Cell Biol., 72 (1977) 194.

37. Holley, R.W., and Kiernan, J.A., In: G.E.W. Wolstenholme and J. Knight (eds.), Growth Control in Cell Cultures, Churchill Livingstone, London, (1971) 33.

38. Huberman, A.A., Firshein, W., Hobart, P., and Murray, L., Biochemistry, 15 (1976) 4810.

39. Infante, A.A., Firshein, W., Hobart, P., and Murray, L., Biochemistry 15 (1976) 4810.

40. Iwamura, Y., Ono, T., and Morris, H.P., Cancer Res., 28 (1968) 2466.

41. Johnson, J.D., Douvas, A.S., and Bonner, J., Int. Rev. Cyt., Suppl. 4 (1974) 273.

42. Kay, R.R., Fraser, D., and Johnston, I.R., Eur. J. Biochem., 30 (1972) 145.

43. Keller, J.M., and Riley, D.E., Science, 193 (1976) 399.

44. Kemper, B.W., Pratt, W.B., and Aronow, L., Mol. Pharmacol., 5 (1969) 507.

45. Kidwell, W.R., and Mueller, G.C., Biochem. Biophys. Res. Commun., 36 (1969) 756.

46. Kirsch, W.M., Leitner, J.W., Gainey, M., Schulz, D., Lasher, R., and Nakane, P., Science, 168 (1970) 1592.

47. Lagunoff, D., Exptl. Cell Res., 55 (1969) 53.

48. Levis, A.G., Krsmanovic, V., Miller-Faures, A., and Errera, M., Eur. J. Biochem., 3 (1967) 57.

49. Loeb, L.A., In: P.D. Boyer (ed.), The Enzymes, Vol 10, Academic Press, N.Y., (1974) 173.

50. Lowry, O.H., Rosebrough, N.J., Farr, A.L., and Randall, R.J., J. Biol. Chem., 193 (1951) 265.

51. Lynch, W.E., Brown, R.F., Umeda, T., Langreth, S.G., and Lieberman, I., J. Biol. Chem., 245 (1970) 3911.

52. Lynch, W.E., and Lieberman, I., Biochem, Biophys,
     Res. Commun., 52 (1973) 843.

53. Manzoli, F.A., Muchmore, J.H., Bonora, B., Capitani,
     S., and Bartoli, S., Biochim. Biophys. Acta, 340
     (1974) 1.

54. Manzoli, F.A., Muchmore, J.H., Bonora, B., Sabioni,
     A., and Stefoni, S., Biochim. Biophys. Acta, 277
     (1972) 251.

55. Mejbaum, W., Physiol. Che., 258 (1939) 117.

56. Mizuno, N.A., Stoops, C.E., and Sinha, A.A., Nature
     New Biol., 229 (1971) 22.

58. Monneron, A., Blobel, G., and Palade, G.E., J. Cell
     Biol., 55 (1972) 104.

59. Moolten, F.L., and Bucher, N.L.R., Science, 158
     (1967) 272.

60. Nagai, K., Suzuki, H., Tanaka, N., and Umezawa, H.,
     J. Antibiotics Tokyo Ser. A., 22 (1969) 569.

61. Nagai, K., Yamaki, H., Suzuki, H., Tanaka, N., and
     Umezawa, H., Biochim. Biophys. Acta, 179 (1969) 165.

62. Olson, M.O.J., and Busch, H., In: H. Busch (ed.),
     The Cell Nucleus, Vol. III Academic Press, N.Y.,
     (1974) 212.

63. Ono, T., and Umehara, Y., Gann, 6 (1968) 99.

64. Ord, M.G., and Stocken, L.A., In: Antoni, F., and
     Farago, A. (eds.), Post Synthetic Modification of
     Macromolecules, Elsevier: Amsterdam (1975) 113.

65. Otnaess, A-B., Krokan, H., Bjørkld, E., and Prydz,
     H., Biochim. Biophys. Acta, 454 (1976) 193.

66. Ove, P., Brown, O.E., and Laszlo, J., Cancer Res.,
     29 (1969) 1562.

67. Ove, P., Coetzee, M.L., and Morris, H.P., Cancer
     Res., 31 (1971) 1389.

68. Ove, P., Coetzee, M.L., and Morris, H.P., Cancer
     Res., 33 (1973) 1272.

69. Ove, P., Coetzee, M.L., Obenrader, M., and Short,
     J., Oncology, 29 (1974) 13.

70. Ove, P., Laszlo, J., Jenkins, M.D., and Morris, H.P.,
     Cancer Res., 29 (1969) 1557.

71. Ove, P., Takai, S., Umeda, T., and Lieberman, I.,
     J. Biol. Chem., 242 (1967) 4963.

72. Pardon, J.F., and Wilkins, M.H.F., J. Mol. Biol.,
     68 (1972) 115.

73. Paul, D., Lipton, A., and Klinger, I., Proc. Natl.
     Acad. Sci. U.S., 68 (1971) 645.

74. Phillips, J.L., Arch. Biochem. Biophys., 156 (1973)
     377.

75. Prescott, D.M., and Goldstein,L., Science, 155 (1970)
     469.

76. Richards, B.M., and Pardon, J.F., Exptl. Cell Res.,
     62 (1970) 184.

77. Riley, D.E., Keller, J.M., and Byers, B., Biochemist-
     ry, 14 (1975) 3005.

78. Saito, M., and Andoh, T., Cancer Res., 33 (1973)1696.

79. Sartiano, G.P., Coetzeee, M.L., Klein, K., and Ove,
     P., J. Natl. Cancer Inst., in press (1977).

80. Sartiano, G.P., Lynch, W., Boggs, S.S., and Neil,
     G.L., Proc. Soc. Exper. Biol. Med., 150 (1975) 718.

81. Siebert, G. von, Z. Kliniscge Chemie, 4 (1966) 93.

82. Spadari, S., and Weissbach, A., J. Biol. Chem.,
     249 (1974) 5809.

83. Spangler, M., Coetzee, M.L., Katyal, S.L., Morris,
     H.P., and Ove, P., Cancer Res., 35 (1975) 3131.

84. Spangler, M., Sartiano, G.P., Coetzee, M.L., and
     Ove, P., Cancer Res., 36 (1976) 1339.

85. Stalker, D.M., Probst, G.S., Mosbaugh, D.M., Kunkel,
     T.A., and Meyer, R.R., J. Cell Biol. 63 (1974) 332a.

86.   Stenstrom, M.L., Edelstein, M., and Grisham, J.W.,
      Exptl. Cell Res., 89 (1974) 439.

87.   Stuart, S.E., Clawson, G.A., Rottman, F.M., and
      Patterson, R.J., J. Cell Biol., 72 (1977) 57.

88.   Terasima, T., Yasukawa, M., and Umezawa, H., Gann,
      61 (1970) 513.

89.   Thompson, L.R., and McCarthy, B.J., Biochem. Biophys.
      Res. Commun., 30 (1968) 166.

90.   Thompson, L.R., and Mueller, G.C., Biochim. Biophys.
      Acta, 378 (1975) 344.

91.   Umezawa, H., Biomedicine, 18 (1973) 459.

92.   Weber, G., In: H. Busch (ed.), The Molecular Bio-
      logy of Cancer, Academic Press, New York (1974) 487.

93.   Weissbach, A., Cell 5 (1975) 101.

94.   Widnell, C.C., J. Cell Biol., 52 (1972) 542.

95.   Widnell, C.C., Methods Enzymol., 32 (1974) 368.

96.   Wilkins, M.H.F., Zubay, G., and Wilson, H.R., J.
      Mol. Biol., 1 (1959) 179.

DNA–DEPENDENT RNA POLYMERASES FROM MORRIS HEPATOMAS 3924A AND 7800 AND FROM LIVER TREATED WITH THIOACETAMIDE

Samson T. Jacob, Kathleen M. Rose, Thomas B. Leonard and
Barry W. Duceman

Department of Pharmacology and Specialized Cancer
Research Center
The Milton S. Hershey Medical Center
The Pennsylvania State University, Hershey, PA. 17033

SUMMARY

Nuclear DNA-dependent RNA polymerases were extracted from
Morris hepatomas 3924A and 7800, thioacetamide-treated liver and
normal rat liver. The enzymes were fractionated chromatographically. The levels of nucleolar RNA polymerases, particularly IB, were
several fold higher in the tmors and thioacetamide-treated liver
than in normal liver. The ratios of I/II in liver, thioacetamide-
treated liver, Morris hepatoma 7800 and 3924A were 0.29, 0.58, 0.70
and 6.9, respectively. Detailed investigations on the enzymes derived from thioacetamide-treated liver showed that the increase in
the levels of RNA polymerase was specific to the transcriptionally
active, chromatin-associated form of IB. The available data suggest that the increase in the levels of RNA polymerases IA and IB
is largely due to augmented quantities of enzyme protein. These
studies show that the observed rise in the levels of nucleolar RNA
polymerases is directly related to the degree of neoplasia and suggest that this phenomenon might be one of the early biochemical
events which eventually lead to tumorigenesis.

Unlike RNA polymerase from prokaryotes, the enzyme from eukaryotes exists as multiple species. They are designated as class I
(or A), class II (or B) and class III (or C) enzymes. Class I enzymes (IA and IB) are localized in the nucleolus and are involved
in the synthesis of ribosomal RNA. Class II (IIA, IIB, IIo) and
class III (IIIA, IIIB, IIIo) enzymes are confined to the nucleoplasmic (extranucleolar) compartment. Class I enzymes are believed
to play a role in the synthesis of mRNA, whereas class III enzymes
are involved in the synthesis of 5S and tRNA as well as some of the

273

low molecular weight nuclear RNA species (27). Nucleolar RNA polymerases are generally insensitive to the mushroom toxin α-amanitin.
On the other hand, the nucleoplasmic enzymes II and III are sensi-
tive to low (10^{-9}-10^{-8} M)(14, 15, 18, 20) and high (10^{-5}-10^{-4}M) concentrations (28) of the toxin, respectively. The three classes of
RNA ploymerases are also different with respect to the size of at
least one large subunit (22). Finally, these enzymes bind to and
transcribe different regions of the chromatin. (For general review
on mammalian RNA polymerases, see. ref. 4, 11, 13).

Despite enormous progress made in the characterization of RNA
p olymerases from normal cells, investigations on these enzymes in
cancer cells are relatively few. The major drawback of studies on
RNA polymerases from tumor cells is the lack of the proper control
normal cells for comparison. We have resolved this problem by taking advantage of the availability of Morris hepatomas with different
growth rates and using liver as control tissue. This chapter deals
with the extraction, purification and properties of nuclear DNA-
dependent RNA polymerases from two Morris hepatomas, 3923A and 7800.
Most of the studies were performed on the former tumor strain, a
poorly differentiated, rapidly growing tumor. Concurrently, the
effect of thioacetamide, a hepatocarcinogen, on RNA polymerases was
investigated in order to examine whether the alterations in the
characteristics of RNA polymerases observed in the hepatomas are induced in the early stages of tumorigenesis.

I.   Extraction of RNA Polymerases from Morris hepatomas 3924A and
     7800

     a) Isolation of nuclei

     Quantitative extraction of RNA polymerases from the hepatomas
depended on proper isolation of the nuclei. Although direct homogenization of the tissue in hypertonic sucrose followed by centrifugation resulted in good recovery of nuclei, they were contaminated
with membranous materials which interfered with the subsequent solubilization of RNA polymerase. Large quantities of lipids associated
with these contaminants not only prevented quantitative extraction
of the enzyme, but also caused problems in column chromatographic
fractionations. Three major modifications were made (24) of the
method originally devised for the isolation of liver nuclei (15).
First, the concentration of sucrose was reduced to 2.0 M in order to
achieve maximal recovery of the nuclei. Second, the $MgCl_2$ concentration was reduced from 10-15 mM to 3.3 mM; this was found necessary
to minimize overall contamination with cytoplasmic materials and to
achieve satisfactory nuclear breakage during the subsequent sonica-
tion step. Third, the nuclear pellet obtained after the initial homogenization was washed briefly with 0.3% (v/v) Triton X-100; this
treatment removed the membranous material and other cytoplasmic con-

taminants. This procedure gave high recovery of the tumor nuclei with little or no loss of enzyme activity.

Liver nuclei were isolated as described previously (15) using 2.2-2.3 M sucrose containing 15 $MgCl_2$ and 0.25 mM spermine for initial homogenization of the tissue. The liver nuclear pellet was used as such for extraction of RNA polymerase.

b) Extraction of RNA polymerases

RNA polymerases were extracted from liver and hepatoma nuclei as described previously (23, 24). The nuclei were homogenized in buffer (1 ml/g wet weight of tissue) consisting of 50 mM Tris-HCl (pH 8.9), 1 mM $MgCl_2$, 0.1 mM EDTA, 2 mM dithiothreitol, 50 mM KCl, 0.5 mM phenylmethylsulfonylfluoride and 40% (v/v) glycerol. The homogenate was sonicated at full output in a Branson Sonifier (approximately 90 sec and 60 sec for tumor and liver nuclei, respectively, monitoring the nuclear breakage). The suspension was diluted to 20% (v/v) glycerol by addition of the solubilization buffer without glycerol and the enzyme was precipitated by slowly adding solid $(NH_4)_2SO_4$ (0.42 g/ml). After stirring for 1 hr, the suspension was centrifuged at high speed and the precipitate thus obtained was suspended (1 ml/g tumor and 0.5 ml/g liver) in 50 mM Tris-HCl buffer (pH 7.9) containing 25% (v/v) glycerol, 5 mM $MgCl_2$, 0.1 mM EDTA and 0.5 mM dithiothreitol (TGMED buffer). The suspension was dialyzed against TGMED buffer and centrifuged at 80,000 x g for 40 min. The supernatant was saved. The pellet was resuspended in the same buffer, sonicated for 30 sec and recentrifuged again. The combined supernatants from the two centrifugations were pooled and subjected to DEAE-Sephedex chromatography. This procedure achieved maximal recovery of RNA polymerases. No detectable enzyme activity was observed in the final residue. It should be noted that the bulk of the enzyme was released from liver nuclei in the very first extraction.

c) Purification of RNA polymerases I and II

Unlike other mammalian RNA polymerases, RNA polymerases from hepatoma 3924A were not resolved by a single DEAE-Sephadex chromatography. In fact, at least three chromatographic fractionations were required for complete separation of IA, IB and II. The following sequence of chromatographic steps was employed (Fig 1). Although liver enzymes could easily be separated by a single DEAE-Sephadex chromatography, RNA polymerases from the hepatoma and liver were purified using similar sequences of chromatographic fractionations (Figs 2 and 3). Since the DNA content in the nuclei isolated from the hepatoma was twice that in the liver nuclei, only half as much tumor tissue as liver was used for enzyme extraction. Approximately 100 g of the hepatoma 3924A and 200 g of liver were used for extensive purifica-

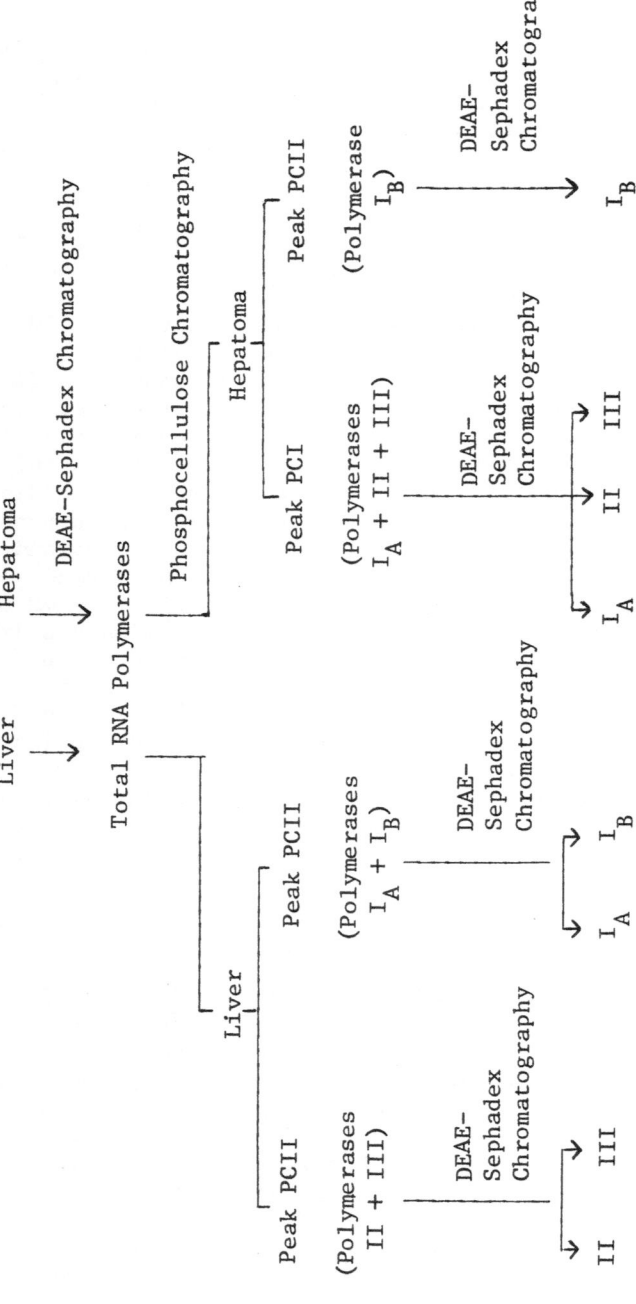

Figure 1

Scheme for the chromatographic fractionation of RNA polymerases from large quantities of liver and hepatomas

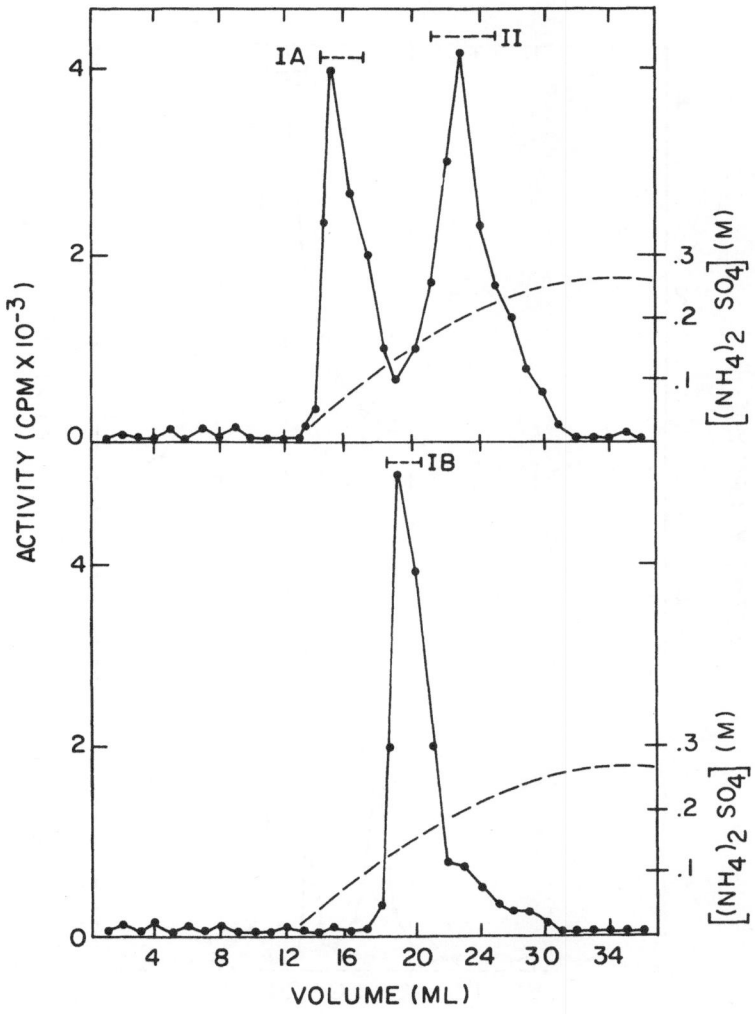

Figure 2
Fractionation of RNA polymerases from Morris hepatoma 3924A.
Enzyme (total RNA polymerases) recovered from the 350 mM $(NH_4)_2SO_4$
elution of the first DEAE-Spehadex column was subjected to phospho-
cellulose column chromatography using a linear (0-0.4 M) $(NH_4)_2SO_4$
gradient. Two peaks of enzyme activity were resolved, which were
then fractionated on a second DEAE-Sephadex column. RNA polymerases
were assayed as described previously (24).

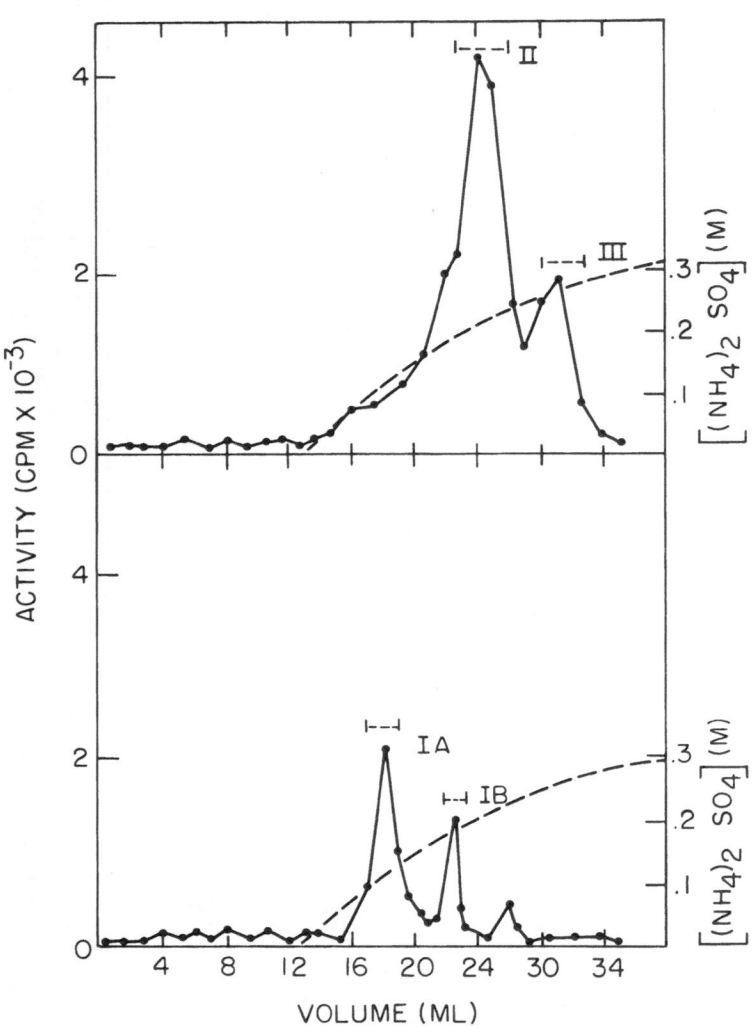

Figure 3
Fractionation of RNA polymerases from rat liver. RNA polymerases from livers of rats carrying Morris hepatoma were fractionated essentially as described in the Legend to Fig. 2. Further
details are given elsewhere (24).

tion of the enzymes. The recovery of IA, IB and II from the hepatoma was 0.21, 0.28 and 0.42 units/mg DNA, respectively, whereas the recovery of the corresponding liver enzymes was 0.07, 0.05 and 0.42 units/mg DNA. Subsequent studies have shown that the levels of RNA polymerase I (A + B) are even higher (at least 10-fold) in the hepatoma as compared to liver. Of the two nucleolar enzymes, the level of IB was elevated more than that of IA. Under these conditions, the level of RNA polymerase II was identical in liver and tumor. Even when the enzyme assay was performed in isolated nuclei or in nuclear lysates, the enzyme activity resistant to high levels (130 µg/ml) of α-amanitin (which represents RNA polymerase I) was higher (at least 3-5-fold) in the hepatoma than in liver. Since the enzyme activity expressed in such crude preparations is hindered by contaminating nucleases and other inhibitors, it is only an approximation of the absolute values of the enzyme activities. Nevertheless, the preferential increase in the levels of RNA polymerases IA and IB in the hepatoma was evident at all stages of enzyme preparation.

The nucleolar enzymes (IA + IB) were recently purified essentially to homogeneity by glycerol density gradient fractionation. The specific activity of the purified enzyme was 300-400 nmoles UMP incorporated/mg protein.

II. Some Properties of the Hepatoma RNA Polymerases I and II

As observed with other mammalian RNA polymerases, RNA polymerase II was completely sensitive to low levels (< 1 µg/ml) of α-amanitin, whereas RNA polymerase I was totally insensitive to the toxin, even at 130 µg/ml. The template requirements for the enzymes were studied and the relevant data are presented in Table 1. The nucleolar enzymes utilized native DNA and denatured DNA equally well as the template. RNA polymerase II used denatured DNA more efficiently (3-4-fold) than native DNA. However, in the presence of spermine, transcription of native DNA by polymerase II was significantly elevated (2-fold for liver enzyme and 6-7-fold for the hepatoma enzyme). In fact, the activity of the hepatoma RNA polymerase II was several times higher with native DNA and spermine than with denatured DNA. Spermine did not stimulate transcription of denatured DNA. These studies have further confirmed our earlier data (12, 27) which indicated that spermine selectively stimulates transcription of native or double-stranded DNA. The activities of all polymerases were higher (2-4-fold) when poly[d(A-T)] was used as the template instead of native DNA.

III. Direct Comparison of the Levels of RNA Polymerases in Morris Hepatomas 7800 and 3924A

If the increase in the levels of RNA polymerases IA and IB is

Table One
Effect of Spermine and Template on RNA Polymerases IA,
IB, and II from Liver and Hepatoma 3924A

Source of enzyme	RNA Polymerase	Template	Activity (pmol UMP incorporated	
			Control	Spermine
Liver	IA	DNA	182	421
		denatured DNA	186	217
		Poly[d(A-T)]	641	666
	IB	DNA	134	228
		denatured DNA	137	176
		Poly{d(A-T)]	271	115
	II	DNA	120	275
		denatured DNA	487	443
		Poly[d(A-T)]	413	238
Hepatoma	IA	DNA	30	93
		denatured DNA	35	16
		Poly[d(A-T)]	95	24
	IB	DNA	88	470
		denatured DNA	87	61
		Poly[d(A-T)]	233	55
	II	DNA	92	600
		denatured DNA	264	306
		Poly[d(A-T)]	348	192

Purified enzymes were analyzed using the optimal $(NH_4)_2SO_4$ concentrations (40 mM for liver IA, IB; 100 mM for liver II; 12 mM for tumor IA, IB; and 50 mM for tumor II). The optimal concentration of spermine was used for each enzyme (1.25 mM for liver IA, IB: 5.0 mM for liver II; 0.6 mM for tumor IA, IB; and 5.0 mM for tumor II). Spermine (12 µl) or glass-distilled water (controls) was added just prior to addition of enzyme which was used to start the reaction. The concentrations of the templates (used in saturating quantities) were 133 µg/ml for native and denatured DNA and 42 µg/ml for poly[d(A-T)].

related to the degree of differentiation and growth rates of the
tumor, it might be expected that the levels of these enzymes in a
well-differentiated hepatoma such as 7800 would be intermediate between the levels in liver and in the poorly differentiated hepatoma
3924A.   To test this correlation, RNA polymerases from the two hepatomas were extracted and subjected to DEAE-Sephadex chromatogarphy
(Fig 4).   By employing a large column size and extended linear
gradients, all three classes of hepatoma RNA polymerases were resolved, As expected, the poorly differentiated, rapidly growing
hepatoma 3924A had higher levels of RNA polymerases IA and IB than
hepatoma 7800.   The levels of the nucleolar enzymes were in the
following order: hepatoma 3924A < hepatoma 7800 < liver (liver data
from ref. 19).   Table 2 summarizes these data.

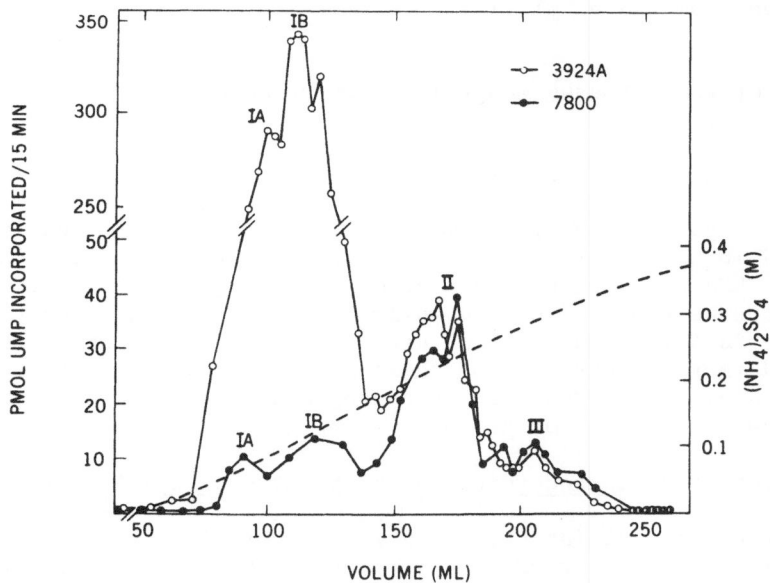

Figure 4

Fractionation of RNA polymerases I, II and III from Morris
hepatomas 3924A and 7800 using smaller quantities of tissue for enzyme extraction.   RNA polymerases were extracted from 12-15 g of the
tumors and fractionated on a DEAE-Sephadex column as described
previously (19).

Table Two
Levels of RNA Polymerases I and II

		RNA Polymerase Activity[a] (pmol/ UMP incorporated/g tissue)		
Enzyme	Liver	Thioacetamide-treated Liver	Hepatomas 7800	3924A
I	137[b]	390	500	5,900[c]
II	473[b]	670	710	860[c]
I/II	0.29	0.58	0.70	6.9

a
RNA polymerase activity was determined after a single DEAE-Sephadex chromatography, as described by Lin et al.(19).

b
Data taken from Lin et al.(19).

c
Recovery of DNA/g tissue was twice that of normal liver.

Relative to polymerase I, polymerases II and III were essentially unaltered in the tumors. These data indicate that the level of nucleolar RNA polymerases is related to the degree of differentiation of the hepatoma. The overwhelming levels of RNA polymerases IA and IB in 3924A could partly explain the technical problems encountered in the separation of these enzymes from polymerases II and III in a single DEAE-Sephadex chromatography when they were extracted from larger quantities of tissues.

IV. Effect of a Hepatocarcinogen on the Levels of RNA Polymerases

Another line of investigation was to correlate the changes in the levels of nucleolar RNA polymerases in the hepatoma with those observed after treatment with a hepatocarcinogen. The idea was to demonstrate whether such biochemical events were triggered early in tumorigenesis. Studies on transcriptional modifications induced by hepatocarcinogens are complicated by the initial deleterious cytotoxic effects of many of these compounds. For example, treatment of rats with ethionine (5), aflatoxin B_1 (25), acetylaminofluorene (8) or dimethylnitrosamine (7) resulted in decreased levels of RNA polymerase II with no significant changes in the levels of RNA poly-

merase I from liver. However, in vivo, these carcinogens selectively inhibited nucleolar RNA synthesis (2). The complete lack of
correlation of in vivo and in vitro data has cast serious doubts
on the validity of the in vitro studies. An alternate approach to
this problem is to select a compound which has limited early cytotoxic effects and yet produces tumors in target tissues after prolonged treatment. One such agent appears to be thioacetamide (9)
which, in the first week of treatment, can induce enlargement of
nucleoli (2) and enhance rRNA synthesis in liver (26), both of
which are characteristics of many solid tumors. Moreover, thioacetamide can produce liver tumors after prolonged treatment (1, 6).

The effect of a single injection of thioacetamide (50 mg/kg)
on the levels of RNA polymerases I and II was investigated. Since
a considerable body of information was available on the effect of
this compound on RNA labeling in vivo after 24 hours of administration (21), this time point was chosen for the present investigation.
Accordingly, rats were sacrificed at the 24 hour time point, RNA
polymerases were extracted from rat liver nuclei and chromatographically resolved. Initial studies showed preferential effects on
'bound' form (29) of RNA polymerase I. Subsequently, attention was
focused on changes in the 'bound' population of RNA polymerases after
thioacetamide treatment. Table 3 shows the activities of 'bound'
and 'free' RNA polymerase I and II from the control and thioacetamide
treated liver. It is evident that the carcinogen produced a preferential increase in the levels of RNA polymerases IA and IB and
this increase was manifested primarily in the bound population of
the enzyme. The increase in the nucleolar RNA polymerases was not
due to preferential recovery of these enzymes after thioacetamide
treatments, as suggested by the following observations:

(a) the stimulatory effect of thioacetamide was evident in the
solubilized enzyme extract (activity resistant to high levels of
(α-amanitin) prior to chromatography;

(b) the total proteins in the thioacetamide-treated liver nuclei or in enzyme extract increased at most 30%, which was not sufficient to account for to 3-4-fold increase in the level of polymerase I;

(c) two additional chromatographic fractionations (not shown)
did not change the extent of stimulation of polymerase I; and

(d) the level of 'bound' RNA polymerase I extracted after mix-
ing equal amounts of liver from the control and thioacetamide-treated rats was very close to the theoretical value.

That the effect of thioacetamide on the 'bound' RNA polymerase
I was due to a preferential increase in the actual amounts of enzyme

Table Three
Effect of Thioacetamide on RNA Polymerases
I and II after a Single DEAE-Sephadex Chromatography

	'Bound'		'Free'	
	I	II	I	II
Control	2.5	9.5	1.0	10.1
Thioacetamide	7.8	13.4	1.5	13.5

Enzymes were extracted from livers of control and thioacetamide
treated (20 g each) rats. Fraction containing the respective RNA
polymerases obtained after a single DEAE-Sephadex column chromatography were pooled separately, dialyzed, and assayed as described
previously (24). The values represent total units of enzyme (1
unit = 1 nmole UMP incorporated/10 min at 30°C) derived from 20 g
each of control and thioacetamide-treated liver.

has been supported by the following observations. In one set of
experiments, RNA polymerase I (IA + IB) fractions were pooled from
the control and the carcinogen-treated samples and fixed aliquots
of the enzymes were assayed with increasing quantities of DNA as
the template. Since enzymes derived from the same DNA-equivalent
nuclei were used for these experiments, limiting quantities of
DNA should give identical values for the control and thioacetamide-
treated enzymes. As shown in Table 4, when 1-2 µg/ml of native
calf thymus DNA were used as the template, no difference in the
activity between the two enzymes was observed. However, when the
DNA concentration was raised further, the difference between the
two enzymes was evident. On the other hand, if the same units
(nmol UMP incorporated/20 min at 37°C) of control and thioacetamide-
treated enzyme (rather than quantities of enzymes derived from fixed
amounts of tissues or DNA-equivalent nuclei) were used and the enzymes assayed with different concentrations of DNA under conditions
which permitted only one round of initiation, there was no difference
in the activity of the two enzymes. Finally, the size of the product synthesized by the two enzymes was identical (6-8S). These
data tend to indicate that thioacetamide treatment produces an increased number of RNA polymerase I molecules which, in turn, may have
resulted from increased synthesis and/or decreased turnover of the
enzyme molecules. Current evidence also seems to suggest that the
increased level of polymerase I observed in hepatomas relative to
liver is due to larger quantities of RNA polymerase I. The levels

Table Four
Effect of In Vivo Administration of Thioacetamide
On the Level of Rat Liver 'Bound' RNA Polymerase I Activity
Assayed with Varying Amounts of DNA

DNA Concentration (μg/ml)	Control Liver	Thioacetamide-treated Liver
1	3.6	3.7
2	10.0	10.5
4	21.2	28.9
8	32.0	68.3

The nuclear fraction containing the bound RNA polymerases
was prepared by gently homogenizing the isolated nuclei in 0.25
M sucrose and centrifuging off the supernatant, which contained
the free enzymes. The bound enzymes were extracted as described
by Rose et al. (23). RNA polymerase I was separated from the
other enzymes as described in the text. The enzyme assay was performed under conditions inhibitory to reinitiation by a modification of the methods originally devised by Hyman and Davidson (10)
and extended to mammalian RNA polymerase II by Cedar (3).

of RNA polymerases I and II in liver, hepatomas 3924A and 7800
and in thioacetamide-treated liver are given in Table 2. The
ratio I/II was in the following order: 3924A ⟨ 7800 ⟨ thioacetamide-
treated liver ⟨ liver.

V. Conclusions

The present studies have clearly demonstrated that relative to
normal liver, Morris hepatomas 3924A and 7800 contain several-fold
higher levels of RNA polymerase I, particularly IB, and that this
increase in the levels of nucleolar RNA polymerase is related to the
degree of neoplasia. It is noteworthy that similar changes were also
observed in the early stages following the administration of a hepatocarcinogen. The available data tend to suggest that the higher
levels of nucleolar RNA polymerase are due to increased quantities
of the enzymes, rather than modification of pre-existing enzyme
molecules. Ultimate proof for such a contention should await immunoprecipitation of the enzymes in these tissues with antiserum against
purified RNA polymerase I. Nevertheless, the present data certainly

point to a preferential increase in the RNA polymerase I molecules at some stage in tumorigenesis. This is consistent with the augmented synthesis of rRNA and with the enlarged size of nucleolus which are characteristics of several tumors. Finally, the selective increase in the 'bound' form of RNA polymerase I is in line with the proposed role of this enzyme population in 'active' transcription. In this context, it should be noted that in other growing tissues or cells such as regenerating liver (29, 30) or lymphocytes treated with phytohaemoglutinin (16), all classes of RNA polymerases are elevated. Thus, the elevation of nucleolar enzymes with negligible changes in the levels of other RNA polymerases seems to be a unique property of neoplastic tissues.

Acknowledgements

This work was supported in part by USPHS Grant CA 16438 and National Science Foundation Grant PCM 76-82224, to S.T.J., a specialized Cancer Research Center Grant I PO 30 CA 18450 and an American Cancer Society Institutional Grant IN-109.

REFERENCES

1. Ahghileri, L.J., Heidlreder, M., Weiler, G. and Dermietzel, R.
    Exp. Cell Biol. 45 (1977) 34

2. Busch, H. and Smetana, K. In: The Nucleolus, Academic Press
    (1970) p. 495

3. Cedar, H. J. Mol. Biol. 95 (1975) 257

4. Chambon, P. Ann. Rev. Biochem. 44 (1975) 613

5. Farber, J.L., Shinozuka, H., Serroni, A. and Farmer, R. Lab.
    Invest. 31 (1974) 465

6. Fitzburgh, O.G. and Nelson, A.A., Science 108 (1948) 626

7. Herzog, J. and Farber, J.L. Cancer Res. 36 (1976) 1761

8. Herzog, J., Serroni, A., Briesmesiter, B.A. and Farber, J.L.
    Cancer Res. 35 (1975) 2138

9. Hunter, A.L., Holscher, M.A. and Nealm R.A. J. Pharmacol. Exp.
    Ther. 200 (1977) 439

10. Hyman, R.W. and Davidson, N. J. Mol. Biol. 50 (1970) 421

11. Jacob, S.T. Prog. Nuc. Acid. Mol. Biol. 13 (1973) 93

12. Jacob, S.T. and Rose, K.M., Biochim. Biophys. Acta 425 (1976)
    125

13. Jacob, S.T. and Rose, K.M. In: Methods in Cancer Research,
    H. Busch (ed), Academic Press, Vol. 14. In press

14. Jacob, S.T., Sajdel, E.M., Muecke, W. amd Munro, H.N. Cold
    Spring Harbor Symp. Quant. Biol. 35 (1970) 681

15. Jacob, S.T., Sajdel, E.M., and Munro, H.N. Biochem. Biophys.
    Res. Comm. 38 (1970) 765

16. Jeahning, J., Stewart, C. and Roeder, R.G. Cell 4 (1975) 51

17. Jänne, O., Bardin, C.W. and Jacob, S.T. Biochemistry 14 (1975)
    3589.

18. Kedinger, C., Gniazdowski, M., Mandel, J.L., Gissinger, F. and
    Chambron, P. Biochem. Biophys. Res. Comm. 38 (1970) 165

19. Lin, Y.C., Rose, K.M. and Jacob, S.T. Biochem. Biophys. Res. Comm. 72 (1976) 114

20. Lindell, T.J., Weinberg, F., Morris, P.W., Roeder, R.G. and Rutter, W.J. Science 170 (1970) 447

21. Ro-Choi, T.S., Raj, N.B.K., Pike, L.M. and Busch, H. Biochemistry 15 (1976) 3823

22. Roeder, R.G., Chou, S., Jeahning, J.A., Schwartz, L.B., Sklar, V.E.F. and Weinman, R. In: Isozymes, C.L. Markert (ed). Academic Press, 3 (1975) 27

23. Rose, K.M., Ruch, P. and Jacob, S.T. Biochemistry 14 (1975) 3598

24. Rose, K.M., Ruch, P., Morris, H.P. and Jacob, S.T., Biochim. Biophys. Acta 432 (1976) 60

25. Saunders, F.C., Barker, E.A. and Smuckler, E.A., Cancer Res. 32 (1972) 2487

26. Steele, W.J. and Busch, H. Biochim. Biophys. Acta 119 (1966) 501

27. Weinman, R., Brendler, T.G., Raskes, H.J. and Roeder, R.G. Cell 7 (1976) 557

28. Weinman, R. and Roeder, R.G. Proc. Natl. Acad. Sci. U.S.A. 71 (1974) 1790

29. Yu, F.L. Biochem. Biophys. Res. Comm. 64 (1975) 1107

30. Yu, F.L. Biochim. Biophys. Acta 395 (1975) 329

REGULATION OF MACROMOLECULAR SYNTHESIS IN MORRIS HEPATOMAS[1]

Michael A. Lea

Department of Biochemistry
New Jersey Medical School
Newark, New Jersey 07103

SUMMARY

In this review, some studies are discussed in which an attempt
has been made to determine the nature of changes in macromolecular
synthesis in Morris hepatomas. The incorporation of isotope labeled
precursors into nucleic acids and proteins has suggested greatly increased rates of DNA synthesis in comparison with rat liver of normal
and tumor bearing rats, but for RNA and proteins the changes may be
impressive for individual macromolecular species but total synthesis
is not greatly changed. Fractionation of nuclear proteins has indicated altered patterns of synthesis which are related to the growth
rates of the tumors and are much more pronounced than in regenerating
liver despite a growth rate similar to that of the most rapidly growing hepatomas. Investigations with drugs which inhibit synthesis of
macromolecules has suggested that liver neoplasia may be accompanied
by changes in response which may make the tumor less sensitive or
more sensitive to regulation than the tissue of origin.

INTRODUCTION

Many investigators have taken advantage of the spectrum of growth
rates provided by the Morris hepatomas to examine the correlation of
molecular changes with growth and this concept has been most vigorous-
ly pursued by George Weber and coworkers (50-52). One of the most
convenient approaches for determining alterations in macromolecular
synthesis is the measurement of the incorporation of isotopically-
labelled precursors into proteins and nucleic acids. This review
considers some of the results which have been obtained in such studies and some of the problems and apparent inconsistencies which such

data reveal. By the use of drugs which regulate growth it may be
possible to probe the reversability of metabolic changes in tumors
and to assess their relative significance for the neoplastic transformation or for accelerated proliferation in all tissues.

MATERIALS AND METHODS

The experiments reviewed here were performed with male Buffalo
strain rats. Morris hepatomas (38-39) were routinely transplanted
bilaterally in a subcutaneous position but have also been studied
in an intra-muscular position or at an intra-hepatic site according
to the procedure of Bullock et al. (7). Regenerating liver was examined 24 hours after partial hepatectomy by the procedure of Higgins
and Anderson (19). In studies on nuclear constituents, tissues
were homogenized in 9 volumes of 0.25 M sucrose, 5mM $MgCl_2$, 25 mM
KCl, 50 mM tris pH 7.4, filtered through cheesecloth and centrifuged
at 800 g for 8 min. The nuclei were suspended in 2.4 M sucrose
3 mM $MgCl_2$ and centrifuged at 25,000 rpm for 60 min in the Beckman
30 rotor. Assay procedures have been described previously (23-36).

RESULTS AND INTERPRETATION

Although the incorporation of ^3H or ^{14}C-labeled thymidine into
DNA is the most widely used measure of DNA synthesis and hepatomas
have more mitotic figures than the normal liver, there are several
factors which could make this a less than optimal approach to the
measurement of relative growth in vivo. These include differences
in blood flow, nucleotide pool sizes and the relative contributions
of the de novo and salvage pathways for thymidylate synthesis. Despite these variables, the observed rates of thymidine incorporation
into DNA do show a positive correlation with growth rate (34). This
work has been extended to show that a closer correlation exists between growth rate of hepatomas and the ratio of thymidine incorporation into DNA and degradation to CO_2 (14). The correlation between
hepatoma growth rate and thymidine incorporation into DNA is greater
if the incorporation is expressed per unit weight of tissue rather
than DNA. This is because the more rapidly growing hepatomas contain
more DNA per gram of tissue than do slowly growing hepatomas and
normal liver (34). It it is assumed that DNA is metabolically stable,
a more satisfactory measure of DNA synthesis is measurement of the
rate of decrease in specific activity of DNA after first labeling
the DNA in vivo with a radioactive precursor. Since this procedure
involves killing groups of rats over a period of days it is time
consuming and expensive but it has the potential to provide an
accurate measure of relative growth rates in different tissues (35).
On the other hand, measurement of the incorporation of ^{14}C-labeled
glycine into DNA has indicated lower rates in the rapidly growing
hepatomas 9618A$_2$ and 7777 than in host livers (Bullock and Lea, unpublished observations). Even more anomalous results are obtained

using orotate as a precursor of RNA synthesis. Weber et al. (53)
found a low rate of incorporation of orotate into RNA of hepatomas.
Subsequent work has suggested that this observation is due to decreased uptake of orotate by hepatomas (Fig 1) rather than arising
from a block in RNA synthesis (24). A similar prehomenon has been
seen in kidney tumors but is not seen with uridine as a precursor
for the synthesis of RNA (32).

     Early work with tissue slices indicated a greater rate of in-
corporation of amino acids into protein of hepatomas than control
liver preparations (49). This pattern has not generally been observed in vivo where similar rates may be seen for incorporation
into total proteins in the normal and neoplastic tissues (31).
Determinations of amino acid nitrogen have revealed similar total
amino acid concentrations in these tissues (26) although measurements of individual amino acids show that they can undergo considerable variation in hepatomas (40) and regenerating liver (47).
Alterations may also be seen in protein fractions. The incorporation of amino acids into histones is increased in hepatomas as would
be anticipated for proliferating tissues (26). The ratio of histone:
DNA concentration is similar in control liver and hepatomas but the
increase in amino acid incorporation into histone is not as great as
for thymidine incorporation. In view of the metabolic stability of
DNA and histones, in vivo incorporation of precursors should be a
measure of synthesis rather than turnover of these macromolecules.
Uptake studies indicated that Morris hepatomas generally have a well-
developed capacity to concentrate amino acids but, as for other precursors of macromolecular synthesis, the uptake is less rapidly growing hepatomas than liver at short intervals after injection (0-30
minutes).   In slowly growing hepatomas there is evidence for decrease uptake of the non-metabolizable amino-acid α-aminoisobutyric
acid (22). It is not possible at present to provide a documented
mechanism for apparent discrepancies in the relative rates of histone
and DNA synthesis in liver and hepatomas as measured by precursor incorporation. In contrast to the histones, a non-histone nuclear protein fraction, which is not extracted by 0.5 M NaCl and 0.24 M HCl,
shows low rates of amino acid incorporation in rapidly growing hepatomas (27). Temporal studies have indicated that incorporation of
amino acids into protein of host liver tends to peak earlier than in
hepatomas as that relative rates are influenced by the observation
time. Differences in blood flow through these tissues (18) should also be considered in the interpretation of the results. Amongst the
side chain modifications to which proteins are subject, phosphorylation of H1 histone has been shown to correlate with the growth rate
of hepatomas (2). Greater phosphorylation of non-histone chromosomal
proteins has frequently been associated with the neoplastic transformation but a decreased phosphate concentration and incorporation of
^{32}P-phosphate into acid-stable phosphate in a low-solubility fraction
of nuclear proteins has been noted in rapidly growing hepatomas (27).

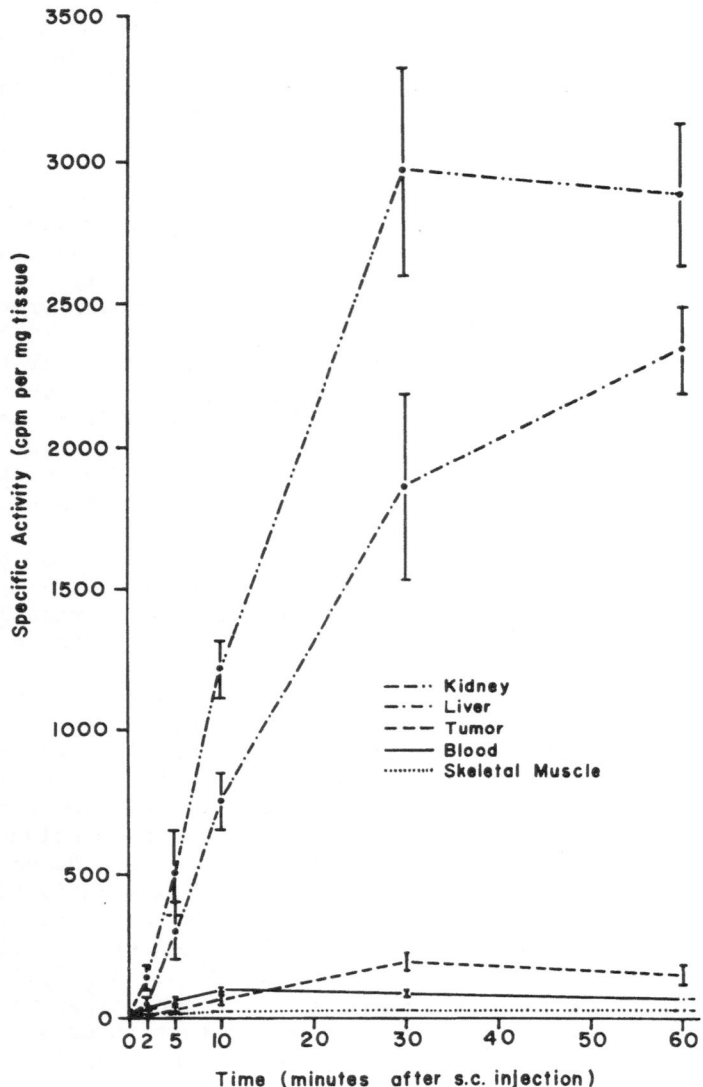

Figure 1
Incorporation of [³H] orotate into acid-soluble fractions of
tissues in rats bearing hepatoma 7777. Radioactivity with respect
to time is shown following the subcutaneous injection of the isotope (25 uCi per 100 g body weight). Means and standard errors
where significant are given for 3 rats. Similar values were obtained with rats bearing hepatoma 9618A$_2$ and the data were discussed
previously (24).

These differences were not seen in regenerating liver or slowly
growing hepatomas (11, 13) and may be a factor in changes in nuclear
protein phosphorylation (9, 10). It is not clear at the present
time to what extent 3'5' - cyclic AMP serves as a modulator of nuclear protein phosphorylation. It may have an indirect role by
causing the dissociation of cytoplasmic protein kinase with subsequent translocation of the catalytic sub-unit to the nucleus (21).
In vitro studies have shown that binding of cyclic AMP to nuclei
is facilitated by a cytoplasmic protein. In our investigations we
have observed that a temperature-dependent activation is required
for rat liver cytosol to function in this fashion (Kallos, Koch and
Lea, unpublished observations). The capacity of a cytosol preparation to increase ^{3}H-cyclic AMP binding by nuclei was reduced with a
cytosol fraction from Morris hepatoma 7777 (Table 1). Crossover
studies revealed that the tumor cytosol did not increase the binding
of ^{3}H-cyclic AMP by normal liver nuclei as much as did the host liver
cytosol but liver cytosol fraction had a similar effect with liver
and hepatoma nuclei which suggested that the deficiency in this hepatoma is in the soluble receptor for cyclic AMP rather than in the
nuclear acceptor site. Up to 10 fold stimulations of nuclear binding were obtained with some liver cytosol preparations but the values
in Table 1 are more typical. Cytosol preparations from the slowly
growing hepatoma 9618A were similar to the liver in their stimulatory
effect. Alterations in cytoplasmic proteins which bind cyclic AMP
have been reported in the HTC cell line (16, 37). There are inconsistencies in reported levels of total cyclic nucleotides in Morris hepatomas (15, 46) and it remains to be established if there are differences in the concentrations of cyclic nucleotides in nuclei of these
tissues.

Chromosomal proteins are believed to serve an important role not
only in the structure of chromosomes but also in regulating transcriptional activity (4, 12, 41). There is a tendency for the proportion
of non-histone nuclear proteins to increase relative to the histones
in liver tumors. This is seen in the data presented in Table 2 for
two rapidly growing hepatomas and the liver of the tumor-bearing rats.
In addition to examining the incorporation of isotope labeled precursors nuclear proteins have been studied by electrophoretic techniques with the object of identifying changes in neoplasia. The major
histone fractions from hepatomas and normal liver show similar qualitative and quantitative properties on polyacrylamide gel electrophoresis (36). The minor histone fraction H1° which was identified by
Panyim and Chalkley (43) as being associated with non-dividing cells,
can be readily identified in slowly growing hepatomas (36). It is
greatly decreased in rapidly growing hepatomas. In comparisons between hepatoma and liver the cellular heterogeneity of the latter tissue makes it possible that the changes observed arise from the contribution of non-parenchymal cells to biochemical parameters rather
than from the neoplastic transformation in hepatocytes. One approach

Table One

Influence of Liver and Hepatoma Cytosol on Binding of
[^{3}H] cAMP by Nuclei

| | Nuclear binding (cpm/10 ug DNA) | |
| | Host liver | Hepatoma 7777 |
Source of Cytosol	nuclei	nuclei
Liver	12	130
Hepatoma	71	82
None	24	35

The cytosol fraction was prepared by precipitation of cytosol from a 10% (w/v) tissue homogenate with 50% saturated ammonium sulfate and was dissolved in its original volume of 25 mM NaCl, 1 mM EDTA, 3 mM 2-mercaptoethanol, 15% glycerol, 20 mM tris, pH 7.4 followed by dialysis against 100 volumes of this buffer. A preincubation was performed at 25° C for 20 min with 0.35 ml cytosol fraction or buffer together with 0.01 ml [^{3}H] cyclic AMP (0.25 mCi/ml of specific activity 23 Ci/mMole) and 0.5 ml 0.32 M sucrose, 50 mM KCl. 3 mM 2-mercaptoethanol, 1 mM EDTA, 1 mM CaCl$_2$, 0.02% bovine serum albumin, 25 mM tris pH 7.4. Nuclei (0.1 ml containing 0.5 mg DNA) were then added and incubated at 25° C for 30 min. The nuclei were centrifuged, washed three times with the incubation buffer and radioactivity was determined. (Kallos, Koch and Lea, unpublished observations).

Table Two
Distribution of Nuclear Proteins in Fractions from Rapidly
Growing Hepatomas and Host Livers

| | Nuclear Protein Fraction | | | |
Tissue	0.14 M NaCl extract	0.35 M NaCl extract	Histones	Residual nuclear protein
Hepatoma 7777	19 + 2	17 + 1	24 + 2	39 + 2
7777 Host Liver	26 + 2	20 + 1	34 + 1	20 + 1
Hepatoma 9618A$_2$	26 + 3	15 + 1	23 + 1	36 + 3
9618A$_2$ Host Liver	26 + 2	20 + 1	36 + 1	19 + 1

The nuclear protein fractions are expressed as percentages of the total nuclear proteins. Means and standard errors are presented for seven rats (Lea and Koch, unpublished observations).

to this problem in studies of the cell nucleus is to fractionate
the nuclei by centrifugation on a sucrose gradient. In an investigation with hepatoma 7777 a large decrease was noted in nuclei corresponding to the stromal diploid nuclei of control or host liver
(54). When histones from three nuclear fractions of liver and of
hepatoma 7777 were examined by polyacrylamide gel electrophoresis,
the $H1^O$ histone was present to a similar extent in all the nuclear
fractions of liver but was greatly decreased or absent in all the
nuclear fractions from hepatoma 7777. In order to clearly identify
the $H1^O$ histone in hepatoma 7777 we have found it advategous to
perform polyacrylamide gel electrophoresis on 5% $HClO_4$ extracts of
nuclei and to overload the gels with respect to the H1 histone
(Fig 2).

The non-histone nuclear proteins have been extracted from nuclei of hepatomas by a variety of techniques and subject to polyacrylamide gel electrophoresis or isoelectric focusing (1, 8, 30,
44). One of the extraction media was 8 M urea - 50 mM phsophate,
H 7.6 which had been shown by Gronow and Griffiths (17) to extract
most of the non-histone proteins from liver nuclei with little extraction of the histones. Isoelectric focusing of these extracts
indicated that with increasing growth rate of the hepatomas there
was a progressive tendency for a decrease in non-histone nuclear
proteins with isoelectric points in the range 7.5 to 8.9 and an increase in the range 5.1 to 6.7 (30). Only a small part of the histones were extracted by 8M urea - 50 mM phosphate pH 7.6 in all tissues examined but the tendency was for more extraction from liver
than hepatoma nuclei. Due to a pH plateau phenomenon on prolonged
isoelectric focusing a 24 hour period was found preferable to a 5-7
hour period for resolution of acidic proteins using ampholytes for
a pH gradient of 3.5 to 10. An increase in certain acidic nuclear
proteins has also been observed in proteins extracted from nuclei
of hepatoma 7777 with 0.35 M NaCl. Concurrent with this change is a
decrease in two basic proteins which are prominent in the host livers
(Dayal and Lea, unpublished observations). Non-histone chromosomal
proteins from regenerating liver and slowly growing hepatomas are
very similar to those of normal liver when separated by one dimensional polyacrylamide gel electrophoresis, but differences have been
established by a two dimensional procedure (55). The proteins obtained from nuclei by the phenol extraction procedure of Teng et al. (45)
form an interesting class of proteins notable for their high degree
of phosphorylation. Sodium dodecyl sulfate polyacrylamide gel electrophoresis of these proteins from hepatoma 7777 and control liver revealed
additional proteins of molecular weight 60,000, 100,000, and 135,000
and the loss of proteins of about 45,000 and 55,000 in the tumor (54).
The different subfractions of liver nuclei had similar complements of
phenol-soluble proteins, but in the hepatoma nuclei several differences were found between the minor slowly sedimenting nuclear fraction, and the two major fractions, while the two latter fractions

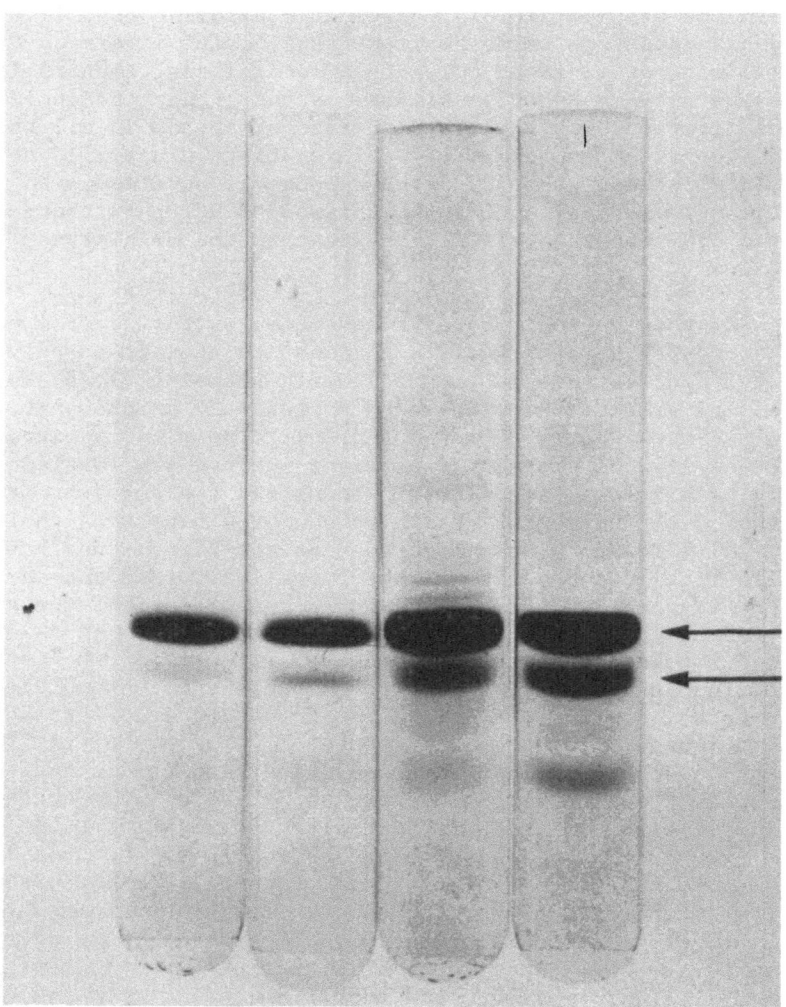

Figure 2
Electrophoresis of H1 histones from hepatoma 7777 and host liver.
H1 histones were extracted with 5% $HClO_4$ from nuclei which had been
washed with 0.35 M NaCl. Polyacrylamide gel electrophoresis by the
procedure of Panyim and Chalkley (42) was performed from left to
right with: 1.10 μg hepatoma 7777 protein, 4.50 μg host liver
protein. The upper arrow indicates the H1 histone and the lower
arrow indicates the H1o histone band which is more prominent in the
host liver preparations.

were very similar in their protein composition.

Studies on inhibitions of macromolecular synthesis have shown
that transplanted hepatomas may show similar sensitivity to that of
the normal liver with some agents but may exhibit decreased or increased sensitivity with other drugs. In measuring DNA synthesis
by the incorporation of isotope-labeled thymidine the low rates in
normal liver make the regenerating liver after partial hepatectomy
a more convenient control tissue. Injection of hydroxyurea (i.p.)
at levels in the range 250-1000 mg/kg body weight causes a virtually complete inhibition of [3H] thymidine incorporation into DNA
in both regenerating rat liver and hepatomas. Formamidoxime
(H_2N-CH=NOHO, a compound structurally related to hydroxyurea
(H_2N-CO-NHOH), also caused a large inhibition of [3H] thymidine
incorporation into DNA of regenerating liver and hepatomas when
administered by i.p. injection to rats (500 mg/kg body weight) and
at the same time had little or no effect on the incorporation of
[3H] orotate into RNA (24). On the other hand certain thiaxanthe-
nones, including Miracil D and hycanthone, were found to have greater effects on precursor incorporation into nucleic acids in regenerating liver than in hepatomas (33). Fractionation of nuclei from regenerating liver after treatment with Miracil D and injection of
[3H] thymidine gave evidence of an equivalent inhibition of incorporation into DNA in the different nuclear classes (Campana and Lea,
unpublished observations). The inhibitory effect of Miracil D on
DNA synthesis was greater in slowly growing than rapidly growing neoplasms (33). The lesser effect on the hepatomas may be related to
decrease drug uptake. This suggestion is supported by uptake studies
with 3H-labeled hycanthone (24). Relatively low uptake was seen in
rapidly growing hepatomas in studies with 3H-labeled 5-fluorouracil
but uptake in the moderately growing hepatoma 5123C was not significantly different from host liver (24). Even in a rapidly growing
hepatoma such as the 9618A$_2$ line, the uptake of a drug may be similar
to that of host liver. Thus, 14C-labeled cyanate showed a similar
uptake in these tissues (28). The action of cyanate on [3H] thymidine
incorporation into DNA provides an example of inhibition in hepatomas
which is greater than that seen with regenerating liver (28) and
similar effects may be seen with thiocyanate (unpublished observation)
and TPCK[2].

In some systems, notably HeLa cells (5, 6), there is a tight
coupling between DNA synthesis and histone synthesis. In cultured
hepatoma cells it has been possible to demonstrate a considerable
degree of uncoupling between the two types of synthesis after inhibition of DNA synthesis with hydroxyurea (3). After treatment of
rats with 500 mg formamidoxime (i.p.) per kg body weight there was
an approximately 50% inhibition of incorporation of [3H] amino acids
into histone fractions of regenerating liver and hepatomas but a
greater than 75% inhibition of DNA synthesis (26). Under these

conditions there was no significant effect on amino acid nitrogen concentration and the incorporation of [^{3}H] orotate into RNA and of ^{3}H-labeled amino acids into acid soluble material, cytoplasmic proteins and acid-insoluble nuclear proteins were either unaffected or showed only small changes in the tissues examined. A similar pattern of response was seen in regenerating liver when Miracil D or hycanthone were injected i.p. (50 mg per kg body weight) 8 hours after partial hepatectomy (25). Again the effects were largely on histone and DNA synthesis with DNA synthesis showing the greater inhibition. At the same time hycanthone was observed to inhibit the increased incorporation of [^{32}P] phosphate into H1 histone which is normally seen in regenerating liver.

With some drugs which inhibit amino acid incorporation into protein there may be little discrimination between effects on histone synthesis and that of other proteins, We observed that sodium cyanate at a dose level of 125 or 25o mg/kg body weight (i.p.) caused an inhibition of incorporation of ^{3}H-labeled amino acids into cytoplasmic and nuclear proteins of the rapidly growing hepatoma 7777 and the slowly growing hepatoma 9618A, but there was no inhibitory effect in the livers of the rats bearing these tumors (31). The action of cyanate on the subcutaneously transplanted hepatomas may, at least in part, be due to an effect on active transport in the tumors. The uptake of the non-metabolizable amino acid, α-aminoisobutyric acid, was found to be inhibited by sodium cyanate in transplanted hepatomas but was increased in the livers of the tumor - bearing rats (29). Assay of individual amino acids after treatment of rats bearing hepatoma 7777 with cyanate revealed a complex pattern of changes but the concentrations of many amino acids were not significantly changed in either tumor or host liver (Table 3). On the other hand there was a significant increase in ammonia in both tumor and host liver. Cyanate showed inhibitory effects on tissue uptake of [^{32}P] phosphate and incorporation into macromolecules (29).

TPCK was found by Vidali et al.(48) to exert selective effects on protein synthesis in HeLa cells with synthesis of non-histone chromosomal proteins being less sensitive than the synthesis of histones and cytoplasmic proteins. We have observed an inhibition of incorporation of [^{3}H] amino acids into protein in several Morris hepatomas and a transplanted colon tumor after rats received 100 mg TPCK i.p. per kg body weight (23). This action was accompanied by decreased uptake of isotope into acid soluble tissue fractions but there was no significant inhibition in regenerating liver and there was an increased uptake of [^{3}H] amino acids in the livers of normal and tumor bearing rats. The inhibitory effects in hepatomas did not appear selective for individual protein fractions being similar for incorporation of [^{3}H] amino acids into cytoplasmic proteins, histones and non-histone nuclear protein fractions (Table 4). The data in Table 4 also illustrate the relatively low incorporation of [^{3}H]

Table Three

Effect of Cyanate on the Concentration of Amino Acids and Ammonia in Hepatoma 7777 and Host Liver

Compound	Control		Cyanate treated	
	Hepatoma 7777 (4)	Host Liver (5)	Hepatoma 7777 (3)	Host Liver (3)
Alanine	131 ± 23	213 ± 37	165 ± 28	349 ± 55
Arginine	10 ± 2	Trace	5 ± 1	Trace
Aspartic acid	90 ± 34	70 ± 26	55 ± 31	288 ± 33
Glutamic acid	187 ± 69	158 ± 40	198 ± 13	225 ± 41
Half-cystine	16 ± 9	Trace	Trace	4 ± 1
Histidine	15 ± 3	45 ± 6	14 ± 3	45 ± 6
Isoleucine	8 ± 2	8 ± 1	9 ± 3	9 ± 1
Leucine	9 ± 1	15 ± 3	20 ± 3	14 ± 2
Lysine	55 ± 8	41 ± 5	77 ± 5	60 ± 5
Methionine	4 ± 1	2	6 ± 1	3
Phenylalanine	7 ± 2	7 ± 1	5	5 ± 1
Proline	68 ± 20	13 ± 2	69 ± 5	21 ± 4
Serine	95 ± 26	430 ± 134	99 ± 20	184 ± 77
Threonine	52 ± 10	29 ± 5	42 ± 4	37 ± 2
Tyrosine	8 ± 1	3 ± 1	10 ± 1	7
Valine	19 ± 1	13 ± 2	24 ± 4	13 ± 2
Ammonia	156 ± 52	139 ± 47	445 ± 80	360 ± 52

Rats were killed one hour after i.p. injection of 250 mg sodium cyanate per kg body weight. Amino acids were assayed with the Beckman 120C amino acid analyzer. Concentrations are expressed as nmoles per 100 mg tissue with the results given as means ± standard errors when significant for the number of rats in parantheses (Lea and Koch, unpublished observations).

Table Four

Effect of TPCK on Incorporation of [³H] Amino Acids in Hepatoma 7777 and Host Liver

Tissue Fraction	Hepatoma 7777		Host Liver	
	Control	TPCK	Control	TPCK
Cytoplasmic protein	104 ± 13	60 ± 8	372 ± 34	418 ± 18
0.14 M NaCl nuclear extract	153 ± 12	99 ± 14	432 ± 35	461 ± 21
0.35 M NaCl nuclear extract	90 ± 9	54 ± 8	183 ± 6	203 ± 14
Histones	60 ± 5	33 ± 4	56 ± 4	72 ± 2
Residual nuclear protein	34 ± 7	14 ± 2	218 ± 33	266 ± 13

Rats received i.p. injections of TPCK solution in dimethylsulfoxide (0.1 ml containing 10 mg per 100 g body weight) or dimethylsulfoxide alone at the same time 100 uCi [³H] amino acids per 100 g body weight. The rats were killed 10 minutes after the injections. Means and standard errors are presented for 4 rats. Incorporation is expressed as cpm per 100 μg protein (Lea and Koch, unpublished observations).

amino acids into hepatomas which is seen at brief time periods after isotope injection. Although chemotherapy with a combination of drugs has been examined in a number of experimental tumors and has been of clinical value, there have been few such studies in hepatomas. The work of Jackson and Weber (20) suggests that this approach may be of value and can be undertaken on a systematic basis in the light of our extensive knowledge of enzyme activities in these tissues. Where two drugs have similar effects on macromolecular synthesis but differ in toxicity their combined effects may merit investigation. Such may be the case with the effects of cyanate and TPCK on hepatoma metabolism.

ACKNOWLEDGEMENTS

The work from the author's laboratory described in this review was performed in collaboration with Drs. Rosemary Barra, John Bullock, Teresa Campana, Erich Hirschberg, John Kallos and Fikry Khalil. The participation of Sr. Catherine Daly, Ms. Veena Dayal, Mr. Frank Perrella, Ms. Maria Rey and Mr. Norman Weeker, and the technical assistance of Mr. Bennett Beres, Mr. Herbert Hicks, Mr. Micheal Koch and Ms. Lynda Youngworth are gratefully acknowledged.

FOOTNOTES

[1] This work was supported in part by NIH grant CA-10729 to Dr. Harold P. Morris, NIH grants CA-11096, CA-12933 and CA-16274, American Cancer Society Institutional grant IN-92 and the Alma Toorock Memorial for Cancer Research.

[2] Abbreviation: TPCK, L-1-tosylamido-2-phenylethyl chloromethyl ketone.

REFERENCES

1. Arnold, E.A., Buksas, M.M., and Young, K.E. Cancer Rès. 33 (1973) 1169.

2. Balhorn, R., Balhorn, M., Morris, H.P., and Chalkley, R. Cancer Res 32 (1972) 1775.

3. Balhorn, R., Tanphaichitr, N., Chalkley, R., and Granner, D.K. Biochemistry 12 (1973) 5146.

4. Baserga, R., and Nicolini, C., Biochim. Biophys. Acta, 458 (1976) 109.

5. Borun, T.W., Gabrielli, F., Ajiro, K., Zweidler, A., and Balioni, C. Cell 4 (1975) 59.

6. Breindl, M., and Gallwitz, D. Eur. J. Biochem. 45 (1974) 91.

7. Bullock, J., Khan, M.Y., and Ianzano, J.A. Neoplasma 23 (1976) 277.

8. Chae, C.B., Smith, M.C., and Morris, H.P. Biochem. Biophys. Res. Comm. 60 (1974) 1468.

9. Chiu, J.F., Brade, W.P., Thomson, J., Tsai, Y.H., and Hnilica, L.S. Exper. Cell Res. 91 (1975) 200.

10. Chiu, J.F., Craddock, C., Getz, S., and Hnilica, L.S., FEBS Letters 33 (1973) 247.

11. Criss, W.E., and Morris, H.P. Biochem. Biophys. Res. Comm. 54 (1973) 380.

12. Elgin, S.C.R., and Weintraub, H. Ann. Rev. Biochem. 22 (1975) 725.

13. Farron-Furstenthal, F., Biochem. Biophys. Res. Comm. 67 (1975) 307.

14. Ferdinandaus, J.A., Morris, H.P., and Weber, G. Cancer Res. 31 (1971) 550.

15. Goldberg, M.L., Burke, G.C., and Morris, H.P. Biochem. Biophys. Res. Comm. 62 (1975) 320.

16. Granner, D. K. Biochem. Biophys. Res. Comm. 46 (1972) 1516.

17. Gronow, M., and Griffiths, G. FEBS Letters 15 (1971) 340.

18. Gullino,P. M., Prog. Exp. Tumor Res. 8 (1966) 1.

19. Higgins, G.N., and Anderson, R.M. Arch. Pathol. 12 (1931) 186.

20. Jackson, R.C., and Weber, G. Biochem. Pharmacol. 25 (1976) 2613.

21. Jungmann, R.A., Lee S., and DeAngelo, A.B. Adv. Cyclic Nucleotide Res. 5 (1975) 281.

22. Kelly, D.D., and Potter, V.R. Biochem. Biophys. Res. Comm. 75 (1977) 219.

23. Lea, M.A., Barra, R., Koch, M.R., Hicks, H., and Daly, C. Biochem. Biophys. Res. Comm. 75 (1977) 519.

24. Lea, M.A., Khalil, F.L., and Morris, H.P. Cancer Res 34 (1974) 3414.

25. Lea, M.A., Khalil, F.L., Rey, M.L., and Morris, H.P. Chem. Biol. Interactions 7 (1973) 367.

26. Lea, M.A., Khalil, F.L., Rey, M.L., and Morris, H.P. Chem. Biol. Interactions 6 (1973) 339.

27. Lea, M.A., and Koch, M.R. Int. J. Biochem., in press.

28. Lea, M.A., Koch, M.R., Allfrey, V.G., and Morris, H.P. Cancer Biochem. Biophys. 1 (1975) 129.

29. Lea, M.A., Koch, M.R.,Beres, B., and Dayal, V. Biochim. Biophys Acta 474 (1977) 321.

30. Lea, M.A., Koch, M.R., and Morris, H.P. Cancer Res 35 (1975) 2321.

31. Lea, M.A., Koch, M.R., and Morris, H.P. Cancer Res 35 (1975) 1693.

32. Lea, M.A., Koch, M.R., and Morris, H.P. Cancer Biochem. Biophys. 1 (1976) 265.

33. Lea, M.A., Miller, S., Mackauf, I., Hirschberg, E., and Morris, H.P. Int. J. Cancer 9 (1972) 484.

34. Lea, M.A., Morris, H.P., and Weber, G. Cancer Res 26 (1966) 465.

35. Lea, M.A., Morris, H.P., and Weber, G. Cancer Res 28 (1968) 71.

36. Lea, M.A., Youngworth, L.A., and Morris, H.P. Biochem. Biophys.

Res. Comm. 58 (1974) 862.

37. Mackenzie, C.W., and Stellwagen, R.H. J. Biol. Chem. 249 (1974) 5755.

38. Morris, H.P., and Meranze, D.R. In: Recent Results Cancer Res. E. Grundman (ed). 44 (1974) 102.

39. Morris, H.P., and Wagner, B.P. In: Methods in Cancer Research, H. Busch (ed). Academic Press, New York, 4 (1968) 125.

40. Moyer, G.H., and Pitot, H.C. Cancer Res 34 (1974) 2653.

41. Olson, M.O.J., abd Guetzow, K. In: The Molecular Biology of Cancer, H. Busch (ed). Academic Press, New York (1974) 309.

42. Panyim, S., and Chalkley, R. Arch. Biochem. Biophys. 130 (1969) 337.

43. Panyim, S., and Chalkley, R. Biochem. Biophys. Res. Comm. 37 (1969) 1042.

44. Stein, G.S., Criss, W.E., and Morris, H.P. Life Sciences, 14 (1974) 95.

45. Teng, C.S., Teng, C.T., and Allfrey, V.G. J. Biol. Chem. 246 (1971) 3957.

46. Thomas, E.W., Murad, F., Looney, W.B., and Morris, H.P. Biochim. Biophys. Acta 297 (1973) 564.

47. Tidwell, T., Bruce, B.J., and Griffin, A.C. Cancer Res 32 (1972) 1002.

48. Vidali, G., Karn, J., and Allfrey, V.G. Proc. Natl. Acad. Sci. U.S.A. 72 (1975) 4450.

49. Wagle, S.R., Morris, H.P., and Weber, G. Cancer Res 23 (1963) 1003.

50. Weber, G., New England J. Med., 296 (1977) 486.

51. Weberm G., New England J. Med., 296 (1977) 541.

52. Weber, G., and Lea, M.A. In: Methods in Cancer Research, H. Busch (ed). Academic Press, New York 2 (1967) 523.

53. Weber, G., Singhal, R.L., and Srivastava, S.K. Adv. Enzyme Reg. 3 (1965) 369.

54. Wilson, B., Lea, M.A., Vidali, G., and Allfrey, V.G. Cancer
    Res 35 (1975) 2954.

55. Yeoman, L.C., Taylor, C.W., and Busch, H. Cancer Res 34 (1974)
    424.

CONTROL OF SPECIFIC MESSENGER RNA SPECIES IN

LIVER AND HEPATOMA

Philip Feigelson and Linda W. DeLap

The Institute of Cancer Research and the
Department of Biochemistry
College of Physicians and Surgeons
Columbia University, New York, N.Y. 10032

SUMMARY

Two liver proteins subject to hormonal induction,
α2u-globulin and tryptophan oxygenase, were absent from
well-differentiated Morris hepatomas. Pulse [^{3}H]-leucine
incorporation studies in vivo demonstrated that in Morris
hepatoma 5123D no synthesis of α2u-globulin occurs while
the host liver synthesizes this protein at a normal rate.
Using an in vitro translation system and polyadenylate-
containing RNA isolated from host livers or hepatomas,
the level of specific mRNA functionally capable of coding
for α2u-globulin was determined. Host liver was found to
contain α2u-globulin mRNA at normal levels whereas hepatoma tissue was devoid of functionally competent mRNA
coding for this protein.

Similarly, levels of specific mRNA coding for tryptophan oxygenase were determined for host livers and hepatomas from control rats and rats administered an inducing
dose of hydrocortisone. The hormonal induction of tryptophan oxygenase activity in the host livers was accompanied by a proportionate increase in the level of its mRNA.
Tryptophan oxygenase catalytic activity and functional
mRNA for this enzyme were undetectable in hepatomas from
either control or glucocorticoid-induced animals. The
hepatomas contained normal levels of cytoplasmic glucocorticoid receptor that could bind glucocorticoids, undergo
normal "activation" and translocate both normal and hepatoma nuclei. Thus, the hepatomas failed to synthesize

tryptophan oxygenase due to some pretranslational defect
despite the presence of functional glucocorticoid receptor
and nuclear binding sites.

The deletion of α2u-globulin and tryptophan oxygenase
in these hepatomas is a consequence of a lack of specific
mRNA species coding for these two proteins. These findings support the view that hepatomas differ from liver in
patterns of gene expression.

INTRODUCTION

Tumors often lack some of the specialized proteins
associated with the differentiated normal tissues from
which they arise. For example, many thyroid tumors do not
synthesize thyroid hormone, and certain skin cancers do
not produce keratin. Many hepatomas do not synthesize
plasma proteins (1, 20) and lack certain enzymes found in
normal liver cells, such as urea cycle enzymes and those
involved in gluconeogenesis or amino acid metabolism (9).
In place of specialized liver isoenzymes which are subject
to dietary and hormonal control, most hepatomas contain
what seem to be prototypic isoenzymes; for example, aldolase B, pyruvate kinase L and glucokinase may be replaced
by aldolase A, pyruvate kinase K and a form of hexokinase
(27). In addition, many tumors produce proteins characteristic of early developmental stages, such as α - fetoprotein, placental alkaline phosphatase, fetal forms of
thymidine kinase and ferritin (6) and a number of proteins
recognized as carcinofetal antigens (3). The striking
examples of the etopic production of various polypeptide
hormones by some non-endocrine human tumors (12) indicate
that alterations in patterns of protein synthesis have
occurred in these tumor cells. Abnormalities in the regulation of gene expression in neoplastic cells could be
responsible for their altered phenotypes and could be involved in the transformation process itself.

It has been difficult to identify the mechanism responsible for the absence of some of the characteristic
liver proteins in hepatomas. One approach to this problem
is to compare the level of functional mRNA (coding for a
liver protein not found in hepatoma) in hepatoma to that
in normal liver, in order to determine whether the deletion
of that protein is a pre- or post-translational event.
This review describes the results of such experiments for
two proteins produced in rat liver, α 2u-globulin and tryptophan oxygenase. α2u-globulin, first described by Roy and
Neuhaus (17), is synthesized by the livers of male rats,

secreted into the serum, and excreted in the urine. Its
function is this far unknown. The hepatic synthesis of
this protein is under complex hormonal control by sex
hormones, glucocorticoids, thyroid hormones, and pituitary hormones (11, 16, 18, 25). In various endocrine
states there is a direct correlation between the level
of a α2u-globulin mRNA (assayed by methods developed in
this laboratory) in male rat liver and level of this
protein in liver, serum and urine (11, 25). Studies of
in vivo synthesis rates of α2u-globulin and levels of
its functional mRNA in Morris hepatomas and host livers,
reported previously (26), are described here.

        Like α 2u-globulin, tryptophan oxygenase is subject
to complex biological controls involving hormonal regulation of its rate of synthesis (5), as well as substrate
mediated control of its rate of degredation (19) and
allosteric control of its catalytic activity (4). Previous results from this laboratory (24) have demonstrated
that induction of hepatic tryptophan oxygenase by glucocorticoids is accompanied by a proportional increase in
the level of its mRNA. However, induction by its substrate tryptophan and superinduction by actinomycin D are
not accompanied by parallel increases in tryptophan oxygenase mRNA.

        Other workers have found low or negligible tryptophan
oxygenase activity in the rat hepatomas they examined.
The low catalytic activity found in several well-differentiated hepatomas either failed to respond or responded
abnormally to tryptophan and glucocorticoids, which caused increases in tryptophan oxygenase activity in normal
and host livers (2, 14). Studies done in this laboratory
did not detect any tryptophan oxygenase activity in three
well-differentiated Morris hepatomas, even in rats treated
with hydro-cortisone. The results presented here help to
locate the defect in hepatomas which results in the deletion of tryptophan oxygenase (15).

                            METHODS

In vivo Labeling of Hepatic and Hepatoma Proteins and
Measurement of the Rate of α2u-globulin Synthesis

        Non-tumor bearing rats were given i.v. injections of
[^{3}H]-leucine, (50 Ci/mmole), 0.5 mCi/100g body weight, and
hepatoma carrying animals received 1.0 mCi/100g body
weight. Twelve minutes after injection the animals were
sacrificed and the livers and/or tumors were excised.

Polysome-free supernatant fractions (S100s) were prepared, TCA-precipitable radioactivity was determined in
the supernatants, and SDS polyacrylamide gel electrophoresis of TCA-precipitable material from these fractions
was performed as described (26). α2u-globulin synthesis
was determined by specific immunoprecipitates of 2u-
globulin from the liver or hepatoma S100s. Immunoprecipitates were washed thoroughly and subjected to SDS
gel electrophoresis and the amount of radioactivity incorporated into the α2u-globulin peak was estimated.

Isolation of mRNA fractions

Total RNA was prepared from frozen liver, hepatoma
and kidney by phenol-chloroform extraction (21). Polyadenylate-containing RNA was isolated as described (21).

In vitro Protein Synthesis and Quantitation of α2u-globulin and tryptophan oxygenase mRNA Activity

For mRNA-directed in vitro protein synthesis, a
Krebs II ascites mRNA dependent cell-free translational
system, supplemented with tRNA and rabbit reticulocyte
initiation factors, was used (22). After incubation, the
total amount of radioactivity incorporated into the newly
synthesized released polypeptide chains and the SDS polyacrylamide gel electrophoretic profile of total proteins
were determined. mRNA dependent synthesis of a α2u-
globulin or tryptophan oxygenase was measured by isolation
of these de novo labeled proteins by immunoprecipitation
with mono-specific antibodies following the addition of
carrier levels of the respective proteins. The immunoprecipitates were then subjected to SDS polyacrylamide
gel electrophoresis. Radioactive peaks were evident at
positions of the gel corresponding to the protomeric molecular weights of tryptophan oxygenase and α2u-globulin.
The amount of radioactivity in these peaks was taken to
reflect the amount of the corresponding functional mRNA
(5, 10, 25, 26).

Glucocorticoid Receptor Studies

The methods used for these studies have been described (15). Cytosol was prepared from homogenates of perfused rat liver or hepatoma. The amount of glucocorticoid
receptor present in the cytosol was determined from binding of [^{3}H]-triamcinolone acetonide (16 Ci/mmole, 20 n$\underline{M}$)
after incubation for 2 hours at 0. After correction for
non-specific binding the specific macromolecular bound

fraction was determined using the dextran-coated charcoal adsorption technique. DNA-cellulose was used to measure the degree to which glucocorticoidal-receptor complex of hepatomas was capable of activation. To evaluate the ability of nuclei of host livers and hepatomas to bind activated glucocorticoid-receptor complex, purified nuclei were prepared and incubated at 25° for 25 min with cytosol containing activated [^{3}H]-triamcinolone-saturated glucocorticoid receptor. The nuclei were then washed and their radioactivity was measured.

Experimental Studies on α2u-globulin in Rat Liver and Morris Hepatoma 5123D

The rate of α2u-globulin synthesis in vivo can be evaluated by specific immunoprecipitation of this protein from male rat liver cytosol after pulse incorporation of labeled amino acids into newly synthesized hepatic proteins. SDS polyacrylamide gel electrophoresis of the immunoprecipitate reveals the presence of a single radioactive species of the same electrophoretic mobility as α2u-globulin(Fig 1). No corresponding radioactive material was found in the immunoprecipitate from female rat liver, as expected since females do not synthesize α2u-globulin (25). Data from this experiment permit calculation of the amount of α2u-globulin synthesized by male rat liver as a percentage of total hepatic protein synthesis in vivo. The validity of the calculation depends on complete recovery of radioactive α2u-globulin in the immunoprecipitate. A second immunoprecipitation with added carrier gave no additional radioactive α2u-globulin. Also, the short in vivo labeling time (12 min) ensured that newly synthesized radioactive α2u-globulin would not be secreted into the blood. As shown in Table 1, about 0.9% of the total [^{3}H]-leucine incorporated into S100 protein was found in α2u-globulin.

Following measurement of α2u-globulin synthesis rates in vivo, levels of functional mRNA for this protein were quantitated by translational analysis in an heterologous cell free system. Polyadenylate-containing RNA from male rat liver directed the synthesis of α2u-globulin and many other proteins in the Krebs IIascites cell free system (Fig 2). The α2u-globulin synthesized, isolated by specific immunoprecipitation, was calculated to represent about 1.5% of total [^{3}H]-leucine incorporation into proteins in vitro (Table 1). As expected, female liver or male kidney mRNA preparations effectively stimulated total protein syn-

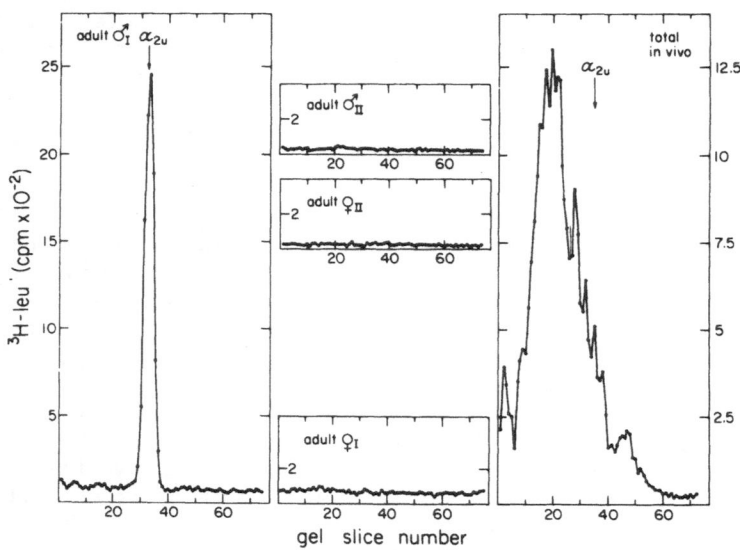

Figure 1
SDS-polyacrylamide gel electrophoretic profile of
total S100 proteins and immunoprecipitated α2u-globulin
synthesized in rat liver in vivo. Male and female rats
were injected with [3H]-leucine as described in Methods.
Right panel: Electrophoretic pattern of 25 ul total S100
protein. Left panel: α2u-globulin immunoprecipitated from
1 ml of the labeled S100 derived from male liver. Bottom
center: Immunoprecipitate derived from 1 ml of labeled
S100 from female liver. The two top center panels verify
that no labeled α2u-globulin could be found with a second
round of immunoprecipitation. Arrows mark position of
authentic α2u-globulin.

Table One

Comparison of in vivo and in vitro α2u-globulin Synthesis

A. in vivo incorporation [a]

	[³H]-leucine (cpm)	%
Total protein	22,000,000	119
S100 protein	18,500,000	100
α2u-globulin	163,000	0.88

B. in vitro incorporation [b]

	[³H]-leucine (pmol)	%
Total protein	1,580	284
Released chains	564	100
α2u-globulin	8.34	1.49

[a]
Values for 5 g male liver, calculated from experiment outlined in the legend to Chart 1.

[b]
Values for 500ul assay volume, calculated from experiment outlined in the legend to Chart 2.

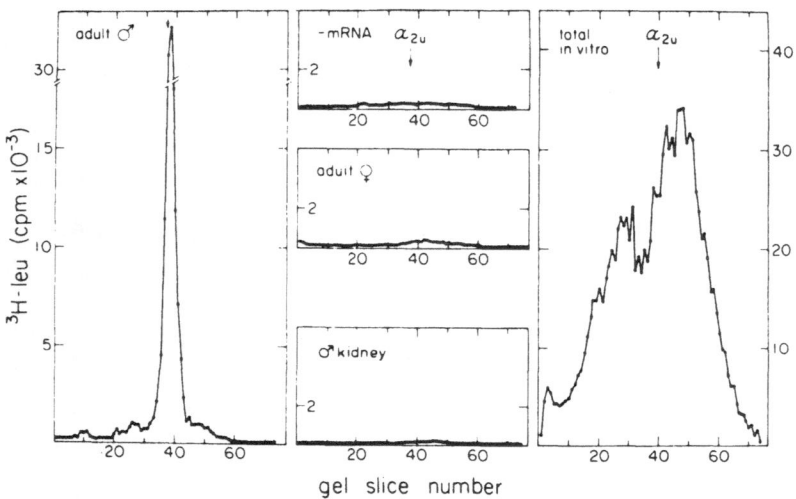

Figure 2
        SDS-polyacrylamide gel electrophoretic profile in
total protein and immunoprecipitated α2u-globulin synthesized in vitro. Protein synthesis performed as described in Methods. Right panel: electrophoretic profile of 70µl of the released chain fraction of the Krebs
IIascites system following incubation for 90 min with
5 µg male rat liver mRNA. Left panel: immunoprecipitated α2u-globulin synthesized in 350 µl of the Krebs system containing 35 ug male liver mRNA. To center panel:
same as left; no exogenous mRNA added. Middle center:
same as left; 35 µg female liver mRNA added. Bottom
center: same as left; 37.5 µg male kidney mRNA added.

thesis but did not detectably direct synthesis of α 2u-
globulin.

To determine whether α2u-globulin is synthesized by
hepatoma 5123D, male rats bearing this tumor intramuscularly were injected with [^{3}H]-leucine. Due perhaps to
differences in protein synthesis rate, amino acid uptake,
or pool size, incorporation of [^{3}H]-leucine into S100
protein of the hepatoma was only one third that incorporated into hepatic protein (Table 2). However, the amount of
radioactivity incorporated was sufficient for detection of
a protein representing as little as 0.1% of the total protein synthesis. Figure 3 shows that no α2u-globulin synthesis could be detected in this hepatoma whereas the liver
of the tumor bearing rat synthesized α2u-globulin at a
normal rate (Table 2). Synthesis of α2u-globulin by rat
liver is dependent on a number of hormones. The possibility existed that absence of α 2u-globulin synthesis in hepatoma 5123D was due to an alteration in the endocrine
state of the tumor bearing animal. However, the normal
level of α 2u-globulin synthesis in the liver of the tumor
bearing animal makes this impossible.

To determine if the failure of hepatoma 5123D to synthesize α2u-globulin _in vivo_ was due to absence of functional mRNA for this protein, polyadenylate-containing RNA
was prepared from hepatomas. This mRNA preparation directed incorporation of [^{3}H]-leucine into total protein in the
ascites system as efficiently as did that derived from
host liver (Table 2). In contrast to host liver, mRNA derived from the hepatomas did not direct detectable synthesis of α2u-globulin (Fig 4). Thus, hepatoma 5123D
lacks functional mRNA for α2u-globulin.

Experimental Studies on the Control of Tryptophan
Oxygenase Levels in Morris Hepatomas and Host Livers

Morris hepatomas 7793, 5123C and livers of rats bearing these tumors were examined for trypthan oxygenase
catalytic activity (Table 3). The host livers were comparable to normal rat liver in tryptophan oxygenase activity and in induction of the enzyme by hydrocortisone,
while the hepatomas contained no detectable activity (15).

To determine whether these hepatomas contained mRNA
coding for tryptophan oxygenase, polyadenylate-containing
RNA was prepared from them and translated in the ascites
system. In earlier experiments with normal rat liver mRNA
(24) specific immunoprecipitation of the translation

Table Two

α2u-globulin Synthesis in vivo and α2u-globulin mRNA
Activity in Hepatoma and
Host Liver

Tissue		[³H]-leucine incorporation			
		In vivo [a]		In vitro [b]	
		cpm	%	pmoles	%
Male host liver	Total protein	406,000	100	111.1	100
	α2u-globulin	4,100	1.2	1.92	1.7
Hepatoma 5123D	Total protein	146,000	100	106.7	100
	α2u-globulin	0	0	0	0

[a] Values are derived from 1 ml of S-100 prepared from host liver and hepatoma from rats given [³H]-leucine in vivo.

[b] Values are derived from 250μl of the released chain fraction of the Krebs IIascites system translating liver and hepatoma mRNA.

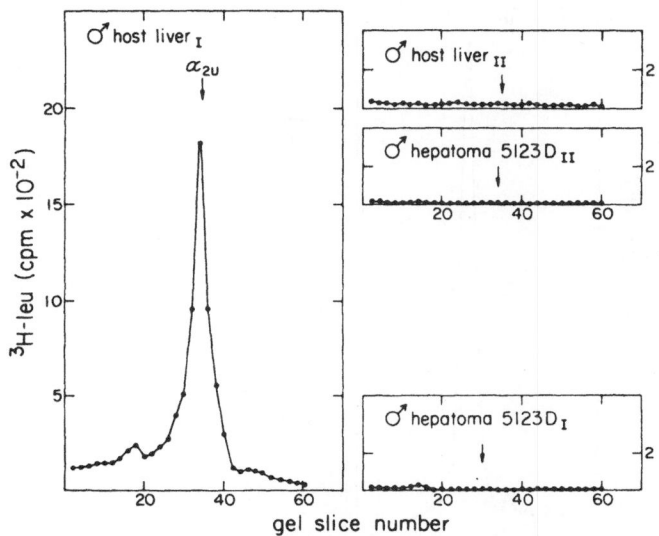

Figure 3

SDS-polyacrylamide gel electrophoretic profile of
immunoprecipitated α2u-globulin synthesized <u>in</u> <u>vivo</u> in
hepatoma 5123D and male host liver. A tumor bearing animal was injected with [^{3}H]leucine as described in Methods.
Left panel: α2u-globulin immunoprecipitated from 1 ml of
labeled S100 derived from host liver. Bottom right panel:
immunoprecipitate derived from 1 ml of labeled S100 derived from hepatoma tissue. The two top right panels
verify that no labeled α2u-globulin could be found with
a second round of immunoprecipitation.

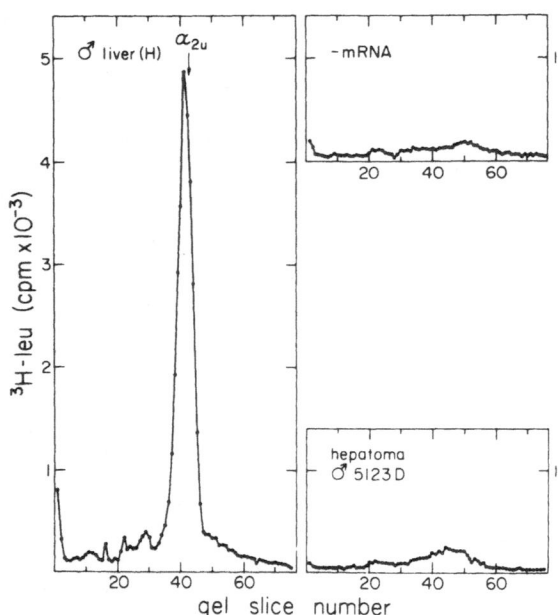

Figure 4
SDS-polyacrylamide gel electrophoretic profile of α2u-globulin synthesis in vitro directed by mRNA from hepatoma 5123D and host liver. Protein synthesis performed as described in Methods. Left panel: immunoprecipitated α2u-globulin synthesized in vitro under the direction of 9.5 ug mRNA derived from the liver of a male rat bearing hepatoma 5123D. Bottom right panel: same as left, except that 9.0 μg mRNA derived from hepatoma tissue was added rather than liver mRNA. Top right panel: same as left; no exogenous mRNA added.

Table Three

Levels of Catalytic Activity and mRNA for Tryptophan in Host
Livers and Hepatomas

Experimental details are given in
the legend to Fig. 7.

Tissue	Treatment	Tryptophan Oxygenase catalytic activity (umoles of kynurenine hr/g of tissue)	Translational Assay ($[^3H]$-leucine incorporation)		Tryptophan Oxygenase as % of total protein synthesis
			Total Released chains (cpm x 10^6)	cpm in Tryptophan Oxygenase	
Host Liver 7793	None	3.1	1.35	337	0.025
	Hydrocortisone	10.6	1.89	931	0.069
Hepatoma 7793	None	0	1.90	0	
	Hydrocortisone	0	1.35	0	
Host Liver 5123C	None	4.9	1.31	253	0.019
	Hydrocortisone	15.8	1.45	504	0.034
Hepatoma 5123C	None	0	1.24	0	
	Hydrocortisone	0	1.34	0	
Host Liver 5123D	None	4.5	1.25	261	0.020
	Hydrocortisone	18.0	1.36	453	0.032
Hepatoma 5123D	None	0	1.71	0	
	Hydrocortisone	0	1.91	0	

products gave a major peak of radioactivity on SDS polyacrylamide gels, corresponding in electrophoretic mobility to the promoters of tryptophan oxygenase (molecular
weight 43,000). As previously shown the mRNA from livers
of rats treated with hydrocortisone directed the synthesis
of more tryptophan oxygenase than did mRNA from control
rats (Fig 5) (24). The increase in hepatic tryptophan
oxygenase catalytic activity after hydrocortisone treatment paralleled an increase in mRNA levels of this enzyme
(Fig 6). mRNA from livers of rats bearing Morris hepatoma 7793 directed the synthesis of tryptophan oxygenase,
and there was a several fold increase in this enzyme's
synthesis when mRNA was obtained from livers of these
rats after injection of hydrocortisone (Fig 7). mRNA
isolated from the hepatomas of control or hydrocortisone-
treated rats did not direct detectable synthesis of tryptophan oxygenase. The data in Table 3 demonstrate that
mRNA from this hepatoma and also from two other hepatomas,
5123C and 5123D, was as efficient in directing incorporation of [^{3}H]-leucine into total proteins as was mRNA from
the host livers. However, none of the hepatomas had detectable mRNA functionally capable of directing the synthesis of tryptophan oxygenase.

The lack of tryptophan oxygenase or tryptophan oxygenase mRNA activity in the hepatomas could have been due
to absence of the normal mechanism for induction of this
enzyme by glucocorticoids. To investigate this possibility, the hepatomas were examined for the presence of glucocorticoid receptor. Cytosol fractions were prepared from
hepatoma 7793 and from host liver and incubated with a
saturating concentration of [^{3}H]-triamcinolone (Table 4).
Hepatoma cytosol contained as much glucocorticoid receptor
activity as did liver cytosol from the same rat, from 100
to 200 fmoles of receptor per mg of cytosol protein. This
level of receptor is that expected of steroid target tissues.

Hepatic glucocorticoid receptor undergoes a temperature-dependent conversion enabling it to bind to DNA,
chromatin or nuclei (5). Evidence for similar functional
behavior of the hepatoma glucocorticoid-receptor complex
was sought. It was found that, after incubation at 25°
for 25 min, steroid-receptor complexes from host liver and
from hepatoma 7793 bound equally well to rat liver DNA-
cellulose (Table 5). Similarly, activated glucocorticoid-
receptor complex from host liver and from the hepatoma
bound to nuclei from host liver. When this experiment was
repeated using nuclei from the hepatoma similar results

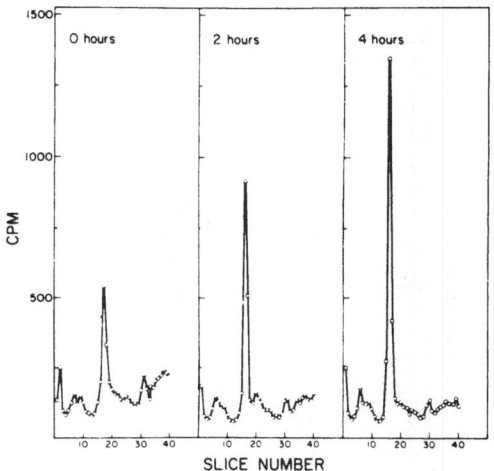

Figure 5
        SDS-polyacrylamide gel electrophoretic profile of
immunoprecipitated tryptophan oxygenase synthesized in
vitro.   Left panel: immunoprecipitated tryptophan oxygenase synthesized in 500 µl of the Krebs IIascites system containing 60 ug of mRNA from the livers of control
rats.   Middle and right panels: same as left except that
mRNA was from livers of rats received 5 mg of hydrocortisone 100 g body weight 2 and 4 hours before they
were killed.

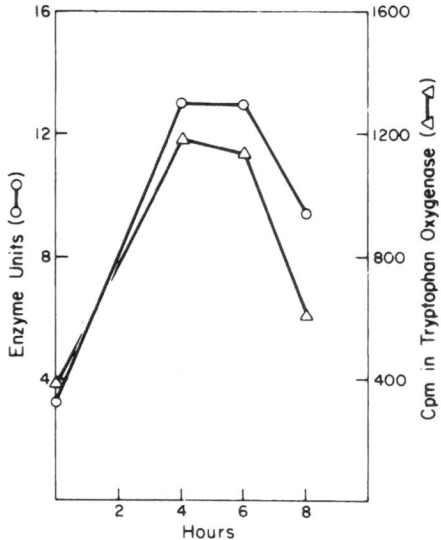

Figure 6
Tryptophan oxygenase activity and mRNA levels for
tryptophan oxygenase in the livers of rats after intra-
peritoenal injection of 2 mg of hydrocortisone/100 g of
body weight.

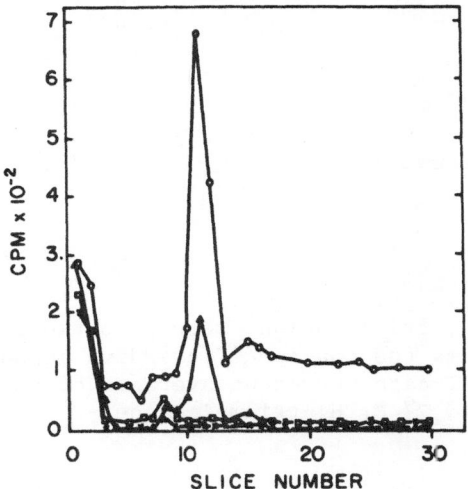

Figure 7
SDS-polyacrylamide gel electrophoretic profiles of
immunoprecipitated tryptophan oxygenase synthesized in
the Krebs IIascites system. The reaction mixture (500
µl) contained 60 µg of mRNA prepared from host livers
(△) or from hepatoma 7793 (◻) of control rats, or from
livers (○) and tumors (X) of rats injected with 5.0
mg of hydrocortisone/100 g of body weight 4 hours before
sacrifice.

Table Four

Glucocorticoid Receptor Activity in Liver and Morris Hepatoma
Cytosols

Source of Cytosol	Specific bound [a] [^{3}H]-triamcinolone (cpm/mg protein)
Host Liver	2286 [b]
Morris Hepatoma 7793	2339 [b]

[a]
Specific bound [^{3}H]-triamcinolone refers to the total macromolecular bound cpm less the non-specific inding measured as described in Methods.   All data represent averages of duplicate determinations at 20 x 10 $^{-9}$ M[^{3}H]-triamcinolone.

[b]
Expressed in molar units: 2286 cpm/mg equals 193 fmoles per mg of cytosol protein;   2339 cpm/mg equals 197 fmoles per mg of cytosol protein.

Table Five

The Binding of Liver and Morris Hepatoma Cytoplasmic Glucocorticoid
Receptor Complexes to Rat Liver DNA-cellulose

Source of Cytosol	Bound [^{3}H]-triamcinolone-receptor Complex (cpm/100µg DNA)
Host Liver	7090
Morris Hepatoma 7793	6966

Table Six

The Binding of Liver and Morris Hepatoma Cytoplasmic Glucocorticoid-receptor
Complexes to Homologous and Heterologous Nuclei

Source of Nuclei	Bound [^{3}H]-triamcinolone Host Liver Receptor Complex		Bound [^{3}H]-triamcinolone- Hepatoma Receptor Complex	
	(cpm/mg DNA)		(cpm/mg DNA)	
Host Liver	57,371		77,214	
Morris Hepatoma 7793	67,143		72,814	

were obtained (Table 6). These experiments indicate
that hepatoma 7793 contains glucocorticoid receptor
which normally binds steroids and undergoes activation
enabling it to bind to DNA and nuclei. Furthermore, nuclei of this hepatoma possess normal binding capacity
for the glucocorticoid-receptor complex.

INTERPRETATION

     The results presented here have helped to elucidate
the mechanism responsible for the absence of two hepatic
proteins, α2u-globulin and tryptophan oxygenase in hepatomas. These proteins are not synthesized in hepatomas
because the tumors are unable to generate the correspon-
ing functional mRNA species. Expression of the genes for
these proteins involves many steps, schematized in Fig 8.
Both α2u-globulin and tryptophan oxygenase are induced
by steroids. The fact that normal levels of these proteins were found in the livers of hepatoma bearing rats
seems to rule out possible endocrine disturbances in
these animals as an explanation for absence of α2u-
globulin and tryptophan oxygenase in the hepatomas. The
upper left hand part of Figure 8 diagrams the binding of
steroid hormones to receptors and translocation of the
activated steroid-receptor complex to the nucleus, where
it binds to DNA. Results presented here suggest that at
least the first several steps by which glucocorticoids
act to induce synthesis of specific proteins (among them
tryptophan oxygenase and α2u-globulin), including binding
of the activated steroid-receptor complex to nuclei and to
DNA, occur normally in Morris hepatoma 7793. Some other
Morris hepatomas have been reported to contain somewhat
lower levels of apparently normal glucocorticoid receptor
(8).

     To gather information about events that take place
within the nucleus, it is necessary to have some means
of detecting specific genes and the nucleic acids that
code for a specific protein but that may not fucntion in
protein synthesis; these might include the initial transcripts of genes and the intermediate precursors (some
probably as yet unknown) of mRNA. The transport of mRNA
from the nucleus to the cytoplasm and its degredation might
also be important points for regulation of gene expression.
The assay of functional mRNA does not provide information
about these processes. However, these results do tell a
good deal about what can occur in the cytoplasm. Obviously, without the corresponding specific functional mRNA
no α2u-globulin or tryptophan oxygenase protein can be

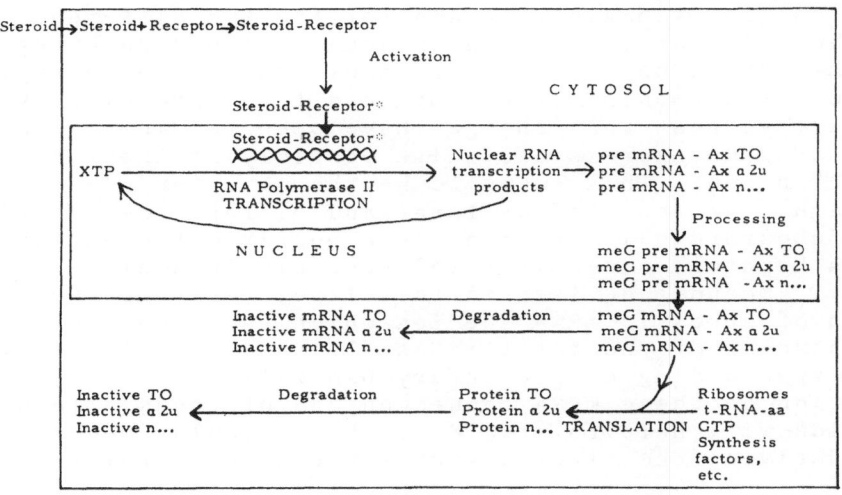

Figure 8
Steps in the expression of the genes for α2u-globulin,
tryptophan oxygenase, and other hepatic proteins.

made. The absence of α2u-globulin and trypton oxygenase
in the hepatomas examined, which do not contain normal
levels of mRNA capable of directing global protein synthesis, must be due to lack of these specific mRNAs and
not to some translational aberration or to increased
degradation of these proteins.

The absence of α2u-globulin and tryptophan oxygenase
mRNAs in the hepatomas examined presumably reflect changes
in transcription patterns. Hepatomas 7793, 5123C and
5123D have more than the diploid number of chromosomes
(13). The possibility of deletion of the genes themselves
has not been excluded, but it seems unlikely that all
three genes (for α2u-globulin and for the two different
protomeric units of tryptophan oxygenase) could have been
lost in all these hepatomas. The many examples of ectopic
production of hormones, isoenzymes and fetal proteins by
tumors (27) suggest that changes have occurred in the regulation of gene expression, quite possibly at the level
of transcription. This seems to be the case for α -
fetoprotein. As reported by Innes and Miller, the mRNA
for α - fetoprotein is abundant in a poorly differentiated Morris hepatoma but almost undetectable in adult rat
liver (6). Methods devised in this laboratory for the
isolation of specific mRNA species which represent only
a small percent of the total mRNAs (17) and preparation
of the corresponding complementary DNA will allow the
quantitation of these mRNA sequences and of genes. This
information will help to elucidate the molecular mechanisms underlying the altered gene expression in tumors.

Abbreviations used are: SDS sodium dodecyl sulfate
                           TCA trichloroacetic acid
                           S100 100,000 g supernatant
                           fraction

REFERENCES

1. Becker, F.F., Klein, K.M., Wolman, S.R., Asofsky, R. and Sell, S. Cancer Res. 33 (1973) 3330.

2. Cho, Y.S., Pitot, H.C. and Morris, H.P. Cancer Res. 24 (1962)52.

3. Coggin, J.H. Jr., Ambrose, K.R. and Anderson, N.G. In: Embryonic and Fetal Antigens in Cancer, N.G. Anderson and J.H. Coggin (eds) Springfield, Va., U.S. Department of Commerce, 1 (1971) 185.

4. Feigelson, P. and Brady, F.O. In: Molecular Mechanisms of Oxygen Activation, O. Hayaishi (ed). Academic Press, New York, (1974) p. 87.

5. Feigelson, P., Beato, M., Colman, P., Kalimi, M., Killewich, L. and Schutz, G., Recent Progress in Cancer Res. 31 (1975) 213.

6. Fishman, W.H. and Singer, R.M. In: Cancer: A Comprehensive Treatise, F.F. Becker (ed). Plenum Press, New York (1975) p. 57.

7. Innis, M.A., and Miller, D.L. Federal Proc. 36 (1977) 818.

8. Kenney, F.T., Lane, S.E., lee, K.L. and Ihle, J.N. In: Control Mechanisms in Cancer, W.E. Criss, T. Onom J.R. Sabine (eds). Raven Press, New York (1976) p. 25.

9. Knox, W.E., Enzyme Patterns in Fetal, Adult and Neoplastic Rat Tissues, second edition, S. Krgaer, New York (1976).

10. Kurtz, D.T. and Feigelson, P. Adv. Enzymol. in press.

11. Kurtz, D.T., Sippel, A.E. and Feigelson, P. Biochemistry 15 (1976) 1031.

12. Levine, R.J. and Metz, S.A. Ann. N.Y. Acad. Sci. 230 (1974) 533.

13. Nowell, P.C., Morris, H.P. and Potter, V.R. Cancer Res. 27 (1967) 1565.

14. Pitot, H.C. Adv. in Enzyme Regul. 1 (1963) 309.

15. Ramanarayanan-Murthy, L., Colman, P.D., Morris, H.P. and Feigelson, P. Cancer Res. 36 (1976) 3594.

16. Roy, A.K. and Leonard, S.J. Endocrinol. 57 (1973) 327.

17. Roy, A.K. and Neuhaus, O.W. Biochim. Biophys. Acta, 127 (1966) 82.

18. Roy, A.K. and Neuhaus, O.W. Nature, 214 (1967) 618.

19. Schimke, R.T. and Doyle, D. Ann. Rev. Biochem. 39 (1970) 929.

20. Schreiber, G., Urban, J., Edwards, K., Dryburgh, H. and Inglis, A.S. Adv. in Enzyme Regul. 14 (1976) 163.

21. Schutz, G., Beato, M. and Feigelson, P. Proc. Natl. Acad. Sci. U.S.A. 70 (1973) 1218.

22. Schutz, G., Beato, M. and Feigelson, P. Methods Enzymol. 30 (1974) 701.

23. Schutz, G., Kieval, S., Groner, B., Sippel, A.E., Kurtz, D.T. and Feigelson, P. Nucleic Scids Res. 4 (1977) 71.

24. Schutz, G., Killewich, L., Chen, G. and Feigelson, P. Proc. Natl. Acad. Sci. U.S.A. 72 (1975) 1017.

25. Sippel, A.E., Feigelson, P. and Roy, A.K. Biochemistry 14 (1975) 825.

26. Sippel, A.E., Kurtz, D.T., Morris, H.P. and Feigelson, P., Cancer Res. 36 (1976) 3588.

27. Weinhouse, S., Shatton, J.B. and Morris, H.P. In: Cancer Enzymology, J. Schultz, F. Ahmad (eds). Academic Press, New York, (1976) p. 41.

ALTERATIONS IN PEROXISOMES OF HEPATOMAS

Hideyuki Tsukada, Yohichi Mochizuki, and Mikio Gotoh

Department of Pathology
Cancer   Research Institute
Sapporo Medical College
Sapporo 060, Japan

SUMMARY

Perixosomes are considered to provide a profitable tool in the study of differentiation of hepatocytes at the level of intracellular organelles. Thus, a review was made on the features of hepatocyte peroxisomes and alterations thereof in hepatomas. The following are suggested as characteristic traits of hepatomas.

(1) Alterations corresponding to the growth rate and/or the degree of differentiation of the tumors. For example, the number of peroxisomes and activity of catalase are approximately inversely related to this parameter of the tumors. Furthermore, it is possible to distinguish highly differentiated hepatomas from well and poorly differentiated tumors with respect to differences of the abnormal response of peroxisomes to peroxisome-proliferating agents.

(2) Alterations relating to retrodifferentiation in the tumors. The multiplicity pattern of catalase of hepatomas resembles closely that of the fetal enzymes, and this fetal pattern appears almost regardless of the growth rate and/or the degree of differentiation of the tumors.

(3) Alterations presumably relevant to cancerization. The inducive proliferation of peroxisomes seems to be strongly impaired in hepatomas, regardless of the growth rate and/or the degree of differentiation, contrasting with fetal as well as newborn livers.

(4) Alterations probably taking place randomly.

Peroxisomes are regarded as phylogenetically primitive organelles and their enzymes may delete progressively through evolutional development. Thus, further studies on peroxisomes may concern phylogenetical aspects of neoplasia.

INTRODUCTION

It is well known that malignant neoplasia are characterized by autonomic cell growth, retrodifferentiation, and metabolic independency from the control mechanisms of their hosts.

Peroxisomes are cytoplasmic organelles of hepatocytes which are easily identifiable histochemically or electron microscopically. The organelles and their enzymes are readily influenced by the state of the cells related to growth or differentiation. They are inducible as whole organelles and as constituent enzymes. In this context, peroxisomes may provide an appropriate tool to study the cellular alterations involved in cancerization of hepatocytes.

Peroxisomes were biochemically characterized by de Duve and his associates (4-6) in rat hepatocytes at first as containing catalase and hydrogen peroxide producing enzymes. At present it is well known that peroxisomes are distributed widely in the animal and plant kingdoms. Morphologically, peroxisomes correspond to microbodies which were identified electron microscopically in renal tubular epithelial cells of mice by Rhodin (49) and the identical cytoplasmic organelles were soon found in rat hepatocytes. Recently, with the development of histochemcial and electron microscopic-cytochemical techniques to demonstrate catalase activity (38), catalase-containing cytoplasmic organelles, namely peroxisomes, were found to distribute in a wide variety of vertebrate cells (16, 37). Conceivably, peroxisomes are now regarded as constituent organelles of animal cells; however, little is known about the metabolic sequences occurring in animal peroxisomes.

PEROXISOMES OF HEPATOCYTES

For an introduction to alterations of peroxisomes in hepatomas, morphological and functional features of the organelles of normal hepatocytes will be described briefly. For details refer to review articles (1, 4-7, 13, 29, 37, 50, 54, 58).

Morphology

Peroxisomes of hepatocytes are generally 300-600 mμ in diameter, are almost round or oval in shape, are bounded by a single limiting membrane of 60-80 Å in width, contain fine granular matrices, and contain highly electron dense crystalloid nucleoids in certain animal species (Fig 1). Occasionally, peroxisomes are seen bearing tubular

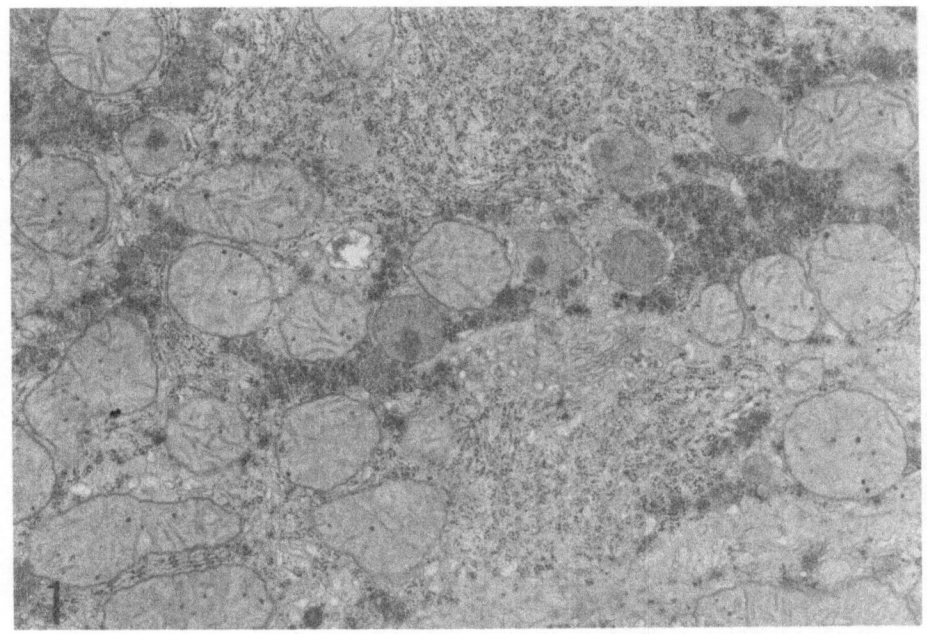

Figure 1
Hepatocyte of Normal Adult Rat. There are seven peroxisomes,
four of which contain electron-dense crystalloid nucleoid. x 15,000

connections with endoplasmic reticulum or tubular protrusions pro-
jecting from the surface of the peroxisomes. Typical peroxisomes
are identified as such in hepatocytes and renal tubular epithelial
cells; however, cytoplasmic organelles containing catalase but
lacking, in general, hydrogen peroxide producing enzymes are distributed in a wide variety of tissue cells. They were designated
as microperoxisomes by Novikoff (37). They are small in size, resemble frequently mere focal dilations of smooth endoplasmic cytochemistry for catalase as shown in Fig 2. It has been suggested
by Novikoff that microperoxisomes are also present in hepatocytes
and serve as progenitors of typical peroxisomes. However, it is
rather difficult to observe microperoxisomes in normal hepatocytes.

Biochemistry

     According to Leighton et al. (26), matrix of rat hepatocyte
peroxisomes occupies about 90% of peroxisomal proteins, while crystalloid nucleoid constitutes 10% thereof. As to the enzyme profile
catalase, d-amino acid oxidase, 1-α-hydroxy acid oxidase, and iso-
citrate dehydrogenase constitutes about 16%, 2%, 3%, and 25% of
the matrical proteins, respectively. Urate oxidase binds firmly
to crystalloid nucleoid and this enzyme constitutes no more than
25% of the nucleoid proteins in rat hepatocyte peroxisomes. This
enzyme is absent in peroxisomes lacking crystalloid nucleoids.
Carnitine acetyl transferase of rat liver is distributed to mitochondria, peroxisomes and a yet undetermined fraction at 52%, 14%
and 34%, respectively (28). Proteins that make up between one-half
and two-thirds of peroxisomal proteins have not been determined as
yet. From the biochemical and immunological studies of Hokama et
al. (10), it is suggested that a protein like C-reactive protein
may be one of the probable candidates for the unknown peroxisomal
proteins. The assumption that hepatic synthesis of acute-phase
serum protein occurs at the expense of peroxisomal proteins is considered along this line.

     As to the probable role of peroxisomal function in animal cell
metabolism, virtually no unifying hypothesis has been proposed since
the view of de Duve and his associates (1, 4-6). Peroxisomes are
suggested as an intracellular compartment of the peroxide forming
flavin oxidases and catalase, to play a role in reoxidation of reduced nicotinamide-adenine dinucleotide, in urate metabolism, and
in protection of the cells from hydrogen peroxide. Desert rats
(Meriones crassus) are known to utilize oxidation water for their
life, and peroxisomes present numerously in their liver may contribute to the removal of intermediates produced by active fatty acid
oxidation (50). The relation of peroxisomes to lipid and cholesterol
metabolism has been suggested on the basis that peroxisomes are present abundantly in the cells where lipid metabolism takes place actively, or that they exist spatially in close relation to lipid granules.

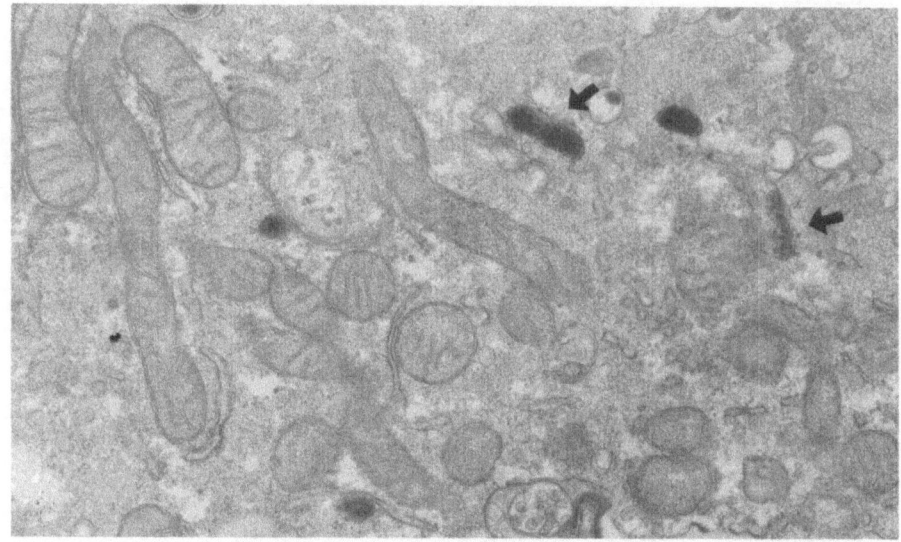

Figure 2
Electron Microscopic Cytochemistry for Catalase of Morris
7316A Hepatoma Cultured _in vitro_ for 3 months. There are five
peroxisomes of microperoxisome type. Note elongate shape of peroxisomes (arrows). x 20,000.

The role of peroxisomal carnitine acetyl transferase in lipid metabolism has not been clarified as yet. The hypolipidemic effects of ethyl-α-p-chlorophenoxyiso-butyrate (CPIB) and its analogs might not be directly linked with the capacity of the agents to induce peroxisomal proliferation and synthesis of liver catalase.

As to the intracellular distribution of catalase in the liver, the activity is recovered from both peroxisomal and extraparticulate fractions. The ratios of peroxisomal to the extraparticulate enzyme are various depending on the animal species (11).

Multiplicity of catalase of the liver is found in rats, mice and rabbits. It has been defined with respect to characteristics revealed by immunoelectrophoresis, polyacrylamide or starch gel electrophoresis, DEAE-cellulose column chromatography, or isoelectric focusing using Ampholine. Although opinions about the exact nature of the multiplicity are still in controversy, investigations hitherto reported seem to favor the assumption that the multiplicity results from an epigenetic modification of the enzyme but does not represent a true isoenzyme. According to the observations of Jones and Masters on the mouse liver catalase (20), electrophoretically fast moving acidic catalase is peroxisomal and is a sialated form, whereas slow moving neutral catalase is extraparticulate and is a desialated form. Furthermore, the desialated form is considered as being produced from the sialated form and more labile the latter. However, as to the enzyme in other animal species there have been no investigations of this sort.

Biogenesis and Destruction of Peroxisomes

Based on morphological observations that peroxisomes are occasionally connected with endoplasmic reticulum, it is appropriately suggested that peroxisomes are formed as the budding outgrowth probably of the specialized regions of the endoplasmic reticulum. On the other hand, from the biochemical point of view, it is also possible that peroxisomes do not exist as independent entities but continuously or intermittently exchange materials with one another (41). Reddy and Svoboda (47) surmised that peroxisomes are merely focal dilatations of endoplasmic reticulum, thus providing a scheme that the changes in the amount of peroxisomal proteins may readily reflect the numerical and volumetrical changes of peroxisomes. Microperoxisomes seem to be focal dilatations of endoplasmic reticulum where catalase and presumably other yet unidentified materials accumulate transiently; however, peroxisomes with crystalloid nucleoids are dubiously regarded morphologically as mere focal dilatations of endoplasmic reticulum.

As to the intracellular pathway of catalase, Lawarow and de Duve (24) reported that the newly synthesized catalase in the form of apo-subunits is discharged from polysomes into cytosol, then it is taken up into peroxisomes where insertion of the heme prosthetic group takes place and catalase molecules are assembled. This might be contrasted with a hypothesis that the enzyme synthesized on the bound ribosomes is discharged intracisternally and transported to peroxisomes through the channel of endoplasmic reticulum. There is no concrete evidence as to which concept is convincing. As mentioned above, there is a possibility that peroxisomal catalase is a sialated form; however, no information is available where in the cells the sialation process takes place.

As for the intracellular degradation of peroxisomes, biochemical data on the turnover of peroxisomal proteins favor the assumption that peroxisomes are degraded in autophagic vacuoles. However, peroxisomes are virtually very rarely found in autophagic vacuoles even in a state in which a rapid removal of once proliferated peroxisomes takes place. Thus, another possibility which might exist is that peroxisomal proteins can be degradated by flowing backward to endoplasmic reticulum cisternae through the interconnecting channel between the cisternae and peroxisomes, or that alternatively they enter directly into hyaloplasm across the limiting membranes of peroxisomes. Observations that peroxisomes with scanty matrices and wrinkled cantour increase in number when the proliferation and degradation of peroxisomes are enhanced simultaneously, make it a likely assumption that peroxisomal proteins leak out from the organelles to be degradated.

Induction of Peroxisomal Proliferation and Catalase Synthesis

It has been repeatedly reported that CPIB and several other hypolipidemic agents induce a striking numerical increase of hepatocyte peroxisomes with a significant elevation of catalase activity due to the enhanced synthesis (8, 12, 25, 45, 46, 55, 56) (Figs 3a and 3b). It is worthy of note that the volumetric increase of the total peroxisomal compartment in the cells exceeds the increase of catalase activity, suggesting that an increase of yet unidentified proteins contributes to the volumetric increase of peroxisomes to a considerable extent. Carnitine acetyl transferase activity increases several times in both peroxisomes and mitochondria by treatment with CPIB (8). D-amino acid oxidase activity is greatly diminished, although the mechanisms involved are unknown. Furthermore, the proliferated peroxisomes lack crystalloid nucleoids indicating a qualitative difference from the peroxisomes originally present. The induction of peroxisomes occurs in hepatocytes as well as in renal tubular epithelial cells; however, it is not known what influences the inducers have on microperoxisomes in the tissues other than the liver and kidney.

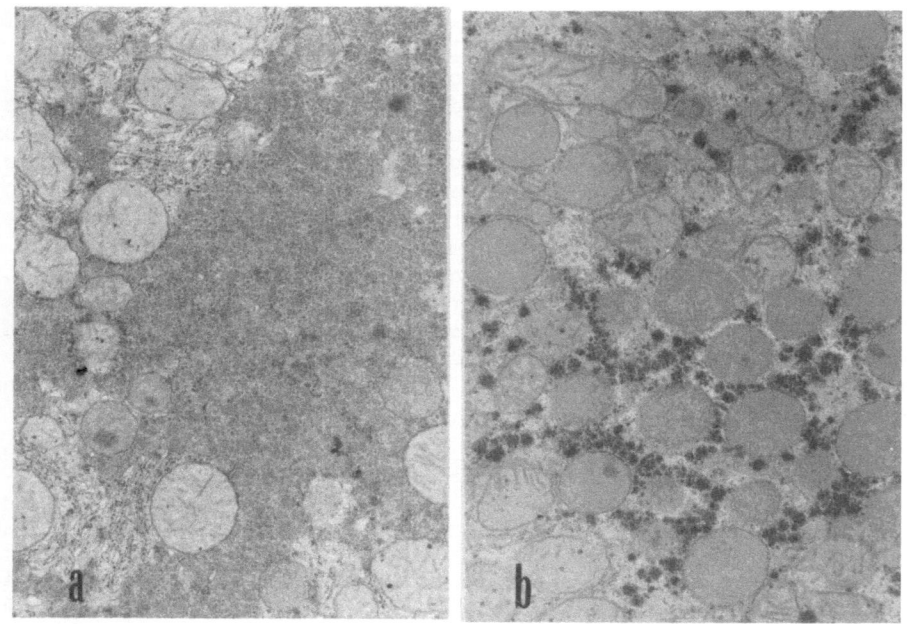

Figure 3
Hepatocyte of Rat Treated with CPIB. a: Control; b: Rat fed
diet containing 1% CPIB for 4 weeks. Numerical and volumetrical
increases of peroxisomes are remarkable. x 12,500.

CHANGES OF PEROXISOMES RELATED TO GROWTH, REGENERATION AND
DIFFERENTIATION

Fetal and Postnatal Growth

As to the numerical changes of peroxisomes during ontogenetic
development of rats, an appearance on or around the 15th day of
gestation and an increase during the late fetal and early postnatal periods were reported (62). Increases in catalase activity
are also obvious in the late fetal period. In rat and mouse hepatocytes, crystalloid nucleoids are rare in peroxisomes in the early
fetal stages; whereas in human and chicken livers, the nucleoids
are present during the fetal period but diminish as the animals
grow postnatally.

Proliferations of peroxisomes and elevation of catalase activity in the liver of fetal rats are inducible by the above-mentioned
hypolipidemic agents that are given to the mother animals, although
the degree of the induction is lower than in adult animals (56, 61)
as shown in Fig 4.

As to the multiplicity of catalase, Koyama (22) reported that
the enzyme of the liver of fetal and newborn rats showed alkaline
and neutral pIs in isoelectric focusing experiments. The acidic
enzyme components appeared while the basic components disappeared
during the third to fourth week after birth. On the other hand,
Patton and Nishimura (40) reported in their immunoelectrophoretic
study that anodic subcomponents of catalase are characteristic of
the enzyme in fetal and early postnatal periods, and that the enzyme
of the adult liver contained cathodic subcomponents in addition to
the anodic ones. These changes in the catalase multiplicity pattern
have relevance to the ontogenic differentiation of hepatocytes.

Partial Hepatectomy

There are at least two conflicting groups of reports concerning
numerical changes of peroxisomes in regenerating hepatocytes after
partial hepatectomy. Saito et al. (53) and we (33) reported the
decrease in early stages after hepatectomy. It is suggested that
the decrease is ascribed to a decreased formation of peroxisomes in
addition to an enhanced elimination of peroxisomes from the cells.
The number of peroxisomes is restored as the cells grow to maturity.
The pI-multiplicity of catalase in the regenerating liver is characterized by a decrease in the acidic components of the enzyme presumably corresponding to the less differentiated state of the cells (22).

Tissue Culture

Descriptions of the changes in peroxisomes in hepatocytes

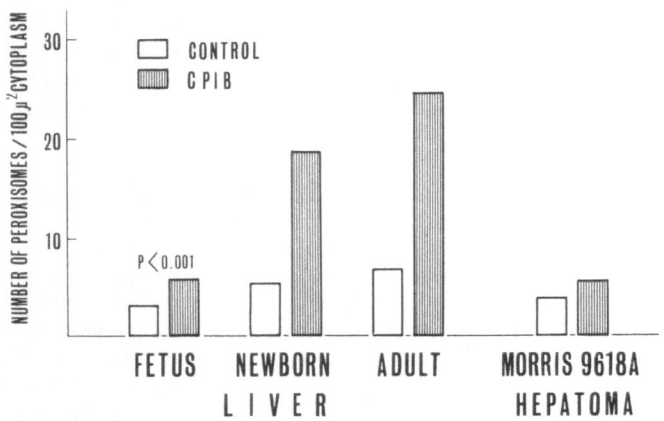

Figure 4
Effects of CPIB on Number of Peroxisomes of Rat Hepatocytes
and Morris 9618A Hepatoma (61).

cultured in vitro are relatively few. In the primary culture of
adult hepatocytes, peroxisomes are found in the relatively early
days of the culture and they disappear in the later days. In the
circumfusion culture of fetal and newborn livers, however, Rose
et al.(52) reported that peroxisomes lacking crystalloid nucleoids
were formed during the initial 1-2 weeks, and those containing the
nucleoids appeared during the subsequent periods of the culture indicating a progression toward maturity. Clonal cultures of hepatocytes generally do not show peroxisomes. However, as reported by
Williams et al. (66), peroxisomes that once diminished in the growing culture of hepatocytes appeared again in the confluent culture,
suggesting that the disappearance implied dedifferentiation and
simplification that occurred during the cell·multiplication.
Furthermore, a tumorigenic cell line isolated from a long term
culture of adult hepatocytes by Karasaki et al. (21) did not show
peroxisomes in vitro but showed in the cells grown in vivo following implantation of the cells in animals. It is conceivably assumed
that the absence of peroxisomes in cultured hepatocytes might not
necessarily imply the lack of capacity to form the organelles. The
problems of peroxisomes make a considerable donation to the evaluation of the nature of differentiation and maturation of hepatocytes.

PEROXISOMES OF HEPATOMAS

Peroxisomes are easily identifiable by their characteristic
ultrastructures. Thus, a number of electron microscopic studies
on hepatomas have referred to alterations of peroxisomes, although
only a little attention has been paid to the significance of the
alterations in tumors. A greater emphasis should be paid to peroxisomes to provide a greater amount of information on hepatomas, as
Malik (27) assumed that peroxisomes were virtually sole cytoplasmic
organelles which reflect most sensitively the degree of dedifferentiation of hepatomas.

Hruban et al. (14) reported that peroxisomes were absent in
fast-growing Novikoff and Morris 3683 hepatomas, while present in
slow-growing Reuber H-35 and Morris 5123 hepatomas. As to Morris
hepatomas, observations of Mochizuki et al. (30) cover a great number
of the tumor lines of various growth rates. Fast-growing, poorly
differentiated hepatomas contain none or a very small number of
peroxisomes which are small in size, scanty in matrices and usually
lacking crystalloid nucleoids. Frequently, peroxisomes in these
tumors are only identifiable by electron microscopic cytochemistry
(Figs 5a, 5b). Dalton (2) also reported that the size and complexity
of peroxisomes of hepatomas were inversely proportional to the growth
rate of the tumors. There might be general agreement that peroxisomes
of fast-growing, poorly differentiated hepatomas are very few, in
number or virtually absent, regardless of whether the tumors are
primarily induced or transplantable. Furthermore, adenocarcinomas

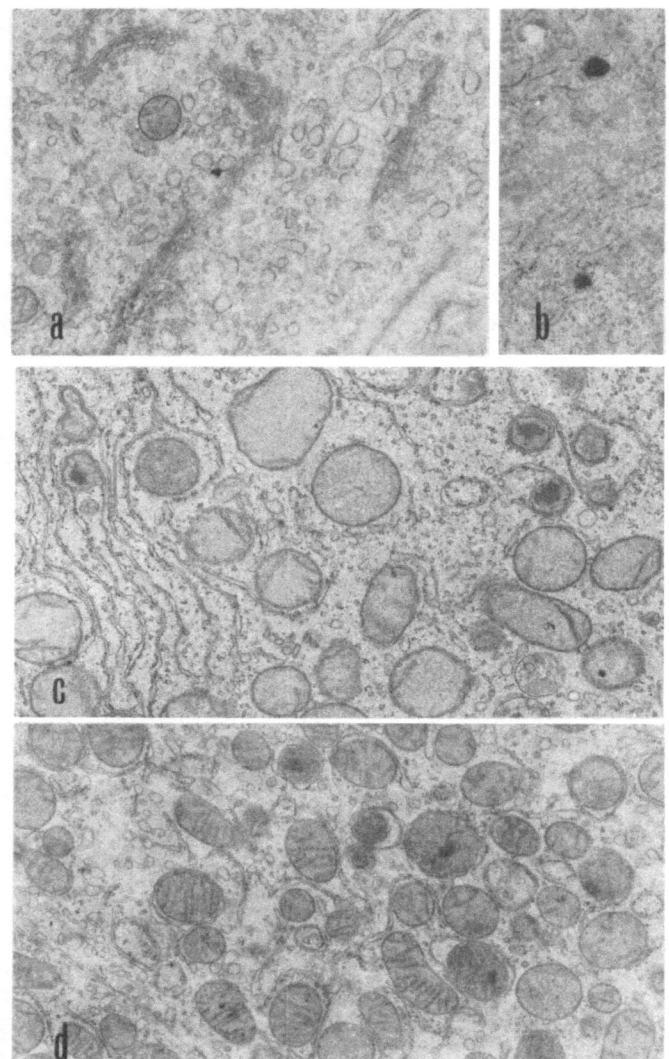

Figure 5
Poorly Differentiated (8994), Well Differentiated (7316A), and
Higly Differentiated (9618B) Morris Hepatomas. a: 8994, No peroxisomes are seen in this figure. b: 8994, electron microscopic cytochemistry for catalase. Two peroxisomes are stained positively,
c: 7316A. Note prominent crystalloid nucleoids in peroxisomes.
d: 9618B. Peroxisomes are rich in matrices. x 15,000 (reduced
25% for reproduction).

primarily induced in the liver contain none or very few peroxisomes in general.

Peroxisomes in well differentiated primary hepatomas have mostly been described as normal in hitherto published electron microscopic studies. However, a detailed description of Morris hepatomas (30) showed a certain tendency of alterations in well and highly differentiated hepatomas (Figs 5c, 5d). The incidence of peroxisomes in these hepatomas is occasional to as frequent as in normal hepatocytes, with a tendency for the number and size in the amount of their matrices to be generally greater in highly differentiated tumors than in well differentiated ones, although individual variations among the tumor lines are seen to a considerable extent. The difference between peroxisomes of well and highly differentiated hepatomas appears more notably in the size and the amount of matrices than in the number. On the other hand, the frequency of crystalloid nucleoids was found to be higher in well than in highly differentiated hepatomas, although no appropriate explanation is at present available for this phenomenon. It is well known that crystalloid nucleoids in human hepatocyte peroxisomes are present in the fetal stages but absent in the adult stages. Our observations and those previously reported could not demonstrate the occurrence of crystalloid nucleoids in peroxisomes in human hepatomas, despite the fact that fetal phenotypic expression is one of the characteristics of neoplasia.

There are some exceptions with respect to the relation between the features of peroxisomes and the degree of differentiation of hepatomas. Morris 16 hepatoma contains numerous peroxisomes rich in matrices but poor in crystalloid nucleoids, morphologically closely resembling but biochemically different from peroxisomes of hepatocytes after induction treatment with peroxisome-proliferating agents (Fig 6). On the other hand, as shown in Figs 4a and 4b, Morris 7794A hepatoma contains no peroxisomes, but considerable catalase activity is observed histochemically in the nuclei as well as in the hyaloplasm of the cells. As an exceptional ultrastructural alteration of peroxisomes, Dalton (3) reported the occurrence of tubular inclusions of Morris 7787 hepatoma, but Mochizuki et al. (30) could not find them in the tumor cells of later transplant generations. Electron microscopic investigations of a large number of Morris hepatomas and the primary hepatomas of various animal species have been reported but without description of the abnormal inclusion structures of peroxisomes including the above-mentioned tubular structures.

Acceleration of the growth rate of transplantable hepatomas during serial transplantation occurs on occasion accompanying alterations of peroxisomes. A decrease in the number and size of peroxisomes accompanying the loss of crystalloid nucleoids was reported in Morris 9A hepatoma during the serial transplantation as an indication

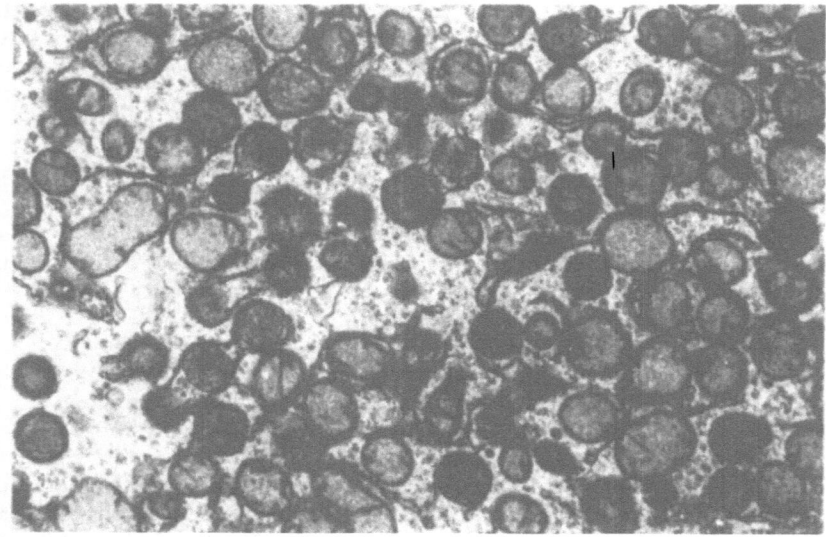

Figure 6
Morris 16 hepatoma. Note numerous peroxisomes rich in matrices,
but lacking crystalloid nucleoids. x 15,000

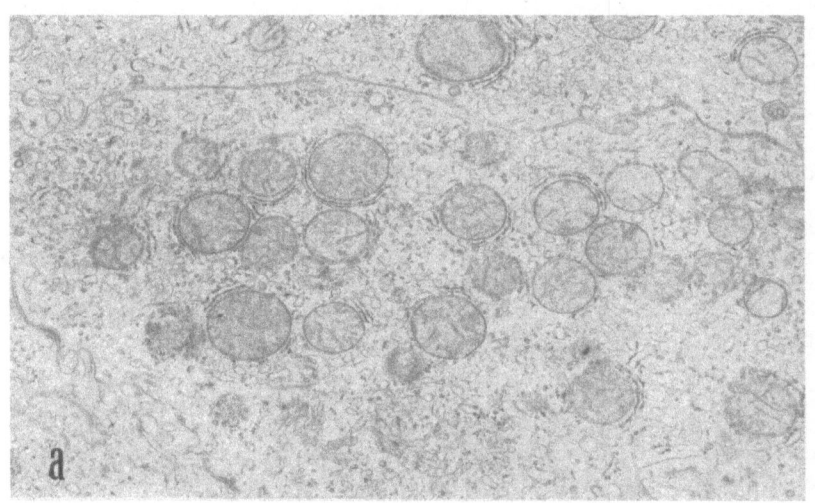

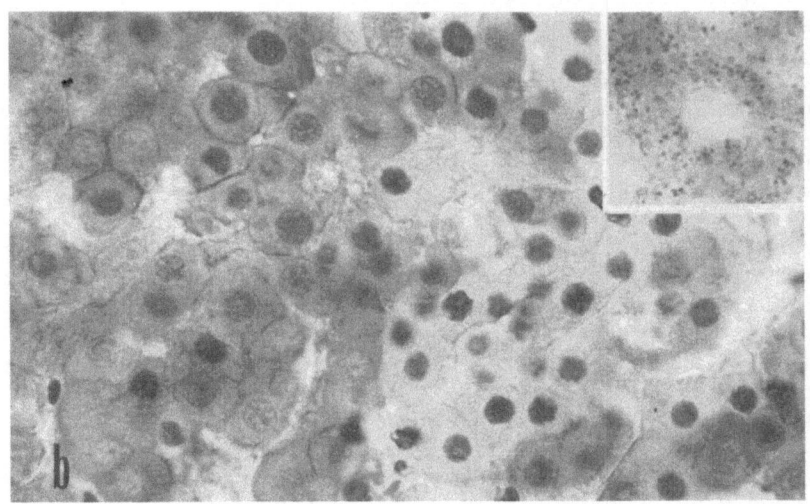

Figure 7
Morris 7794A Hepatoma. a: Electron microscopy. No peroxisomes
are seen in this figure. x 10,000. b: Light microscopic histo-
chemistry of catalase. Nuclei, cytoplasm, or both of the tumor cells
are stained diffusely in contrast to normal hepatocyte (inset,
x 1,000) in which peroxisomes are stained as cytoplasmic granules.
x 625 (reduced 10% for reproduction).

of further dedifferentiation of the tumor (30).

As to hepatomas grown in vitro, Watanabe and Essner (64) found that Morris 5123tc hepatoma contained peroxisomes in vivo, while it showed none after cultivation, although they decreased in number and size and usually lacked crystalloid nucleoids (Fig 7). They frequently showed an elongated shape, closely resembling microperoxisomes. This may convey an information concerning the mechanisms involved in the formation of microperoxisomes.

In any event, numerical changes and ultrastructural alterations of peroxisomes in hepatomas are considered to be intimately correlated with the rate of growth, the degree of differentiation, and to some extent with environmental conditions, but may not necessarily reflect the process of malignant transformation of the cells itself.

PEROXISOMAL ENZYMES OF HEPATOMAS

Since the emphasis in the early studies of Greenstein and his associates (9) that tumor tissues had in general no or negligible activity of catalase, a number of investigations have been made on catalase of hepatomas. In particular, the isolation of two transplantable hepatoma lines each having a high and low catalase activity according to Rechcigl and Sidransky (44) has prompted further studies on a large number of primary and transplantable hepatomas (30, 34, 39). Furthermore, since the identification of peroxisomal enzymes has been attained, studies on tumor catalase have been made considering its intracellular localization. There is general agreement that fast growing hepatomas essentially have no catalase activity, while there is a wide diversity of opinions regarding the correlation between catalase activity and the growth rate of hepatomas of intermediate and slow growth rates. Morris et al. (34) suggested that catalase activity is not always related to the growth rate of hepatomas. On the other hand, studies of Ono (39) and Mochizuki et al. (30) on a large number of Morris hepatomas asserted that the level of catalase activity was inversely related to the growth rate of the tumors, although with inevitable exceptions (Fig 8).

In contrast to catalase, other peroxisomal enzymes in hepatomas have not been studied extensively. It was reported that fast-growing hepatomas or poorly differentiated hepatomas did not contain or contained only a low activity of urate oxidase, d-amino acid oxidase and 1-α-hydroxy acid oxidase (14, 30, 31). However, in hepatomas of intermediate and slow growth rate, there seems to be no distinct parallel correlation between the growth rate and the activities of these enzymes. It might be worthy of mention that urate oxidase activity in hepatomas of intermediate growth rate (well-differentiated hepatomas) is generally much higher than that in the tumors of slow growth rate (highly differentiated tumors), and is frequently even higher than the

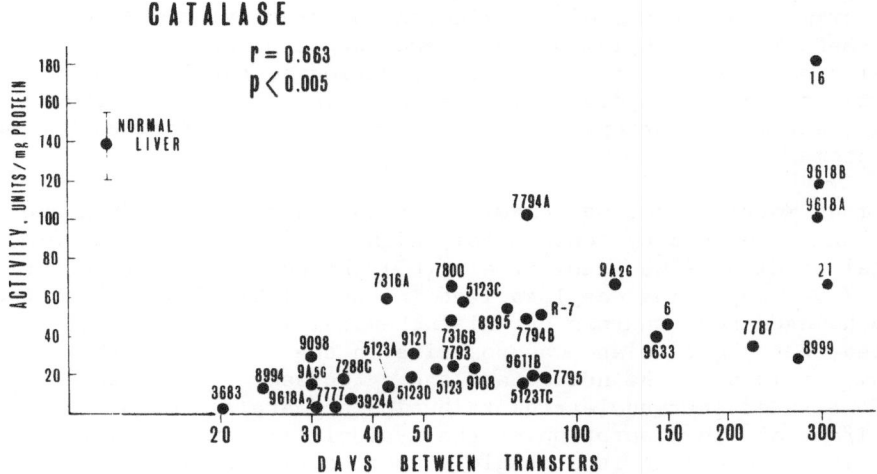

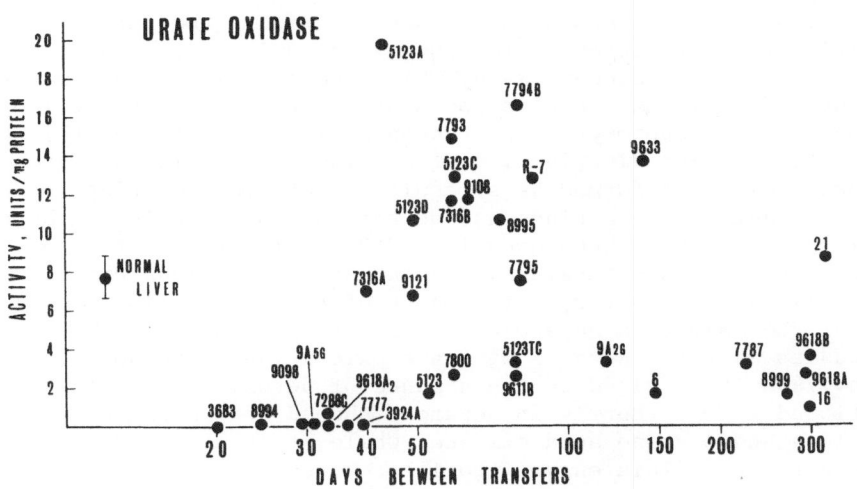

Figure 8
Correlation between growth rate of Morris hepatomas and
activities of catalase and urate oxidase (30).

activity in the normal liver (Fig 8). The higher activity of
urate oxidase accompanies the more prominent crystalloid nucleoids
of peroxisomes, However, the significance of high urate oxidase
activity in the tumor cell metabolism is not known. Our experiments
on the primary hepatomas of rats induced by 2-acetylaminofluorene
and 3'-methyl-p-dimethylaminoazobenzene suggest that there is
virtually no correlation among the activities of catalase, d-amino
acid oxidase and l-α-hydroxy acid oxidase, indicating that the individual enzymes of peroxisomes change independently form each other
in hepatomas.

Among Morris hepatomas examined in our laboratory, 7794A and
16 are characterized by considerably high catalase activity. Biochemical studies of Wattiaux et al. (65) showed that catalase activity of 7794A hepatomas was localized in the soluble fraction of the
tissue homogenates, whereas our histochemical investigation (32)
revealed that the catalase was positive in the nuclei, in the cytoplasm, or in both the nuclei and the cytoplasm. The histochemically demonstrated intranuclear distribution of catalase might not be
an artifact due to adsorption of the hyaloplasmic enzyme to the nuclei. This assumption is strongly supported by the findings of
Roels (51) on the sheep liver enzyme. Conversely, the enzyme in the
nuclei may leak out to the soluble fraction giving rise to the results of Wattiaux et al. It is tempting to regard the catalase in
the nuclei of 7794A hepatoma as synthesized within the nuclei unless
a specific transport channel from the cytoplasmic site of synthesis
to the nuclei or the mechanisms by which the nuclei take up selectively the hyaloplasmic catalase is postulated. During hepatocarcinogenesis, occasional hepatocytes in preneoplastic stages showed this abnormal intracellular distribution of catalase (19). It is suggested
that these cells are formed as a result of mutation occuring incident-
ally by the action of carcinogens and some of these cells can be ancestral cells of later hepatomas like 7794A. The ratio of peroxisomal extraparticulate catalase is outstandingly various among animal
species (11, 51). However, differences of the intracellular distribution of the enzyme in hepatomas between animal species have not
been studies as yet. Absence of urate oxidase and d-amino acid oxidase in 7794A is ascribed to the absence of peroxisomes in this tumor
as mentioned above. Morris 16 hepatoma showed very high activities
of catalase and d-amino acid oxidase, while it showed very low urate
oxidase activity. This enzyme profile corresponds to the fact that
this tumor contains numerous peroxisomes rich in matrices but deficient in crystalloid nucleoids. HC-hepatoma also contains catalase
activity comparable to that of the normal liver but none or very low
activity of urate and d-amino acid oxidase (14, 65). However, a
detailed description of the peroxisomes in relation to the enzyme
pattern is not available.

Investigations of the multiplicity of tumor catalase have been

reported on various Morris hepatomas, 3'-methyl-p-dimethylamino-
azobenzene induced hepatomas of rats, human hepatomas, and myelo-
genous leukemia (23, 31, 36, 57). In isoelectric focusing experiments on catalase of Morris hepatomas, disappearance of the
catalase components having isoelectric points at acidic pHs (acidic
catalase) and appearance of those having isoelectric points at
alkaline pHs (basic catalase) are characteristic of hepatomas, regardless of the growth rate and/or the degree of differentiation of
the tumors (Figs 9a and 9b). This multiplicity pattern of the enzyme of hepatomas resembles closely the profiles of fetal and newborn livers, but obviously differs from that of the adult liver.
The multiplicity of catalase in hepatomas seems to correlate neither
with intracellular distribution nor stability of the enzyme. A decrease of acidic catalase components was also found in the livers
of tumor-bearing hosts, probably as a result of synchronization of
the host liver metabolism with the tumor, and in the regenerating
liver of rats after partial hepatectomy, presumably being ascribed
to a dedifferentiated state of cells (22, 35). However, an appearance of basic catalase components was not demonstrated in these two
conditions.

Multiplicity of mouse liver catalase was assumed to result from
a sialation-desialation phenomenon of the enzyme (20). However, no
information is available about the relation betweeen this phenomenon
and the changes in the multiplicity pattern of the hepatoma catalase.
Sialyl transferase activity was reported to be various among Morris
7777, 7800 and 5123D hepatomas (17). Thus, it is suggested that a
decrease in this enzyme activity at least cannot explain the occurrence of basic catalase components in hepatomas, even though the
sialation-diasialation process is assumed to play a role in the
occurrence of the tumor catalase.

D-amino acid oxidase is present in rat liver and rat hepatomas;
however, it is absent in mouse liver as well as in mouse hepatomas.
No information has been provided on carnitine acetyl transferase of
hepatomas.

REGULATION OF PEROXISOMES AND PEROXISOMAL ENZYMES IN HEPATOMAS

Regulation of hepatocyte peroxisomes and its alterations brought
about by cancerization have not been clearly understood yet. Concerning regulation of peroxisomal enzymes, several studies were reported on catalase. Turnover of catalase in Morris hepatomas was
examined by Rechcigl et al. (42). The rates of destruction of catalase of hepatoma 5123C and 7316A did not differ much from each other
or from that of the host liver. Furthermore, our observations on
Morris 7794A and 7316A hepatomas suggest that catalase of these hepatomas is not necessarily more labile, regardless of the intracellular
distribution and pIs of the enzyme, as compared to the enzyme of the

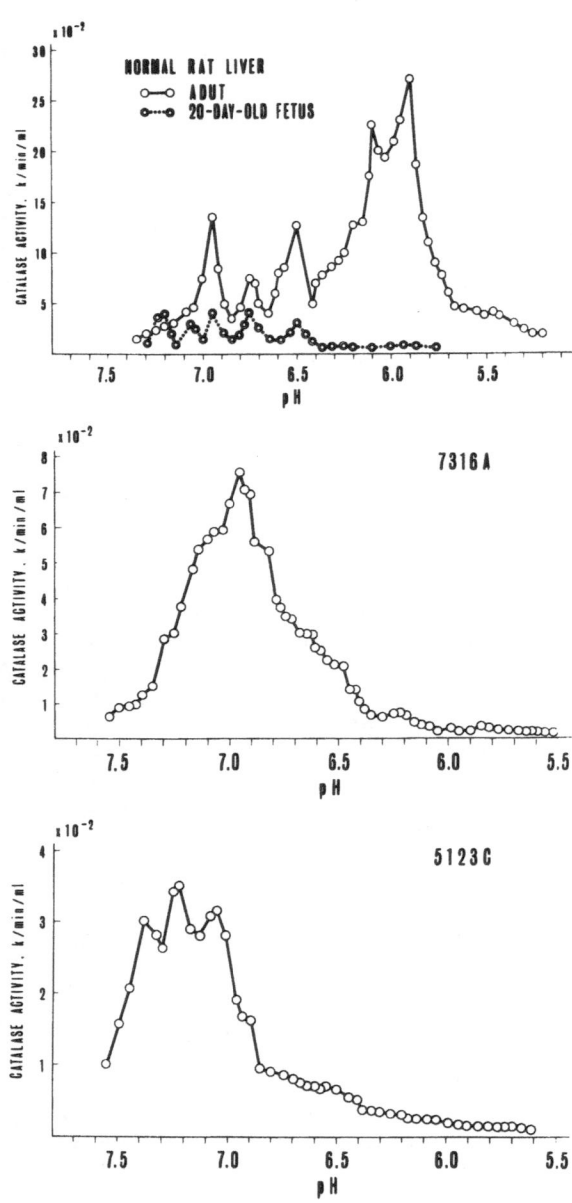

Figure 9a
Isoelectric focusing pattern of catalase of normal liver and
Morris hepatomas 7316A and 5123C (57).

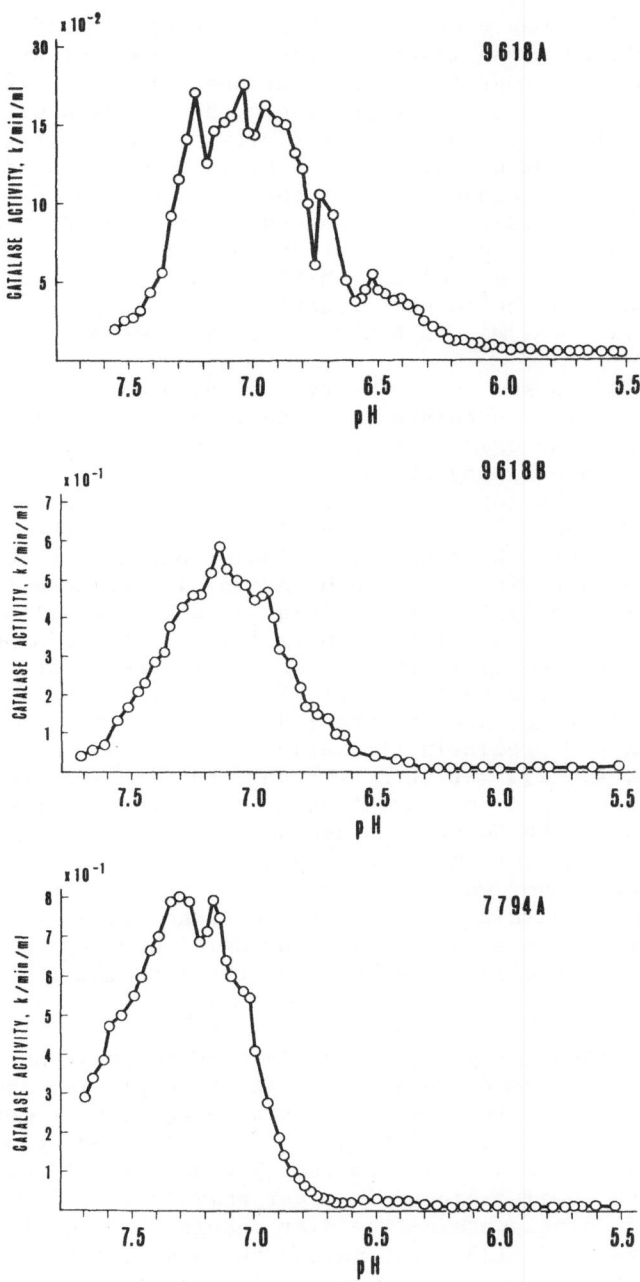

Figure 9b
Isoelectric focusing pattern of catalase of Morris hepatomas
9618A, 9618B, and 7794A (57).

normal liver. This may contrast with the assumption made by Jones
and Masters (20) on mouse liver catalase. The rate of synthesis
of catalase, on the other hand, is about one fifth for 5123C and
one half for 7316A hepatoma, respectively, as compared with that
of the host liver (42). Thus, low activity of the tumor catalase
results from low rates of enzyme synthesis. Mechanisms responsible
for the decrease of the synthesis of the tumor catalase were analyzed
by Uenoyama and Ono (63). It was suggested that the decrease was due
to an inhibition of the synthesis at the post-transcriptional level
occurring from an increase of an inhibitor and a decrease of an activator both present in the soluble fraction of the cells. Turnover of
other peroxisomal enzymes in hepatomas is not known.

As already discussed, proliferation of hepatocyte peroxisomes
and synthesis of liver catalase are inducible by several hypolipidemic agents such as CPIB. We examined morphologically and biochemically the inducibility of peroxisomes of Morris hepatomas,
particularly of 9618A hepatoma (61), and the primary hepatomas of
rats induced by 2-acetylaminofluorene (60), and 3'-methyl-p-dimethyl-
aminoazobenzene (18). Both proliferation of peroxisomes and elevation of catalase activity in these hepatomas in response to CPIB
were lost or strikingly impaired. This is contrasted with peroxisomes and catalase in the liver of normal fetal, newborn and adult
animals, although a possibility may not be excluded that the impaired
inducibility of the tumors is comparable to that in the liver at a
particular fetal stage, because the induction treatment might not
allow us to analyze precisely the various fetal stages (Figs 3a, b,
10a, b, 11a, b, 4, 12). It is noteworthy that the impairment of the
inducibility appears to be brought about regardless of the degree of
differentiation of the tumors. Likewise, d-amino acid oxidase activity of hepatomas was not influenced by CPIB, while the enzyme activity of the normal liver was strongly lowered by this agent. As
already mentioned, carnitine acetyl transferase activity in both mitochondria and peroxisomes is inducible by CPIB; however, no investigation has been reported on the changes of the inducibility in hepatomas.

Unresponsiveness of metabolic activities to environmental stimuli is also a salient characteristic trait of neoplasia, and it was
reported on hepatomas with respect to a wide variety of metabolic
activities. Liver catalase is known to be influenced by age, sex and
nutritional conditions of the animals. The activity is higher in the
male than in the female, higher in older animals than in younger ones.
Starvation or feeding protein-free diet results in lowering the activity. A comparison of 5123 hepatoma and the host liver was reported
revealing that these factors did not influence the tumor catalase,
while they markedly affected the host liver catalase (43). In our
experiments on 7316A hepatoma, it was observed that peroxisomal enzyme
other than catalase of the host liver were also decreased, while those

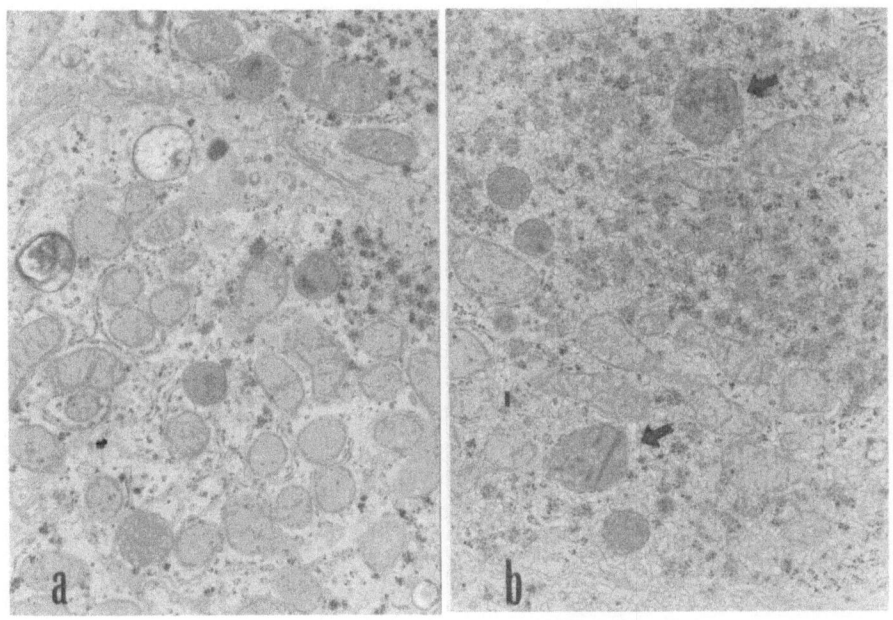

Figure 10
Morris 9618A hepatoma from rat treated with CPIB. a: control;
b: rat fed diet containing 1% CPIB for 4 weeks. Numerical increase
of peroxisomes is not evident. Note peroxisomes containing matrical
plates (arrows). x 12,500

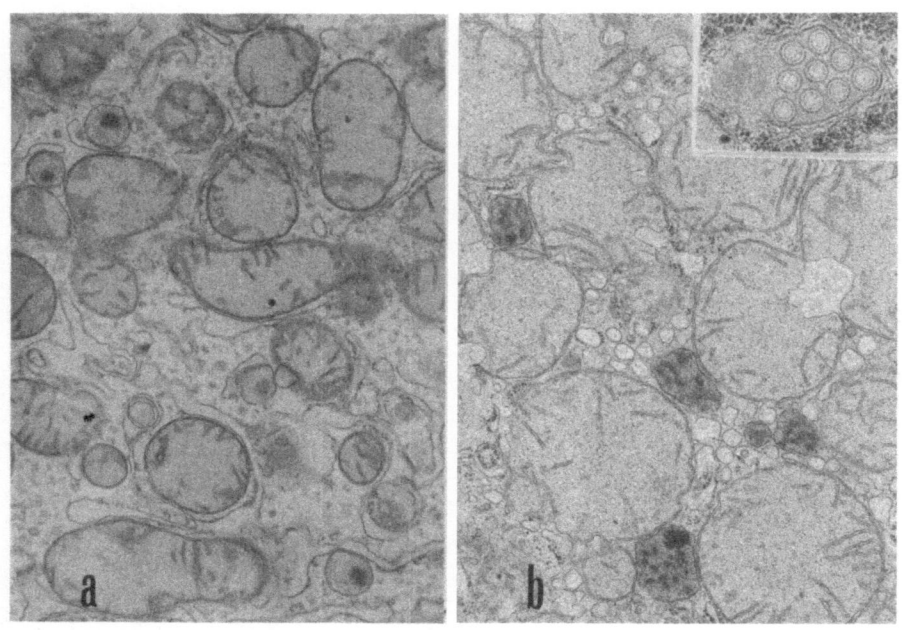

Figure 11
Hepatoma of rats fed diet containing 1% CPIB for 4 weeks.
a: Morris 7316A hepatoma. Almost no response of peroxisomes to
CPIB. x 15,000. b: highly differentiated primary hepatoma induced
by 2-acetylaminofluorene. Note abundant matrical plates in peroxisomes. x 15,000 Inset: Matrical tubules in peroxisomes formed in
response to CPIB. x 30,000

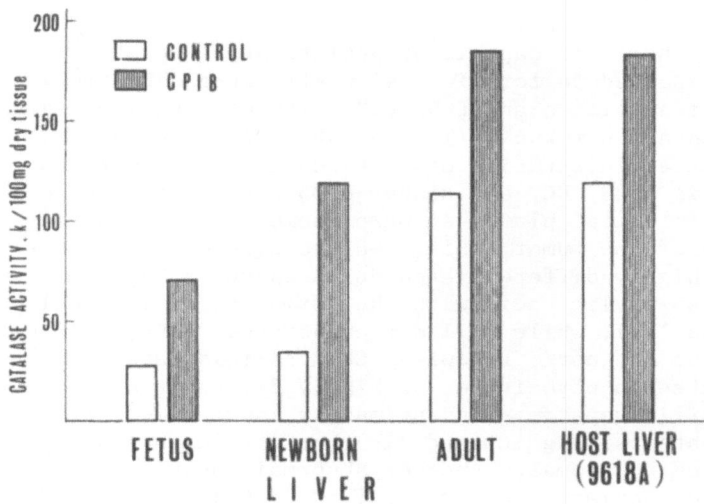

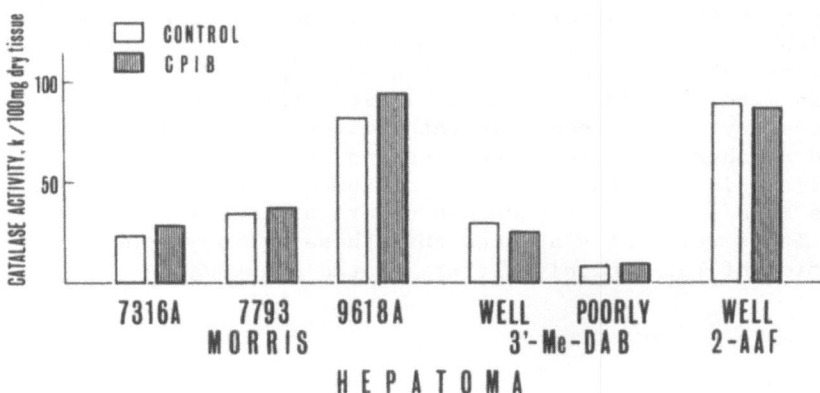

Figure 12
Effects of CPIB on catalase activity of rat liver, Morris
hepatomas and primary hepatomas induced by 3'-methyl-dimethylamino-
azobenzene and 2-acetylaminofluorene.

of the tumor were not, in the feeding on protein-free diet for 7
days (Fig 13). In the host liver, the number of peroxisomes decreased strikingly and matrices thereof became electron-lucent,
whereas peroxisomes of the tumor were not altered electron-micro-
scopically.

Certain chemicals capable of proliferating hepatocyte peroxisomes were reported to form inclusion structures in peroxisomes
called "matrical plates and tubules", although the mechanisms of
the formation are not known (12, 15, 48, 59). Hruban et al. (15)
reported that administration of acetylsalicylic acid to rats
bearing Morris 5123, HC, and Reuber H-35 hepatomas resulted in the
formation of matrical plates in peroxisomes of the host liver, but
not in those of the tumor cells. Our results on Morris hepatomas
showed that highly differentiated 9618A and9618B hepatomas responded to acetylsalicylic acid with the formation of matrical plates
(Figs 14a and 14b), while well differentiated 7316A, 5123C and
7800 hepatomas did not. Likewise, CPIB administration also induced
matrical plates in peroxisomes of highly differentiated hepatomas
including Morris hepatomas and primarily induced 2-acetylamino-
fluorene hepatomas (Fig 10b and 11b) but not in well and poorly
differentiated hepatomas. Another abnormal inclusion structure is
double-walled tubular structures called "matrical tubules" (12, 48,
59). In contrast to matrical plates, matrical tubules in hepatomas
were only rarely found in highly differentiated hepatomas treated
heavily with CPIB. Nevertheless, the induction of these abnormal
inclusion structures of peroxisomes may provide parameters relevant
to distinguish highly differentiated hepatomas from well and poorly
differentiated tumors. Furthermore, it might be worthy of mention
that hepatocyte peroxisomes in rats in certain preneoplastic stages
induced by chemical carcinogens respond to CPIB as well as to acetylsalicylic acid with the formation of abundant matrical plates and
tubules in addition to a moderate numerical increase of peroxisomes
(59). It is relevantly assumed that these cells are an ancestral
population of later highly differentiated hepatomas.

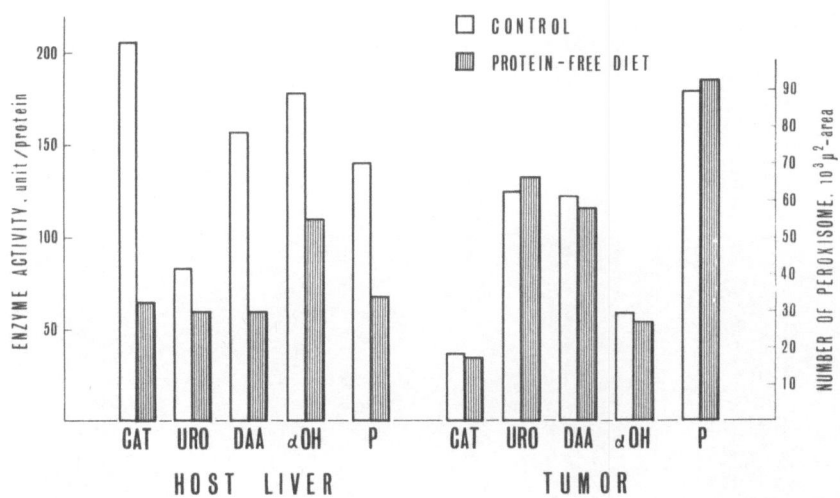

Figure 13
Effects of protein-free diet on peroxisomes and peroxisomal
enzymes of Morris 7316A hepatoma and host liver. CAT: catalase,
URO: urate oxidase, DAA: d-amino acid oxidase, α OH: 1-α-hydroxy
acid oxidase, P: peroxisome.

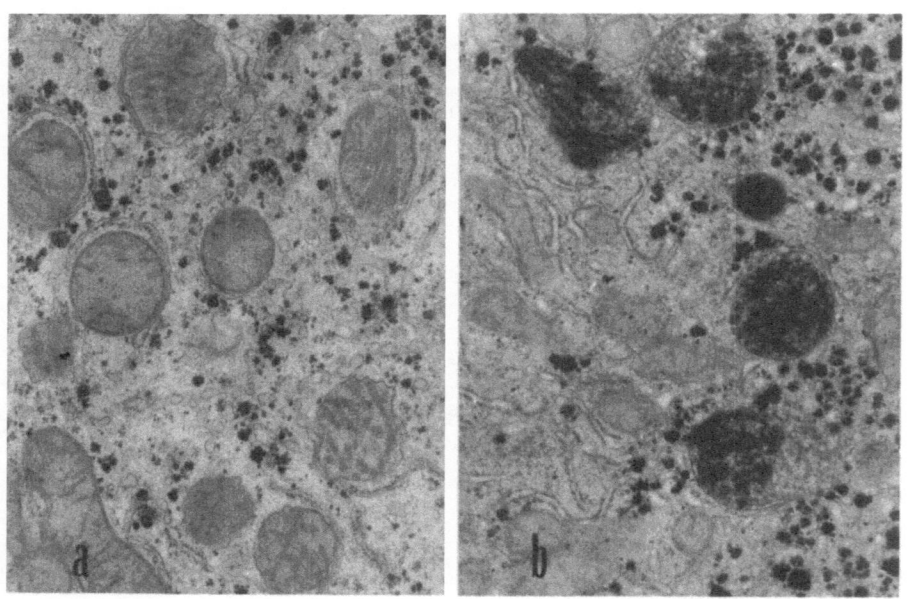

Figure 14
     Morris 9618B hepatoma from rat fed diet containing 1% acetyl-
salicylic acid for 4 weeks. a: electron microscopy; b: electron
microscopic cytochemistry for catalase. x 15,000
Note abundant matrical plates in peroxisomes. Fig 14b shows
positive cytochemistry of the plates.

REFERENCES

1. Baudhuin, P. Ann. N.Y. Acad. Sci. 168 (1969) 214.

2. Dalton, A.J. In: Cellular Control Mechanisms and Cancer,
    P. Emmelot and O. Muhlbock (eds)., Elsevier Press, Inc.,
    Amsterdam (1964) pp. 211-225.

3. Dalton, A.J. In: Primary Hepatoma, W. Burdette (ed). University
    of Utah Press, Salt Lake City (1965) pp. 51-64.

4. DeDuve, C. Ann. N.Y. Acad. Sci. 168 (1969) 369.

5. DeDuve, C. J. Histochem. Cytochem. 21 (1973) 941.

6. DeDuve, C. and Baudhuin, P. Physiol. Rev. 46 (1966) 323.

7. De la Iglesia, F.A. Acta Hepato-Splenol. 16 (1969) 141.

8. Golderberg, H., Huttinger, M., Kampfer, P., Kramer, R. and
    Pavelka, M. Histochemistry, 46 (1976) 189.

9. Greenstein, J.P. Biochemistry of Cancer, Academic Press, New
    York 2 (1954)

10. Hokama, Y., Yamada, K. and Kimura, L. Res. Comm. Chem. Pathol.
    Pharmacol. 4 (1972) 359.

11. Holmes, R.S. and Masters, C.J. Int. J. Biochem. 1 (1970) 474.

12. Hruban, Z., Gotoh, M., Slesers, A. and Chou, S.F. Lab. Invest.
    30 (1974) 64.

13. Hruban, Z. and Rechcigl, M. In: Microbodies and Related Particles,
    Morphology, Biochemistry and Physiology, Int. Rev. Cytol. New
    York Academic Press Inc. Suppl. 1. 1969.

14. Hruban, Z., Swift, H. and Rechcigl, M. J. Natl. Cancer Inst. 35
    (1965) 459.

15. Hruban, Z., Swift, H. and Slesers, A. Lab. Invest. 15 (1966) 1884.

16. Hruban, Z., Vigil, E.L., Slesers, A. and Hopkins, E. Lab. Invest.
    27 (1972) 184.

17. Hudgin, R.L., Murray, R.K., Pinteric, L., Morris, H.P. and
    Schachter, H. Can. J. Biochem. 49 (1971) 61.

18. Itabashi, M., Mochizuki, Y. and Tsukada, H. Cancer Res. 37 (1977)
    1035.

19. Itabashi, M., Mochizuki, Y. and Tsukada, H. Gann, 66 (1975) 463.

20. Jones, G.L. and Masters, C.J. Arch. Biochem. Biophys. 169 (1975) 7.

21. Karasaki, S., Simard, A. and Lamirande, G. Europ. J. Cancer 12 (1976) 527.

22. Koyama, S. Tumor Res. 6 (1971) 81.

23. Koyama, S., Hattori, N., Okazaki, N., Onho, T. and Kanda, Y. Jap. J. Clin. Oncol. 6 (1974) 47.

24. Lazarow, P.B. and DeDuve, C. J. Cell Biol. 59 (1973) 507.

25. Leighton, F., Coloma, L. and Koenig, C. J. Cell Biol. 67 (1975) 281.

26. Leighton, F., Poole, B., Lazarow, P.B. and DeDuve, C. J. Cell Biol. 41 (1969) 521.

27. Malick, L.E. J. Natl. Cancer Inst. 49 (1972) 1039.

28. Markwell, M.A.K., McGroarty, E.J., Bieber, L.L. and Tolbert, N.E. J. Biol. Chem. 248 (1973) 3426.

29. McGroarty, E. and Tolbert, N.E. J. Histochem. Cytochem. 21 (1973) 949.

30. Mochizuki, Y., Hruban, Z., Morris, H.P., Slesers, A. and Vigil, E.L. Cancer Res. 31 (1971) 763.

31. Mochizuki, Y., Itabashi, M. and Haga, H. Tumor Res. 11 (1976) 38.

32. Mochizuki, Y., Itabashi, M. and Tsukada, H. Med. and Biol. 87 (1973) 361.

33. Mochizuki, Y. and Tsukada, H. Tumor Res. 5 (1970) 1.

34. Morris, H.P., Dyer, H.M., Wagner, B.P., Miyaji, H. and Rechcigl, M. Adv. Enzy. Reg. 2 (1964) 321.

35. Nakamura, T., Matuo, Y., Nishikawa, K., Horio, T. and Okunuki, K. Gann 59 (1968) 317.

36. Nishimura, E.T., Hokama, Y. and Jim, R. Cancer Res. 32 (1972) 2353.

37. Novikoff, A.B. and Novikoff, P.M. J. Histochem. Cytochem. 21 (1973) 963.

38. Novikoff, A.B., Novikoff, P.M., Davis, C. and Quintana, N.
    J. Histochem. Cytochem. 20 (1972) 1006.

39. Ono, T. Gann Monograph, 1 (1966) 189.

40. Patton, G.W. and Nishimura, E.T. Cancer Res. 27 (1967) 117.

41. Poole, B., Higashi, T. and DeDuve, C. J. Cell Biol. 45 (1970) 408.

42. Rechcigl, M., Hruban, Z. and Morris, H.P. Enzym. Biol. Clin.
    10 (1969) 161.

43. Rechcigl, M.,Price, V.E. and Morris, H.P. Cancer Res. 22 (1962)
    874.

44. Rechcigl, M. and Sidransky, H. J. Natl. Cancer Inst. 28 (1962)
    1411.

45. Reddy, J., Chiga, M. and Svoboda, D. Biochem. Biophys. Res.
    Comm. 43 (1971) 318.

46. Reddy, J.K. and Krishnakantha, T.P. Science 190 (1975) 787.

47. Reddy, J. and Svoboda, D. Am. J. Pathol. 70 (1973) 421.

48. Reddy, J. and Svoboda, D. Virchow Arch. Abt. B. Zellpath. 14
    (1973) 83.

49. Rhodin, J. Correlation of Unltrastructural Organization and
    Function in Normal and Experimentally Changed Proximal Convoluted
    Tubule Cells of Mouse Kidney, Aktiebolaget Godvil, Stockholm
    (1954).

50. Riede, U.N. and Rohr, H.P. Beitr. Pathol. 151 (1974) 111.

51. Roels, F. J. Histochem. Cytochem. 24 (1976) 713.

52. Rose, G.G., Kumegawa, M. and Cattoni, M. J. Cell Biol. 39 (1968)
    430.

53. Saito, T., Iwata, K. and Ogawa, K. Acta Histochem. Cytochem. 6
    (1973) 212.

54. Sies, H. Agnew. Chem. 86 (1974) 789.

55. Staubli, W. and Hess, R. Handb. Exp. Pharm. 41 (1975) 229.

56. Svoboda, D., Azarnoff, D. and Reddy, J. J. Cell Biol. 40 (1969)
    734.

57. Tsukada, H., Koyama, S., Mochizuki, Y. and Morris, H.P. Gann, 64 (1973) 599.

58. Tsukada, H., Mochizuki, Y. and Gotoh, M. Symposia Cell Biol. 21 (1970) 263.

59. Tsukada, H., Mochizuki, Y. and Gotoh, M. J. Natl. Cancer Inst. 54 (1975) 519.

60. Tsukada, H., Mochizuki, Y., Itabashi, M., Gotoh, M. and Morris, H.P. J. Natl. Cancer Inst. 55 (1975) 153.

61. Tsukada, H., Mochizuki, Y. and Itabashi, M. Proc. Japanese Cancer Assoc. 31 (1972) 39.

62. Tsukada, H., Mochizuki, Y. and Konishi, T. J. Cell Biol. 37 (1968) 231.

63. Uenoyama, K. and Ono, T. Intl. J. Cancer 9 (1972) 608.

64. Watanabe, H. and Essner, E. Cancer Res. 29 (1969) 631.

65. Wattiaux, R., Wattiaux-De Conick, S., Van Dijck, J.M. and Morris, H.P. Eur. J. Cancer 6 (1970) 261.

66. Williams, G.M., Stromberg, K. and Kroes, R. Lab. Invest. 29 (1973) 293.

HEXOKINASE: THE DIRECT LINK BETWEEN MITOCHONDRIAL AND GLYCOLYTIC REACTIONS IN RAPIDLY GROWING CANCER CELLS[1]

Ernesto Bustamante[2], Harold P. Morris, and Peter L. Pedersen

Department of Physiological Chemistry
Johns Hopkins University School of Medicine
725 N. Wolfe St., Baltimore, MD 21205 [E.B., P.L.P.]
                    and
Department of Biochemistry, Howard University
School of Medicine
Washington, D.C. 20001 [H.P.M]

SUMMARY

Studies of glycolytic and respiratory activities of a hepatoma cell line (H-91) in culture are consistent with the view that a form of hexokinase concentrated in the mitochondrial fraction provides a "direct link" between mitochondrial and glycolytic reactions. The activity of hexokinase is found to be about 20-fold higher in H-91 cells than in control and regenerating rat liver, and to be insensitive to inhibition by glucose-6-phosphate. Mitochondria isolated from these cells contain about 50% of the total cell hexokinase activity. The mitochondrial fraction is 3-fold enriched in hexokinase activity relative to the homogenate and 4-fold enriched relative to the nuclear and post-mitochondrial fractions. Addition of glucose to respiring H-91 mitochondria (after a burst of ATP synthesis) results in a stimulation of respiration. Oligomycin, a specific inhibitor of ATP synthesis in mitochondria, inhibits respiration stimulated by glucose. Mitochondria isolated from several other rapidly growing tumors are shown to contain bound hexokinase, whereas mitochondria isolated from the two slowly growing Morris hepatomas 44 and 8995 are without detectable activity. It is suggested that an elevated form of mitochondrially-bound hexokinase may promote a high rate of lactic acid production in rapidly growing tumor cells by providing enhanced levels of the glycolytic substrate Glc-6-$\underline{P}$ and ADP, and/or by reducing the concentration of Pi at the site of oxidative phosphorylation. Consistent in part with the "aberrant ATPase" theory to account for high tumor glycolysis (Racker, E., Am. Sci. 60 (1972) 56), it may be noted that mitochondrially-bound hexokinase functions as a partial ATPase.

INTRODUCTION

Past work from this laboratory has been concerned primarily with elucidating the molecular events involved in ATP synthesis, ATP utilization, and in the regulation of these processes in mitochondria. To this end we have purified and characterized the catalytic unit (F_1) of the enzyme involved in ATP synthesis and ATP hydrolysis in rat liver mitochondria (6, 19), and we have purified and characterized a regulatory peptide inhibitor of F_1 (7). We have also purified and characterized the complete proton translocating ATPase (OS-F_1) of rat liver which consists of F_1 and an oligomycin-sensitivity conferring unit called F_0 (28, 29). In addition, we have characterized the Pi transport system of liver mitochondria in some detail since the operation of this system is essential for ATP synthesis (8).

While studies on mitochondrial ATPase and Pi transport were in progress, we also undertook a project concerned with the isolation and characterization of mitochondria from cancer cells in collaboration with Dr. Harold P. Morris of Howard University. This project proved successful in providing experimental procedures for the isolation of intact mitochondria from slow, intermediate, and rapidly growing tumors, and in providing information about the morphology and enzymatic composition of tumor mitochondria (20, 22, 23). The project also revealed that under certain conditions of assay the ATPase activity of many tumor mitochondria (regardless of the growth rate of the tumor) is more resistant to activation by uncoupling agents than the ATPase activity of normal mitochondria (23).

In studies described in this paper we have expanded our research horizons to consider the interaction of mitochondria with the glycolytic enzymes. The impetus for these studies was provided by two unexplained experimental observations in the literature. The first was the observation by Eagle et al. (11) in 1958 that certain animal cell lines in culture grow equally well in medium supplemented with either galactose or glucose, but produce high amounts of lactic acid only when grown on glucose-containing medium. Among the various explanations to account for these observations Eagle and his associates (11) suggested that the enzymatic steps involved in the phosphorylation of glucose and galactose may be different in activity and/or regulation. The second observation, which dates back to 1955, was the finding that in some tissues a large fraction of the total cellular activity of hexokinase is associated with the mitochondrial fraction (3, 13, 18, 24, 25, 36). It seemed to us that these two sets of observations might be related and help explain the high glycolytic activity of rapidly growing cancer cells. Experiments described below were carried out with the purpose of testing this possibility.

RESULTS

A. <u>Establishment and Characteristics of a Hepatoma Cell Line in Culture</u>

The experimental system that we have used throughout much of these studies is an azo-dye induced hepatoma cell line which has been adapted in our laboratory for growth in tissue culture (4). As indicated in Table 1, this cell line was induced originally in the livers of Sprague-Dawley rats by feeding the carcinogen dimethyl-aminoazobenzene(27). The tumor was then adapted to grow in the peritoneal cavity of Sprague-Dawley rats (27), and subsequently in our studies in tissue culture (4). The general characteristics of the hepatoma cell line in culture, referred to hereafter as H-91 cells, are summarized in Table 1. Significantly, the H-91 cell

Table One
Properties of the H-91 Cell Line

Carcinogen of Origin	Dimethylaminoazobenzene
Tumor of Origin	Rat Ascites Hepatoma (AS-30D)
Mean Diameter	20 μm
Karyotype	40 ± 3 Chromosomes
Growth Requirements	L-15 medium + 5% fetal bovine serum
Doubling Time	24 hrs at 37°
Attachment to Plates	2-3 points of anchorage[b]
Tumorigenicity	Yes, in Sprauge-Dawley rats

a
L-15 Leibovitz medium, Osmolality of complete growth medium = 320 m OSm/Kg, pH = 7.4

b
Tends to revert to floater behavior when culture is overcrowded.

line is not markedly deviated from normal rat liver in terms of karyotype, and it is as tumorigenic as the original cell line. Thus, H-91 cells reinjected into the peritoneal cavity of Sprague-Dawley rats proliferate and kill the host in about 1-2 weeks.

In terms of bioenergetic properties the H-91 cell line is characterized by a high rate of glycolysis. As shown in Table 2 the H-91 cell line produces about 120 µmoles lactic acid/gm wet tissue/hr, a value which is about 10-fold greater than liver tissue and about 2-fold greater than that reported for the more rapidly growing Morris hepatomas (30). As might be predicted the rate of lactic acid production of H-91 cells is less than the rate reported for Ehrlich ascites cells, which usually represent the extreme case of a highly glycolytic tumor. The values in Table 1 should be considered only approximate since they have been measured by different investigators and under different experimental conditions. Nevertheless, they do serve to show that the H-91 cell line which we have adapted to grow in tissue culture is characteristic of the rapidly growing, highly glycolytic class of tumors.

Table Two
Lactic Acid Production by H-91 Cells Relative to that of Some Other Well-Established Tumor Lines

Tissue	Growth Rate Time between transfers	Lactic Acid Production µmoles/gm wet tissue/hr
Liver slices	–	9.6 – 16.2
Hepatoma 16	10 months	20
Hepatoma 3924A	1 month	36
Hepatoma 3683	2 weeks	62
H-91 Hepatoma	1 week	120[a]
Erlich Ascites	1 week	270

a
The experimentally measured value was 0.6 µmole/mg protein/hr. To convert to the value tabulated the number was multiplied by 200 mg protein/g wet tissue.

Lactic acid production by H-91 cells was measured at 5 mM

glucose in Leibovitz L-15 medium supplemented with 5% fetal bovine serum (pH 7.4, 37°), (4). Values for lactic acid production by other tumor lines are those reported in References 1, 17 and 30.

B. Growth Properties of H-91 Cells in Galactose or Glucose-
    Supplemented Media

    Results of experiments summarized in Table 3 show that H-91 cells, similar to the animal cell lines studies earlier by Eagle et al. (11), grow equally well at 37° in growth medium supplemented with 5 mM glucose or 5 mM galactose. In both media the cells double in number in about 24 hours. However, only in the case of cells growing in glucose-supplemented medium is a high amount of lactic acid produced. About 3 times more lactic acid is formed when glucose is present in the growth medium than when galactose is present. Significantly also, cells growing in glucose utilize about 3 times as much hexose as cells growing in galactose. The enhanced capacity of H-91 cells to produce lactic acid when grown in glucose- rather than galactose- containing media is observed over hexose concentrations ranging from 5 to 30 mM. In fact, at high concentrations of hexose the differential effect in lactic acid production is even more pronounced.

Table Three
Glycolytic Activity of H-91 Cells in Glucose
and Galactose-Containing Media

Hexose in Growth Medium	Initial Concentration	Cell Number (x10^{-6}) Initial	Cell Number (x10^{-6}) After 24hr	Hexose Utilized	Lactic Acid Formed	%Hexose Utilized Converted Lactic Acid
				μmoles/24 hours		
Glucose	5 mM	5.0	10.1	11.2	20.8	92
Galactose	5 mM	5.0	9.7	4.0	7.2	90

    Cells were grown in L-15 medium containing 5% fetal bovine serum (pH 7.4, 37°). Medium was supplemented with glucose or galactose as indicated. For details of growth conditions see reference 4.

C. Transport of Glucose and Galactose by H-91 Cells

    The observation that H-91 cells utilize more hexose and produce more lactic acid when grown in glucose- than in galactose- supplemented medium could not be accounted for by the differences in transport of these two hexoses. As shown in Table 4, the rates of glucose and galactose entry into H-91 cells at 37⁰ and 5mM hexose are identical when uptake measurements are made within 10 seconds. At this early time point transport studies of glucose and galactose are not complicated by metabolism. This is verified by assays conducted with 3-0-methyl-glucose, a nonmetabolizable sugar, which as indicated in Table 4 enters H-91 cells at the same rate as glucose and galactose.

Table Four
Hexose Transport by Intact H-91 Cells

Hexose	Amount Transported ($nmoles/10^6$ cells)	
	In 10 sec	In 1 min
Glucose	3	6.5
Galactose	3	6.5
3-0-methyl-glucose	3	6.2

Hexose transport was measured at 37⁰ and pH 7.4 in a 0.1 ml system containing 140 mM NaCl, 2.7 mM KCl, 10 mM KPi, and 10^6 to 4×10^6 cells. The process was started by adding 5 mM hexose containing 0.1 μCi [^{14}C] hexose. In order to correct for nonspecific trapping and adsorption 5 mM unlabelled hexose containing 0.1 uCi [^{14}C] sucrose was substituted for the radioactive hexose in control experiments. For assay details see reference 4.

D.   Activity and Regulation of Hexokinase in H-91 Cells

The finding that transport of glucose and galactose into H-91 cells occurred at similar rates led us to consider the possibility that the phosphorylation of glucose in H-91 cells might be greatly enhanced relative to the phosphorylation of galactose. In this regard it is important to note that phosphorylation of these two sugars does not involve the same enzymatic mechanism. Glucose upon entering animal cells is phosphorylated directly by hexokinase (or glucokinase in liver) whereas galactose is phosphorylated and then converted to Glc-6-P via a series of enzymatic steps (Leloir pathway) which bypass the hexokinase step. Thus, as noted below Glc-6-P derived from galactose enters the glycolytic mainstream without the involvement of hexokinase.

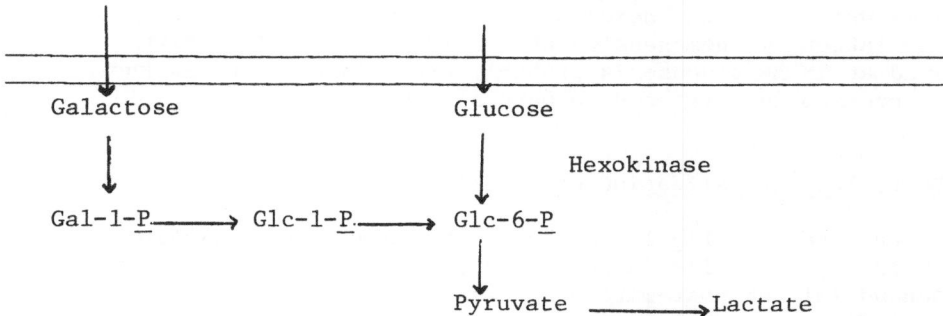

It is noteworthy then as emphasized by the data summarized in Table 5 that the activity of hexokinase in H-91 cells is more than 20 times greater than the activity observed in regenerating rat liver. In the latter two cases the glucose phosphorylation activity measured may actually be that of glucokinase since 13 mM glucose had to be used in the assay to see significant rates.

Results presented in Table 5 show therefore that H-91 cells contain markedly elevated levels of hexokinase which is not readily regulated by the reaction product Glc-6-P.

Table Five
Hexokinase Specific Activity In Homogenates of Rat Liver
and H-91 Cells

Homogenate	Specific Activity (units/mg protein)[a]
Rat Liver	4.6
Regenerating Rat Liver	10.8
H-91 Hepatoma	124
+ 0.1 mM Glc-6-P	124
+ 0.6 mM Glc-6-P	124

a
    One unit = One nmole of Glc-6-P formed/min

Hexokinase activity was measured at 340 nm in a 1 ml coupled system containing 40 mM Tris-HCO$_3$ buffer, 10 mM MgCl$_2$, 5 mM KCN, 0.2 mM NADH, 0.64 mM phosphoenolpruyvate, 2 mM ATP, 55 units pyruvate kinase, and 6 units lactic dehydrogenase, at pH 7.9 and 22°. 0.5 mM glucose was present when H-91 homogenates were assayed and 13 mM glucose was present when rat liver and regenerating rat liver homo-

genates were assayed. Hexokinase activity could not be detected
in the latter two homogenates at 0.5 mM glucose. The enzyme
assayed at 13 mM glucose is probably glucokinase which is known
to be present in liver and to have a high K_m for glucose (35).

F. Subcellular Localization of Hexokinase

     The insert in Fig 1 shows that the bulk of the hexokinase
activity of H-91 cells is shared in about equal proportion by the
mitochondrial and post-mitochondrial fractions. The activity
found in the nuclear fraction correlates well with the percentage
of unbroken cells present in H-91 homogenates and, consequently,
can be most likely ascribed to unbroken cells sedimenting in the
nuclear fraction. Fig 1 shows the same experimental data in the
"insert" presented in the form of a De Duve plot (2). The figure
emphasizes that the specific activity of the mitochondrial fraction is 3-fold higher than that of the homogenate, and 4-fold
higher than the activities of the nuclear and post-mitochondrial
fractions. These results indicate that although the hexokinase
activity of H-91 cells is equally distributed among the mitochondrial and post-mitochondrial fractions, the former is 4-fold
more enriched in hexokinase activity than the latter. These findings are consistent with earlier reports of hexokinase bound to
the mitochondrial fraction in other systems (3, 13, 18, 25, 36).

     There have been several reports in the literature which in-
dicate that some hexokinase activity may be associated with the
plasma membrane fraction in tumor cells (10, 12). Such plasma
membrane fractions are prepared from the nuclear fraction which is
known to be highly contaminated in liver with mitochondria (5).
Nevertheless, it was of concern to us to ascertain whether plasma
or microsomal membrane contamination could account for the hexokinase activity observed in the mitochondrial fraction. In preliminary studies less than 20% of the total cell activity of 5'-
nucleotidase, a plasma membrane marker, and glucose-6-phosphatase,
a microsomal membrane marker has been found in the mitochondrial
fraction of H-91 cells. Thus, it seems unlikely that the hexokinase
activity associated with the mitochondrial fraction of H-91 cells
is due to contamination by other membrane fractions. We emphasize,
however, that this is a difficult question to resolve rigorously
since there may be intimate and perhaps physiologically significant
contact points between the mitochondria and other cellular membranes
in the intact cell.

G. Coupling of Mitochondrially-bound Hexokinase to Oxidative
    Phosphorylation

     Figure 2B shows that after a burst of ATP synthesis, glucose

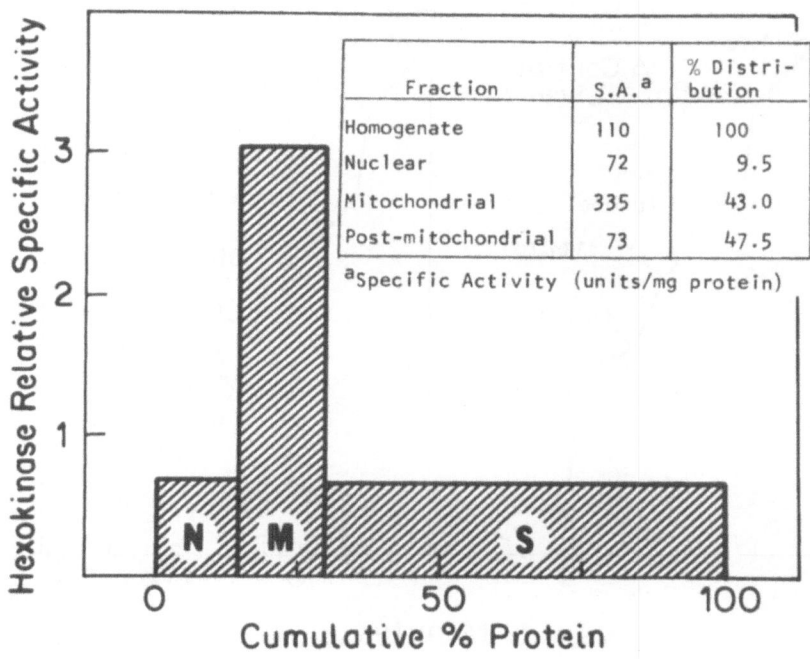

Figure 12

Subcellular distribution of hexokinase activity in H-91 hepatoma cells. The cells were fractionated by a differential centrifugation scheme described by previously (4). The subcellular fractions were assayed for hexokinase by following the formation of NADP at 340 nm in a 1 ml system containing 32 mM HEPES buffer, 12 mM $MgCl_2$, 6.5 mM ATP, 0.9 mM $NADP^+$, 1 unit Glc-6-P dehydrogenase, and 0.5 mM D-glucose at pH 7.6 and 22o.

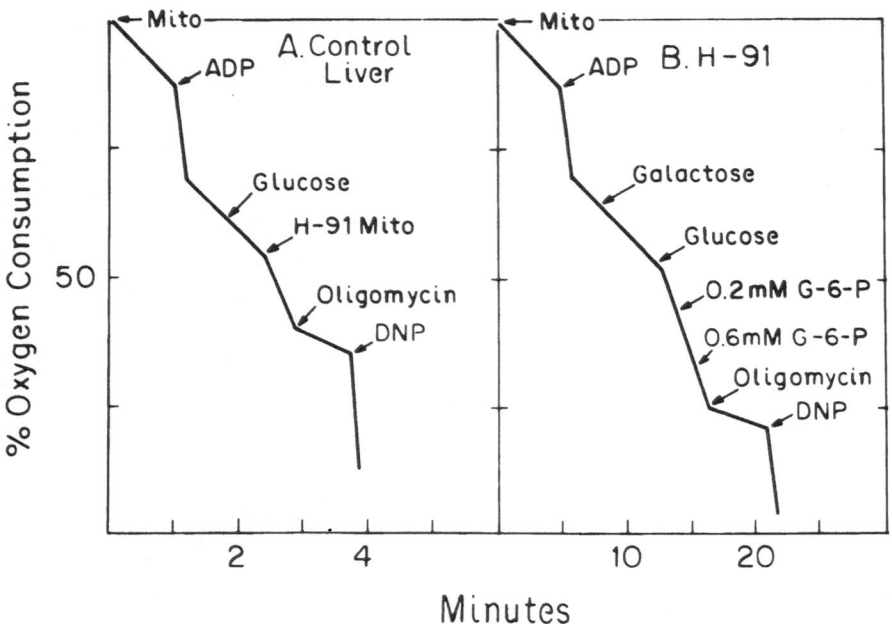

Figure 2
Polarographic traces of control rat liver mitochondria and H-91
mitochondria. Note glucose stimulates respiration (after a burst of
ATP synthesis) only in H-91 mitochondria. A. Control liver. Indicated
additions were: 2.5 mg control liver mitochondria, 0.25 μmoles ADP,
0.5 μmoles glucose, 0.1 mg H-91 mitochondria, 1 μg oligomycin, 0.1
μmoles DNP. B. H-91 Hepatomas. Indicated additions were: 1.2 mg
H-91 mitochondria, 0.25 μmoles ADP, 0.5 μmoles galactose, 0.5 μmoles
glucose, 1 μg oligomycin, and 0.1 μmoles DNP.

significantly stimulates the respiration of coupled hepatoma mitochondria, a result that should be obtained only if the hexokinase
reaction (Glucose + ATP $\rightleftharpoons$ Glc-6-$\underline{P}$ + ADP) occurs at the expense of mitochondrially-synthesized ATP. Significantly, this
glucose-stimulated respiration is inhibited by oligomycin, and in
turn enhanced by the uncoupler 2, 4-dinitrophenol to a maximal
rate, indicating coupling of the hexokinase reaction with the
oxidative phosphorylation system. The glucose-stimulated respiration of H-91 mitochondria is not subject to inhibition by up to
0.6 mM Glc-6-$\underline{P}$ in analogy to the lack of inhibition of hexokinase
activity in H-91 homogenates.

Fig 2A shows that glucose is unable to stimulate the respiratory rate of mitochondria from control liver. The respiratory
rate of regenerating liver mitochondria also was unaffected by
glucose addition (data not shown). However, when small amounts of
tumor mitochondria (which would not detectably increase oxygen
consumption via their own respiration) are added to respiring
normal mitochondria, glucose is now able to stimulate respiration.
These results emphasize that hexokinase bound to the mitochondria
of H-91 cells is characteristic of the neoplastic state and not a
property of the tissue of origin or of rapidly dividing normal
liver cells.

H. Ubiquity of Mitochondrially-bound Hexokinase

Results summarized in Table 6 show that all highly glycolytic,
rapidly growing tumors examined to date have a significant portion
of the total cell hexokinase activity associated with the mitochondrial fraction. Tumor lines examined include Ehrlich ascites,
H-91 hepatoma (in ascites form and in tissue culture), Novikoff
hepatoma, L-1210 ascites, Krebs-2 ascites, and S-91 melanoma.
Significantly, we have very recently isolated intact mitochondria
(acceptor control ratios 5) from the very slowly growing Morris
hepatomas 44 and 8995. These mitochondria have no detectable
mitochondrial hexokinase activity. Thus, to date it seems that
mitochondrially-associated hexokinase is preferentially associated
with rapidly growing, highly glycolytic tumor lines. Studies are
currently under way in our laboratory to ascertain the extent to
which mitochondrially-bound hexokinase activity correlates with
the growth and glycolytic characteristics of the Morris hepatoma
lines.

Results presented in Table 6 also show that mitochondrially-
associated hexokinase activity is not solely a characteristic of
the neoplastic state. Mitochondrially-associated hexokinase is
found also in other glycolytic tissues including brain, kidney,
heart and intestinal mucosa. What has not been established about
the activity of hexokinase in these normal tissues, however, is

whether the mitochondrial form of the enzyme increases during
transformation. Thus, as indicated previously in this report,
transformation of liver tissue to give a rapidly growing hepatoma,
results in the elevation of mitochondrially-associated hexokinase
from a value near zero to at least 50% of the total cell activity.
Transformation of other tissues may be found to result in a basal
mitochondrial hexokinase activity increasing to a much higher
level.

Table Six
Ubiquity of Mitochondrially-Associated Hexokinase

Tumors	Normal Tissues
Ehrlich Ascites (3, 36)	Brain (9, 14)
H-91 Hepatoma	Kidney (9)
Novikoff Hepatoma	Heart (9)
L-1210 Ascites	Intestinal Mucosa (9)
Krebs-2 Ascites (18)	
S-91 Melanoma (13)	
Sarcoma 37 (25)	

Evidence for the association of hexokinase with the mitochondrial fraction of Ehrlich ascites cells, H-91 hepatoma,
Novikoff hepatoma and L-1210 ascites cells has been obtained in
our laboratory. Evidence for the association of hexokinase with
the mitochondrial fraction of some of the tissues listed above
has been obtained in other laboratories. See references indicated
in parantheses.

DISCUSSION

Results of experiments summarized in this report show that
the hexokinase activity of H-91 hepatoma cells in culture is 20-
fold higher than that found in control liver; that this activity
is insensitive to inhibition by Glc-6-$\underline{P}$; and that about 50% of
the total cell activity is localized in the mitochondrial fraction.
(DeDuve plots actually suggest a mitochondrial localization for
the hexokinase of H-91 cells). The localization of hexokinase in
mitochondria of H-91 cells is not unique to this tumor line but it

is characteristic also of all rapidly growing, highly glycolytic tumors examined to date. These findings, together with the additional finding that H-91 cells are highly glycolytic when grown on glucose but not galactose, strongly suggest that mitochondrially-bound hexokinase may be responsible in part, for the high glycolytic activity of H-91 cells (and perhaps other rapidly growing cancer cells as well).

Localization of elevated amounts of hexokinase in the outer mitochondrial compartment might promote glycolysis in at least three different ways (Fig 3). First, hexokinase bound to the outer mitochondrial compartment is coupled directly to ATP synthesis in the inner compartment and should efficiently convert glucose to Glc-6-P, the initial substrate for the glycolytic pathway. Secondly, mitochondrially-bound hexokinase should rapidly and efficiently regenerate ADP which is essential for maximal glycolytic rates. In this respect the enzyme would function as a "partial ATPase" converting ATP to ADP, Third, bound hexokinase may reduce the concentration of P_i at or near the site of oxidative phosphorylation in mitochondria as suggested earlier by Koobs (16) (See below).

$$\text{ADP} + P_i \xrightarrow{\text{oxidative phosphorylation}} \text{ATP} + \text{HOH}$$

$$\text{Glucose} + \text{ATP} \xrightarrow[\text{(mitochondrially-bound)}]{\text{hexokinase}} \text{Glc-6-P} + \text{ADP}$$

$$\text{Net: } \text{Glucose} + P_i \xrightarrow{} \text{Glc-6-P} + \text{HOH}$$

The latter effect would prevent the attainment of maximal rates of respiration in the presence of excess pyruvate and therefore promote reduction of pyruvate (formed from glucose) to lactate in the cytoplasm.

Several workers have suggested that an elevated, aberrant or unregulated form of hexokinase may play a key role in the high glycolytic activity of rapidly growing cancer cells (16, 26, 33, 34). However, most workers have not seriously emphasized the possible relationship that mitochondrially-bound hexokinase may play in promoting high tumor glycolysis. This is despite the fact that the mitochondrially-bound form of hexokinase has been rather extensively studied in ascites tumors (24). It would be of interest therefore to establish to what extent mitochondrially-bound hexokinase correlates with the glycolytic and growth patterns of tumor cells. Such studies are currently under way in our laboratory.

Finally, it would seem that every investigator searching for a molecular explanation for the high glycolytic activity of cancer

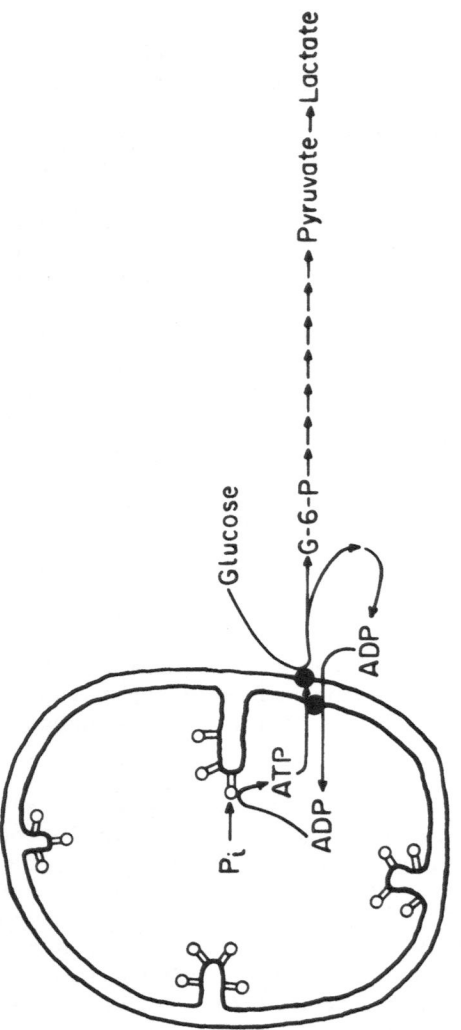

Figure 3

Model depicting how hexokinase associated with tumor mitochondria might allow for a direct and efficient phosphorylation mechanism. In this model the hexokinase reaction (proceeding in the outer mitochondrial compartment) is shown to be coupled directly to ATP synthesis occurring at the level of the F_1 ATPase in the inner mitochondrial compartment. Rose and Warms (25) have suggested a similar type of model to account for the possible role of the mitochondrially-bound hexokinase in the retinal rod.

A SOME SLOWLY GROWING TUMORS & MANY NORMAL TISSUES
(LOW LACTATE PRODUCTION)

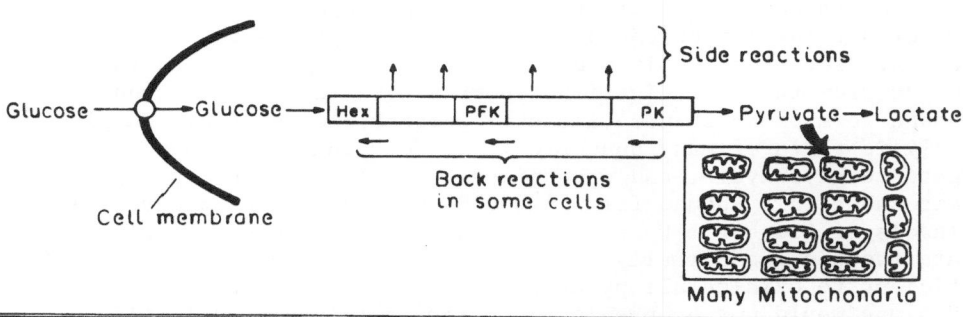

B RAPIDLY GROWING TUMORS & SOME NORMAL TISSUES
(HIGH LACTATE PRODUCTION)

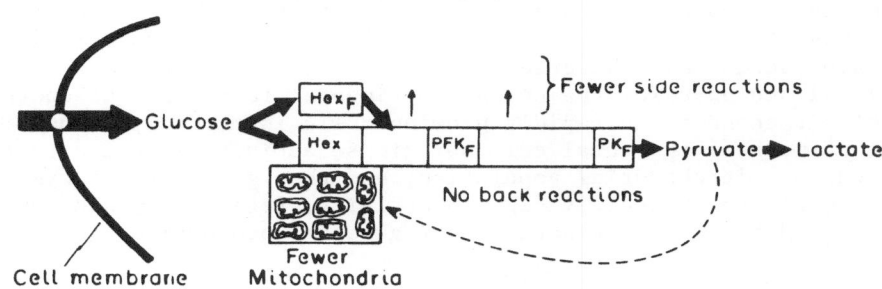

Hex = Hexokinase
PFK = Phosphofructokinase
PK = Pyruvate Kinase
F = Fetal

Figure 4

Model indicating that in addition to an aberrant hexokinase type reaction, other genetically programmed alterations, both at the level of mitochondria and glycolysis, may favor high lactic acid production in certain tissues. In particular some glycolytic enzymes are high in activity, fetal-like, and have altered kinetic and regulating properties. Moreover, mitochondria are reduced in number in highly glycolytic tumors by 50% or more relative to appropriate controls (21). Thus, the glycolytic activity/mitochondrial activity ratio is very high in such tissues and most likely favors the consumption of elevated amounts of pyruvate. Under such conditions, and for reasons discussed in the text, the oxidative capacity of the mitochondria for pyruvate becomes limiting. Lactic acid production in the cytoplasm is favored. For a more detailed discussion of this "Unifying Hypothesis" for the high lactic acid production of certain tissues, see reference 4.

cells has a "pet theory" which usually involves a single enzymatic step or a single type of process. It would seem to us that this type of thinking is extremely narrow in scope and ignores many important investigations of the high glycolytic activity of cancer cells. For example, it would be very presumptuous of us to conclude from the investigation reported here that a mitochondrially-bound form of hexokinase alone is responsible for the high glycolytic rates of many cancer cells. Certainly hexokinase is the gate to glycolysis, and when present in elevated, unregulated, and mitochondrially-bound form it would be predicted to produce high levels of Glc-6-$\underline{P}$. However, if other control points in glycolysis are functioning normally, or if the mitochondrial content is sufficient to oxidize all pyruvate formed, elevated levels of Glc-6-$\underline{P}$ alone would not be predicted to result in enhanced lactic acid production. In Fig 4 we summarize what we believe to be a more unifying concept for the high glycolytic rates of many cancer cells, a concept which not only accounts for some of the original views of Warburg (31, 32) but the views of those who believe they have successfully discredited him. It will be noted that the model accounts for the known experimental fact that the content of mitochondria in rapidly growing cells is markedly reduced; that much of the total cell hexokinase activity is bound to this reduced mitochondrial population; and that glycolytic enzymes in general are frequently high in activity, fetal-like, and characterized by altered kinetic and regulatory properties.

ACKNOWLEDGEMENTS

The authors are grateful to Drs. A. Clark Griffin and E. Walborg of the Department of Biochemistry, M.D. Anderson Hospital and Tumor Institute for supplying us with the AS-30D hepatoma line which we used as starting material to develop the H-91 cell line.

[1]

This project was funded by grants from the National Cancer Institute (CA 10951) and the National Science Foundation (PCM 76-11024) to PLP and by a grant from the National Cancer Institute (CA 10729) to HPM.

[2]

Ernesto Bustamante, who was supported by fellowships from the Lilly Research Laboratories, the DuPont Company, and the Ford Foundation, is on leave from the Universidad Peruana Cayetano Heredia (Lima, Peru).

REFERENCES

1. Aisenberg, A.C. In: The Glycolysis and Respiration of Tumors, Academic Press, New York (1961) p. 5.

2. Appelmans, F., Wattiaux, R., DeDuve, C. Biochem. J. 59 (1955) 438.

3. Asc, G., Garzo, T., Grosz, G., Molnar, J., Stephaneck, O., and Staub, F.B. Acta Physiol. Acad. Sci. Hung. 8 (1955) 269.

4. Bustamante, E. and Pedersen, P.L. Proc. Natl. Acad. Sci. US.A. (1977) submitted.

5. Bustamante, E., Soper, J.W. and Pedersen, P.L. Anal. Biochem. (1977) In Press.

6. Catterall, W.A. and Pedersen, P.L. Biochem. Soc. Spec. Publ. 4 (1974) 63.

7. Cintron, N.M. and Pedersen, P.L. Methods in Enzymol. (1977) In Press.

8. Coty, W.A. and Pedersen, P.L. Mol. and Cell. Biochem. 9 (1975) 109.

9. Crane, R.K. and Sols, A. J. Biol. Chem. 230 (1953) 273.

10. Davidova, S.Y., Shapot, V.S. and Solowjeva, A.A. Biochim. Biophys. Acta 158 (1968) 303.

11. Eagle, H., Barban, S., Levy, M. and Schulze, H.O. J. Biol. Chem. 233 (1958) 551.

12. Emmelot, P. and Bos, C.J. Biochem. Biophys. Acta 158 (1968) 434.

13. Giger, K. Annals. N.Y. Acad. Sci. 100 (1963) 866.

14. Johnson, M.K. Biochem. J. 77 (1960) 610.

15. Knull, H.R., Taylor, W.F. and Wells, W.W. J. Biol. Chem. 249 (1974) 6930.

16. Koobs, D.H. Science 178 (1972) 127.

17. LaNoue, K.F., Hemington, J.G., Ohnishi, T., Morris, H.P. and Williamson, J.R. In: Hormones and Cancer, Academic Press, New York (1974) 131.

18. McComb, R.B. and Yushok, W.D. Biochim. Biophys. Acta 34 (1959) 515.

19. Pedersen, P.L. Bioenergetics, 6 (1975) 243.

20. Pedersen, P.L. Gann Mono. in Cancer Res. 13 (1972) 251.

21. Pedersen, P.L. Prog. Exp. Tumor Res. (1977) In Press.

22. Pedersen, P.L., Greenwalt, J.W., Chan, T.L. and Morris, H.P. Cancer Res. 30 (1970) 2620.

23. Pedersen, P.L. and Morris, H.P. J. Biol. Chem. 249 (1974) 3327.

24. Purich, D.L., Fromm, H.J. and Rudolph, F.B. Adv. Enzymol. 39 (1973) 249.

25. Rose, I.A. and Warms, J.V.B. J. Biol. Chem. 242 (1967) 1635.

26. Singh, V.N., Singh, M., August, J.T. and Horecker, B.L. Proc. Natl. Acad. Sci. U.S.A. 71 (1974) 4129.

27. Smith, D., Walborg, E. and Chang, J. Cancer Res. 30 (1970) 2306.

28. Soper, J.W. and Pedersen, P.L. Biochem. 15 (1976) 2682.

29. Soper, J.W. and Pedersen, P.L. Methods in Enzymol. (1977) In Press.

30. Sweeney, M.M., Ashmore, J., Morris, H.P. and Weber, G. Cancer Res. 23 (1963) 995.

31. Warburg, O., Posener, K. and Negelein, E. Biochem. Z. 152 (1924) 309.

32. Warburg, O. In: The Metabolism of Tumors, Constable, London (1930).

33. Weinhouse, S. Gann Mono. in Cancer Res. 1 (1966) 99.

34. Weinhouse, S. In: Glycolysis and Enzyme Alterations in Liver Neoplasms, Miami Winter Symposia 2 (1970) 462.

35. Weinhouse, S. Cancer Res. 32 (1972) 2007.

36. Wu, R. and Racker, E. J. Biol. 234 (1959) 1029.

THE COMPOSITION AND METABOLISM OF MICROSOMAL AND MITOCHONDRIAL

MEMBRANE LIPIDS IN THE MORRIS 7777 HEPATOMA[1]

Richard Morton, Moseley Waite[2], John W. Hartz, Carol
Cunningham and Harold P. Morris

Departments of Biochemistry (RM, MW, CC) and Pathology
(JWH), Bowman Gray School of Medicine
Winston-Salem, North Carolina 27103   and
Biochemical Cancer Research Unit (HPM) Howard University
Washington, D.C. 20001

SUMMARY

Mitochondria and microsomes isolated from the Morris 7777
hepatoma demonstrated a markedly different phospholipid composition
from the control organelle both with respect to the types present
and the fatty acid composition. Hepatoma mitochondria contained
lower amounts of cardiolipin than control liver (3.7% versus 5.2%).
Some compensation in the amount of acidic phospholipids in the hepatoma mitochondria was made by an increase in phosphatidylserine
(4.9% versus 1.3%). The major difference in microsomal phospholipids was an increase in the hepatoma sphingomyelin content. The
level of polyunsaturated fatty acids in both hepatoma organelles
was lowered, concomitant with an increase in the level of monoun-
saturated fatty acid. Moreover, the usual distribution of saturated
fatty acids at position 1 and polyunsaturated fatty acids at position 2 was not observed in hepatoma mitochondrial phospholipids.
Force-area curves of the hepatoma phospholipids spread on a monomolecular film demonstrated a smaller area per molecule than those
from control liver mitochondria. The zeta potential of liposomes
of the hepatoma mitochondria phospholipids (-45) was less than that
of control mitochondria (-81) as determined by microelectrophoresis.
In studies of phosphoglyceride metabolism, the calcium-stimulated
phospholipase A activity of the hepatoma mitochondria appeared to
be more readily expressed than the same activity in the liver organelle. The maximal activity was lower, however, than that in liver
mitochondria. Hepatoma microsomes incorporated free fatty acids into
monoacyl phospholipids, in the presence of an acyl-CoA generating
system, to a lesser degree than liver microsomes. Additionally,

frozen and thawed microsomes from the hepatoma 7777 had little
capacity to incorporate free fatty acids, whereas, such treatment
had no effect on liver microsomes. These results indicate that
the fatty acid activating enzyme of hepatoma microsomes is more
labile than that of liver. Both microsomal samples had phospho-
lipase(s) which were active on membrane phospholipids, yet the hepatoma microsomes demonstrated no accumulation of the monoacylphos-
phoglyceride product, unlike liver where one half of the product
accumulated. This indicates that the precursor for reacylation in
the Lands' cycle is decreased in the hepatoma. The hepatoma
stearoyl-CoA desaturate activity was elevated with respect to the
liver microsomal enzyme. Moreover, the $^6\Delta$desaturase was significantly decreased in hepatoma. We conclude from these results that
the alterations in hepatoma phospholipid composition, both quantitatively and qualitatively, may be accounted for, in part, by the
metabolic aberrations described here.

INTRODUCTION

Interest in the role of lipids in biological membranes has
grown considerably over recent years and most significantly since
the development of the fluid-mosiac model of membrane structure
(35). This model suggests that membrane lipids exist as a bimole-
cular layer containing globular proteins. On the basis of this
membrane model, several functions have been attributed to membrane
lipids. First, the lipid bilayer provides a point of attachment
and thus a potential means of regulation of membrane protein function. This occurs both at the level of electrostatic interactions
between charged protein groups and the polar head region of the
membrane phsopholipid, and at the level of hydrophobic interaction
between membrane phospholipid fatty acid chains and exposed apolar
residues on proteins penetrating into the lipid bilayer. Second,
the lipid bilayer defines the permeability of the biological membrane to a wide variety of ions and compounds, thus regulating the
chemical environment enclosed by the membrane. The effects that
membrane lipids impart on membrane structure and function are influenced by several lipid characteristics, 1) the ratio of lipid to
protein within the membrane, 2) the membrane cholesterol content relative to the phospholipid present, 3) the phospholipid composition,
and 4) the fatty acid content of the phosphoglycerides.

Since many cellular functions are dependent upon the nature of
the cellular lipids, it has become imperative to determine the nature
and causes of membrane aberrations that occur in neoplasias. Many
laboratories are devoting their efforts to such studies with the
result that some key characteristics of neoplastic membranes have
been elucidated.

It is well established that there are alterations in the phos-

pholipid and fatty acid composition of hepatoma-derived organelles
(3, 4, 8, 16, 30, 32, 41). Moreover, isolated hepatoma diacyl-
GPC[3], when spread into monomolecular films, occupied more area per
molecule at a fixed pressure than normal liver lecithin (7, 8).
The effect altered lipid packing could have on membrane permeability to ions, lipid-protein interactions, and bilayer stability within the intact hepatoma membrane has been discussed (2). Additionally, there are two hallmarks of neoplasia that contribute to altered membrane character. First, nearly all hepatomas studied to
date show a loss of cholesterol regulation (33) which leads to increased membrane cholesterol content (38, 40, 41). Second, elevated levels of ether glycerolipids in cancer have been correlated with
the rate of neoplastic growth and thus to the degree of tumor dedifferentiation (36). Together, these modifications in lipid composition form a strong basis for an abnormal membrane character.

Some of the most dramatic changes noted in neoplastic cell
function have been plasma membrane associated events (27). Characteristically, cancer cells demonstrate increased agglutinability
by plant lectins (17, 27) which has been associated with the loss
in cell-cell communication (1), both of which are dependent on the
integrity of membrane function. Furthermore, decreases in the membrane associated nutrient uptake (11) and membrane bound $Na^+K^+ATPase$
(43) have been detected in cells lacking contact inhibition, whereas
the reported activity of adenylate cyclase varies considerably in
these cells (29, 43).

Despite the numerous aberrations that have been detected in neoplastic cell function and metabolism, the search for a common underlying affector is difficult. It has been our basic approach to study
the changes in one factor that many membrane associated fractions
have in common, the lipids. We feel that future investigations of
membrane associated properties in neoplasia should be carefully
analyzed with the altered membrane lipid environment in mind. The
importance of this approach is even more apparent when the close
interaction between lipid and protein observed in normal cell membranes is considered.

The transport of some cationic molecules across the biological
membrane by membrane bound enzymes has been shown to depend absolutely on membrane lipids. Delipidated and therefore inactivated preparations of $Na^+K^+ATPase$ could be fully reactivated by diacyl-GPS and
diacyl-GPG that were above their phase transition temperatures (19).
The same study showed that the presence of cholesterol in the reconstituted system decreased $Na^+K^+ATPase$ activity which is consistent
with the requirement for membrane fluidity. Similarly, the permeability properties of phospholipid membranes to Na^+, K^+, Cl^-, and glucose
decreased with increasing cholesterol to phospholipid ratios (28).
Furthermore, alterations in fatty acid composition and cholesterol

content of membranes have been correlated with changes in the
kinetic parameters for several membrane bound enzymes including
$Na^+K^+ATPase$, Mg^{2+} $Ca^{2+}ATPase$ and the bacterial $Ca^{2+}ATPase$ (9).

The importance of membrane lipids in hormone interaction has
been investigated recently by Limbrid and Lefkowitz (22). Studying
the coupling of the β-adrenergic receptor and adenylate cyclase of
frog erythrocyte plasma membranes, they demonstrated that the
stimulation of adenylate cyclase by receptor bound molecules was
sensitive to perturbation of the membrane hydrophobic region. This
indicated that the coupling of the hormone binding site and adenylate cyclase is mediated by lipids. Other studies have demonstrated
that specific lipids are required for the normal interaction of the
hormone binding site with adenylate cyclase. Cat ventricular myo-
cardium, when solubilized by Lubrol PX, was unresponsive to hormone
stimulation (21). However, the addition of monophosphatidylinositol
led to specific reactivation of catecholamine responsiveness of
adenylate cyclase.

Numerous investigations have been carried out to characterize
the nature of lipid-protein interaction within the mitochondrion.
Isolated inactive β-hyroxybutyrate dehydrogenase has been shown to
have an absolute requirement for lecithin molecules containing long
chain polyunsaturated fatty acid (10). The mitochondrial ATPase,
studied in reconstituted systems, was reactivated by a wide variety
of phospholipids but most effectively by cardiolipin (6). Using
synthetic diacyl-GPC, Bruni et al. (5) showed that long chain unsaturated diacyl-GPC confers oligomycin sensitive ATPase activity
and the presence of cholesterol decreased this activity. Additionally, reconstituted vesicles catalyzing P_i-ATP exchange and ATP driven
proton translocation showed a specific requirement for the presence
of a mixture of diacyl-GPE and diacyl-GPC, with the activity found
dependent on the diacyl-GPE to diacyl-GPC ratio (18). The presence
of cardiolipin facilitated the reactivation achieved by the phosphoglycerides.

In addition to the research above which has centered on normal
tissue, some classic observations also have been made on neoplastic
cells. For example, increased cell agglutination, a common characteristic of neoplastic cells, can be rationalized by a number of cell
membrane alterations (27). Many of these alterations involve factors
that affect the distribution and mobility of the lectin receptors
(glycoproteins) in the plasma membrane. Studies modifying membrane
fatty acid composition in cultured cell systems have related the
agglutinability of cells with fatty acid composition and membrane
fluidity (14, 31). The results of these studies are consistent with
the predictions of the fluid-mosiac membrane model, that is, the
mobility of proteins within the membrane are dependent on the physical state of the membrane lipids.

With the growing awareness that membrane lipids are vitally important for many membrane functions, the observed variations in neoplastic lipid composition are becoming increasingly appreciated as one of the underlying causes of the numerous metabolic and functional changes in neoplasias. Equally important then are the metabolic alterations which lead to the observed lipid compositional changes. Our experimental approach to date has been to investigate one neoplastic cell type, the Morris 7777 hepatoma, in detail. We feel this approach is basic to understanding the modifications seen in lipid composition within this hepatoma. We have fractionated the Morris 7777 hepatoma organelles into mitochondrial and microsomal rich fractions. Furthermore, a quantitative and qualitative evaluation of the phosphoglycerides from these fractions has allowed us to establish the phospholipid composition, and the fatty acid content of the membrane phospholipids. Microelectrophoresis and lipid monolayer studies have allowed an evaluation of the effect altered hepatoma lipid composition has on membrane lipid packing and ionic charge. In addition, initial studies in the systematic elucidation of hepatoma phosphoglyceride metabolism have involved the mitochondrial phospholipase and the microsome deacylation-reacylation (Land's) cycle.

RESULTS

Cell Fractionation. Classically, the purity of isolated cellular fractions is monitored by two techniques, electron microscopy and marker enzyme analysis. Electron microscopy of organelles isolated from various neoplasia reveals dramatic alterations in ultrastructure, indicating that the organelles derived from neoplastic tissue are significantly changed in shape and size. The difficulty in identifying modified neoplastic organelles, coupled with the physical limits of the instrumentation, prevents electron microscopy from being suitable for quantitative analyses. Marker enzyme analysis is an extremely useful tool in evaluating fractions isolated from comparable cell types. However, in view of the ultrastructural changes noted above, the validity and usefulness of such analyses are predicated on the assumption that redistribution of marker enzymes does not accompany the neoplastic state.

Tables 1 and 2 show the percentage distribution and specific activity of marker enzymes from normal and host liver, and the Morris 7777 hepatoma. The capacity of the isolation procedures employed to select for a particular organelle is illustrated in Table 1. In mitochondrial preparations, 66.5 and 72.1% of the total cytochrome oxidase activity is recovered from the hepatoma and control liver, respectively. Likewise, microsomal preparations contain 60.2 and 63.8% of the total NADPH cytochrome C reductase activity when isolated from hepatoma and control liver. Interestingly, the total units of all three marker enzymes analyzed are significantly de-

Table One

% Distribution of Marker Enzymes in the Fractionated Morris 7777 Hepatoma, Host Liver, and Control Liver

Enzyme	Fraction				
	Mitochondria	Lysosomes	Microsomes	Soluble Fraction	Total Units
Cytochrome Oxidase					
Control Liver	72.1	17.7	9.6	0.7	20.9
Host Liver	80.3	13.7	4.6	1.4	28.4
Hepatoma	66.5	24.5	7.4	1.6	5.7
Acid Phosphatase*					
Control Liver	38.5	27.5	20.8	13.2	1.64
Host Liver	43.7	30.2	15.5	10.6	2.08
Hepatoma	27.7	13.8	30.2	28.3	0.85
NADPH Cytochrome C Reductase					
Control Liver	15.5	9.7	63.8	10.9	4.12
Host Liver	16.6	13.0	59.0	11.4	3.32
Hepatoma	6.8	1.25	60.2	20.5	0.88

Total Units are from 4g of tissue wet weight.
Unit = μmoles substrate utilized/min/mg protein.
The cell organelles were prepared and marker enzyme measurements performed as indicated by Morton et al. (26) and Waite et al. (42).

* Acid phosphatase activity = nmoles substrate/min/mg protein.

creased in the hepatoma. This decrease probably reflects the
lower protein content of the hepatoma observed when quantitated
on a wet weight basis.

Contamination of each fraction by other organelles has been
estimated by marker enzyme specific activities (Table 2). Mitochondrial fractions (26) from control and host liver, and hepatoma
contain moderate microsomal and lysosomal contamination. Washing
the mitochondrial fraction after isolation lowers lysosomal and
microsomal contamination in both liver and hepatoma derived organelles (data not shown). This modification yields hepatoma mitochondria enriched 19 fold with respect to cytochrome oxidase as
compared to a 4 fold enrichment in liver. The final specific activities are comparable, however. This indicates that the hepatoma
homogenate has higher amounts of non-mitochondrial protein than
does liver.

Hepatoma and liver microsome preparations (42) are equally
contaminated by mitochondria (Table 2). The cytochrome oxidase
specific activity is about 3% of that present in washed mitochondria.
Lysosomal contamination, however, is higher in the hepatoma microsomes. The data suggest hepatoma cells contain a population of
either lighter or smaller lysosomes than liver; further investigations will be required to verify this supposition. In both preparations at least 60% of the total NADPH cytochrome C reducatse
activity is recovered in the microsomes. This latter observation
is similar to analyses obtained for Novikoff hepatomas (24).

Lipid Composition. The percentage phospholipid composition of the
isolated mitochondrial and microsomal fractions is presented in
Table 3. The hepatoma mitochondria contain lower amounts of cardiolipin than host liver. Conversely, the hepatoma contains about 4
times more diacyl-GPS and monoacyl-GPE than host liver. Also there
is a slight increase in the relative amounts of diacyl-GPE concomitant with a decrease in diacyl-GPC. The host liver phospholipid content is not significantly different than that reported for control
animals (4). Similar changes in cardiolipin and the diacyl-GPS/
diacyl-GPI fraction have been reported in this hepatoma (16), as
well as in others (4).

The changes in mitochondrial phospholipid composition in the
hepatoma suggest alterations in both mitochondrial and microsomal
phospholipid metabolism. The lower levels of cardiolipin probably
reflect changes in the phospholipid metabolism within the mitochondrion itself since this is the reported site of cardiolipin biosynthesis (15). Additionally, the higher levels of monoacyl-GPE
suggest that there are alterations in the relative rates of the mitochondrial reacylation and the deacylation systems. In contrast, the
elevated diacyl-GPS probably reflects alterations in microsomal meta-

Table Two

Specific Activity of Marker Enzymes in the Fractionated Morris 7777 Hepatoma,
Host Liver and Control Liver

µMoles Substrate Utilized/min/mg Protein

Enzyme	Mitochondria	Lysosomes	Microsomes	Soluble Fraction
Cytochrome Oxidase				
Control Liver	0.26 ± 0.10[a]	0.20 ± 0.11	0.04 ± 0.02	0
Host Liver	0.41 ± 0.14	0.23 ± 0.09	0.02 ± 0.0005	0.0003 ± 0.0003
Hepatoma	0.11 ± 0.02[d]	0.08 ± 0.02	0.02 ± 0.0004	0
Acid Phosphatase*				
Control Liver	10.0 ± 2.7	27.5 ± 3.4	6.5 ± 0.3	1.5 ± 0.4
Host Liver	15.3 ± 1.6	39.3 ± 5.6	6.8 ± 0.4	1.5 ± 0.3
Hepatoma	8.4 ± 1.7[c]	23.0 ± 7.6	10.6 ± 0.9[b,c]	2.4 ± 0.5
NADPH Cytochrome C Reductase				
Control Liver	0.010 ± 0.0002	0.023 ± 0.0004	0.050 ± 0.007	0.006 ± 0.004
Host Liver	0.009 ± 0.001	0.022 ± 0.003	0.037 ± 0.011	0.002 ± 0.002
Hepatoma	0.002 ± 0.001[b,c]	0.010 ± 0.002[b,c]	0.021 ± 0.002[b]	0.002 ± 0

[a] Mean ± S.E. of 5 preparations

[b] Significantly different than control liver $P < 0.05$.

[c] Significantly different than host liver $P < 0.05$.

[d] Compared to host liver $0.1 > P > 0.05$.

* Acid Phosphatase Activity = nmoles substrate/min/mg protein

bolism at the level of biosynthesis (25) or the specificity of the
phospholipid exchange mechanism between the 2 organelles (12).
The modest increase in the diacyl-GPE to diacyl-GPC ratio we find
was not noted by Hostetler et al. (16).

The only significant alterations in hepatoma microsomal phospholipid composition are increases in the sphingomyelin content
and in the diacyl-GPE to diacyl-GPC ratio (Table 3). However, when
expressed as nmoles lipid phosphorus/mg protein, a decrease in the
total phosphoglyceride content of the hepatoma microsomes is observed (145 vs. 441), yet the sphingomyelin content remains near
normal. This emphasizes that the abnormal phospholipid content is
class specific rather than a general effect on all lipids. Similar
changes in the phospholipid to protein ratio have been reported by
Hostetler et al. (16).

The most striking change in fatty acid composition in the hepatoma mitochondria and microsomes is the drastic increase in mono-
unsaturate content coupled with a decrease in polyunsaturated fatty
acids. Fatty acids from the total mitochondrial phosphoglyceride
pool (Table 4) contain a 3-4 fold increase in monounsaturates. This
pattern is also found in the isolated major phosphoglycerides, diacyl-GPC and diacyl-GPE (data shown for diacyl-GPC only, Table 4).
Hepatoma phospholipids contain 31% of C16:1 and C18:1 fatty acids
compared to 8% for host and 10.6% for control liver mitochondria.
Concomitantly, hepatoma phosphoglycerides contain only 34% of C18:2,
C20:4, and C22:6, whereas the liver mitochondria contained 50% more
of these unsaturated fatty acids. The total double index, a reflection of total fatty acid unsaturation, is 33% higher in liver mitochondria than hepatoma. Microsomes show similar changes in double
bond content (42). The changes observed in these studies are consistent with those described in several neoplasia (4, 30, 32). This
suggests that there may be some common metabolic alterations in
lipid metabolism. The metabolic processes responsible for the phosphoglyceride acyl content reflect the activities of 2 pathways, the
desaturation-elongation system involved in the modification of de
novo and dietary fatty acids, and the phosphoglyceride metabolism
pathways involving the incorporation of fatty acids into the cellular
phospholipid. Experiments concerning the contribution of these pathways to the altered acyl composition of the hepatoma are presented
in a later section (Metabolic alterations - Microsomes).

The decreased polyene content of hepatoma membranes should cause
dramatic changes in the physical characteristics of the phospholipid
molecule within the biological membrane. The lower number of double
bonds or "bends" in the acyl chains will facilitate closer association of phospholipid acyl chains. As a result, the membrane phospholipids should be less mobile within the bilayer due to tighter packing of the lipid molecules; therefore, membrane fluidity would be

Table Three
Phospholipid Composition Based on Phosphorus Content

Fraction	Tissue	CL	diacyl GPA	diacyl GPE	diacyl GPC	diacyl GPS[a]	monoacyl GPE	monoacyl GPC	SM
Mitochondria	Host Liver	5.2	0.0[b]	36.0	50.9	1.3	0.9	0.0	2.8
	Hepatoma	3.7	0.0	40.1	43.7	4.9	4.0	0.5	2.4
Microsomes	Host Liver	0.6	0.9	18.0	61.1	12.0	1.2	2.9	3.3
	Hepatoma	0.3	0.2	24.4	48.0	14.6	1.2	2.1	9.2

Values are the mean of 4-5 determinations and represent the percentage of total phospholipid present.

[a] PS and PI are not separated by this TLC procedure.

[b] No detectable amount present.

Table Four
Fatty Acids of Membrane Phosphoglycerides

Mole %

	16:0	16:1	18:0	18:1	18:2	20:1,2,3,	20:4	22:4,5	22:6
Total Phosphoglycerides									
Hepatoma	14.1	5.7	17.1	25.3	17.8	3.6	12.3	0	3.8
Host Liver	16.0	0	23.8	8.0	23.1	0	23.3	0	5.7
Control Liver	16.4	1.6	17.4	9.0	25.3	0	22.2	1.8	6.0
Diacyl GPC									
Hepatoma	15.4	5.3	19.0	27.5	15.3	3.3	12.1	0	1.9
Host Liver	14.5	0	30.0	5.9	12.8	0	30.0	2.1	5.6
Control Liver	14.3	0	25.9	6.8	11.0	1.1	32.1	1.3	6.2

Pooled mitochondria phospholipids from the hepatomas and livers of 12 tumor-bearing animals, as well as 4 control animal livers, were utilized in this experiment.

decreased.

The alterations in fatty acid composition are accompanied by changes in the distribution of the acyl chains on the glycerol backbone. The normal fatty acid distribution of position #1 saturate, position #2 unsaturate is perturbed in the hepatoma with significant amounts of monounsaturates present in both positions and a decrease in position #2 polyunsaturates. The presence of unsaturated fatty acids in both positions has been shown to have an expanding effect on lecithin monomolecular films (8).

Physical membrane properties. Microelectrophoresis is useful in evaluating the effect alterations in phospholipid composition have on surface charge of the lipid. Liposomes are prepared from total phosphoglycerides extracted from the mitochondrial fraction. Both control and host liver, and the hepatoma liposomes, exhibit a net negative zeta potential, and thus a net negative surface charge. Hepatoma liposomes have a zeta potential of −45, considerably less negative than either liver liposomes (control −71 and host −81). This drastic change in surface charge is not readily explained in terms of phospholipid composition (Table 3), but may reflect an asymmteric distribution of liposomal phospholipids. For example, if cardiolipin is preferentially distributed along the liposome-water interphase and diacyl-GPS associates with the interior half of the bilayer, then the changes in phospholipid content associated with the hepatoma mitochondria could generate the lower surface charge. Although speculative in this case, such asymmetric distributions have been observed (23). If similar asymmetry does exist in the biological membrane, then altered surface charge could affect both electrostatic lipid-protein interactions and the permeability of the membrane to ionic metabolites.

The effect of altered phospholipid and fatty acid composition on lipid-lipid interaction is best evaluated by monomolecular films. In Fig 1, the force-area curve shows that for any given surface pressure applied to a monomolecular film derived from hepatoma mitochondrial phospholipid, a smaller area per molecule is occupied than for host or control liver. This appears to be a reflection of 2 parameters, 1) reduced zeta potential thus decreasing phospholipid polar head group repulsion in the hepatoma phosphoglyceride and 2) closer packing of fatty acyl chains facilitated by the decrease in the polyenoic fatty acid content. The correlation of fatty acid unsaturation to molecular packing is consistent with similar results obtained in monomolecular studies of unsaturated lecithins (7) and diacyl-GPC (8). Monomolecular films of hepatoma and liver diacyl-GPE show similar force-area characteristics. However, isolated hepatoma diacyl-GPC demonstrates a larger area per molecule than liver lecithin (8, 26). This characteristic is not easily related to the fatty acid composition of the diacyl-GPC (Table 3). It has been sug-

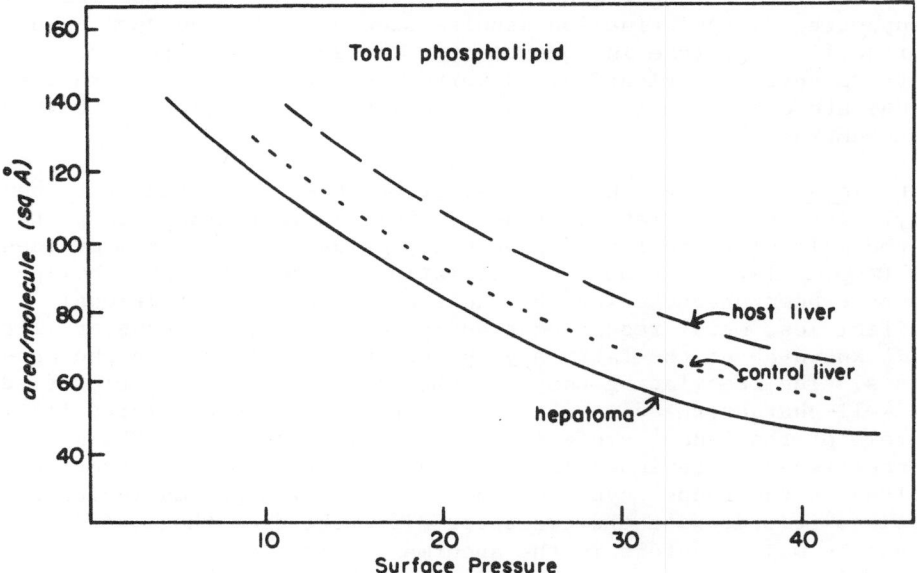

Figure 1
Force-area curves of monomolecular films constructed of mitochondria phospholipids from hepatoma and liver. The curves were
constructed as described in <u>Materials and Methods</u> (26).

gested that the presence of diacyl-GPC species containing two unsaturated fatty acids in the hepatoma does contribute an expanding
effect on lecithin monomolecular films, however (8).

     The correlation of monolayer data to the physical state of the
biological membrane must be applied with caution until measurements
of membrane surface pressure can be made. If it is assumed that
the hepatoma and liver membranes possess similar surface pressures
in vivo, then the hepatoma membrane lipids would occupy less area
per molecule than liver (Fig 1). However, if the in vivo hepatoma
membrane surface pressure is less than that of liver then the lipids
may demonstrate a larger area per molecule. The latter possibility
is supported by agglutination studies showing increased neoplasia
membrane fluidity (see Introduction). The solution to this problem
awaits further investigation. Nevertheless, the monolayer studies
do indicate dramatically altered lipid-lipid interaction in the hepatoma membranes.

Metabolic alterations - Microsomes. It has been suggested that the
deacylation and reacylation (Lands') cycle is responsible in part
for the molecular species of phosphoglycerides present in membranes
(13) (Figure 1). Some of the deacylating enzymes, the phospholipases have been characterized by their base group and positional
specificities, metal requirement and pH optimum (39). However, little in known about the fatty acyl group specificity of the phospholipases. The reacylating enzymes, the acyl-CoA-acyltransferases, do
have well-characterized acyl group and positional specificity (13).
The role of the Lands' cycle in the metabolism of diacyl-GPC species
has been recently reviewed (39). Studies of the various reactions
involved in the Lands' cycle of the Morris 7777 hepatoma indicate 2
reactions related with the cycle are different from those of liver
and can be major factors in the abnormal lipid composition of hepatoma membranes. First, our studies on microsomal phospholipase
activity (Fig 3) demonstrate two major differences between hepatoma
and liver: 1) an increased methanol-water soluble radioactivity
(radiolabel resides in the phospholipid head group), and 2) no accumulation of monoacyl phosphoglycerides in the presence of Ca^{2+}.
Both of these alterations suggest the presence of a highly-active
lysophospholipase (reaction 4, Scheme 1). Lumb and Allen found
elevated lysophospholipase activity in Novikoff hepatomas as well
(24). The elevated lysophospholipase activity does account for, in
part, the decreased amount of diacyl phosphoglycerides containing
C20:4 in hepatoma membranes, since this species is thought to be
produced by monoacyl-GPC reacylation in the Lands' cycle (13).
Furthermore, the loss of phosphoglycerides via an elevated lysophospholipase could contribute significantly to the lower phospholipid
content of hepatoma microsomes.

     Second, the decrease in hepatoma micorosmal phosphoglycerides

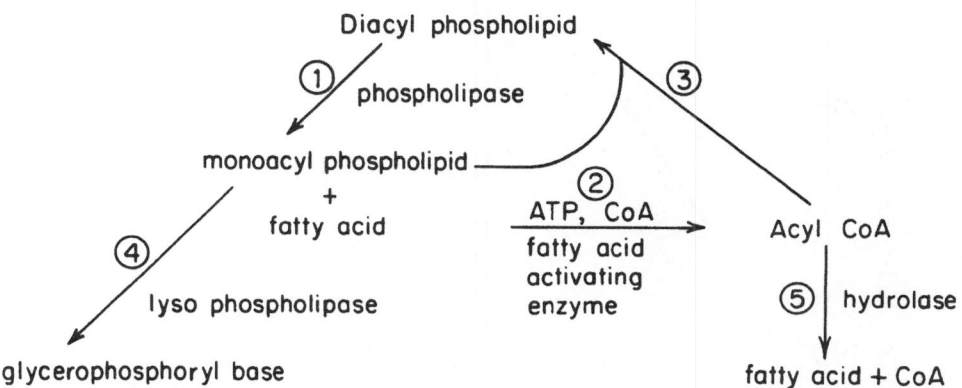

Figure 2
This scheme indicates the steps in the Lands' (deacylation-reacylation)
cycle considered in this study (42). They are: 1) deacylation by
the phospholipase(s) (without specification of positional attack),
2) activation of free fatty acid by the fatty acid activating enzyme,
3) transfer of the active acyl group to the monoacylphospholipid
from reaction one which reforms the diacylphospholipid; two additional
reactions are considered that are related to this cycle which are
catabolic, 4) lysophospholipase which deacylates the monoacylphospholipid and thereby removes the lipid from the cycle, and 5) hydrolysis
of the acyl-CoA by the acyl-CoA hydrolase which removes the acyl-
CoA from the cycle.

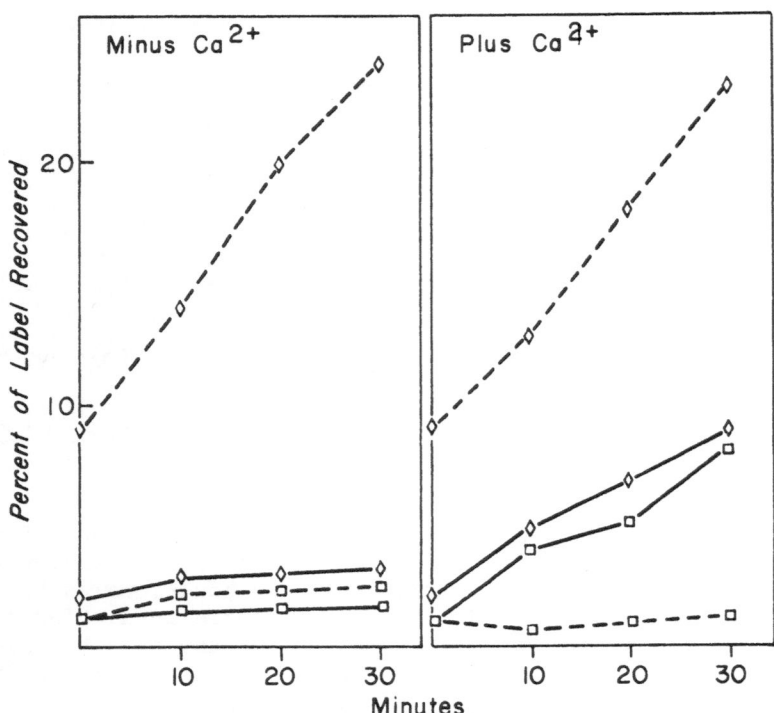

Figure 3
The hydrolysis of membrane phospholipids labeled in the polar
head group was measured at different time intervals. An aliquot
of the methanol-H_2O layer was counted ($\diamond$) and the products in the
chloroform layer, monacyl-GPE and monoacyl-GPC fractions ($\square$) were
isolated by thin-layer chromatography and combined for counting.

could be the result of lower fatty acid activating enzyme activities (reaction 2, Figure 1). Decreased activating enzyme activity is observed when the incorporation of oleic acid and oleoyl-CoA into diacyl-GPC is compared. The results indicate comparable incorporation of oleoyl-CoA by both hepatoma and control liver microsomes, whereas the hepatoma incorporates oleic acid to a lesser degree than does liver. Since the fatty acid activating enzyme is membrane associated, we believe that the lower activity could be the result of an alteration of the membrane lipid surrounding this enzyme. This is based in part on our observation that freezing and thawing completely inactivates the system that incorporates free fatty acids into hepatoma monoacyl phosphoglycerides.

Analysis of free fatty acid pool of microsomes indicates that the hepatoma contains higher levels of free fatty acids than liver (17.0 vs. 11.4 nmoles/mg protein). This increase is consistent with the observed decrease in fatty acid activating enzyme. Furthermore, the content of the hepatoma pool (42) is not a complete reflection of the acyl composition of the phosphoglycerides. This difference may reflect alterations in the specificity of the fatty acid activating system or changes in the relative activities of the Lands' cycle enzymes, such as the acyl-CoA-acyltransferase (30).

Since the microsomal desaturates are responsible in part for defining the content of the free fatty acid pool, we have initiated studies in our laboratory to determine the relative rates of desaturate activites. Preliminary results indicate an elevated $^9\Delta$ stearoyl-CoA desaturase and a decreased $^6\Delta$ desaturase in the hepatoma microsomes (unpublished data). The elevated $^9\Delta$ activity is in contrast to the observations made by Lee et al. (20), however, this difference may be explained by our observation that the hepatoma $^9\Delta$ desaturase activity is cold labile. These changes in $^9\Delta$ and $^6\Delta$ desaturase activities are consistent with the elevated moneonic and decreased polyenoic content of the hepatoma phospholipids. Interestingly, cytochrome b_5, a component of the electron transport chain providing reducing equivalents to the desaturases, has been shown to be dramatically decreased in the Morris 7777 hepatoma (Table 5). However, this decrease is not related to the observed desaturase activities since cytochrome b_5 participates in both $^9\Delta$ and $^6\Delta$ pathways. Similar decreases have been found in rapidly growing Yoshida ascitic hepatomas (34, 37). The decrease in cytochrome b_5 content suggests that the desaturase enzymes may utilize electrons from other sources; however, this awaits further investigation. Interestingly, cytochrome P_{450}, another heme-containing microsomal enzyme, is also greatly reduced in the Morris 7777 hepatoma, however, NADPH cytochrome C reducatse is decreased to only 20% of that found in the control liver microsomes. These observations suggest significant differences exist between the hepatoma and liver microsomal electron transport systems. The significance of these alterations is not

Table Five

Average Results of Microsomal Cytochrome b5 Analyses

Tissue source of microsomes[b]	nmoles cytochrome b5 per mg of microsomal protein[c]	nmoles of cytochrome b5 per g wet weight of liver
Normal Liver (4)[a]	0.40	5.3
Tumor-bearing host liver (6)[a]	0.33	4.2
Morris hepatoma 7777 (4)[a]	0.00[d]	0.00

a

The figure in parenthesis is the number of animals studied.

b

Microsomes were prepared by the procedure of Mitoma et al. [Arch. Biochem. Biophys. 61 (1956) 431.].

c

Activities were determined by difference in spectra according to Klingenberg, M. [Arch. Biochem. Biophys. 75 (1958) 376].

d

Technical problems limit sensitivity to approximately 10% of control values.

known.

Metabolic alterations - Mitochondria. The mitochondrial phospholipase A_2 has been implicated as a mechanism by which the mitochondria effects changes in phospholipid composition. Fig 4 contains a time course study of the mitochondrial phospholipase A on
endogenous diacyl-GPE. In brief, the experimental procedure is
to isolate mitochondria from rats fed [^{3}H] ethanolamine and in-
cubate them at 18°. Periodically, aliquots are incubated at 37°
for 30 min in the presence of Ca^{2+} to measure phospholipase A
activity. Zero time values for the 18° incubations reflect the
in vivo activity of the phospholipase A. The higher zero time
value for the hepatoma is consistent with the elevated monoacyl-
GPE content in phospholipid composition studies (Table 3). Most
significant, however, is the lack of a lag time of phospholipase
A activity expression in the hepatoma mitochondria compared to
control liver (lag $\simeq$ 1 hr). Although the hepatoma demonstrates
lower total phospholipase A activity, there appears to be no mechanism for delaying and thereby controlling the expression of its
activity. Due to the lower, yet less regulated, phospholipase A
activity in the hepatoma, we suggest that the high levels of monoacyl-GPE present in hepatoma mitochondria membranes may reflect
the relative steady-state activities of the phospholipase A and
the reacylation system.

INTERPRETATION

We have taken as our working model that there are aberrations
in membrane lipids of neoplastic cells that are held in common and
produce a pathologic state. Our approach in studying this hypothesis has been to identify changes in phosphoglyceride composition and the metabolic alterations responsible for these changes
in the Morris 7777 hepatoma. We describe here a number of qualitative and quantitative changes in the phospholipid pool from the
hepatoma microsomes and mitochondria. Furthermore, these changes
were found to create alterations in the physical characteristics
of the lipids.

In our endeavor to determine the metabolic alterations responsible for these changes our initial studies have identified
several significantly modified metabolic events which may account
for the compositional changes noted. Obviously, much more time is
needed to better understand the full realm of metabolic alterations that accompany the neoplastic state. Nonetheless, our initial observations have made it clear that metabolic changes within
the hepatoma itself can be responsible for the lipid alterations
present in the hepatoma, at least in part.

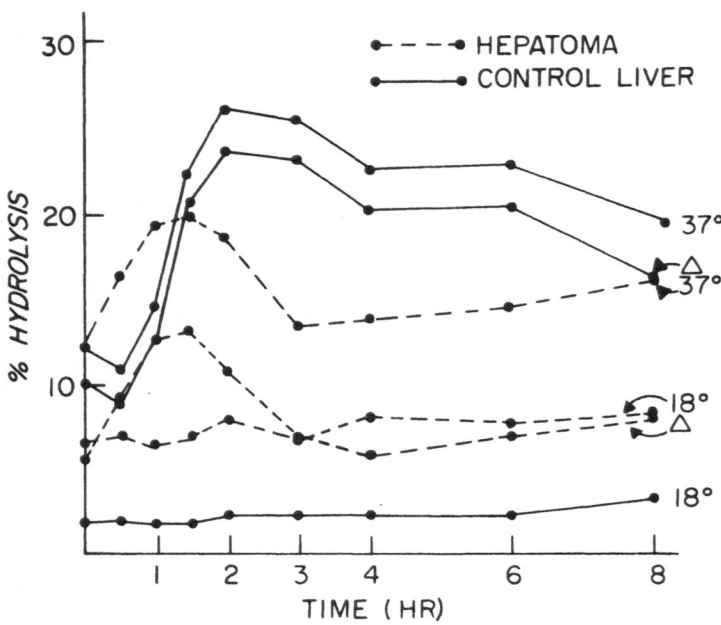

Figure 4
Activity of the mitochondrial phospholipase A on endogenous
diacyl-GPE (radiolabeled in the ethanolamine moiety) in hepatoma
and control mitochondria. The phospholipase A assay was carried
out as described in Materials and Methods (26). The percent hydrolysis of diacyl-GPE was calculated by dividing the cpm found in
monoacyl-GPE by the sum of the cpm of monoacyl-GPE and diacyl-GPE
which were recovered from the thin-layer chromatography plate utilized to separate the products of the reaction; this value was multiplied by 100 to obtain percent hydrolysis. The △ values were
derived by subtracting the % hydrolysis at 18° from that obtained
after incubation at 37° for 30 min in the presence of additional
calcium. Host liver mitochondria demonstrated activities similar
to those shown here for control mitochondria.

[1] Supported by USPH Grants CA 14318 and CA 10729, and by the Forsyth Cancer Service.

[2] Recipient of NIH Career Development Award AM 17392.

[3] Abbreviations: GPC, glycerophosphorylcholine; GPS, glycerophosphorylserine; GPG, glycerophosphorylglycerol; GPI, glycerophosphorylinositol; CL, cardioplipin; GPE, glycerophosphorylethanolamine; SM, sphingomyelin.

REFERENCES

1. Abercombie, H.N. and Heaysman, J.E.M. Exp. Cell Res. 6 (1954) 293.

2. Bergelson, L.D. and Dyatlovitskaya, E.V. In: Tumor Lipids: Biochemistry and Metabolism, R. Wood (ed). (1973) 111.

3. Bergelson, L.D., Dyatlovistkaya, E.V., Sorokina, I.B. and Gorkova, N.P. BBA 360 (1974) 361.

4. Bergelson, L.D., Dyatlovitskaya, E.V., Torkhovskaya, T.I., Sorokina, I.B. and Gorkova, N.P. BBA, 210 (1970) 287.

5. Bruni, A., van Dijck, P.W.M. and DeGier, J. BBA, 406 (1975) 315.

6. Cunningham, C.C. and George, D.T. JBC, 250 (1975) 2036.

7. Demel, R.A., van Deenen, L.L.M. and Pethica, B.A. BBA 135 (1967) 11.

8. Dyatlovitskaya, E.V., Yanchevskaya, G.V. and Bergelson, L.D. Chem. Phys. Lipids 12 (1974) 132.

9. Farias, R.N., Bloj, B., Morero, R.D., Siñeriz, F. and Trucco, R.E., BBA 415 (1975) 231.

10. Gazzotti, P., Bock, H., and Fleischer, S. JBC, 250 (1975) 5782.

11. Griffiths, J.B. J. Cell Sci. 10 (1972) 515.

12. Harvey, M.S., Wirtz, K.W.A., Kamp, H.H., Zegers, B.J.M. and van Deenen, L.L.M. BBA 323 (1973) 234.

13. Hill, E.E. and Lands, W.E.M. In: Lipid Metabolism, S.J. Wakil (ed)., (1970) 185.

14. Horwitz, A.F., Hatten, M.E. and Burger, M.M. PNAS 71 (1974) 3115.

15. Hostetler, K.Y., van den Bosch, H. and van Deenen, L.L.M. BBA, 239 (1971) 113.

16. Hostetler, K.Y., Zenner, B.D. and Morris, H.P. BBA 441 (1976) 231.

17. Inbar, M. and Sachs, L. PNAS, 63 (1969) 1418.

18. Kagawa, Y., Kandrach, A. and Racker, E. JBC, 248 (1973) 676.

19. Kimelberg, H.K. and Papahadjopoulos, D. BBA, 282 (1972) 277.

20. Lee, T.C., Stephens, N. and Snyder, F. Cancer Res. 34 (1974) 3270.

21. Levey, G.S. and Klein, I. J. Clin. Invest. 51 (1972) 1578.

22. Limbrid, L.E. and Lefkowitz, R.J. Mol. Phar. 12 (1976) 559.

23. Litman, B.J. Biochemistry, 13 (1974) 2844.

24. Lumb, R. and Allen, K.F. BBA 450 (1976) 175.

25. McMurry, W.C. and Magee, W.L. Ann. Rev. Biochem. 41 (1972) 129.

26. Morton, R., Cunningham, C., Jester, R., Waite, M., Miller, N. and Morris, H.P., Cancer Res. 36 (1976) 3246.

27. Nicolson, G.L. BBA, 458 (1976) 1.

28. Papahadjopoulos, D., Nir, S. and Ohki, S. BBA, 266 (1971) 561.

29. Peery, C.V., Johnson, G.S. and Pastan, I. JBC, 246 (1971) 5785.

30. Reitz, R.C., Thompson, J.A. and Morris, H.P. Cancer Res. 37 (1977) 561.

31. Rittenhouse, H.G., Williams, R.E., Wisnieski, B. and Fox, C.F. BBRC, 58 (1974) 222.

32. Ruggieri, S. and Fallini, A. In: Tumor Lipids, Biochemistry and Metabolism, R. Wood (ed). (1973) 89.

33. Sabine, J.R. Prog. Biochem. Pharmacol. 10 (1975) 269.

34. Sato, N. and Hagihara, B. Cancer Res. 30 (1970) 2061.

35. Singer, S.J. and Nicolson, G.L. Science, 175 (1972) 720.

36. Snyder, F. and Snyder, C. Prog. Biochem. Phar. 10 (1975) 1.

37. Sugimura, T., Ikeda, K., Hirota, K., Hozumi, M. and Morris,
    H.P. Cancer Res. 26 (1966) 1711.

38. Teise, H. and Bielka, H. Arch. Geshwulstforch, 32 (1968) 11.

39. van den Bosch, H. Ann. Rev. Biochem. 43 (1974) 243.

40. van Hoeven, R.P. and Emmelot, P. J. Memb. Biol. 9 (1972) 105.

41. van Hoeven, R.P. and Emmelot, P. In: Tumor Lipids: Biochemistry
    and Metabolism, R. Wood (ed). (1973) 126.

42. Waite, M., Parce, B., Morton, R., Cunningham, C. and Morris,
    H.P. Cancer Res. (1977) In Press.

43. Yoshikawa-Fukada, M. and Nojima, T. J. Cell Phys. 80 (1972)
    421.

TERMINAL SUGARS IN GLYCOCONJUGATES: METABOLISM OF FREE AND PROTEIN-
BOUND L-FUCOSE, N-ACETYLNEURAMINIC ACID AND D-GALACTOSE IN LIVER
AND MORRIS HEPATOMAS

W. Reutter and C. Bauer

Biochemisches Institut, Universitat

D-7800 Freiburg, Germany

SUMMARY

1. In Morris hepatomas the activity of UDP-N-acetyl-glucosamine
2'-epimerase, the key enzyme for the synthesis of N-acetylneuraminic
acid, was always decreased to about 10%. 2. In all tumors investigated the activity of ADP-galactose 4-epimerase was raised between 2
to 28-fold, whereas the level of galactose 1-phosphate uridyltransferase was lowered. 3. The specific activity of GDP-fucose:
glycoprotein fucosyltransferase was elevated between 2 to 3-fold;
conversely, the activity of sialyltransferase was generally decreased.
4. In fast growing tumors the content of GDP-fucose was raised between 2 to 3-fold, the concentration of CMP-N-acetylneuraminic acid was
more or less unchanged and the content of UDP-galactose markedly decreased. 5. Measurement of the protein-bound carbohydrate content
of plasma membranes revealed that none of the neutral sugars showed
a significant difference, except for L-fucose, which was greatly increased from 6.1 ± 1.7 nmoles/mg of protein in host or normal liver
to 26.1 ± 2.7 nmoles/mg of protein in hepatoma 7777. 6. The specific activity of α-L-fucosidase in hepatomas with a short or intermediate growth rate was 2 to 7-fold higher than in normal liver, the
level of neuraminidase and galactosidase lowered or at least remained
unchanged. 7. A fucoprotein with a molecular weight of about 130,000
has been isolated from both liver and hepatoma plasma membranes.

The results indicate that specific alterations of free and protein-bound sugars are a characteristic feature of Morris hepatomas.

INTRODUCTION

Already in 1944 it had been shown by Coman (31) and later on
by Abercombie and Ambrose (1) that changes of cell surface properties
might be connected with malignancy, but only during the last ten years
studies on the organization and composition of plasma membranes have
expanded greatly. A number of recent observations have altered our
view of the cell surface (78, 111) and evidence is accumulating indicating that changes in the carbohydrate content of glycoproteins
and glycolipids is associated with malignant transformation (37, 78,
100). Sugars and the equivalent glycosyltransferases may have important functions in surface adhesiveness, contact inhibition and
antigenicity (28, 89, 102). The use of phytohemagglutinins revealed specific alterations of terminal sugars during stimulated growth
(102). Moreover, Buck et al.(27) have described a fucose-containing
sialoprotein that is increased in the plasma membrane of Rous sarcoma
virus-transformed hamster cells and Bryant et al. (25) demonstrated
that human lung tumor cells synthesize elevated amounts of fucoproteins.

Single cells have been the favorable object for many years and
still are quite valuable when investigating specific problems. However, for our studies we have chosen Morris hepatomas in preference
to cell culture because:

(a) these hepatomas are solid tumors, (b) most of them still
have a closer relationship to hepatocytes than the other frequently
used hepatoma cells (85).

L-fucose, N-acetylneuraminic acid and D-galactose are important
terminal (or subterminal) sugars of glycoconjugates and the evidence
available leaves little doubt that some of the observed changes after
malignant transformation are intimately connected with these carbohydrates. Hence, comparative investigations on their metabolism in
liver and Morris hepatomas may contribute to a better understanding
of plasma memberane alterations found in malignant cells.

METABOLISM OF N-ACETYLNEURAMINIC ACID

N-Acetylneuraminic acid (NANA) is an outstanding amino sugar
derivative endowed with a carboxyl group which contributes substantially to a negative charge of glycoconjugates. The metabolic route leading to the biosynthesis of NANA and CMP-NANA was established primarily
by the groups of Roseman and Warren (for review see 72, 113). This
most complex pathway may be divided into two sections: (a) the steps
between transamidation of fructose 6-P to glucosamine 6-P and the
synthesis of UDP-N-acetylglucosamine from N-acetylglucosamine 1-P
(Fig 1). The first enzyme of this pathway, L-glutamine: D-fructose
6-P-aminotransferase is under feedback regulation of UDP-N-acetylgluco-

samine (65). (b) steps between the epimerization of UDP-N-acetyl-glucosamine to N-acetylmannosamine and the activation of NANA to CMP-NANA. The 5 reactions of this second area are irreversible, utilizing 4 energy-rich phosphate-bondings. In liver, the biosynthesis of CMP-NANA virtually begins by the epimerization of UDP-N-acetylglucosamine to N-acetylmannosamine. The significance of UDP-N-acetyl-glucosamine 2'-epimerase as the key enzyme for the synthesis of CMP-NANA could be demonstrated by Kornfeld et al. (65), showing that the activity of this allosteric enzyme is controlled by the level of CMP-NANA in vitro. An epimerization of N-acetylglucosamine to N-acetylmannosamine as occurring in kidney (41) or the epimerization of N-acetylglucosamine 6-P to N-acetylmannosamine 6-P as shown in some bacteria (42) could not be ascertained for rat liver (54). Applying the cell-free system of Hultsch et al. (54) to Morris hepatomas a greatly diminished synthesis of NANA was observed due to a decreased activity of UDP-N-acetylglucosamine 2'-epimerase (48, 60, 88). Therefore, the activity of this key enzyme, the content of UDP-N-acetylhexosamines, NANA and CMP-NANA as well as the conversion of radioactive labelled precursors ($[1-^{14}C]$glucosamine, N-acetyl-$[U-^{14}C]$mannosamine) to NANA have been investigated more thoroughly in vivo. The results reveal the existence of the same metabolic pathway for NANA synthesis in liver and hepatoma (48). However, the amount of NANA deriving from $[1-^{14}C]$ glucosamine is diminished to about 15% in hepatoma when compared with liver, whereas the synthesis of UDP-N-acetylglucosamine is unchanged. It is remarkable that the formation of NANA, using N-acetyl-mannosamine as precursor, is not lowered, but slightly increased (Table 1). These findings demonstrate the important role of the UDP-N-acetylglucosamine 2'-epimerase for the regulation of NANA biosynthesis in hepatomas. Measurements of enzyme activity in several Morris hepatoma lines show a uniform decrease to 6 to 13% (Table 2). For comparison, in different fast growing tissues in the regenerating and neonatal rat liver, no decrease was observed. Hence, the low activity of this key enzyme can be regarded as a characteristic of Morris hepatoma. The possible alternative pathway, synthesis of N-acetylmannosamine by a direct epimerisation of N-acetylglucosamine, mentioned above for kidney, is devoid of any importance in vivo or in vitro. This fact, as well as the low concentration of free N-acetylhexosamines (48) and the high K_M-value of the N-acetylglucosamine 2-epimerase (41) argue against a physiological role of this route for NANA synthesis in liver and hepatoma. Conversely, the K_M-value of UDP-N-acetyl-glucosamine 2'-epimerase for UDP-N-acetylglucosamine is fairly low in both liver (17 µM) and hepatoma (12 µM). Furthermore, the concentration of this amino sugar nucleotide is 20- (liver) or 10-fold (hepatoma) higher than the respective K_M-value.

These findings show quite clearly that the UDP-N-acetylglucosamine 2'-epimerase is indeed the key enzyme for NANA synthesis in Morris hepatomas (48).

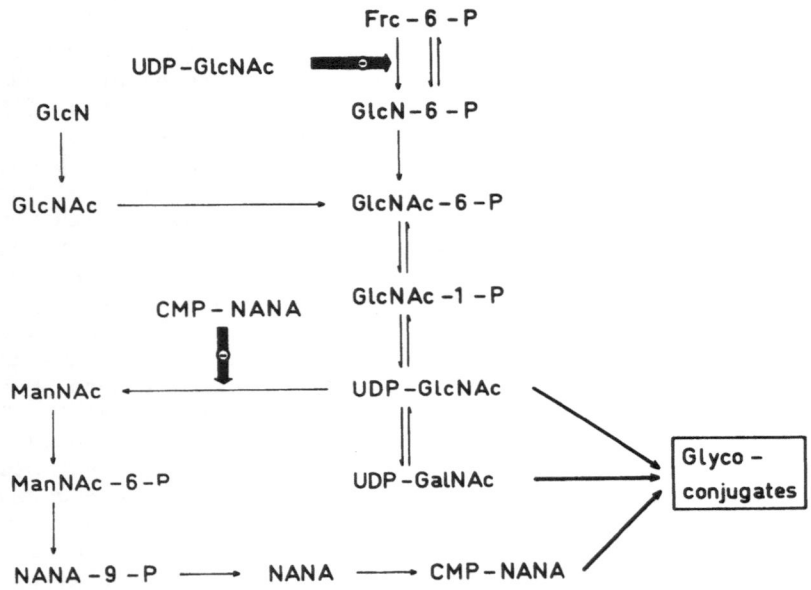

Figure 1
Major hepatic reactions leading to the synthesis of N-acetylneuraminic acid and sialoglycoconjugates.

Table 1

Specific Radioactivity of Aminosugar Nucleotides

Tissue	$[1-^{14}C]$glucosamine		N-acetyl-$[U-^{14}C]$mannosamine	
	Liver	Hepatoma 7777	Liver	Hepatoma 7777
	mCi/mmol			
UDP-N-acetylglucosamine	0.256	0.225	—	—
UDP-N-acetylgalactosamine	0.249	0.227	—	—
NANA + CMP-NANA	0.224	0.047	0.252	0.320

(NANA, N-acetylneuraminic acid)

Specific radioactivities of UDP-N-acetylhexosamines and NANA+CMP-NANA were determined 2 hours after the injection of $[1-^{14}C]$glucosamine (0.1 mCi/kg body weight) or N-acetyl-$[U-^{14}C]$mannosamine (0.3 mCi/kg body weight) in host liver and Morris hepatoma 7777. For the preparation and determination of acid soluble radioactivity see Harms et al. (48).

Table Two

Specific Activity of UDP-N-acetylglucosamine 2'-epimerase in Liver and Morris Hepatomas

Tissue	Specific activity nmoles/min/mg prot.	Tissue	Specific activity nmoles/min/mg prot.
Hepatoma 7777	0.158 ± 0.039	Control	
Host Liver	1.94 ± 0.26	(a) Normal adult liver (buffalo strain)	1.94 ± 0.063
Hepatoma 5123 TC	0.190	(b) Neonatal liver,	
Host Liver	2.17	1st day	1.60
Hepatoma 5123 C	0.208	(c) Neonatal liver,	
Host Liver	1.74	10th day	2.16
Hepatoma 5123 D	0.181	(d) Regenerating liver,	
Host Liver	1.65	6 hr	2.14 ± 0.12
Hepatoma 7800	0.231	1st day	2.09 ± 0.17
Host Liver	2.04	3rd day	2.32 ± 0.03
Hepatoma 7795	0.088	5th day	2.54 ± 0.12
Host Liver	1.22	9th day	2.41 ± 0.23
Hepatoma 9121	0.200		
Host Liver	1.50		
Hepatoma 9618 A	0.202		
Host Liver	1.83		

Activity was measured in a radiochemical assay (48). Units of specific activity are given as nmoles N-acetylmannosamine formed/min/mg protein.

Despite the decreased conversion of UDP-N-acetylglucosamine into N-acetylmannosamine, the concentration of CMP-NANA in hepatoma is in the same range as in liver (Table 3). In order to explain this remarkable discrepancy it should be pointed out that the remaining 2'-epimerase activity of 0.2 mU/mg of protein is still sufficient to synthesize 40 nmoles of CMP-NANA/hr, assuming a turnover time of about 1 hr. (46). Moreover, it should be considered that Morris hepatomas are characterized by a lack of secretion of plasma proteins (94). The deletion of this specific function decreases the requirement for NANA, because most plasma proteins are sialoglycoproteins. A prolongation of the half-life of protein-bound NANA, as a further possible explanation can also be excluded. In total homogenate as well as in the plasma membrane of liver and Morris hepatoma quite similar half-lives of protein-bound NANA have been described (49).

ENZYMES OF THE LELOIR PATHWAY

Galactose is a major constituent of glycoproteins and glycolipids. Significant amounts of this sugar are only available in the postnatal period when lactose is essentially the only carbohydrate nutrient in milk. Lactose is split by enzymatic hydrolysis in the intestinal mucosa and the galactose liberated is then absorbed and phosphorylated by galactokinase. In the following step the enzyme galactose 1-phosphate uridyl-transferase catalyzes the reversible transformation to UDP-galactose. However, in adult animals the necessary supply of this sugar nucleotide is provided by the interconversion of UDP-glucose to UDP-galactose, a reaction which is catalyzed by UDP-galactose 4-epimerase (for review see 30).

Only minor changes of galactokinase activity were found in Morris hepatomas when compared with normal adult liver (Table 4). Yet, in all tumors investigated the UDP-galactose 4-epimerase was elevated by 2 to 28-fold. Moreover, a striking correlation between the enzyme level and the growth rate of the hepatoma was observed (7). Contrary to this, the activity of galactose 1-phosphate uridyltransferase was diminished by 15 to 50%.

Uridine nucleotides are important metabolites regulating the activity of uridyltransferase and 4-epimerase. It is known that galactose 1-phosphate uridyltransferase is inhibited by UDP-glucose, if the concentration exceeds the K_M-value of 0.1 to 0.2 mM (95). UTP and UDP are potent inhibitors of the UDP-glucose binding to the enzyme with K_i-values in the low nanomolar range. UMP is far less effective. In all Morris hepatomas except line 7800 substantially decreased levels of UDP-glucose, UTP and UDP have been determined (data not shown). For that reason the lowered uridyltransferase activity cannot be explained by a possible substrate inhibition. Preliminary studies on UDP-galactose 4-epimerase indicate that the elevated activity is due to an increased synthesis of enzyme protein and not the result of a

Table Three

Concentration of Sugar Nucleotides

Tissue	GDP-fucose	CMP-N-acetylneuraminic acid	UDP-galactose
		nmoles/g wet weight of tissue	
Hepatoma 9618 A$_2$	10.2 ± 1.4		47 ± 3
Host Liver	14.4 ± 5.0		175 ± 18
Hepatoma 3924 A	21.9 ± 1.0	55.3 ± 6.0	48 ± 12
Host Liver	14.6 ± 0.8	52.5 ± 7.0	148 ± 15
Hepatoma 7777	12.1 ± 1.0	61.9 ± 5.7	69 ± 6
Host Liver	6.2 ± 0.5	41.2 ± 3.2	145 ± 18
Hepatoma 66	6.5 ± 3.0		76 ± 12
Host Liver	8.1 ± 1.4		188 ± 48
Hepatoma 7800	--		147 ± 8
Host Liver			304 ± 37
Hepatoma 9121	20.3 ± 6.5		--
Host Liver	9.9 ± 0.7		
Hepatoma 20	5.6 ± 1.9		58 ± 17
Host Liver	4.8 ± 0.8		142 ± 19
Control (normal adult liver)			
Buffalo strain	6.5 ± 0.8	42.8 ± 7.0	92 ± 7
ACI strain	9.5 ± 1.1	40.3 ± 8.8	--
Regenerating Liver (maximal concentration)	7.2 ± 1.1 (72 hr)	44.4 ± 3.9)72 hr)	108 ± 9 (24 hr)

Hepatoma tissue and liver lobes were instantly frozen in situ between metal tongs precooled in liquid N$_2$. GDP-fucose and CMP-N-acetylneuraminic acid were isolated by repeated ethanol extractions and determined by the isotope dilution technique (10). UDP-galactose was determined enzymatically in neutralized HClO$_4$ extracts. Values are means ± S.D. from five rats.

Table Four

Specific Activity of Galactokinase, Galactose 1-Phosphate Uridyltransferase and UDP-galactose 4-Epimerase

Tissue	Galactokinase	Uridyltranferase	4-Epimerase
	μmoles metabolized/hr/mg protein		
Hepatoma 9618 A$_2$	0.32 ± 0.04	0.18 ± 0.06	7.68 ± 1.32
Host Liver	0.44 ± 0.04	0.56 ± 0.04	0.36 ± 0.06
Hepatoma 3924 A	—	0.22 ± 0.02	2.46 ± 0.22
Host Liver		0.52 ± 0.05	0.31 ± 0.04
Hepatoma 7777	0.39 ± 0.02	0.18 ± 0.02	1.54 ± 0.13
Host Liver	0.44 ± 0.05	0.44 ± 0.04	0.29 ± 0.02
Hepatoma 66	0.47 ± 0.05	0.28 ± 0.02	0.73 ± 0.05
Host Liver	0.49 ± 0.04	0.50 ± 0.02	0.25 ± 0.03
Hepatoma 7800	0.40 ± 0.06	0.26 ± 0.04	0.69 ± 0.09
Host Liver	0.55 ± 0.06	0.45 ± 0.06	0.27 ± 0.04
Hepatoma 9618 A	0.38 ± 0.04	0.17 ± 0.03	0.57 ± 0.07
Host Liver	0.49 ± 0.02	0.53 ± 0.03	0.26 ± 0.03
Hepatoma 20	0.51 ± 0.07	0.21 ± 0.02	0.47 ± 0.02
Host Liver	0.60 ± 0.02	0.43 ± 0.02	0.25 ± 0.04
Control			
(a) normal adult liver	0.38 ± 0.03	0.32 ± 0.03	0.27 ± 0.04
(b) regenerating liver (maximal activity)	0.90 ± 0.10 (24 hr)	0.48 ± 0.04 (36 hr)	0.92 ± 0.14 (96 hr)

The activity of galactokinase, uridyltransferase was measured either in a radiochemical assay (15, 98, 110) or spectrophotometrically (70, 71). UDP-galactose 4-epimerase activity was determined by following the formation of NADH (6). Values are means ± S.D. from 4 to 6 animals.

positive allosteric effector. To sum up the findings it is fairly
certain that at least in adult animals the enzymes of the Leloir
pathway are not regulated in a coordinate fashion. In favor of this
conclusion are observations of Stern and Krooth (101) who have shown
that the activities of galactokinase, uridyltransferase and 4-
epimerase change substantially during the growth of mammalian cells,
but there was no consistent correlation between the specific activities of the individual enzymes.

CONCENTRATION OF GDP-FUCOSE, CMP-NANA AND UDP-GALACTOSE

Only recently data on the concentration of GDP-fucose and CMP-
NANA became available due to the extreme acid lability of these
metabolites (11, 48). It should be stressed that the level of GDP-
fucose does normally not exceed 7 to 10 nmoles/g wet weight of liver,
thus representing the lowest concentration of a sugar nucleotide
measured hitherto in solid tissue (108, 109). The data in Table 3
shows that the content of GDP-fucose in rapidly growing hepatomas is
twice as high as in liver, whereas the concentration and that of GDP-
galactose is decreased. The comparatively high level of GDP-fucose
may be regarded as a characteristic feature of Morris hepatomas,
because in the rapid proliferating liver after partial hepatectomy
no increase of the GDP-fucose pool was determined. In some cases
the host liver also had elevated levels of GDP-fucose, a finding
worth considering for further studies on the interrelation between
hepatoma and liver. In this respect, quite an interesting phenomenon should be mentioned. When measuring the turnover of GDP-fucose
in host liver at different times after the inoculation of hepatoma
7777, Dr. Vischer (108) observed at the 13th day a greater turnover
rate than 10 days later. Probably, the organism secretes more fucose-
containing plasma proteins during a defined period of malignant growth.
Further work is in progress to elucidate the significance of this
finding.

No data is available on the activity of enzymes catalyzing the
reactions between GDP-mannose and GDP-L-fucose. It should be noted
that the level of GDP-fucose cannot be increased by intraperitoneal
injections of mannose (108). Conversely, administration of fucose up
to a dose of 0.5 moles/kg body weight leads to a rise of GDP-fucose
from 6 to 300 nmoles/g liver wet weight. A similar elevation could
be observed in hepatomas.

In contrast to regenerating liver which shows a slight increase
of UDP-galactose concentration (6), most Morris hepatomas exhibited
lowered levels. This finding might be explained (a) by a lack of
glycoprotein secretion and (b) by an enhanced flux of UDP-galactose
via UDP-glucose into glycogen, because glycolysis is substantially
increased in tumors (112, 115, 116).

CONTENT OF PROTEIN-BOUND FUCOSE, N-ACETYLNEURAMINIC ACID AND
GALACTOSE

N-Acetylneuraminic Acid

As outlined in the section "Metabolism of N-acetylneuraminic acid" the amount of radioactive labelled NANA incorporated into proteins and membranes is decisively dependent on the precursor employed (Table 5). From the data it can be concluded that the metabolization of N-acetylmannosamine into protein-bound NANA is not disturbed, although the activity of N-acetylmannosamine kinase is greatly decreased (60). Despite the low activity of sialytransferase in Morris hepatomas (Table 6) the concentration of protein-bound NANA in total homogenate (48) and plasma membranes is even slightly elevated (Table 7). A higher content of NANA has also been described for the Walker sarcoma 256 (67). These findings contrast with studies dealing with virally transformed cells (44, 47, 68, 80, 118), showing a decreased content of NANA in the membrane fraction. However, the latter result is not a general characteristic of single cells because Polyoma-transformed Swiss 3T3 cells are endowed with a normal content of NANA (45). The controversial observations of a raised NANA concentration in solid tumors and an almost decreased NANA level in virally transformed single cells should remind us to be cautious with any generalization on this point. Similar contradictory results have been gained in the field of cyclic nucleotides, e.g. the concentration of cyclic AMP is increased in some solid tumors (29) but substantially reduced in single cells after malignant transformation (50, 97). The transfer of surface-specific alterations from single cells to solid tissue and vice versa in order to establish a common conception of malignancy is apparently not possible, at least not with respect to the metabolism of NANA.

Fucose

In Morris hepatoma 7777 the content of L-fucose in total homogenate (108) and particularly in the plasma membrane is greatly increased when compared to host liver (Table 7). This can be explained as follows: (a) by an increased activity of the fucosyltransferases in hepatomas (10, 11), though this elevation is probably of minor importance. One should bear in mind that enzyme activities were measured in vitro and therefore do not necessarily represent the in vivo level, which may be modified by effectors or protein-protein interactions, (b) by the increased content of GDP-fucose. This finding is of importance because the K_M-value of the fucosyltransferase is in the low nanmolar range. A rise of GDP-fucose from 6 µM to 12 µM might lead to an enhanced incorporation of fucose into glycoproteins, provided that sufficient suitable acceptor molecules are present. This assumption could be verified unequivocally by measuring the incorporation rate of different doses of fucose (up to 0.5 moles/kg body weight).

Table Five

Content of Protein-bound [1-^{14}C]N-acetylneuraminic
Acid in Total Homogenate

Tissue	[1-^{14}C]glucosamine		N-acetyl-[U-^{14}C]mannosamine	
	Liver	Hepatoma 7777	Liver	Hepatoma 7777
nCi/mg Protein	0.95	0.49	0.17	0.55
nCi/mmol NANA	39.9	8.8	19.1	74.7

Two hours before sacrifice the rats received a single injection of [1-^{14}C] glucosamine or N-acetyl[U-^{14}C]mannosamine (same dosage as in Table 1). Protein-bound radioactivity and specific radioactivity of N-acetylneuraminic acid were determined according to Harms et al. (48).

Table Six

Specific Activity of Fucosyl-, Sialyl- and
Galactosyltransferase

Tissue	Fucosyltransferase	Sialyltransferase	Galactosyltransferase
	nmoles of sugar transferred/hr/mg protein		
Hepatoma 9618 A$_2$	0.20 ± 0.01	0.36 ± 0.09	4.26 ± 0.60
Host Liver	0.13 ± 0.01	4.48 ± 0.62	5.88 ± 0.12
Hepatoma 3924 A	0.40 ± 0.01	0.62 ± 0.14	8.04 ± 0.42
Host Liver	0.21 ± 0.06	3.33 ± 0.25	6.60 ± 0.24
Hepatoma 7777	0.43 ± 0.08	3.34 ± 0.28	6.12 ± 0.33
Host Liver	0.19 ± 0.01	5.30 ± 0.30	7.02 ± 0.57
Hepatoma 66	0.58 ± 0.02	3.02 ± 0.10	
Host Liver	0.22 ± 0.01	3.15 ± 0.43	
Hepatoma 7800	0.26 ± 0.01	3.39 ± 0.12	8.58 ± 0.62
Host Liver	0.15 ± 0.02	6.32 ± 0.37	7.80 ± 0.25
Hepatoma 20	0.30 ± 0.01	0.35 ± 0.06	7.26 ± 0.51
Host Liver	0.14 ± 0.01	3.59 ± 0.15	6.42 ± 0.37
Hepatoma 47 C	0.29 ± 0.01	4.91 ± 0.34	4.26 ± 0.31
Host Liver	0.15 ± 0.02	5.71 ± 0.05	5.28 ± 0.49
Control			
(a) normal adult liver	0.16 ± 0.02	5.02 ± 0.33	4.92 ± 0.28
(b) regenerating liver (maximal activity)	--	12.04 ± 0.45 (36 hr)	9.66 ± 0.36 (72 hr)

Activity was measured in a radiochemical assay by measuring the transfer of [^{14}C]fucose or [^{14}C] N-acetylneuraminic acid to desialo-fetuin. Fetuin from which both N-acetylneuraminic acid and galactose had been removed was used as acceptor for the incorporation of [^{14}C]galactose (6, 10, 55). Values are means ± S.D. from 4 to 6 rats.

Table Seven
Membrane-bound Carbohydrate Content of
Liver and Hepatoma Membranes

Tissue	Membrane Type	Fucose	N-acetyl-neuraminic acid	Galactose	Mannose	N-acetyl-glucosamine	N-acetyl-galatosamine	Glucose
				nmoles/mg/protein				
Hepatoma 7777	PM	26.1 ± 3.7	60.7 ± 8.7	100.3 ± 9.1	44.6 ± 4.2	127.4 ± 32.9	78.4 ± 32.9	N.D
Host Liver	PM	6.1 ± 1.7	50.1 ± 8.7	81.4 ± 8.4	35.2 ± 2.5	95.8 ± 8.8	49.8 ± 6.6	N.D.
Hepatoma 7800[a]	MM	N.D.	13.2 ± 0.7	21.0 ± 0.3	73.4 ± 2.3	36.0 ± 1.5	6.5 ± 0.7	10.9 ± 0.2
Liver[a]	MM	N.D.	10.5 ± 0.4	15.3 ± 1.5	70.1 ± 4.0	36.6 ± 1.8	12.0 ± 1.1	4.7 ± 0.4
Novikoff[b] Hepatoma AG 7974 F	PM	34.0	29.0	97.0	57.0	N.D.	N.D.	56.0
Liver[c]	PM	13.4	58.0	134.9	73.3	103.3		19.4
Liver[c]	MM	3.0	6.0	18.3	52.2	34.0		6.1

PM, plasmamembranes; MM, microsomal membranes, [a]Phillips (1973); [b]Leblond-Larouche, L. (1975); [c]adapted from Franke et al. (1976).

Before liberating the carbohydrates by acid hydrolysis internal standards for the individual sugars were added. Fucose was determined according to Dische and Shettles (35), N-acetylneuraminic acid by the resorcinol method of Jourdian et al. (56), mannose and galactose enzymatically. N-acetylglucos-amine and N-acetylgalactosamine were separated by using an automatic amino acid analyser (5, 13). Phillips (82) and Franke et al. (39), however, determined neutral sugars and hexosamines by gas-liquid chromatography.

Actually the plasma membranes of Morris hepatoma possess 3 times
as much free acceptor molecules than the plasma membranes of host
liver (108).   There is a further observation which fits quite well
in this concept.   When analyzing the plasma membranes by SDS-polyacrylamide gel electrophoresis, it could be demonstrated that hepatoma 7777 exhibits qualitatively and quantitatively more [^{14}C]
fucose labelled glycoprotein bands ([^{14}C] fucose was injected two
hours before sacrifice).   This finding may draw our attention to
those incomplete acceptor molecules in surface membranes.   (c) a
reduced degradation of fucoproteins may also be involved.   Measurements indeed revealed a prolongation of the turnover of protein-
bound L-fucose in the plasma membrane of Morris hepatoma 7777 from
24 to 34 hours.   However, in hepatomas cells in culture a half-
life about 100 hours has been determined for fucose-labelled glycoproteins of the plasma membrane (104), but nevertheless in both
systems, cells in culture and solid Morris hepatoma, an apparent
hete:ogeneity in the degradation rates of fucoproteins has been described (36, 108).   The observation of elevated α-L-fucosidase in
Morris hepatomas (Table 8) may be regarded as inconsistent with the
latter finding (10).   However, these measurements were performed
with an artifical substrate.   Moreover, we determined the activity
of lysosomal α-L-fucosidase, whereas it is likely that membrane
fucoproteins are degraded by neutral hydrolases.

     Conversely, comparative measurements of the half-life of pro-
tein-bound NANA in total homogenate and plasma membrane did not
elicit any difference between host liver and Morris hepatoma 7777
(49).

Galactose

     Besides L-fucose, the content of galactose in the plasma mem-
barne of Morris hepatoma 7777 is slightly increased.   The difference
between liver and hepatoma (about 19 nmoles/mg) corresponds well
with the difference of L-fucose (about 20 nmoles/mg).   The other
sugars measured do not show significant differences between liver
and hepatoma.

Glycosyltransferases

     Glycosyltransferases have gained increasing interest during the
last years and much attention has been focused on their potential
role in tumor cells.   Evidence indicating that the activity of these
enzymes does change substantially in the course of malignant transformation is accumulating (for review see 77).   Of particular interest
are those transferases which attach the terminal sugars L-fucose and
N-acetylneuraminic acid to nascent glycoconjugate, because it is well
established that these carbohydrates participate in intercellular
adhesion, cellular recognition (28, 37, 89, 114, 117) and affect the

Table Eight

Specific Activity of α-L-Fucoside, Neuraminidase and β-Galactoside

Tissue	α-L-Fucosidase nmoles p-nitrophenol/ hr/mg protein	Neuraminidase nmoles N-acetylneuraminic acid/hr/mg protein	β-Galactosidase nmoles p-nitrophenol/ hr/mg protein
Hepatoma 9618 A$_2$	351.2 ± 12.5	2.8 ± 0.2	283 ± 26
Host Liver	50.5 ± 2.6	5.3 ± 0.3	534 ± 24
Hepatoma 7777	114.8 ± 4.2	4.4 ± 0.5	271 ± 18
Host Liver	68.6 ± 2.1	6.6 ± 0.2	419 ± 39
Hepatoma 66	125.5 ± 3.4	7.2 ± 0.3	416 ± 22
Host Liver	67.2 ± 3.7	6.9 ± 0.2	425 ± 36
Hepatoma 3924 A	107.2 ± 5.6	4.5 ± 0.2	638 ± 48
Host Liver	46.2 ± 3.5	14.8 ± 0.6	639 ± 38
Hepatoma 7800	121.1 ± 4.4	6.9 ± 0.3	
Host Liver	67.9 ± 0.6	6.7 ± 0.3	
Hepatoma 47 C	84.8 ± 4.5	6.7 ± 0.3	318 ± 31
Host Liver	70.1 ± 1.8	6.5 ± 0.2	474 ± 38
Control (normal liver)			
(a) Buffalo strain	64.9 ± 2.8	7.8 ± 0.1	402 ± 31
(b) ACI strain	60.5 ± 2.1	11.5 ± 0.5	615 ± 42

Fucosidase was determined by measuring the liberated p-nitrophenol at 405 nm. The activity of neuraminidase was measured spectrophotometrically in a linked assay system (10, 107).

Values are means ± S.D. from five rats.

half-life of serum glycoproteins (23, 106). In addition, investigations on the galactosyltransferase are necessary since terminal
galactose residues serve as the point of attachment of L-fucose
and N-acetylneuraminic acid (43).

As shown in Table 6, the specific activity of GDP-fucose:
glycoprotein fucosyltransferase is raised between 1.6 to 3.6-fold
in all hepatomas investigated (10). However, it should be pointed
out that this increase is lowered by about one third when the activity is expressed in nmoles/g wet wt. of tissue instead of nmole/mg
of protein, a result of the decreased protein concentration in Morris
hepatomas. In general poorly differentiated hepatomas exhibit the
highest fucosyltransferase activity except for the tumor 9618 A_2.
Though this line belongs to this group, only a slight elevation of
the transferase level was found. These and other findings make it
more difficult to fit the observed enzymatic and metabolic alterations into a general scheme. Increased levels of intracellular
fucosyltransferase (and GDP-fucose) favor the incorporation of fucose
into glycoconjugates thus changing the properties and possibly the
half-lives of tumor specific humoral glycoproteins. In the serum of
patients with metastasizing tumors (38) or progressive breast cancer
(76) elevated ratios of focuse to protein have been determined whereas in cases of "responsive" malignancy a decrease of protein-bound
fucose was found and Mrochek et al. (76) showed that the serum concentration of fucose correlates fairly well with the clinical status
of the patient. According to the endomembrane concept (75) the Golgi
apparatus is the source of vesicles capable of fusing with the plasma
membrane. By this route increasing amounts of fucose can become part
of this subcellular structure and it is conceivable that this change
of the surface property facilitates uncontrolled proliferation of the
tumor cell, escape from immune destruction or spreading of metastases.

In contrast to the results just summarized the specific activity
of CMP-N-acetylneuraminic acid: glycoprotein sialylstransferase was
greatly decreased in all hepatomas with a short or intermediate growth
rate, e.g., in the most rapidly growing hepatoma 9618 A_2 the activity
is reduced to 7% (10). Of interest is the observation that the sialyltransferase activity in the predominantly poorly differentiated hepatoma 7777 is decreased by only 35% though a markedly lower enzyme
activity has been reported a few years ago (52). Moreover, a 2-fold
higher level was described for the host liver, whereas our measurements show no increase indicating that stability and the degree of
metabolic imbalance has changed in line 7777.

In order to find an explanation for the low sialyltransferase
activity in most Morris hepatomas, Hudgin et al. (52) assume that
the Golgi function may be shifted from a secretory mode to a predominantly nonsecretory membrane-generating mode. Morris hepatomas
of minimal deviation incorporate significant amounts of radioactive

amino acids into protein within the tumor, but fail to secrete any
serum proteins into the blood stream (94). This observation might
explain the low level of sialyltransferase but nevertheless the
question is still unsolved why Morris hepatomas possess substantially higher fucosyltransferase activities. It is conceivable that
both transferases compete for the same binding site, because in
vitro studies have shown that desialo-fetuin or lacto-N-neotetrasyl-
ceramide (obtained from lactosialo-N-neotrasylceramide after removal of N-acetylneuraminic acid with neuraminidase) serve as excellent acceptors for both fucose or N-acetylneuraminic acid (20,
81). From these results it may be concluded that the low activity
of the sialyltransferase is compensated to some extent by an increase of the fucosyltransferase. This conclusion is supported by
findings of Dische (34) who described an inverse relationship of the
fucose and N-acetylneuraminic acid content in urinary and some other
mammalian glycoproteins. Table 6 also represents data for the UDP-
galactose: glycoprotein galactosyltransferase and in most tumors the
activity was elevated by about 50% on an average. It should be added that the N-acetylglucosaminyltransferase does show normal activity in Morris hepatomas (7777, 7800, 5123 D) and it has been suggested that the level of this transferase is more resistant to changes
in the metabolic function of the Golgi apparatus (52). Alternatively,
unchanged N-acetylglucosaminyltransferase levels can be explained
either by a different localization of glycosyltransferases within the
endomembrane system (a major site for the transfer of N-acetyl-glucos-
amine is not only the Golgi apparatus but the endoplasmic reticulum
(73)) or by a selective mechanism responsible for controlling the activity of the individual glycosyltransferase. Moreover it should be taken
into account that several fucosyl-, (55, 92), sialyl- (53) and N-
acetylglycosaminyltransferases exist which may be controlled independently and specifier proteins may change the activity and specificity
of glycosyltransferases (22, 24). While considering regulatory
mechanisms it is worth recalling the stimulatory effect of lysophosphatides on glycosyltransferase activities. Recent studies have shown
that several transferases are very sensitive to exogenously added lysophosphatidylcholine (4, 63, 74, 99). A similar stimulation was observed by carrying out preincubations with phospholipase A suggesting
that this lipase releases lysophosphatides from endogenous phospholipids (4, 74). There is evidence that the observed stimulation is mainly due to the detergent-like effect of lysophosphatidylcholine (51),
though it cannot be entirely ruled out that lysolecithin acts as a
positive allosteric effector (32). About 2.2 % of total phospholipid
in rat liver is lysophosphatidylcholine (87) and assuming a uniform
distribution within the cell a final concentration of 3 mM has been
calculated (74). Mookerjea and Yung (74) have shown that lysophosphatidylcholine is already very effective in vitro at a concentration
of 1 to 3 mM, with maximal stimulation at 7.5 mM. Since lysophosphatidylcholine is a constituent of membranes a much higher concentration is to be expected in the Golgi cisternae. It is therefore in-

telligible that lysophosphatidylcholine is able to increase or decrease glycosyltransferase activity in vivo.

    Determination of serum glycosyltransferases may become an im-
portant aid for the clinician. The fucosyltransferase (8, 59),
sialyltransferase (12, 58) and even the galactosyltransferase (83,
84) are of value to facilitate the diagnosis of neoplasia and to
control the success of chemotherapy or radiation. The levels of
these enzymes have not been studied in detail in the serum of Morris
hepatomas, but in the lines investigated (7777, 9121) the activity
of sialyltransferase is increased between 2 to 3-fold (data is not
shown). It has been observed that elevated activity of serum sialyltransferase in rats bearing mammary tumors is paralleled by a higher
content of N-acetylneuraminic acid (14). The function of serum
transferases is still open to question. A sialylation of external
substrates is unlikely, because CMP-N-acetylneuraminic acid is rapidly hydrolyzed in the serum and no free N-acetylneuraminic acid was
detectable in the blood (14). As to the origin of the sialyltransferase most studies favor the concept that glycosyltransferases are
either secreted by neoplastic cells or released by degradation of
cells (21, 58). We believe that a substantial increase of serum
glycosyltransferases is due to proliferative and secretory processes
of neoplastic (or even normal) cells. This assumption is supported
by the observation of elevated sialyltransferase activity after
partial hepatectomy (Table 6). Within 36 hours after operation the
specific activity of the liver enzyme increased by 200 % and it is
quite remarkable that this elevation was accompanied by a nearly 2-
fold higher level of serum sialyltransferase. Therefore the increased
activity of glycosyltransferases in the serum should be mainly due to
an increased synthesis and/or secretion; the release of glycosyltransferases can also rise with the deterioration of liver function (62).
At the moment it is most convincing to assume that serum glycosyltransferases do not have any physiological role at all. They just
appear due to a certain "leakage" of the surface membrane and will be
degraded within a few days.

    Glycosyltransferases are associated with membrane structures and
can normally only be released by the aid of a detergent as Triton X-
100, which is believed to cause unfolding of proteins and thereby
also promoting the access of substrates to the active site. Vesicles
which arise by blebbing of the Golgi cesternae migrate to the cell
periphery carrying a few transferase molecules on their inner surface.
When fusing with the plasma membrane the vesicle is turned inside out
thus exposing the glycosyltransferases to the blood stream and some
enzyme molecules are loosened or "escape" their binding, others might
be inactivated in situ or will be degraded (Fig 2). In the case of
enhanced enzyme synthesis an increased number of glycosyltransferase
molecules will be transported and finally released to the circulation.
Moreover, the exposure of proteins on the cell surface after malignant

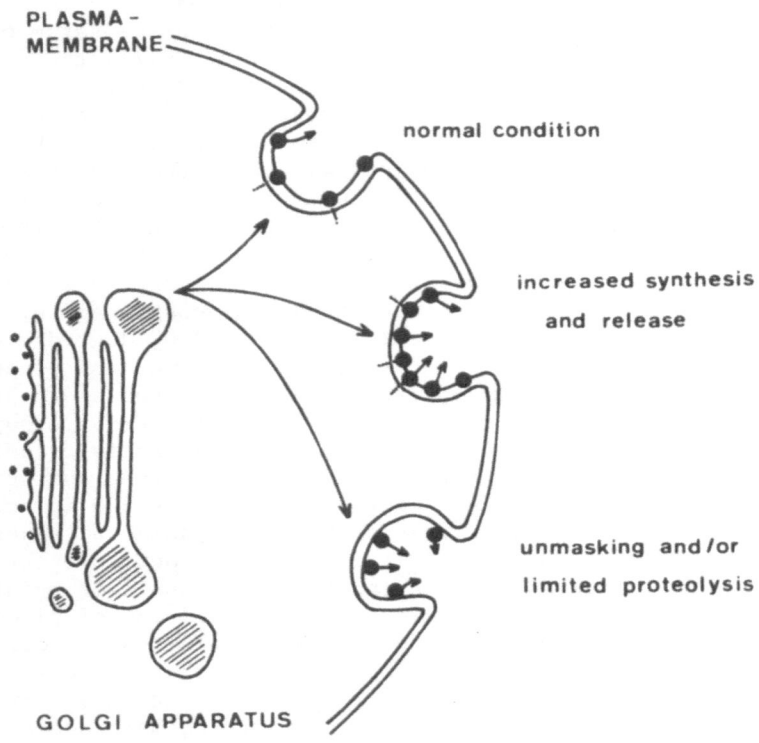

Figure 2
Diagram summarizing the possible mechanisms leading to an increased release of glycosyltransferases. The black circles represent glycosyltransferase molecules, the short dotted line inactivation or degradation processes.

transformation and the appearance of degradative enzymes (18, 77, 105) may also account for elevated levels of glycosyltransferases in the serum.   These alterations of the outer surface may no longer "mask" certain enzyme molecules and/or facilitate the liberation of glycosyltransferases by a limited proteolysis.   Furthermore, the observation that LETS protein is removed from transformed cells by proteases secreted by the cells themselves is in favor of this hypothesis and cleavage of the enzymes' catalytic property (16).

Glycosidases

It is generally assumed that lysosomes play an important role in the pathogenesis of cancer and it has been suggested that carcinogenic chemicals, radiation and oncogenic viruses damage the lysosomal membrane thus causing the release of enzymes (3).   Lysosomes are responsible for most of the intracellular hydrolytic and digestive processes and therefore they are quite abundant in tumor cells.   In malignant tissue an increase of lysosomal enzymes can be anticipated because due to multiple necroses and tumor regression a large amount of material accumulates and has to be degraded.

Among the enzymes detected in the lysosomes are α-L-fucosidase, neuraminidase and β-galatosidase and it is believed that these glycohydrolases are involved in the ultimate breakdown of glycoproteins, glycoplipids and mucopolysaccharides(Fig 3).   In recent years attention has been drawn to α-L-fucosidase, because fucose is an integral constituent of biological molecules (43) and deficiency of this enzyme results in the storage of fucose containing acid mucopolysaccharides and glycolipids (107).   Lysosomal α-L-fucosidases from liver (2, 79) are only active on glycopeptides not on native glycoproteins, which also has been confirmed for most of the other glycosidases.   Therefore, p-nitrophenyl glycosides or trisaccharides are mostly used to determine enzyme activity.   The level of α-L-fucosidase in crude homogenates from Morris hepatomas, host liver and normal adult liver are shown in Table 8.   In all hepatomas with a short or intermediate growth rate the specific activity was nearly twice as high as in normal liver, except for the hepatoma 9618 A_2. In this tumor an even 7-fold elevation of fucosidase activity was measured.   Furthermore, the level of fucosidase elevates substantially during tumor progression.   Within two weeks after inoculation the activity increased 2.6-fold (9618 A_2), reaching a maximum at the 18th day and slowly declining thereafter (10).   Fucosidase activity in host liver was not altered significantly from control values, although enzyme activity had the tendency to increase with age of the tumor.   Conversely, neuraminidase showed only a negligible increase in specific activity during tumor progression.   Unlike α-L-fucosidase the activity of neuraminidase in hepatomas was not raised but lowered or at least remained unchanged (Table 8).   Similar low or unchanged levels have been observed for β-galactosidase.   However,

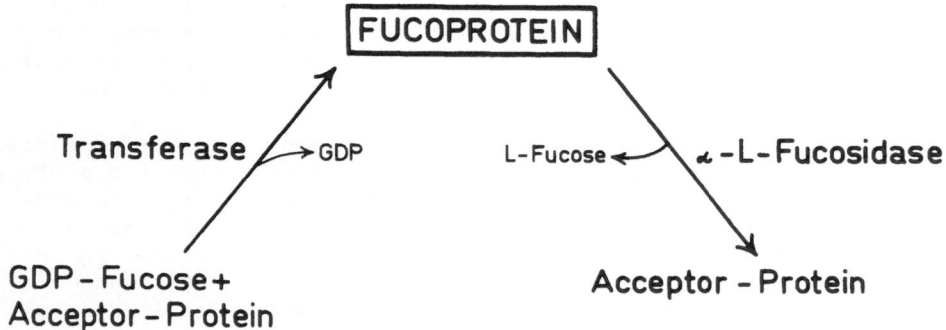

Figure 3
Hepatic fucoprotein metabolism.

studies of Shamberger et al. (96) have shown that certain Morris hepatomas exhibited elevated galactosidase activity. Particularly high levels (increase between 4 to 6-fold) have been described for line 5123 tc, 5123 tcf and 7794 A. Quite interesting in this respect is a possible correlation between growth rate, degree of differentiation, chromosome number and lysosomal activity. The highest level of β-galactosidase has been measured in poorly differentiated hepatomas (5123 tcf, 5123 tc, H-35-tc-1) with a high number of chromosomes (between 47 to 52) and from these findings it has been concluded that poorly differentiated tumors may be a result from excess-free lysosomal enzymes not separated from the cell interior by a membrane (96). A high percentage of β-galactosidase (and of other enzymes) seems to be free in the inner necrotic region of tumors (57), though it should be considered that this so-called free activity does mainly reflect increased lysosomal fragility during the fractionation procedure.

It is worth mentioning that the level of β-galactosidase and neuraminidase in control animals of the ACI strain were markedly higher than those of the Buffalo strain, indicating that a comparison should preferentially be made within a strain.

Summing up the findings it appears that no general conclusion can be drawn with respect to glycosidase activity in Morris hepatomas. One reason may be that several glycosidases are present in the cell. For example at least four different neuraminidases have been discovered in rat liver (64, 91, 103): one is firmly bound to lysosomes (pH optimum 4.4), the second occurs in soluble form in the cytosol (pH optimum 5.8), the third has been detected in the Golgi apparatus (fairly broad maximum between 4.0 to 4.4) and the fourth is associated with the plasma membrane (pH optimum about 4.2). Though the neuraminidase of the Golgi apparatus has specific properties it is conceivable that a functional interrelationship exists between the glycosidase of this organelle and the lysosomes. An intrinsic structural change or alteration in the microenvironment during the differentiation from Golgi vesicles to lysosomes may account for the change of the enzymes specificity (64). It should be added that only one lysosomal α-L-fucosidase and β-galactosidase has been described so far. However, a bimodale localization of β-galactosidase has been discussed.

ISOLATION OF A FUCOPROTEIN

It has been proposed a few years ago that membrane proteins can be divided into two groups, integral and peripheral(100). Integral proteins are believed to be embedded by their hydrophobic portion into the lipid bilayer while their hydrophilic "tail" - most likely the glycopeptide portion of the molecule - protrudes into the aqueous phase. Conversely, peripheral proteins are not inserted into the

membrane matrix, but instead are loosely attached to the surface
by noncovalent bondings.

It is widely agreed that especially glycoconjugates play an
important role in mediating cell interactions and in view of the
increasing interest of glycoproteins as indicators of neoplastic
transformation, a fucoprotein has been isolated from both liver
and hepatoma plasma membranes (7777). Lithium diiodosalicylate
was used as solubilizer (Fig 4) because by the aid of this salt,
proteins can be isolated in a biologically active and water-soluble
form (69). The results show that both fucoproteins (11) have a
molecular weight of about 130,000, a low isoelectric point of about
4, but probably differ in their content of L-fucose. At the moment,
no exact data is available because the analysis of the carbohydrate
composition is still in progress.

Alterations in the synthesis or in the content of cell surface
fucoproteins have been described for transformed or mutated fibroblasts (27, 86) and the results indicate the presence of additional
or altered fucoproteins on the cell surface. From these and other
findings (93) it appears increasingly likely that the protein core
is remarkably resistant to oncogenic alterations and consequently
only the side chains are subject to modifications in the carbohydrate composition.

CONCLUDING REMARKS

Differences in glycosyltransferase activities of normal and
malignant cells are still a matter of controversy because either
reduced (33, 44, 90), increased (17, 19, 114) or unchanged (61)
enzyme activities have been described in neoplastic tissue or transformed cells and the significance of these changes are not entirely
clear. Therefore it is absolutely necessary to investigate always
different metabolic parameters using different tumor lines because
no single solid tumor or cell line can provide all the information
necessary to distinguish between specific and unspecific changes of
the malignant cell. Comparing the parameters studied, it is evident
that specific alterations of the fucose- and to a minor extent of
the galactose metabolism are a characteristic feature of Morris hepatomas (Table 9). Contrary to this finding the metabolism of N-
acetylneuraminic acid does not show a uniform behavior, except for
UDP-N-acetylglycosamine 2'-epimerase. This key enzyme was decreased
to about 10% in all hepatomas investigated.

On the level of plasma membranes the most striking finding was
the increased content and the lowered turnover of protein-bound
fucose (hepatoma 7777). From these results it can be concluded that
a higher number of free binding sites for fucose are present in the
surface membrane. Moreover, when considering the physiological signi-

ficance of the increased fucose content, the more hydrophobic character of this methylpentose in contrast to the hydophylic N-acetylneuraminic acid, may be partly responsible for disturbed cellular interaction and adhesiveness.

This work was supported by the Deutsche Forschungsgemeinschaft, Bonn-Bad Godesberg, Germany.

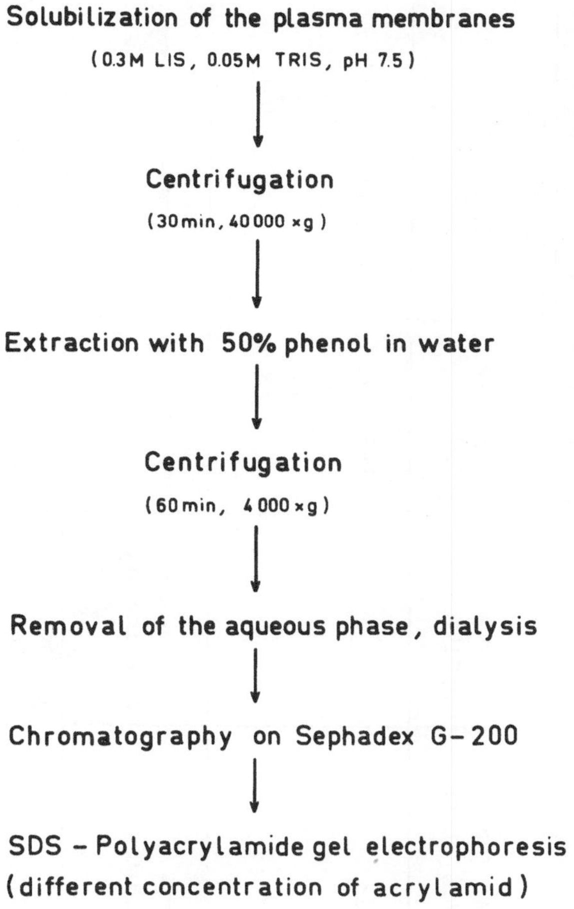

Solubilization of the plasma membranes

(0.3M LIS, 0.05M TRIS, pH 7.5)

↓

Centrifugation

(30min, 40000 ×g)

↓

Extraction with 50% phenol in water

↓

Centrifugation

(60min, 4000 ×g)

↓

Removal of the aqueous phase, dialysis

↓

Chromatography on Sephadex G-200

↓

SDS – Polyacrylamide gel electrophoresis
(different concentration of acrylamid)

Figure 4
Isolation procedure for fucoproteins

Table Nine

Typical Alterations of Glycoprotein Metabolism
in Morris Hepatomas

TERMINAL (OR SUB-TERMINAL) SUGAR	ENZYME ACTIVITIES	NUCLEOTIDE SUGARS	GLYCOSYLTRANSFERASES	PLASMA MEMBRANE-BOUND SUGARS
L-FUCOSE	—	GDP-Fucose ▲	Fucosyltransferase ▲	Fucose ▲▲ Increase of acceptor molecules; decreased turnover
N-ACETYL-NEURAMINIC ACID	UDP-N-acetyl 2'-epimerase ▼▼ ▲	CPM-NANA ± 0	Sialyltransferase ▼	NANA ± 0
D-GALACTOSE	UDP-galactose 4'-epimerase ▼	UDP-galactose ▼	Galactosyltransferase ▲	Galactose ▲

REFERENCES

1. Abercombie, M. and Ambrose, E.J. Cancer Res. 22 (1962) 525

2. Alhadeff, J.A., Miller, A.L., Wenaas, H., Vedvick, T. and O'Brien, J.S. J. Biol. Chem. 250 (1975) 7107

3. Allison, A.C. Lectures Delivered at Symposia on Perspectives in Virology, N.Y. Gustave Stern and Roy. Med. Soc. (1968)

4. Anttinen, H. Biochem. J. 160 (1976) 29

5. Bauer, C., Bachmann, W. and Reutter, W. Hoppe Seyler's Z. Physiol. Chem. 353 (1972) 1053

6. Bauer, C., Hassels, B.F. and Reutter, W. Biochem. J. 154 (1976) 141.

7. Bauer, C., Hassels, B. and Reutter, W. Fed. Eur. Biochem. Soc. Intl. Con. Biochem. 10 (1976) 528.

8. Bauer, C., Köttgen, E. and Reutter, W. Biochem. Biophys. Res. Comm. In press.

9. Bauer, C., Lukaschek, R. and Reutter, W. Biochem. J. 142 (1974) 221.

10. Bauer, C., Vischer, P., Grünholz, H.J. and Reutter, W. Cancer Res. 37 (1977) 1513

11. Bauer, C., Vischer, P., Morris, H.P. and Reutter, W. In: Membrane Alterations as Basis of Liver Injury, H. Popper, L. Bianchi and W. Reutter (eds). MTP Press, Lancaster (1977).

12. Bayer, P.M., Ganzinger, U., Burger, C., Gergely, T. and Moser, K. Wiener Klin. Wschr. 89 (1977) 16

13. Benson, J.V., Gordon, M.J. and Patterson, J.A. Anal. Biochem. 18 (1967) 228

14. Bernacki, R.J. and Kim, U. Science 195 (1977) 577

15. Bertoli, D. and Segal, S. J. Biol. Chem. 241 (1966) 4023

16. Bischoff, E., Tran-Thi, Thuy-Anh, and Decker, K. Eur. J. Biochem. 51 (1975) 353

17. Bosmann, H.B. Biochem. Biophys. Res. Comm. 48 (1972) 523

18. Bosmann, H.B. and Hall, T.H. Biochem. Biophys. Res. Comm. 265 (1972) 339

19. Bosmann, H.B. and Hall, T.H. Proc. Natl. Acad. Sci. U.S.A. 71 (1974) 1833

20. Bosmann, H.B., Hargopian, A. and Eylar, E.H. Arch. Biochem. Biophys. 128 (1968) 470

21. Bosmann, H.B. and Hilf, R. FEBS Letters, 44 (1974) 313

22. Brew, K., Vanaman, T.C. and Hill, R.L. Proc. Natl. Acad. Sci. U.S.A. 59 (1968) 491

23. Briggs, D.W., Fischer, J.W. and Gerorge, W.J. Am. J. Physiol. 227 (1974) 1385

24. Brodbeck, U., Denton, W.L., Tanahashi, N. and Ebner, K.E. J. Biol. Chem. 242 (1967) 1391

25. Bryant, M.L., Stoner, G.D. and Metzger, R.P. Biochim. Biophys. Acta 343 (1974) 226

26. Buck, C.A., Fuhrer, J.P., Soslau, G. and Warren, L. J. Biol. Chem. 249 (1974) 1541

27. Buck, C.A., Glick, M.C. and Warren, L.A. Biochemistry, 9 (1970) 4567

28. Burger, M.M. Curr. Top. Cell. Reg. 3 (1971) 135

29. Chayoth, R., Epstein, S. and Field, J. Biochem. Biophys. Res. Comm. 49 (1972) 1663

30. Cohn, R.M. and Segal, S. Metabolism, 22 (1973) 627

31. Coman, D.R. Cancer Res. 4 (1944) 625

32. Cunningham, C.C. and Hager, L.P. J. Biol. Chem. 246 (1971) 1583

33. Den, H., Schultz, A.M., Basu, M. and Roseman, S. J. Biol. Chem. 246 (1971) 2721

34. Dische, Z. Ann. N.Y. Acad. Sci. 106 (1963) 259

35. Dische, Z. and Shettles, L.B. J. Biol. Chem. 175 (1948) 595

36. Doyle, D., England, B., Friedman, E., Hou, E. and Tweto, J. In: Membrane Alterations as Basis of Liver Injury, H. Popper,

    L. Bianchi and W. Reutter (eds). MTP Press, Lancaster (1977)

37. Emmelot, P. Eur. J. Cancer 9 (1973) 319

38. Evans, A.S., Dolan, M.F., Sobocinski, P.Z. and Quinn, F.A. Cancer Res. 34 (1974) 538

39. Franke, W.W., Keenan, T.W., Stadler, J., Genz, R., Jarasch, E.D. and Kartembeck, J. Cytobiologie, 13 (1976) 28

40. Gesner, B.M. and Gisberg, V. Proc. Natl. Acad. Sci. U.S.A. 52 (1964) 750

41. Gosh, S. and Roseman, S. J. Biol. Chem. 240 (1965) 1531

42. Gosh, S. and Roseman, S. J. Biol. Chem. 240 (1965) 1525

43. Gottschalk, A. In: Glycoproteins, A. Gottschalk (ed). Elsevier Publishing Co. Amsterdam 5 (1972) pp. 860, 1232, 1820

44. Grimes, W.J. Biochemistry, 9 (1970) 5083

45. Grimes, W.J. Biochemistry, 12 (1973) 990

46. Grünholz, H.J., Lehmer, G., Bauer, C. and Reutter, W. Fed. Eur. Biochem. Soc. Intl. Con. Biochem. 10 (1976) 500

47. Hakomori, S. and Murakami, W.T. Proc. Natl. Acad. Sci. U.S. 59 (1968) 254

48. Harms, E., Kreisel, W., Morris, H.P. and Reutter, W. Eur. J. Biochem. 32 (1973) 254

49. Harms, E. and Reutter, W. Cancer Res. 34 (1974) 3165

50. Heidrick, L.H. and Ryan, L.W. Cancer Res. 31 (1971) 1313

51. Helenius, A. and Simons, K. Biochim. Biophys. Acta 415 (1975) 29

52. Hudgin, R.L., Murray, R.K., Pinteric, L., Morris, H.P. and Schachter, H. Canadian J. Biochem. 49 (1971) 61

53. Hudgin, R.L. and Schachter, H. Canadian J. Biochem. 50 (1972) 1024

54. Hultsch, E., Reutter, W. and Decker, K. Biochim. Biophys. Acta 237 (1972) 132

55. Jabbal, I.and Schachter, H. J. Biol. Chem. 246 (1971) 5154

56. Jourdian, G.W., Dean, L. and Roseman, S. J. Biol. Chem. 246
    (1971) 430

57. Kampschmidt, R.F. and Wells, D. Cancer Res. 28 (1968) 1938

58. Kessel, D. and Allen, J. Cancer Res. 35 (1975) 670

59. Kessel, D. and Chou, H.T. Fed. Proc. 35 (1976) 1442

60. Kikuchi, K., Kikuchi, H. and Tsuiki, S. Biochim. Biophys.
    Acta 252 (1971) 357

61. Kim, Y.S., Isaacs, R. and Perdomo, J.M. Proc. Natl. Acad. Sci.
    U.S.A. 71 (1974) 4869

62. Kim, Y.S., Perdomo, J., Whitehead, J.S. and Curtis, K.J. J.
    Clin. Invest. 51 (1972) 2033

63. Kirschbaum, B.B. and Bosmann, H.B. FEBS Letters, 34 (1973) 129

64. Kishore, G.S., Tulsiani, D.R., Bhavanandan, V.P. and Carubelli,
    R. J. Biol. Chem. 250 (1975) 2655

65. Kornfeld, S., Kornfeld, R., Neufeld, E. and O'Brien, P.J. Proc.
    Natl. Acad. Sci. U.S.A. 52 (1964) 371

66. Leblond-Larouche, L., Morais, R., Nigam, V.N. and Karasaki, S.
    Arch. Biochem. Biophys. 167 (1975) 1

67. Macbeth, R.A.L. and Bekesi, J.G. Cancer Res. 24 (1964) 614

68. Makita, A. and Seyama, Y. Biochim. Biophys. Acta 241 (1971) 403

69. Marchesi, V.T. and Andrews, E. Science, 174 (1971) 1247

70. Maxwell, E.S., Kurashi, K. and Kalckar, H.M. In: Methods in
    Enzymology, S.P. Colowick and N.O. Kaplan (eds). 5 (1962) 176

71. Mayes, J.S. and Hansen, R.R. In: Methods in Enzymology, S.P.
    Colowick and N.O. Kaplan (eds). 9 (1966) 708

72. McGuire, E.J. In: Biological Roles of Sialic Acid, A. Rosenberg
    and C.L. Schengrund (eds). Plenum Press, Amsterdam, New York,
    (1976) pp. 123-158

73. Molnar, J. Molecular & Cellular Biochem. 6 (1975) 3

74. Mookerjea, S. and Yung, J.W. Biochem. Biophys. Res. Comm. 57
    (1974) 815

75. Morré, D.J., Mollenhauer, H. and Bracker, C.E. In: Origin and Continuity of Cell Organelles, J. Reinert and H. Ursprung (eds). Springer-Verlag, Heidelberg (1971) pp. 81-126

76. Mrochek, J.E., Dinsmore, S.R., Tormey, D.C. and Waalkes, T.P. Clin. Chem. 22 (1976) 1516

77. Nicholson, G.L. Biochim. Biophys. Acta 458 (1976) 1

78. Nicholson, G.L. and Poste, G. New Eng. J. Med. 295 (1976) 197

79. Opheim, D.J. and Trouser, O. J. Biol. Chem. 252 (1977) 739

80. Otha, N., Pardee, A.B., McAuslan, B.R. and Burger, M.M. Biochim. Biophys. Acta 158 (1968) 98

81. Pacuszka, T. and Kóscielak, J. Eur. J. Biochem. 64 (1976) 499

82. Phillips, J.L. Arch. Biochem. Biophys. 56 (1973) 377

83. Podolsky, D.K. and Weiser, M.M. Biochem. Biophys. Res. Comm. 65 (1975) 545

84. Podolsky, D.K., Weiser, M.M., Westwood, J.C. and Cammon, M. J. Biol. Chem. 252 (1977) 1807

85. Potter, V.R. and Watanabe, M. In: Proc. Intl. Conf. Leukemia-Lymphoma, C.J. Zarafonetics (ed). Lea and Febiger, Philadelphia (1968) pp. 33-46

86. Pouysségur, J. and Pastan, I. J. Biol. Chem. 252 (1977) 1639

87. Ray, T.K., Skipski, V.P., Barclay, M., Essner, E. and Archibald, F.M. J. Biol. Chem. 244 (1969) 5528

88. Reutter, W., Kreisel, W. and Lesch, R. Hoppe Seyler's Physiol. Chem. 351 (1970) 1320

89. Roseman, S. Chem. Phys. Lipids, 5 (1970) 270

90. Saito, M., Satoh, H. and Ukita, T. Biochim. Biophys. Acta, 362 (1974) 549

91. Schengrund, C.L., Jensen, D.S. and Rosenberg, A. J. Biol. Chem. 247 (1972) 2742

92. Schenkel-Brunner, H., Chester, M.A. and Watkins, W. Eur. J. Biochem. 30 (1972) 269

93. Schrager, J. and Oates, M.D. Gut, 14 (1973) 324

94. Schreiber, G., Boutwell, R.K., Potter, V.R. and Morris, H.P. Cancer Res. 26 (1966) 2357

95. Segal, S. and Rogers, S. Biochim. Biophys. Acta 250 (1971) 351

96. Shamberger, R.J., Hozumi, M. and Morris, H.P. Cancer Res. 31 (1971) 1632

97. Sheppard, J.R. Nature New Biol. 236 (1972) 14

98. Sherman, J.R. and Adler, J. J. Biol. Chem. 238 (1963) 873

99. Shier, W.T. and Trotter, J.T. FEBS Letters, 62 (1976) 165

100. Singer, S.J. In: Structure and Function of Biological Membranes, L.I. Rothfield (ed). Academic Press, New York (1971) pp. 145-222

101. Stern, E.S. and Krooth, R.S. Cell. Physiol. 86 (1975) 105

102. Talmadge, K.W. and Burger, M.M. In: Biochemsitry of Carbohydrates, W.J. Whelan (ed). Butterworths, London 5 (1975) pp. 42-93

103. Tulsiani, D.R. and Carubelli, R. J. Biol. Chem. 245 (1970) 1821

104. Tweto, J. and Doyle, D. J. Biol. Chem. 251 (1976) 872

105. Unkeless, J.C., Dano, K., Kellerman, G.M. and Reich, E. J. Biol. Chem. 249 (1974) 4295

106. Van den Hamer, C.J., Morell, A.G., Scheinberg, I.H., Hickmann, J. and Ashwell, G. J. Biol. Chem. 245 (1970) 4397

107. Van Hoof, F. and Hers, H.G. Eur. J. Biochem. 7 (1968) 34

108. Vischer, P., Dissertation. Universität Freiburg, (1977)

109. Vischer, P., Bauer, C., Grünholz, H.J. and Reutter, W. Fed. Eur. Biochem. Soc. Intl. Con. Biochem. 10 (1976) 276

110. Walker, D.G. and Khan, H.H. Biochem. J. 108 (1968) 169

111. Wallach, D.F.H. Proc. Natl. Acad. Sci. U.S.A. 61 (1968) 368

112. Warburg, O. The Metabolism of Tumors R.N. Smith and Co. New

York (1931)

113. Warren, L. In: <u>Glycoproteins</u>, A. Gottschalk (ed). Elsevier
     Publishing Co. Amsterdam 5B (1972) pp. 1097-1126

114. Warren, L., Fuhrer, J.P. and Buck, C.A. Proc. Natl. Acad.
     Sci. U.S.A. 69 (1972) 1838

115. Weber, G. New Eng. J. Med. 296 (1977) 541

116. Weinhouse, S. Cancer Res. 32 (1972) 2007

117. Winzler, R.J. Int. Rev. Cyt. 29 (1970) 77

118. Wu, H.C., Meezan, E., Black, P.H. and Robbins, P.W. Biochem-
     istry, 8 (1969) 2509

SURFACE MEMBRANES AND BIOLOGICAL REGULATION IN DIFFERENTIATED HEPATOMA CELLS IN VITRO*

Carmia Borek

Departments of Radiology and Pathology
College of Physicians & Surgeons
Columbia University, New York, N.Y. 10032

The variety of Morris hepatomas with their properties ranging from minimal deviation, slow growing tumors to undifferentiated, fast replicating carcinomas have been invaluable in their contribution to the understanding of basic mechanisms in cellular biology and biochemistry. The ability to culture (Fig 1) and clone many of these tumors have enhanced their value since under conditions in vitro genetically homogeneous populations, derived from single cells, could be readily studied.

In this presentation I shall relate some of our studies on "minimal deviation" hepatoma cells in culture as compared to cultures derived from normal liver. These studies have involved the surface properties of the cells, cell-cell interactions among them and the effect of corticosteroid hormones and vitamin A on the synthesis of macromolecules in them.

Liver Cell Lines In Culture

Hepatoma cells in culture, to varying degrees depending on the tumor, are able to form multilayers and replicate to higher densities under conditions where normal hepatocytes remain as seemingly contact inhibited monolayers (1-4). In earlier studies we set out to characterize some of the biological properties of the normal and tumor liver cells in culture and addressed ourselves to the question whether the loss of contact inhibition in the hepatoma cells as compared to the normal could be related to an impairment in cell-cell communication which took place in the process of neoplastic transformation. We proceeded to investigate this problem using ionic communication as our probe (4).

439

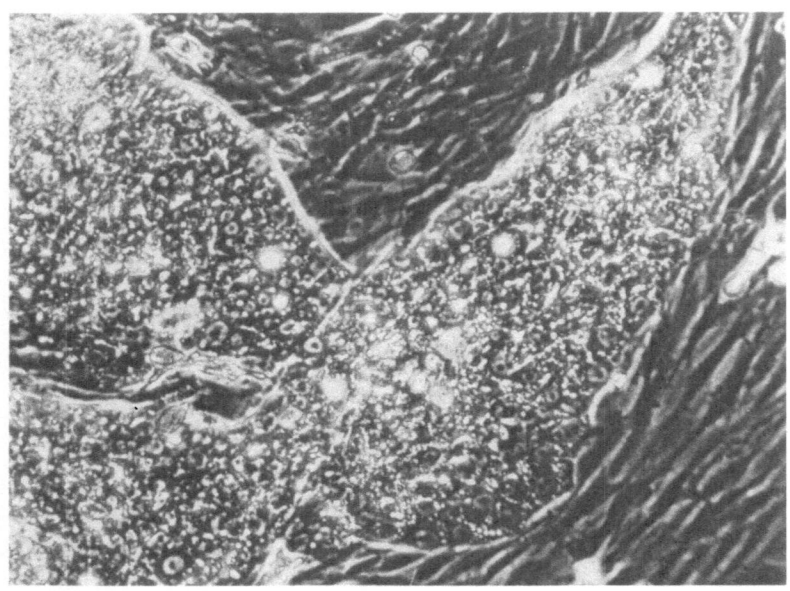

Figure 1
A primary culture of Morris hepatoma H5123. Note the islands
of epthelial cells markedly separated from the mesenchymol derived
fibroblasts in the cultures. Phase contrast x 125 (reduced 21% for
reproduction).

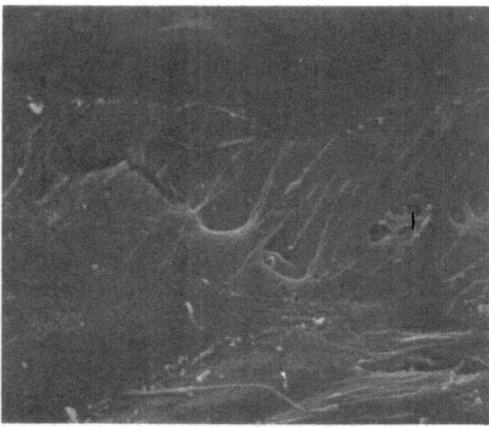

Figure 2
Normal rat liver cells in culture (RLB). Note the flatness
and smoothness of the cells. Small microvilli present near the
cell edge. Note the tight contact between adjacent cells. SEM
x 3000 (reduced 26% for reproduction).

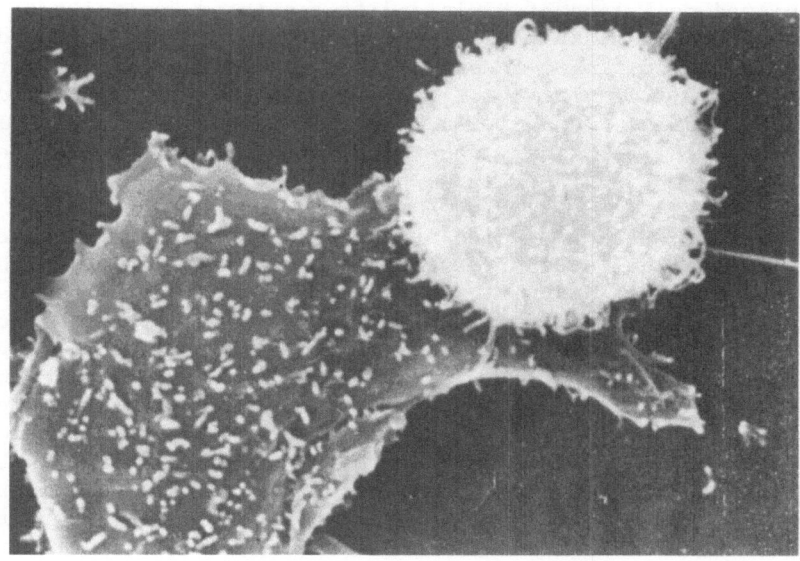

Figure 3
H_4IIEC_3 cells (H_4) in culture. Note few microvilli on the
surface of the interphase cell. Note the abundance of surface
features in the rounded mitotic cell. SEM x 3000 (reduced 31% for
reproduction).

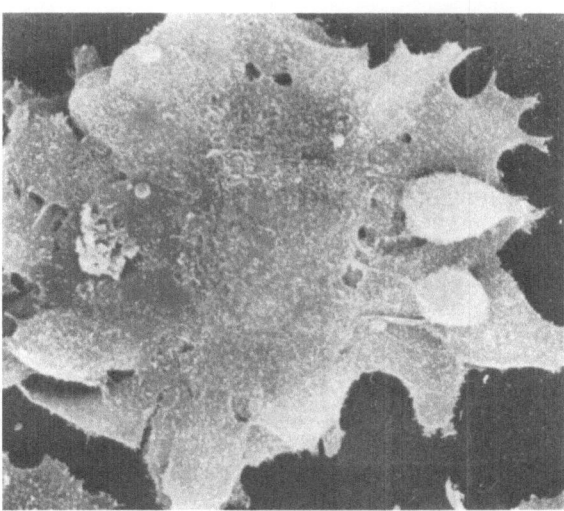

Figure 4
A cluster of H4 cells. Note the cells piled up, the increased
number of surface microvilli. SEM x 900 (reduced 35% for reproduction).

A cloned cell line of diploid differentiated hepatocytes (RLB) was established from adult rat liver(1, 4). Similarly a cloned line was cultured from a freshly dissected differentiated Morris hepatoma H5123 (12). The tumor bearing rats were kindly provided by Dr. H.P. Morris. In addition, the differentiated cloned H_4IIEC_3 cell lines (H_4) (12), kindly donated by Dr. V.R. Potter was used in our studies.

The normal RLB cells which produced serum protein (1) were flat, epithelial cells adhered strongly to the surface on which they grew and to one another. They proliferated into tight sheets of cells (2). Transmission electron microscopy ascertained the epithelial nature of the cells (2). RLB cells were unable to grow in suspension cultures or in semi-solid medium of 0.33% agar and were not tumorigenic. Scanning electron microscopy (SEM) indicated flat smooth cells (Fig 2). The hepatoma cells of both lines were epithelioid and were less adhesive than the normal. They initially grew as monolayers; however, as cell density increased discrete foci of cells appeared in various areas of the dishes and overtook the culture. The hepatoma cells grew in suspension and were tumorigenic when injected back into the appropriate hosts. Scanning electron microscopy of the differentiated hepatoma cells showed single interphase cells to be flat with few microvilli (Fig 3). As cultures increased in density and piled up the number of microvilli increased (Fig 4).

When comparing maximal saturation densities of the three cell lines in F_{12} medium supplemented with 5% fetal calf serum we found that RLB showed a maximum density of 6×10^4 cell/cm^2. The H_4 6×10^5 cells/cm^2 and H5123 reached a maximal saturation of 8×10^5/cm^2.

Karyotype analysis of the cells using Giensa Quinocrine fluorescent banding methods (11) indicated that the normal cells were mostly diploid with 5% tetraploid, (11) the H5123 Pseudodiploid (2) and the H_4 cell line heteroploid with a number of specific chromosome markers (11).

Ionic Communication

Junctional communication between cells was measured electrically, (4) by pulsing currents with a microelectrode between one cell interior and the exterior (grounded) and by recording the resulting voltage with a second microelectrode inside a contiguous cell. We found that the RLB cells, both in sparse cultures where groups of two or three cells were in contact and in confluent monolayers, demonstrated ionic communication. In the latter this communication was detectable over a distance of several diameters from the current sources and any given cell was in communication with its neighbors.

In contrast to the RLB both the H5123 and the H4 cells studied under the same condition as RLB showed no junctional communication between cells in contact. The patterns of communication found in the homogeneous cell cultures were retained in cultures where the normal cells were cocultivated with the hepatoma (2, 4). No communication was found between the normal and the H_4 or the normal and H5123 cells in these heterogeneous cultures. The tumor cells were able to grow over the normal indicating a lack of contact inhibition between the normal and the tumor cells. Transformation in vitro of the normal cells resulted in a loss of intercellular communication between them (1).

Electron Microscopy

Electron microscopic studies of the RLB and the H5123 cell (2) indicated the presence of tight and intermediate junctions and desmosomes in the normal RLB cells. These were present in fixed sequences along the junction. In the H5123 cells in culture there was a marked decrease in mutual cell contact. No tight junctions were observed. Desmosomes and intermediate junctions were sometimes present though less cemented together.

Further studies on the cell surface involved glycolipid composition of the cells, their agglutinability by plant lectins and the production of a macrophage inhibiting factor (MIF).

Gangliosides

Gangliosides are acid containing glycolipids which are largely found in cellular plasma membranes (8). A study of the ganglioside content of the RLB and hepatoma cultures (6) indicated a marked difference between the chemical composition of the cells. The mean molar ratio of the gangliosides GD1a: GM_1: GM_3 in the normal RLB were 1: 0.5: 2.6, respectively, while in the H5123 cell line the ratios were 1: 12: 117. The total concentration of gangliosides in the H5123 cells was about sixfold over that in the RLB in terms of equivalent amount of cell proteins. Using plant agglutinins as surface probes (6) we proceeded to investigate whether the surface microstructure of hepatoma cells differed from that of the normal RLB, and if so, whether the degree of change could be correlated with loss of differentiation in the tumor cell lines (3). The hepatoma cell lines used were the differentiated H_4, the line derived from H5123 tumor, which had partly differentiated in culture, a liver cell line transformed in vitro (1) and the undifferentiated Novikoff hepatoma. These were compared to the normal RLB and to newly suspended liver cells from newborn and adult rat liver. The agglutinins used were wheat germ agglutinin (WGA) Concavalin A (ConA), Phytohemagglutinin (PHA), Ricinus Communis, Great Northern bean (GNB) and Lens Culinaris. We found that both in stationary and growing phase cells the hepatoma cells were significantly more agglutinable than the normal cells sug-

gesting that surface changes had taken place. The fact that
these changes resulting in agglutinability were specific and agglutination was not spontaneous or due to nonspecific adhesion was judged
by the competitive inhibition of the reaction by appropriate carbohydrates (3). Differences in agglutinability of the hepatoma cells
with respect to their degrees of dedifferentiattion were seen with
WGA and PHA. Among the neoplastic liver cell lines H_4 cells the
"most normal" and most contact inhibited were least agglutinable
while the Novikoff which are undifferentiated and have minimal inhibition by contact, (most cells go into suspension having lost
anchorage dependence), were the most agglutinable.

Normal cells were not agglutinable with the low concentration
of lectins used. They were however potentially agglutinable when
treated with proteases or when in mitosis suggesting that under
those conditions their surface architecture mimicks that of the hepatoma cells. Lens culinaris agglutinin reacted unexpectedly well
with the normal cells but not with the tumor cell lines. In ongoing experiments (G. Poste and C. Borek in preparation) we have
found that the H5123 cells in culture produce and release macrophase
inhibitory factor (14) while the normal RLB cells do not.

Glucocorticoid Effects on Normal Liver and Hepatoma Cells in Culture

In view of the known inhibitory effects of glucocorticoid hormones on liver growth in vivo we investigated the effect of these
hormones on cell proliferation and cell morphology in the more isolated and controlled systems of cells in culture (10). We found
using hydrocortisone and dexamethasone that the addition of these
hormones is capable of producing profound suppression of DNA synthesis in the normal RLB cells and in the H5123 cell line. At low
concentration of the hormone (3×10^{-7}M hydrocortisone or 3×10^{-8}M
dexamethasone) the incorporation of radioactive thymidine fell to 50%
of control level by 36 hours and at a higher concentration of the
hormone (5×10^{-5}M) inhibition could be noted as early as twelve
hours and was completed by 24 hours. This inhibition of incorporation
(Table 1) reflected a true suppression of DNA synthesis, was accompanied by an inhibition of cell proliferation and by a marked change in
surface morphology as seen by scanning electron microscopy (9).
While the morphology of the treated RLB cells was not dramatically
changed following hydrocortisone administration, the change in the
hepatoma cells was striking. H5123 cells exhibited in control culture numerous microvilli over the cell surface. The cells were irregular in shape and spherical. Within 24 hrs after the administration
of hydrocortisone the cells assumed a flat form, similar to the skirt-
ed ruffles at their edge and assumed a contact inhibited mode of
growth.

Table One*
Effects of Hydrocortisone on Thymidine Incorporation in
Two Different Cell Lines of Liver
Origin

Cell Line	(^{3}H) Thymidine Incorporation (dpm/µg of DNA)
Normal RLB	
Control	$12,600 \pm 1,100$
Hydrocortisone	$1,540 \pm 60$
% of control	12%
Morris Hepatoma #5123	
Control	$43,100 \pm 700$
Hydrocortisone	$4,180 \pm 70$
% of control	10%

Five to seven plates of each of the above cell lines were treated with either hydrocortisone in ethanol (final concentration of hormone 50 µM) or with an equal volume of ethanol alone ("control"). After 36 hr 10 µCi of (^{3}H) thymidine was added to each plate, and the cells in each plate were harvested 3 hr later and assayed both for incorporation of isotope into DNA. The addition of steroid results in a striking suppression of isotope incorporation.

* Derived from Loeb et al. 1973.

The effects of the corticosteroids on DNA suppression are reversible upon removal of the hormones (10). No cell lysis or degradation of preformed DNA were observed and even when ^{3}H thymidine incorporated into DNA was inhibited by 90% or more, incorporation of ^{14}C uridine into RNA proceeded with little change.

Stimulation of Retinol Binding Protein by Vitamin A

Using the $H_4 IIEC_3$ hepatoma cell line and a line MH_1C_1 derived from the Morris hepatoma 7795(15) we have been investigating in collaboration with Drs. D.W. Goodman and J.E. Smith the effects of vitamin A on the production and secretion of retinol binding proteins (RBP) in the cells.

These studies in vitro have been an extension of the findings in vivo (16) that in the vitamin A deficient rat RBP secretion from the liver into the serum is reduced, while the liver pool of RBP is expanded three to five times the normal level. Upon injection of retinol the expanded liver pool is rapidly depleted, the RBP being secreted into the serum. The hepatoma cell lines of both H_4 and MH_1C_1, grown in vitamin A deficient medium represent the vitamin A deficient liver. While a large number of studies has been carried out with both lines H_4 was decided as the line of choice because of its 24 hr doubling time (in contrast to the 5 day doubling time of the MH_1C_1). We have found that under specific conditions of growth, medium and cell number the addition of retinol as low as 0.1 mg/ml stimulates the hepatoma in vitro to secrete RBP into the medium, the effect is significant as compared to the controls (p<0.005). Rat serum albumin was assayed as a marker protein. Retinol did not influence the albumin level either in its total amount in the cells and the medium indicating the specificity of vitamin A action on the RBP. These studies are being continued and details will be published elsewhere.

Discussion

When differentiated hepatomas are explanted in vitro into primary cultures the cells sort themselves and assume a particular pattern of growth. This pattern consists of islands of closely adhering refractile tumor cells proliferating within a "matrix" of fibroblasts derived from the normal mesenchymal tissue (Fig 1). These islands can be isolated and cloned. Cell lines can be propagated for further investigations from these clones.

The studies described here have dealt in part with a number of membrane associated phenomena and have addressed themselves to the question: How do the "minimal deviation" hepatoma cells which though differentiated are still malignant and have escaped growth control mechanisms, differ from differentiated normal epithelial cells deriv-

ed from the same tissue of origin? The normal cells used in these
studies were diploid epithelial cells cloned from Buffalo adult rat
liver. Their epithelial nature characterized by electronmicroscopy
and their ability to synthesize serum proteins strongly deem them
hepatocytes. The hepatoma cells studied were freshly cloned from
a Morris H5123 tumor and in addition the established H_4IIEC_3 cell
line was used. The cultures H5123 were near diploid; the H_4IIEC_3
were heteropoid.

Table 2 presents a comparison between the normal and neoplastic
liver cells. A variety of biological characteristics which are
hereditary appear to be associated with the malignant nature of the
hepatoma cells. While we still do not know the underlying genetic
or epigenetic regulatory mechanism underlying these phenomena the
association among these phenotypic expressions is striking.

Loss of contact inhibition and escape from growth control coincide with absence of tight junctions, with a loss of intercellular
communications between the cells, with changes in surface microstructure as detected by the agglutinability of the cells by plant
lectins, with a dramatic change in cellular ganglioside composition
and with the ability of the cells to synthesize a macrophage inhibitory factor with protease like activity (13). Scanning electro-
microscopy indicated that differentiated hepatoma cells had few
surface features on single interphase cells (5). In contrast hepatoma cells which had partly dedifferentiated in culture (9) exhibited an abundance of surface excrescences which were dramatically
decreased following treatment with hydrocortisone.

There is insufficient evidence to state whether intercellular
communication in these neoplastic epithelial cells is a consequence
of altered membrane permeability resulting from the changes in the
biochemical composition of the membrane and to what extent decreased
cell adhesion and modified cell typography play a role. Neoplastic
fibroblasts which have a variety of these associated phenomena do
communicate electrically (4). A striking coincidence was found between the potential agglutinability by plant lectins of the normal
liver cells after protease treatment or following vitamin A treatment (3), reversible within 6 hrs after removing the agent, and the
temporary loss of ionic communication in normal cells after trypsin
treatment, which was also recovered 6 hrs later. Methods of restor-
ing ionic communication to the non-communicating cells could shed
light on the underlying mechanisms and on the membrane phenomena associated with these cell-cell interaction.

Our work on the effects of corticosteroids on the synthesis of
cellular macromolecules have shown that DNA synthesis and cell proliferation are markedly inhibited in cultured hepatoma cells and to
a somewhat less extent in the normal liver cells. None of the cell

Table Two
Properties of a Cell Line Cultured from Rat Hepatoma 5123
Compared with Cultured Epithelial Cells from Rat Liver

	Normal Liver (RLB)	Hepatoma Cells (H5123)
Morphology	Epithelial	Epitheliloia
Cell Generation Time	28 hr	18 hr
Karyotype	Diploid	Pseudodiploid
Ability to manufacture serum protein	Yes	Low
Contact inhibition of replication	Yes	No
Pattern of growth in culture	Monolayers	Multilayers
Saturation density (cells/cm^2)	6×10^4	8×10^5
Ability to grow in suspension cultures	No	Yes
Colony formation in 0.33% agar	No	Yes
Agglutinability of the cells by concanavalin A and what-germ agglutinin	No	Yes
Communication at permeable intercellular junctions	Yes	No
Tight junctions	Yes	None
Average total gangliosides (moles/mg protein)	0.53	3.03
Ability to replicate over normal cells	No	Yes
Tumor production in vivo	No	Yes
Suppression of cell proliferation by glucocorticoids	Yes	Yes
Surface features (SEM) of interphase single cells	Few	Few. Increased when cells lose differentiation
Production of MIF	No	Yes
Surface features (SEM) following corticosteroid treatment	Slightly modified	Greatly decreased

lines were inducible for tyrosine amino transferase (10).   Thus
the two "steroid sensitive" phenomena can be dissociated.   The correlation between the surface modifying effect of the steroids concomitant with their inhibition of DNA synthesis are being pursued.

In ongoing studies we find a dramatic stimulating retinol binding protein, a specific liver protein, in two hepatoma cell lines
following exposure to vitamin A. The findings are similar to those
obtained in studies on normal liver in the intact animals, affirming
once again the minimal deviation hepatomas can serve as excellent
models for reproducible and long term studies on biological control
mechanisms in mammalian cells.

* This investigation was supported in part by Grant Number CA 12536
  awarded by the National Cancer Institute, DHEW.

REFERENCES

1. Borek, C. Proc. Nat. Acad. Sci. U.S.A. 69 (1972) 956.

2. Borek, C. In: Gene Expression and Carcinogenesis in Cultured
    Liver, L.E. Gerschenson and E.B. Thompson (eds). Academic Press,
    New York (1975) 62.

3. Borek, C., Grob, M. and Burger, M.M. Exp. Cell Res. 77 (1973)
    207.

4. Borek, C., Higashino, S. and Lowenstein, W.R. J. Mem. Biol. 1
    (1969) 274.

5. Borek, C. and Pain, C. Proc. Am. Assoc. Cancer Res. 18 (1977)
    193.

6. Brady, R.O., Borek, C. and Bradley, R.M. J. Biol. Chem. 244
    (1969) 6552.

7. Burger, M.M. Proc. Nat. Acad. Sci. U.S.A. 62 (1969) 994.

8. Fishman, P.H., Brady, R.O., Bradley, R.M., Aaronson, S.A. and
    Todaro, G.J. Proc. Nat. Acad. Sci. U.S.A. 71 (1974) 298.

9. Freund, J.S., Dempsey, E.W., Loeb, J.N. and Borek, C. Proc. of
    the Soc. for Exp. Biol. and Med. 150 (1975) 14.

10. Loeb, J.N., Borek, C. and Yeung, L.L. Proc. Nat. Acad. Sci.
    U.S.A. 70 (1973) 3852.

11. Miller, D.A., Dev, V.G., Borek, C. and Miller, O.J. Cancer Res.
    32 (1972) 2375.

12. Morris, H.P., Sydransky, H., Wagner, B.P. and Dyer, H.H. Cancer
    Res. 20 (1960) 1252.

13. Pitot, H.C., Periano, C., Morse, P.S. and Potter, V.R. Nat.
    Cancer Inst. Monog. 13 (1964) 229.

14. Poste, G. Cancer Res. 35 (1976) 2558.

15. Richardson, V.I., Tashjian, A.H. Jr. and Levine, L. J. Cell
    Biol. 40 (1969) 236.

16. Smith, J.E., Muto, Y., Milch, P.O., Goodman, D.W. J. Biol. Chem.
    248 (1973) 1544.

REGULATION OF CYCLIC AMP AND CYCLIC GMP

IN MORRIS HEPATOMAS AND LIVER

Robert A. Hickie

Department of Pharmacology, Faculty of Medicine
University of Saskatchewan
Saskatoon, Sask., Canada   S7N 0W0

SUMMARY

Studies on the regulation of tissue levels and action of
adenosine 3':5'-monophosphate (cyclic AMP) and cyclic guanosine
3':5'-monophosphate (cyclic GMP) in Morris hepatomas and liver
have been reviewed. Though the data is incomplete in some areas,
the following generalizations can be made. A prominent difference between Morris hepatomas and normal liver, in relation to
cyclic AMP formation, is the decreased responsiveness of tumor
adenylyl cyclase to glucagon. This characteristic is most
marked in rapidly growing hepatomas and appears to be associated
with diminished plasma membrane binding of glucagon; regenerating
liver and fetal liver resemble hepatomas in their responsiveness
to glucagon. The responsiveness of adenylyl cyclase to epinephrine is, in contrast, generally enhanced in hepatomas as well
as in regenerating and fetal liver. Marked increases in particulate guanylyl cyclase activities, relative to corresponding
soluble activities, are seen consistently in Morris hepatomas
and in regenerating and fetal liver; in the latter tissues, increases in plasma membrane guanylyl cyclase activities can be
correlated with increased proliferative activity. Although the
total cyclic AMP phosphodiesterase activities are significantly
reduced in all Morris hepatomas examined, the activities of the
high affinity (low K_m) cyclic AMP phosphodiesterase in plasma
membranes from some Morris hepatomas are higher than those of
normal liver. The degradation of cyclic GMP by Morris hepatomas
is also impaired, most notably in the particulate fractions. In
regenerating and fetal liver the activities of cyclic AMP and
cyclic GMP phosphodiesterases are, in contrast, not changed
appreciably. The ratios of cyclic GMP levels, relative to cyclic

AMP, tend to be higher in Morris hepatomas than in normal liver. Though these ratios are highest in rapidly growing hepatomas, the correlation between cyclic nucleotide levels and tumor growth rate is not strong. The correlation between cyclic GMP/cyclic AMP ratios and hepatocyte proliferation is controversial at this time; the most recent studies on regenerating liver suggest that these ratios are increased prior to the proliferative phase. Only a few studies have been carried out on cyclic nucleotide binding proteins and kinases. These studies indicate that: cytosols from rapidly growing hepatomas have a reduced ability to bind cyclic AMP with   increased (?) binding of cyclic GMP; there is a positive correlation between cyclic AMP binding and tumor sensitivity to growth inhibition by dibutyryl cyclic AMP; cytosol fractions from rapidly growing hepatomas generally have reduced cyclic AMP dependent protein kinase activities and increased endogenous (cyclic AMP independent) kinase activities.

INTRODUCTION

During the past 7-8 years, a great deal of interest has been shown in the role that cyclic nucleotides may have in regulating basic biological processes such as cell proliferation and differentiation (13, 30, 65, 66, 69, 142, 157, 169, 171, 186, 205).

A variety of in vitro and in vivo tissue models have been utilized to investigate changes in cyclic nucleotide metabolism and action in hyperproliferative disease states such as cancer. Morris hepatomas represent a useful in vivo model for studies of this nature, because there are available, a broad spectrum of stable hepatoma sublines with varying growth rates and degrees of differentiation; also the morphological, biochemical and cell kinetic characteristics are well defined for many of these tumors (114, 115, 128-130, 152, 210-212, refer also to appropriate chapters in this book).

The aim of this chapter is to review studies carried out in Morris hepatomas on cyclic AMP and cyclic GMP synthesis, degradation, levels and action (see Figure 1). These findings will be contrasted with those of normal liver, proliferating hepatocytes (regenerating liver, fetal liver) and other tumors where appropriate.

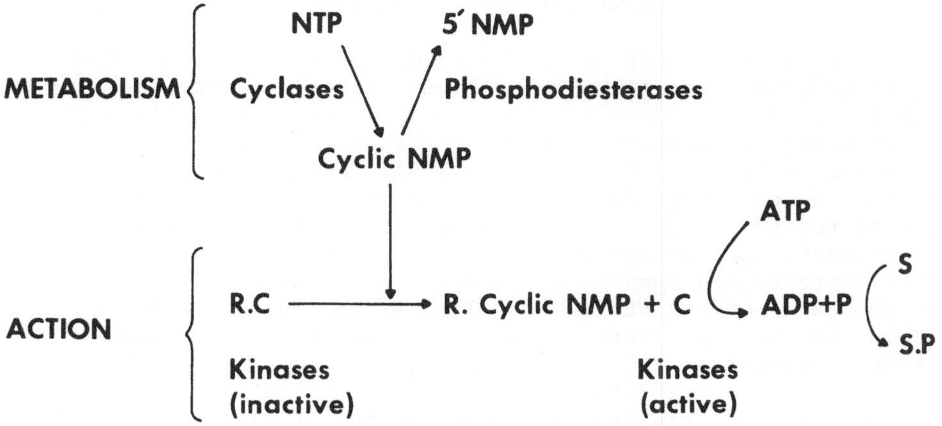

Figure 1. Metabolism and action of cyclic nucleotides.
Cyclic AMP and cyclic GMP are formed from the corresponding nucleotide triphosphate (NTP) by adenylyl
cyclase and guanylyl cyclase respectively. Degradation of the cyclic nucleotides (cyclic NMP) to the
nucleotide monophosphate derivatives (5' NMP) are
catalyzed by the corresponding phosphodiesterases.
Cyclic AMP activates kinases by combining with the
regulatory subunit (R) of the holoenzyme complex
(R.C); this interaction releases a catalytic subunit (C) which, in turn, catalyzes transfer of the
gamma phosphate (P) from ATP to specific substrates
(S). In this scheme it is assumed that the activation of cyclic GMP kinases is by a mechanism
analogous to cyclic AMP kinases; this has not yet
been established.

METABOLISM OF CYCLIC NUCLEOTIDES

SYNTHESIS

ADENYLYL CYCLASE STUDIES

This enzyme catalyzes the formation of cyclic AMP from ATP (Figure 1). In liver, as well as in most other tissues examined, adenylyl cyclase is associated almost exclusively with the particulate fraction and is considered to be localized mainly in plasma membranes (79, 145, 149, 194). Adenylyl cyclase is situated on the inner surface of plasma membranes (145, 161) and is referred to as the catalytic component; other components of the adenylyl cyclase system include: the regulatory (discriminatory or receptor) component, located on the outer surface of the plasma membrane, and the coupling (transducer) component within the membrane, interposed between the regulatory and catalytic subunits.

Extensive studies on the properties of liver adenylyl cyclase have been carried out (14, 15, 76, 77, 90, 91, 110, 111, 113, 150, 151, 158, 162-166, 170, 193); however, a detailed discussion of this aspect is not within the scope of the present review. Suffice it to say briefly that the activity of adenylyl cyclase can be affected by agents acting on any one of the components of the adenylyl cyclase system. For example, glucagon or epinephrine increase the cyclic AMP levels in hepatocytes by interacting with the receptor component of the membrane to activate the adenylyl cyclase; although both hormones interact with specific receptors, only the epinephrine receptor has been well characterized as being a β-adrenergic receptor (108), likely of the β_1 type (103). Cholera toxin produces irreversible stimulation of adenylyl cylcase in vivo by interacting with receptors on the membrane surface (63), but in order for this agent to activate liver adenylyl cyclase in vitro, the addition of nicotinamide adenine dinucleotide (NAD) is required (64). Sodium fluoride stimulates adenylyl cyclase only in broken cell preparations and is therefore considered to act directly on the catalytic subunit. The activity of the catalytic subunit is also modulated physiologically by other ions. For example, Mg++ is essential for optimal adenylyl cyclase activity; Ca++ appears necessary in trace amounts, but in larger concentrations is inhibitory. It is also likely that other endogenous substances such as the inhibitors reported by Ho et al (86) and Levey et al (112) also modulate the physiological activity of adenylyl cyclase and its responsiveness to hormones. The nature of the coupling mechanism is not clear at present, however, specific phospholipids and the guanylyl nucleotides (eg. GTP) appear to be involved in maintaining the proper

functioning of this component. Detergents and phospholipases
markedly affect the responsiveness of adenylyl cyclase to hormones without any significant effect on the fluoride responsiveness. Prostaglandins have also been shown to influence adenylyl
cyclase activity, likely by altering the lipid:lipid interaction
in the cell membrane (153). Storage of membrane preparations,
even for brief periods, at room temperature or at 4°C results
in a marked decrease in adenylyl cyclase activity and hormone
responsiveness, however the fluoride stimulatable activity
remains essentially unaltered. Significant changes in the
hormone responsiveness of adenylyl cyclase are also evident in
regenerating and fetal liver preparations, usually characterized
by increased responsiveness to epinephrine and decreased responsiveness to glucagon. The adenylyl cyclase activity and its
hormone responsiveness has also been shown to be altered (usually decreased) in transformed cell lines in culture (3, 4, 22,
142).

        To examine whether defined changes in adenylyl cyclase
take place in malignant cells in vivo a number of transplantable
Morris hepatomas, with varying growth rates, have been investigated.

        Brown et al (20) and Pennington et al (144) investigated
the adenylyl cyclase activities (in the presence of sodium
fluoride) for 20,000 x g pellets of hepatomas 7777 (rapidly
growing), 7794A and 9618A (slow growing) and found that the
hepatoma cyclase activity was greater than that of normal liver.
Epinephrine (4.4×10^{-5}M) stimulation of hepatoma adenylyl cyclase was reported to be less than normal liver, however these
results are questionable since the sodium fluoride in the assay
medium masks the hormone effect. These workers also reported
that the fluoride-stimulated cyclase activities were higher in
host liver than in normal liver, suggesting a tumor-host effect.

        Allen et al (1) examined the adenylyl cyclase activity
in homogenates from the following Morris hepatomas: 9618B and
7787 (slow growing), 5123tc (intermediate growth rate) and
7288C, 3924A, $9618A_2$ (rapidly growing). The basal and fluoride-
stimulated cyclase activities of all hepatomas were found to be
similar to those of normal and regenerating liver. In contrast,
the responsiveness of adenylyl cyclase to glucagon (1 μM) stimulation was reduced considerably in rapidly growing tumors,
while in slow growing hepatomas the glucagon responsiveness
approximated that of normal and regenerating liver. These findings prompted Weber (210, 211) to place adenylyl cyclase in
Group 1 of his postulated "molecular correlation concept of
neoplasia"; this group includes biochemical parameters that
correlate either positively or negatively with hepatoma growth

rates. Subsequent studies by Weber and coworkers on plasma
membranes (212) indicated that the adenylyl cyclase activities
of the slow growing hepatomas (66 and 7794A) were similar to
normal liver, whereas the cyclase activities of the rapidly
growing hepatomas (3683F, $9618A_2$, 7777 and 3924A) were all
markedly lower than the liver. The adenylyl cyclase activities
in plasma membranes from rapidly growing tumors are considerably
lower than the homogenate preparations reported previously by
this group.

Particulate (10,000 rpm) fractions were studied by
Klein et al (97) for rapidly growing (3924A) and intermediate
growth rate (9121) Morris hepatomas. The basal particulate
adenylyl cyclase activities of both hepatomas were slightly
higher than normal liver. The glucagon responsiveness of these
tumors was lower than liver at high concentrations (10^{-5} and
10^{-6}M) but were similar or even slightly higher at low glucagon
concentrations (10^{-8} and 10^{-9}M). The half-maximal enzyme
stimulation was found to occur at similar glucagon concentrations
for the tumors and liver; similarly, the binding of I^{125}-glucagon
to washed membrane particles was essentially the same for hepatoma and liver. In contrast, these workers found that epinephrine (10^{-5}M) and sodium fluoride (8×10^{-3}M) enhanced hepatoma
adenylyl cyclase activity to a greater extent than that of liver.

For an intermediate growth rate hepatoma (5123tc(h)),
Hickie et al (81) reported that the basal adenylyl cyclase
activities in homogenate and plasma membrane fractions were
similar to normal liver; the glucagon (5.6 µM) responsiveness
of the tumor fractions were considerably less than normal liver,
while the responsiveness of the hepatoma preparations to sodium
fluoride (10 mM) was equivalent to liver; epinephrine (100 µM)
stimulated homogenate activities in both hepatoma and liver,
however with plasma membrane fractions only the hepatoma activities were enhanced. Prostaglandin E_1 (56.6 µM) significantly
increased the adenylyl cyclase activities in liver and hepatoma
homogenates but not the plasma membrane preparations; insulin
(0.7 µM) had no measurable effect on any of the preparations.
It should be noted that the hepatoma used in this study differs
from 5123tc reported by other workers in that 5123tc(h) was
grown subcutaneously and generated by serial inoculations for
more than a decade (84). Recent additional studies have been
carried out by Hickie et al (83) on soluble and particulate
fractions of various Morris hepatomas: 7288ctc (rapidly growing),
5123tc(h) and 5123C (intermediate growth rate) and 7794A (slow
growing). As with liver, more than 95% of all hepatoma adenylyl
cyclase activities was associated with the particulate fractions;
this is in contrast to the findings of Tomasi et al (201)
indicating that the 100,000 x g supernatant from a rapidly

growing hepatoma (Yoshida ascites) contains roughly 70% of the
total adenylyl cyclase activity. The particulate cyclase
activities (fluoride stimulated) for hepatomas 7288ctc and
5123C were lower than normal liver, while 5123tc(h) activity
was similar and 7794A consistently higher than liver. The
preparations from livers of all tumor bearing animals had
higher fluoride stimulated adenylyl cyclase activities than
normal liver, in keeping with a previous report (20). The
glucagon responsiveness of adenylyl cyclase in tumor homogenate and plasma membrane-enriched fractions was lowest in the
more rapidly growing hepatomas but approached that of liver in
the slow growing tumor, supporting the report of Allan et al
(1). Epinephrine responsiveness of tumor homogenates was as
high as liver, however in the plasma membrane enriched fractions,
responsiveness to this hormone was less than homogenates from
liver and tumors.

     Criss and Morris (46) recently investigated the adeny-
lyl cyclase system in plasma membranes from several Morris
hepatomas: 20, 21, 9633F (slow growing), 5123tc (intermediate
growth rate) and 3924A, 7777, 9618A$_2$ (fast growing). All tumor
membrane preparations were found to have lower specific activities than liver preparations. These preparations were,
however, stimulated by fluoride and Gpp(NH)p (an analog of GTP
that appears to act on the catalytic subunit). Glucagon responsiveness of the slow growing tumors was similar to liver,
however that of the rapidly growing hepatomas was very poor;
this was seen at various concentrations of glucagon ranging
from 10^{-5} to 10^{-10}M. These workers also found that I^{125}
glucagon binding to the tumor plasma membranes paralleled,
with one exception, the responsiveness to glucagon, though the
total glucagon binding was generally lower in tumor than liver;
these findings are not in agreement with the previous report of
Klein et al (97). Epinephrine was found to have negligible
effects on the hepatoma membrane preparations. Criss and Morris
(46) also carried out additional kinetic studies on plasma membranes from hepatoma 21 and 3924A using glucagon in the absence
and presence of Gpp(NH)p and various temperatures and Mg:ATP
ratios. The results suggest that the hepatomas are defective
not only in binding glucagon but also show changes in the catalytic subunit. Pradhan, Criss and Morris (153) recently
studied the effect of various prostaglandins on plasma membrane
cyclase activities of several Morris hepatomas: slow growing
(20, 21, 9633F), intermediate growing (5123tc) and rapidly
growing (3924A, 9618A$_2$, 7777). Prostaglandin E$_1$ was the most
effective in stimulating adenylyl cyclase in liver and the
majority of the hepatomas; the only tumors not stimulated were
5123tc and 9618A$_2$. Interestingly, these two tumors were inhibited by prostaglandin A$_1$, A$_2$, and F$_{2\alpha}$ whereas the other tumors
and liver were stimulated.

The adenylyl cyclase system has also been studied with
various other transplantable tumors and carcinogen-induced
primary hepatomas such as: 484A (rapidly growing) and 147042
(slow growing) (59); Ehrlich ascites (11); Zajdela ascites (103);
Yoshida ascites (201); ascites hepatomas 7974, 371A, 130 (139);
2-acetylaminofluorene-induced (37-40); 3-methyl-4-dimethyl-
aminoazobenzene-induced (17, 18); and ethionine-induced (28,52).
Most of these tumors also demonstrated a decrease in glucagon
responsiveness and an increase in epinephrine responsiveness.

The formation of cyclic GMP from GTP is catalyzed by
guanylyl cyclase (Figure 1). This enzyme is present in liver
in both soluble and particulate fractions including the plasma
membrane (83, 96, 190, 192). In regenerating and fetal liver,
the activity of guanylyl cyclase in the particulate fraction
increases substantially (70, 71, 96, 191), with the highest
enzyme activity closely associated with the period of greatest
mitotic activity (191); in contrast, the soluble enzyme activity
is decreased in these tissues. Interestingly, the activity of
this enzyme also increases significantly in liver plasma membranes of pregnant rats (191); again, the increased activity was
found to correspond to the period of highest mitotic activity
in the liver. Recently, immunohistochemical studies (58, 98)
demonstrated the presence of guanylyl cyclase activity in liver
nuclei; this activity was also increased in regenerating liver
nuclei. The above results suggest that there is a strong positive correlation between hepatocyte proliferation and particulate guanylyl cyclase activity. The activity of liver guanylyl
cyclase can also be influenced by various agents (93, 94, 95
125, 192). With regard to ions, Mn^{++} is the most effective sole
cation for both soluble and particulate optimal enzyme activity,
however, Mg^{++} can stimulate guanylyl cyclase in the presence of
low concentrations of Mn^{++}. Ca^{++} stimulates soluble guanylyl
cyclase activity (in the presence of low concentrations of Mn^{++})
however Ca^{++} tends to inhibit particulate guanylyl cyclase
activity. The detergent, Triton X-100 markedly increases the
activity of the particulate enzyme and to a lesser, but significant degree, also the soluble enzyme activity. ATP inhibits
soluble and particulate guanylyl cyclase. Sodium azide stimulates soluble liver guanylyl cyclase activity; this effect
appears to require the presence of a protein activator factor.
In the presence of sodium azide, the Mg^{++} effect on guanylyl
cyclase becomes similar to that of Mn^{++}. In contrast to adenylyl cyclase, both soluble and particulate guanylyl cyclase
activities are reasonably stable (190). Recent studies (58)
indicate that liver nuclear guanylyl cyclase activity is increased
significantly either by injecting glucagon or incubating nuclei

in presence of cyclic AMP (10^{-5}M); these workers suggest that cyclic AMP may be an endogenous regulator for nuclear guanylyl cyclase.

In Morris hepatomas, the earliest study on guanylyl cyclase was carried out by Northup et al (137); for this study, 37,000 x g supernatants were assayed from 9618A$_2$ (rapidly growing), 7800 and 7795 (intermediate growth rate) and 7787 (slow growing). The activity of this enzyme was markedly reduced in all hepatomas ie. not detectable in hepatomas 7795, 7800 and 9618A$_2$ and only 20% of the normal liver activity in 7787. In host livers from rats bearing 7787 and 9618A$_2$, the soluble guanylyl cyclase activity was significantly higher than that of normal liver.

Goridis and Reutter (70) examined the guanylyl cyclase activity in four Morris hepatomas: 7777 and 9618A$_2$ (rapidly growing); 7800 and 9121 (intermediate growth rate). The activities of this enzyme in 7777, 9618A$_2$ and 7800 were not detectable, whereas the activity of tumor 9121 exceeded that of normal liver. Triton X-100 moderately stimulated the enzymes from 9121, but had no effect on the low activities of the other three tumors.

The activities of guanylyl cyclase were studied by Kimura and Murad (96) in homogenates, 105,000 x g supernatants and pellet fractions from hepatoma 3924A (rapidly growing). The specific activity of the tumor enzyme was found to be approximately double that of normal liver in homogenate fractions but close to 10-fold higher in the tumor particulate fraction; in contrast, the tumor soluble activity was less than one-half that of normal liver. Further, the percent recovery of the homogenate activity in the tumor particulate fraction was markedly greater than liver (69% vs 14%). Host liver particulate enzyme activity was almost double that of normal liver.

Criss et al (48) investigated the guanylyl cyclase activity for a number of Morris hepatomas: 3924A, 9618A$_2$ (rapid) and 9633F, 20, 21 (slow). All hepatomas were found to have much higher particulate/soluble ratios than normal liver (ie. between 1.2 - 3.3 for tumors vs 0.24 for liver). In 3924A and 9618A$_2$, the homogenate enzyme activities were significantly lower than normal liver (1.6, 1.2 and 3.2 nmole/min/g respectively). These two tumors were studied further with regard to other properties of the enzyme: Triton X-100 (1%) stimulated the tumor particulate guanylyl cyclase much less than liver (5, 2 and 11-fold respectively); the soluble fractions from normal liver and 3924A were moderately stimulated by Triton while the corresponding fraction from 9618A$_2$ was not

affected. In both tumors, sodium azide (1 mM)did not stimulate
guanylyl cyclase whereas this agent produced 5 and 6-fold
stimulation of the liver particulate and soluble fractions
respectively. These workers suggest that this finding may be
due to the absence of a protein activator factor shown to be
present in liver. Both tumors, like liver, prefer Mn^{++} as the
sole cation but, in contrast to liver, the tumor enzymes were
not stimulated by Mg^{++} in the presence of low Mn^{++} concentrations.
Ca^{++} stimulated all soluble preparations but inhibited the particulate preparations. As with liver, the tumor preparations
were inhibited by ATP. Recent studies by these workers (49) on
transplantable Morris kidney tumors (MK2 and MK3) produced
qualitatively similar results.

Soluble and particulate guanylyl cyclase activities
(Triton stimulated) were studied recently by Hickie et al (83)
for: 7288ctc (rapid), 5123tc(h) and 5123C (medium) and 7794A
(slow). The total guanylyl cyclase activities in all tumor
soluble fractions was markedly less than normal liver; these
activities, expressed as percent of normal liver activity were
as follows: 7288ctc - 2.6%; 5123tc(h) - 11.4%; 5123C - 10.6%;
and 7794A - 24.7%. This confirms the earlier findings of
Northup et al (137). For the particulate fractions, the total
activities for the 3 most rapidly growing tumors were also
lower than normal liver ie. 49% lower for 7288ctc, 28.5% for
5123tc(h) and 16% for 5123C. It should be noted, however, that
with 7288ctc and 5123C the specific activities of the plasma
membrane enriched fractions (fraction 5) were significantly
higher than normal liver suggesting that cyclic GMP synthesis
at the level of the plasma membrane may actually be increased
in these tumors. The particulate activity of the slow growing
7794A was, in contrast to the other tumors, more than 3-fold
higher than liver; further, it is evident that a significant
proportion of the total guanylyl cyclase activity is associated
with the mitochondrial fraction (fraction 9). The particulate/
soluble ratios were also much higher for these tumors than normal
liver ie. 7288ctc -8.8; 5123tc(h) - 2.8; 5123C - 3.5; 7794A - 6.2
vs liver - 0.4. In host livers of animals bearing 7288ctc, 5123C
and 7794A the specific activities of guanylyl cyclase were consistently higher than normal liver, in keeping with the previous
reports (48, 96); the soluble activities for all host livers
were reduced. The latter finding is not in accord with the report of Northup et al (137).

Guanylyl cyclase activities have been investigated in
other hepatomas as well ie. ethionine-induced (54,55) and
nitrosamine-induced (53). Both tumors show increased guanylyl
cyclase activities. The ethionine-induced hepatomas are
stimulated by sodium azide, in contrast to the Morris hepatomas.

DEGRADATION OF CYCLIC NUCLEOTIDES

The hydrolysis of cyclic AMP and cyclic GMP to their corresponding 5'-nucleotide monophosphate derivatives is promoted by
phosphodiesterases (Figure 1). These enzymes are widely distributed in vertebrate and invertebrate cells, being located in
both the soluble and particulate fractions (5-7, 23, 168, 186,187,
197-199, 202). Thompson and Appleman (197) suggested, on the
basis of anomalous kinetic data, that most cells contain at least
two forms of cyclic AMP phosphodiesterases with one form having
a high affinity (low K_m) for cyclic AMP and the other having a
low affinity (high K_m) for this substrate. These enzyme forms
were subsequently separated by agarose gel filtration and characterized by these workers (198). Subsequent studies by Russell
et al (168), using DEAE cellulose chromatography, showed that
rat liver contained three main active cyclic nucleotide phosphodiesterase fractions. One fraction hydrolyzed only cyclic GMP
and had a high affinity for this substrate. The second fraction
degraded both cyclic AMP and cyclic GMP but with a low affinity
for both substrates. The third fraction contained a phosphodiesterase that had a high affinity for cyclic AMP and negatively
cooperative kinetics. These workers also found that the phosphodiesterase activity in the first and second fractions were
mainly associated with the soluble fractions of the cell, whereas
the high affinity cyclic AMP phosphodiesterase activity was associated with the 100,000 x g particulate fraction. The latter
form has been shown to be present in the plasma membranes of rat
liver (85, 212).

The activities of these phosphodiesterases can be modulated by a number of factors (5, 27, 187, 199, 202, 213, 214).
Mg++ and Mn++ will produce optimal activity of these enzymes in
fresh preparations; in stored preparations, Mg++ is more
effective. Ca++ in low concentrations, is necessary for action
of endogenous protein activators of phosphodiesterases (29, 207).
VanInwegen et al (202) has also shown recently that Ca++ markedly
enhances the activation of cyclic AMP hydrolysis by cyclic GMP
with high affinity, kidney membrane cyclic AMP phosphodiesterase.
Prolonged high levels of cyclic AMP have been shown in vitro to
increase phosphodiesterase activity (50, 121). Cyclic AMP
dependent protein kinases appear also to be involved in regulating phosphodiesterase synthesis and activity (16). The following hormones have been reported to increase the activity of
liver particulate cyclic AMP phosphodiesterase activity:
insulin, glucagon and growth hormone; glucocorticoids, in contrast, decrease liver homogenate activity of cyclic AMP and
cyclic GMP phosphodiesterases (199). Various drugs and related
chemicals have been shown to affect phosphodiesterase activity
(27, 160, 213, 214). Examples of inhibitors include: xanthine

derivatives (theophylline, 1-methyl-3-isobutylxanthine (MIX)),
papaverine, sulfonylureas (eg. tolbutamide), phenothiazines
(eg. trifluoperazine) and catecholamines. It is of interest
that some of these agents affect phosphodiesterases by selective
mechanisms. For example, theophylline and papaverine competi-
tively inhibit cyclic AMP phosphodiesterase whereas, trifluoperazine is proposed to inhibit the enzyme by interfering with
the endogenous activation (213). This, therefore, represents
a potentially useful approach to more selective therapy of
appropriate disease states. A start has been made in this direction with the clinical use of phosphodiesterase inhibitors in
neuroblastoma (78, 154) and in psoriasis (206). There are few
chemical agents that stimulate phosphodiesterases; only imidazole
and the ammonium ion have been reported to have this action. Dithiothreitol (DTT) decreases the activity of particulate cyclic
AMP phosphodiesterase, while storage 4°C for several hours will
increase the activity (202).

CYCLIC AMP PHOSPHODIESTERASES IN MORRIS HEPATOMAS

Rhoads et al (159) measured the cyclic AMP phosphodiesterase (substrate concentration, 1 mM) in the 78,000 x g
supernatant fractions of three rapidly growing hepatomas ($9618A_2$,
3924A, 7777); two intermediate growth rate tumors (7800, 5123C)
and two slow growing hepatomas (7794A, 9618A). The resultant
hepatoma activities were 32 to 60% lower than normal liver with
no correlation between activity and tumor growth rate. In contrast, the activities of the regenerating liver (24 hour) and
fetal liver (19 day gestation)were moderately increased. Imidazole produced small increases in the hepatoma activities (8-23%)
while activities with normal, fetal and regenerating livers were
stimulated 24%, 38% and 32% respectively. Kinetic studies indicated that the tumors, like normal liver, contained two types
of phosphodiesterase activities with the K_m for the high
affinity type ranging from 2.5-7.6 μM and the low affinity K_m
being 39-54 μM.

The cyclic AMP phosphodiesterase activies of 100,000 x
g supernatant fractions were studied by Clark et al (41) for
hepatomas 3924A (rapid) and 47C (slow). Analogous to the
previous study, these hepatomas had two apparent K_m's for cyclic
AMP ie. 2-3 μM and 100-600 μM. The activity of the high K_m
phosphodiesterase was decreased substantially in both hepatomas;
in contrast, the activities of the low K_m form in both hepatomas were approximately 2-fold higher than normal liver. The
high and low K_m activities for neonatal liver (5 days after
birth) were not significantly different from normal liver, while
with regenerating liver (24 hour) only the high K_m activity was
significantly altered (ie. increased). Additional studies by

this group (214) on plasma membrane cyclic AMP phosphodiesterases
of hepatomas 3683F, 9618A$_2$, 3924A, 7777 (rapidly growing) and
7794A, 47C and 66 (slow growing) indicated that the low K_m activity was increased to a greater degree in the rapidly growing
tumors than in the more slowly growing tumors. Weber (214)
proposed that these findings suggest that there is a gradual
shift in neoplasia in the isozyme pattern from the high K_m to
the low K_m form; this type of change is classified as Group 2
in the molecular correlation concept. Weber has also suggested
that there is a reciprocal relationship between membrane cAMP
phosphodiesterase and adenylyl cyclase such that the activity
of the phosphodiesterase relative to the cyclase is highest in
rapidly growing tumors, thus favouring a reduction of cellular
cyclic AMP.

        Criss and Morris (45) fractionated cyclic AMP phospho-
diesterases of 7777 (rapid), and 8999, 7787 (slow) using iso-
electrofocusing column chromatography; aliquots of the 100,000
x g supernatant fractions were applied. The two major peaks
seen with liver that represented the high K_m enzyme activity,
were decreased substantially particularly in the rapidly growing
tumor; the two minor peaks (low K_m activity) were increased most
noticeably in 7777.

        Homogenate, 100,000 x g supernatants, and plasma membrane
fractions were investigated by Hickie et al (85) in hepatoma
5123tc(h). The total cyclic AMP phosphodiesterase activities
of tumor homogenate and supernatant fractions were found to be
less than one-half those of normal liver; this was largely due
to a 53% decrease in activity for the hepatoma high K_m enzyme.
On the other hand, the low K_m enzyme activities of the hepatoma
homogenate and plasma membrane fractions were approximately 50%
higher than liver at substrate concentrations of 0.5 and 1 μM;
kinetic studies of these fractions also indicated that the tumor
low K_m enzyme had a lower apparent K_m than liver. Imidazole
(40 mM) increased the low K_m enzyme activity in the hepatoma
plasma membranes to a greater extent than liver; inhibition by
theophylline (5 mM) at 1 μM substrate was about 80% for liver
and tumor plasma membrane enzymes. Recent studies were also
carried out by Hickie et al (83) at low cyclic AMP (0.25 μM)
and high cyclic AMP (200 μM) concentrations on soluble and particulate fractions for hepatomas 7288ctc (rapid), 5123tc(h) and
5123C (intermediate) and 7794A (slow). At low substrate concentrations, the soluble phosphodiesterase activities were reduced
moderately for all hepatomas; the particulate activity was reduced substantially in three of the four tumors - in 5123tc(h),
some particulate fractions had enzyme activities that were
higher than liver supporting our previous studies; hepatoma
7288ctc showed the most marked decrease (88%) in total phospho-

diesterase activity at low substrate concentration. Except for
hepatoma 5123tc(h), the findings with the other hepatomas do not
concur with Weber's findings (212). At high substrate concentrations, the soluble cyclic AMP phosphodiesterase activities
were reduced 10-40%, with the greatest decrease in activity
occuring in hepatoma 7288ctc and least in 7794A; the activities
of this enzyme in the particulate fractions were markedly less
than normal liver in all hepatomas: 7288ctc (98%) reduction;
5123tc(h) (92%); 5123C (86%) and 7794A (87%).

CYCLIC GMP PHOSPHODIESTERASE

The only known study on this enzyme in Morris hepatomas was done by Hickie et al (83). This enzyme was assayed
at 1.25 μM substrate concentration in soluble and particulate
fractions from 7288ctc, 5123tc(h), 5123C and 7794A. In the
soluble fractions, the activities of this enzyme were moderately
reduced (20-48%) in all hepatomas, showing no correlation to
growth rate; the activities in the particulate fractions were
reduced more significantly in all hepatomas: 7288ctc (94%
reduction); 5123tc(h) (52%); 5123C (86%); 7794A (76%).   Therefore, the degradation of cyclic GMP in these hepatomas appears
to be markedly impaired; there is also no correlation between
the degree of impairment and the tumor growth rate.

Cyclic nucleotide phosphodiesterases have also been
carried out in other tumors ie. AAF-induced hepatomas (40);
ethionine-induced hepatomas (53); human mammary carcinoma and,
human colonic carcinoma (52). In contrast to the Morris hepatomas, the phosphodiesterase activities in these tumors were not
reduced, and in some cases they were actually increased.

TISSUE LEVELS OF CYCLIC NUCLEOTIDES

One of the primary reasons for investigating levels of cyclic
AMP and cyclic GMP in cells is to determine if one, or both of
these endogenously synthesized and degraded compounds may be involved in regulating cell growth processes such as proliferation
and differentiation.

During   recent   years a number of studies have accumulated
suggesting that cyclic AMP functions as a negative signal, tending to retard abnormally rapid cell proliferation and to promote
regulated growth and differentiation (3, 4, 22, 140, 142, 169,
176, 177). For example, studies on fibroblasts in culture have
shown that cyclic AMP levels are significantly lower in transformed cells than in the corresponding untransformed cells;
further there appears to be a negative correlation between
cellular cAMP levels and growth rate of fibroblasts (140). If

the cyclic AMP levels are raised in transformed cells by either
growing cells in presence of cyclic AMP analogs or in presence
of phosphodiesterase inhibitors, the transformed cells are
converted to a state resembling the untransformed cells. Some
in vivo hyperplastic tissues have been shown to have decreased
cyclic AMP levels ie. tumors (52, 68, 84, 179) and psoriatic
tissue (206); also, the administration of dibutyryl cyclic AMP
and/or phosphodiesterase inhibitors (aminophylline, papaverine)
has been found to retard the growth of various types of tumors
in vivo (31, 35, 67, 78, 92, 182) and in psoriasis (206). The
levels of cyclic AMP have been shown to fluctuate significantly
during the cell cycle (65, 66, 145, 169); generally, the levels
are decreased during mitosis and increased in the G_1 phase.
There is some disagreement with regard to levels during S and
G_2 phases due mainly to the problem of cell synchrony (66).
Most studies on fibroblasts and lymphocytes suggest that cyclic
AMP or its analogs, arrest cell growth in either the G_1 or G_2
phases (136, 142), however it has also been reported to inhibit in
the S phase in Reuber hepatoma cells (203). It is the opinion
of some workers that cyclic AMP is the only cyclic nucleotide
that is involved in regulating cell proliferation and differentiation; this concept is based on the assumption that the
signal triggering cell proliferation is the low level of cyclic
AMP (ie. negative mitogenic signal).

   A number of studies particularly with in vivo tumors, report
however that cyclic AMP levels may be either similar (24, 68)
or higher (24, 28, 40, 68, 122, 124) than the corresponding
normal tissues. This has prompted other workers to consider
the presence of a positive (mitogenic) signal in cell growth
regulation. Since cyclic GMP has been shown in a number of
physiological systems to act in an opposite manner to cyclic AMP,
it was postulated by Nelson Goldberg that cyclic GMP is the
positive signal in cell growth regulation; this is commonly referred to as the "dualism" or "Yin-Yang" hypothesis (69). Although there is some evidence to the contrary (30, 123, 135, 157)
there is a considerable amount of in vitro and in vivo supportive evidence accumulating to indicate that increased cyclic GMP
levels and/or increased plasma membrane guanylyl cyclase activities are associated with increased proliferative states (47,
53-55, 68-71, 75, 83, 96, 98, 122, 126, 127, 131, 134, 157, 171,
172, 191, 196, 205, 206, 208, 209, 217). In studies where both
cyclic AMP and cyclic GMP were measured, the ratios of cyclic
GMP/cyclic AMP tend to be higher in proliferating than in non-
proliferating cells (54, 55, 83, 179, 206, 208, 209).

   There is relatively little data on changes in cyclic GMP
concentrations during the cell cycle (66). However, a recent
study (217) on fluctuations in cyclic GMP and cyclic AMP of

colcemid synchronized Novikoff hepatoma cells indicate that
the cyclic GMP levels rise and the cyclic AMP levels drop as
the cells enter mitosis. In G_1, the cyclic GMP levels were
low while cyclic AMP levels were high. During the S and early
G_2 phases, the cyclic GMP/cyclic AMP ratios rose initially and
then fell.

Regenerating liver has been studied extensively in relation
to changes occurring in cyclic AMP and cyclic GMP levels at
various stages after partial hepatectomy (61, 71, 119, 120,
126, 127, 180, 200, 215). MacManus , Whitfield et al (119, 120,
215) have shown that significant increases in liver cyclic AMP
levels occur at 4 and 12 hours after hepatectomy, while the
cyclic GMP levels were not noticeably changed. These workers
suggest that cyclic AMP, in concert with calcium, acts as a
positive influence on hepatocyte proliferation. Thrower and
Ord (200) who studied only the cyclic AMP levels, found that in
addition to peak levels occurring at 4 and 12 hours, a third
peak occurs at 22 hours. Short et al (180) showed that an infusion mixture of triiodothyronine, amino acids, glucagon and
heparin (TAGH) increases DNA replication and liver cell mitosis.
Dibutyryl cyclic AMP and theophylline could replace glucagon
in the mixture but cyclic GMP or its butyryl derivatives were
not effective replacements for glucagon. Fausto and Butcher
(61) confirmed the MacManus-Whitfield findings mentioned above
but note an initial rapid drop of cyclic AMP prior to the typical
periodic increases. Miura and coworkers (126, 127) found, after
partial hepatectomy, a transient rise in cyclic GMP within 10-
20 minutes; this rise was accompanied by a corresponding drop
during this time in cyclic AMP. Similarly an increase in cyclic
GMP was noted 15 minutes after infusion with TGH (triiodothyronine, glucagon, and heparin). The addition of prostaglandins
(PGE_1 or $PGF_{2\alpha}$) to the medium for isolated perfused liver increases the cyclic GMP levels. These workers conclude that
cyclic GMP is involved in initiating liver regeneration mediated
through the action of prostaglandins. Recently, Goridis et al
(71) showed that peak liver levels of cyclic GMP and highest
guanylyl cyclase activities occur 8 hours after partial hepatectomy, prior to onset of the proliferative response. It is
of interest that the increased concentrations of cyclic GMP were
found when the animals were sacrificed using pentobarbital
anesthesia, but not when anesthesia was omitted. It would appear
that the increases in cyclic AMP levels in regenerating liver
seen by MacManus, Whitfield et al are not directly involved in
cell proliferation since it was shown by Thrower and Ord (200)
that these increases in cyclic AMP can be prevented by β-adrenergic blocking agents (propranolol, pindolol) without affecting
ornithine decarboxylase induction or DNA synthesis. Therefore
the role of these periodic increases in cyclic AMP in regener-

ating liver is unclear at present and may be, perhaps, related to differentiation and/or changes in intermediary metabolism. In fetal and neonatal liver, cyclic AMP levels have been studied (40, 138); however there are no known studies on cyclic GMP in these tissues. The latter studies indicate that the cyclic AMP levels in fetal liver 7 days before birth are less than one-half those of normal liver; these levels increase gradually and, at the time of birth, exceed those of liver, reaching the maximum peak about 10 days after birth (more than two-fold higher than liver). In approximately one month the levels become similar to adult normal liver. The increase in cyclic AMP levels in the neonate does not appear to be related to hepatocyte proliferation since the mitotic index in the neonate is similar to that of adult liver (191); it would seem that the increased cyclic AMP in the neonate liver may be involved in retarding hepatocyte proliferation and promoting differentiation.

A major problem inherent in attempting to correlate changes in cyclic nucleotide levels with cell growth processes is possible compartmentalization of the cyclic nucleotide within the cell ie. local concentrations of the cyclic nucleotide near cell membranes likely exceed average cell concentrations thus possibly reducing, or even masking, significant changes in the cyclic nucleotide. Some progress has been made recently by Steiner's group (58, 98, 185) in measuring local levels of cyclic nucleotides using an immunocytofluoresence technique. These workers have shown marked increases in cyclic GMP concentrations near membranous structures in regenerating liver corresponding to the increased plasma membrane guanylyl cyclase activities discussed earlier (70, 71, 96, 191).

CYCLIC NUCLEOTIDE LEVELS IN MORRIS HEPATOMAS

Butcher et al (24) measured the cyclic AMP levels in several Morris hepatomas using a protein kinase method: 9121, 7800, 9098, 9108, 5123C (intermediate growth rate) and 7793, 7794B, 7794A, 66, 9618B, 9618A (slow growing). The hepatoma levels, relative to corresponding host liver, were as follows: slightly lower for 5123C and 9618B; essentially the same for 7800, 7793, 7794B, 7794A, 9618A; and slightly higher for 9121, 9098, 9108 and 66. There was no evident correlation between cyclic AMP levels and tumor growth rate. Adrenalectomy had no effect on the tumor cyclic AMP levels. The in vivo glucagon responsiveness of hepatomas 66, 9618A and 9618B was similar to that of normal liver while 9098, 9121, 7794B and 7794A tumor responsiveness exceeded liver; hepatoma 5123C, 7800, 7793 and 9108 were poorly responsive to glucagon. The glucagon responsiveness of the tumors was also compared to the α-amino-isobutyrate (AIB) ratios; this ratio is a measure of amino acid

transport capabilities. Hepatomas with initial AIB ratios less
than 5, like liver, showed significantly increased cyclic AMP
levels after glucagon injection, whereas hepatomas, with AIB
ratios greater than 9, showed poor responsiveness to glucagon.
Isoproterenol responsiveness of all hepatomas was essentially
similar to that of host liver.

Cyclic AMP and cyclic GMP levels were compared by
Thomas et al (196) in various hepatomas: 7288ctc, 3924A
(rapid); 7316B, 9121, 5123tc, 7800 (intermediate); 9633, 16
(slow). The cyclic AMP and cyclic GMP levels of all hepatomas
were higher than normal liver; hepatomas 3924A and 7288ctc had
markedly increased levels of cyclic GMP. There was no apparent
correlation between the cyclic nucleotide levels and the tumor
growth. The calculated GMP/cyclic AMP ratios for these tumors
are greater than liver in 5 of the 8 tumors with the most
marked increase found in the two most rapidly growing tumors
(83). Both cyclic nucleotides in this study were determined
by protein binding assays.

Hickie et al (84) reported cyclic AMP levels measured by
radioimmunoassay for hepatoma 5123tc(h). The basal levels of
this cyclic nucleotide was found to be about one-half that of
liver; this was shown in subsequent studies (85) to be due to
the increased activity of high affinity cyclic AMP phosphodiesterase in plasma membranes of this tumor. The in vivo
glucagon responsiveness of this hepatoma (84) is also significantly decreased in this tumor, in keeping with corresponding
in vitro studies (81).

The concentrations of cyclic GMP and cyclic AMP were
measured by M. Goldberg et al (68) in hepatomas 3924A, 9098
(rapid); 7800, 7316A (intermediate); 7787 (slow). The cyclic
AMP levels for some tumors were lower than normal liver (7800,
7787, 3924A) while in the other tumors the levels were higher;
cyclic GMP levels in the tumors were consistently higher than
normal liver. The corresponding cyclic GMP/cyclic AMP ratios
were higher in four out of the five hepatomas.

Sudilovsky and Gunter (188) found the levels of cyclic
AMP in the slow growing hepatoma 9618A to be the same as that
of normal liver; the glucagon responsiveness of this tumor was
also similar.

Cyclic GMP levels were reported for hepatomas $9618A_2$,
3924A (rapid) and 9633F, 20, 21 (slow) by Criss et al (48).
All hepatomas were found to contain substantially increased
levels of cyclic GMP relative to normal liver ie. usually
between 2-10 fold increase, however the increase in 3924A was
more than 200 fold.

Recent studies were carried out by Hickie et al (83) on the cyclic AMP and cyclic GMP levels in hepatomas 7288ctc (rapid); 5123tc(h), 5123C (intermediate), and 7794A (slow). For hepatoma 7288ctc, the cyclic AMP levels were reduced slightly but the cyclic GMP levels were increased more than four-fold giving a cyclic GMP to cyclic AMP ratio of 20×10^{-2}. With hepatomas 5123tc(h) and 5123C the cyclic AMP levels were significantly less than liver while the cyclic GMP levels were somewhat higher resulting in cyclic GMP to cyclic AMP ratios of 6.2×10^{-2} and 6.0×10^{-2} respectively. Hepatoma 7794A was found to have significantly increased cyclic AMP levels as well as increased cyclic GMP levels. The cyclic GMP/cyclic AMP ratio for this tumor (4.4×10^{-2}) approached that of normal liver (3.6×10^{-2}). Therefore, it would appear that the levels of cyclic GMP relative to cyclic AMP tend to be increased in hepatomas, though a direct correlation between the ratios and tumor growth rate is not evident, particularly for the intermediate and slow growing tumors.

The following two studies have been conducted on the urinary levels of cyclic AMP and cyclic GMP for rats bearing Morris hepatomas (47, 131). These urinary levels are taken by these workers to reflect tumor levels assuming that a similar efflux mechanism exists for each cyclic nucleotide. Murad et al (131) found that the level of cyclic GMP in the urine of a rat bearing 3924A was increased and that the extent of increase correlated closely with the tumor size; removing the tumor surgically resulted in a rapid decrease in urine levels of cyclic GMP to normal. If the growth of the tumor is delayed by radiation therapy or chemotherapy (5-fluoruracil), increases in urinary cyclic GMP are also delayed. Cyclic AMP levels in the urine were not altered in similar experiments. Criss and Murad (47) subsequently showed that rats bearing rapidly growing hepatomas ($9618A_2$, 3924A and a Morris kidney tumor MK3) had significantly increased levels of urinary cyclic GMP while cyclic AMP levels did not change appreciably. Also of interest is the recent report (134) that patients with primary hepatomas had significantly increased levels of urinary cyclic GMP.

GROWTH INHIBITION OF MORRIS HEPATOMAS BY CYCLIC NUCLEOTIDE ANALOGS

The only known report on Morris hepatomas is the work of Cho-Chung and co-workers (31, 32) using hepatoma 5123. This group found that a dose of 8 mg/200 g rat of dibutyryl cyclic AMP produces essentially complete arrest in "responsive" tumors; however some tumors were found to be "unresponsive" to this drug. This was analogous to responses seen in Walker 256 tumor. Subsequent studies on both tumors by Cho-Chung and Clair (33, 34) suggest that the binding of dibutyryl cyclic AMP in the "un-responsive" type of tumor is significantly reduced; this aspect will be discussed in more detail in the section to follow. Other in vivo tumors shown to be inhibited by dibutyryl cyclic AMP and/or a phosphodiesterase inhibitor (aminophylline) include: mammary tumors (35); carcinosarcoma (92); lymphosarcoma (67); and epidermoid carcinoma (182).

ACTION

Although cyclic AMP has been shown to act directly in certain prokaryotic cells (51, 143) it has been postulated (99) that many, if not all, actions of cyclic AMP and cyclic GMP in eukaryotes are mediated through the cyclic nucleotide-dependent protein kinases (Figure 1). Kinases are believed to regulate cell proliferation and growth (36, 42, 87) by promoting phos-phorylation of substrates such as histones (9, 104, 109) and nucleic acid polymerases (2).

Kuo (99) has demonstrated the presence, in a number of tissues, of a protein kinase modulator which depresses the cyclic AMP-dependent kinase activity and enhances the cyclic GMP-dependent activity. The polyamines putrescine, spermidine and spermine have also been shown to inhibit cyclic AMP-dependent protein kinase activity (132). Both cyclic nucleotide kinases require Mg^{++} for optimal activity, however, high concentrations of this cation (50-100 mM) inhibit cyclic AMP-dependent protein kinase activity with little effect on the cyclic GMP-dependent kinase activity (102). Ca^{++} has been reported to inhibit stimulation of protein kinases by both cyclic nucleotides (100, 101). Adenosine also inhibits cyclic AMP-dependent protein kinases (88).

BINDING PROTEIN STUDIES

Most cellular cyclic nucleotide binding proteins appear to be associated with protein kinases (104, 189), though cellular cyclic AMP-binding proteins have been identified recently that are apparently not associated with kinases (155).

To determine whether cyclic nucleotide binding proteins are altered in malignancy, various model systems have been studied. In vivo models include: Morris hepatomas (34, 68, 174); ascites hepatomas (133); and Walker 256 carcinoma (33, 34). Examples of in vitro models studied include: hepatoma cell lines (72, 73, 116-118, 183), and neuroblastoma (154, 155).

M. Goldberg et al (68) measured the cyclic nucleotide bind-ing capacity in the cytosol from various Morris hepatomas: 3924A and 9098 (rapidly growing); 7800 and 7316A (intermediate

growth rate) and 7787 (slow growing). The results suggest that
the rapidly growing hepatomas, which had elevated cyclic GMP
levels, also showed increased cyclic GMP binding; cyclic AMP
binding in the hepatomas was generally lower than that of normal
liver. Similarly, the cytosol fractions from various hepatoma
cell lines, HTC, RLC and H4-II-E had decreased capacities to
bind cyclic AMP at physiological pH (72-74, 116). Recent
studies by Mackenzie and Stellwagen (118) suggest that the
decreased cyclic AMP binding in the HTC cell line is due to the
presence of a macromolecular inhibitory component which possesses
protein kinase activity and appears to be identical to the catalytic subunit of a cyclic AMP-stimulated protein kinase.

    Cho-Chung and Clair (33, 34) have demonstrated the presence
of two cell populations in hepatoma 5123 and Walker 256 ie.
dibutyryl cyclic AMP "responsive" and unresponsive" cells.
Further, these workers have shown that the cytosols from the
dibutyryl cyclic AMP sensitive cells bind cyclic AMP more extensively than do those from resistant cells, suggesting that
defective cyclic AMP-binding proteins may be involved in loss
of growth control by cyclic AMP. This is in keeping with
the report (155) that cytosols from "differentiated" neuroblastoma cells possess higher cyclic AMP binding capacities
than "undifferentiated" neuroblastoma cells. Gene mutation
studies with S49 mouse lymphoma cells (42, 87, 184) have produced a mutant (kin.A) that is less sensitive to cyclic AMP due
primarily to changes in the regulatory subunit.

    Relatively few studies have been carried out on the cyclic
nucleotide binding characteristics of particulate fractions
from malignant tissues. Sharma et al (174) recently investigated this aspect using endoplasmic reticulum membranes from
Morris hepatoma 7777 (rapid) and 5123C (intermediate). The
tumor membranes had two apparent binding sites for cyclic
AMP, in contrast to the single binding site found with normal
liver; the tumor preparations also had a cyclic GMP binding
site which was absent in liver. The cyclic AMP binding of
plasma membranes from three ascites hepatomas (AH-130, AH-
130F(N) and AH-7974) was studied by Nambu and Terayama (133).
These hepatomas were found to have much lower levels of high
affinity cyclic AMP binding activity than did liver.

PROTEIN KINASE STUDIES

    Criss and Morris (44) examined the protein kinase profile of
the cytosol fractions from two rapidly growing Morris hepatomas
(3683F and 7777) and a slowly growing one (8999) using the iso-
electrofocusing technique. The major liver peak, representing
cyclic AMP-dependent protein kinase activity, was decreased
particularly in the rapidly growing tumors. A second liver peak,

insensitive to cyclic AMP stimulation, was found to be increased
in the hepatomas with the greatest increase evident in the
rapidly growing tumors. Studies on various hepatoma cell lines
in culture (72-74, 116) also showed that the cyclic AMP-dependent
kinase activities of these in vitro models are consistently
lower than liver whereas the endogenous (cyclic AMP-independent)
kinase activities are higher.

The subcellular distribution and activities of protein kinases
in a rapidly growing Morris hepatoma (7288C) were compared with
that of adult and fetal liver by Farron-Furstenthal (60). The
protein kinase activities of the cytosol fractions from the
hepatoma and fetal liver were activated by cyclic AMP to only
about 50% that of adult liver. The nuclei from adult liver contained about 3-4% of the homogenate kinase activity, while the
percentages of recovered activities in the nuclear fractions
from hepatoma and fetal liver were 3-5 fold higher. The nuclear
kinase activities of all three tissues were found to be unresponsive to cyclic AMP stimulation.

Sharma et al (175) studied the phosphorylation of proteins in
endoplasmic reticulum membrane preparations from hepatomas 7777
(rapid), 5123C and 7800 (intermediate) and 9618A (slow). As with
liver, the endogenous phosphorylation of smooth endoplasmic reticulum was greater than rough membranes; this phorphorylation
was cyclic AMP-independent. The endogenous kinase activity
tended to be higher in the tumor preparations than in liver. The
addition of histone stimulated phosphorylation; this activity was
cyclic AMP-dependent. Electrophoretic analysis indicated that
smooth membranes from 5123C lacked two phosphoproteins found in
liver. The authors propose that the endogenous protein kinase
in hepatoma is unable to phosphorylate all the membrane proteins
that are normally phosphorylated in liver.

INTERPRETATION

The regulation of cyclic AMP synthesis by glucagon and epinephrine is altered in Morris hepatomas. The responsiveness of
hepatoma adenylyl cyclase to glucagon is reduced, particularly
in the more rapidly growing hepatomas (1, 46, 81, 83); this reduction can be correlated with impaired binding of glucagon by
hepatoma plasma membranes (46). A diminution in glucagon responsiveness is also evident in premalignant and malignant
nodules of carcinogen-induced hepatomas (17, 18, 28, 43) as well
as in regenerating liver (191) and fetal liver (40, 191, 204).
In contrast, the responsiveness to epinephrine is usually increased in hepatomas (17, 18, 37-39, 43, 59, 81, 97), in regenerating liver (191) and in fetal liver (10, 40, 191). Though the
mechanisms underlying the altered hormone responsiveness in these

tissues are not yet known, recent reports suggest that changes in the hormonal milieu may be important in regulating the activity of adenylyl cyclase (21, 43, 52, 106, 107, 178, 204). Leffert et al (106) have shown that partial hepatectomy increases blood glucagon levels. Craven and DeRubertis (43) reported recently that blood glucagon levels are markedly elevated in rats fed the hepatocarcinogen, ethionine; these animals also have a decreased responsiveness to glucagon. These workers also demonstrated that chronic infusion of glucagon produces decreased glucagon responsiveness (52). Shikama and Ui (178) indicate that insulin decreases the responsiveness of liver adenylyl cyclase to epinephrine; if the levels of circulating insulin are reduced, this enhances the elevation of liver cyclic AMP concentrations by epinephrine. Partial hepatectomy decreases the blood insulin levels (21, 106). These studies, as a whole, suggest that the reduced adenylyl cyclase responsiveness of proliferating hepatocytes and hepatomas to glucagon is the result of cyclase desensitization by glucagon, whereas the enhanced enzyme responsiveness to epinephrine is related to the decreased blood insulin levels (191).

The main difference between normal liver and Morris hepatomas with regard to cyclic GMP formation is that the proportion of guanylyl cyclase activity in particulate fractions is much greater than that in soluble fractions (48, 49, 83, 96); this is also the case for regenerating liver, fetal liver and primary (carcinogen-induced) hepatomas (53-55, 70, 71, 96, 191). There is also a positive correlation between plasma membrane guanylyl cyclase activities and mitotic activities in regenerating, fetal and maternal liver (191). These data indicate that the altered subcellular distribution of guanylyl cyclase favours the formation and localization of high cyclic GMP concentrations near membranous structures. This statement is supported by recent immuno-cytofluorescence studies of cyclic GMP localization in regenerating liver (58, 98).

Cyclic AMP and cyclic GMP phosphodiesterase activities in regenerating and fetal livers are not appreciably different than normal liver (41, 159, 191); this, however, is not the case with Morris hepatomas (41, 45, 83, 85, 159, 214). The tumor activities of cyclic GMP phosphodiesterase are markedly reduced, especially in the particulate fractions. Particulate high affinity cyclic AMP phosphodiesterase activities tend to be higher in some of the more rapidly growing hepatomas, however the total cyclic AMP phosphodiesterase activities are reduced substantially in all Morris hepatomas studied. These findings suggest that the degradation of cyclic GMP is impaired in Morris hepatomas,

favouring accumulation of this cyclic nucleotide whereas, the
increased hydrolysis of physiological concentrations of cyclic
AMP by plasma membranes of some Morris hepatomas, favours a
reduction in basal cellular cyclic AMP levels.

Morris hepatomas tend to have higher cyclic GMP/cyclic AMP
ratios than normal liver (68, 83, 196). These ratios are
highest in rapidly growing tumors, however, a strong correlation between cyclic nucleotide levels and growth rate is not
evident in intermediate or slow growing tumors. Rats bearing
rapidly growing Morris hepatomas excrete significantly higher
amounts of cyclic GMP in the urine than normal (47, 131),
possibly reflecting the increased tumor levels of this cyclic
nucleotide. Dibutyryl cyclic AMP has been shown to inhibit
the growth of a Morris hepatoma (31, 32) suggesting that a
deficiency of cyclic AMP, relative to cyclic GMP, exists in
this tumor.

The role of cyclic AMP and cyclic GMP in regulating the
proliferation of hepatocytes is controversial (61, 71, 119, 120,
126, 127, 180, 200, 215). However, more recent studies (71, 126,
127, 191) indicate that increases in cyclic GMP, (relative to
cyclic AMP) occur early in the proliferative phase whereas the
levels of cyclic AMP (relative to cyclic GMP) increase later,
coinciding with the differentiation phase.

Even though studies on the action of cyclic nucleotides, as
expressed through the protein kinase system, have just begun in
Morris hepatomas it is evident that the cyclic nucleotide binding
capacities (33, 34, 68, 174) and the protein kinases (44, 60,
175) are altered signficantly. For example, rapidly growing
hepatomas have an impaired ability to bind cyclic AMP and possibly an increased binding capacity for cyclic GMP; cyclic AMP
dependent protein kinase activities are also reduced but accompanied by increased activities of endogenous (cyclic AMP
independent) kinase activities. These findings imply that the
ability of cyclic nucleotides to regulate cellular processes,
including proliferation and differentiation, is altered in
these tumors. This is supported by the finding that dibutyryl
cyclic AMP inhibits hepatoma growth only if there is adequate
cyclic AMP binding (33, 34).

The metabolism and action of cyclic nucleotides can also
be influenced by a number of other endogenous agents, including:
adenylyl cyclase inhibitors (86, 112); phosphodiesterase activators (29, 207); protein kinase modulator (99); calcium (12,
13, 156, 215); polyamines (25, 26, 132); prostaglandins (89)
and fatty acids (19). The latter four agents have been shown

to be altered in tumors (8, 19, 82, 89, 115, 167, 173, 195, 210-212, 216). However, little is currently known about how any of these agents influence cyclic nucleotides in tumors.

In order to ascertain the exact role of cyclic nucleotides in regulating growth of liver and hepatomas it is essential to establish which components of the pleiotypic response (80, 126) are necessary for hepatocyte proliferation and differentiation. Additional information is also required regarding factors known to influence growth of these tissues (56, 57, 62, 105, 141, 146-148).

REFERENCES

1. Allen, D.O., Munshower, J., Morris, H.P., and Weber, G.,
    Cancer Res., 35 (1971) 557.

2. Anderson, K.M., Differentiation, 4 (1975) 197.

3. Anderson, W.B., Johnson, G.S., and Pastan, I., Proc. Natl.
    Acad. Sci., 70 (1973) 1055.

4. Anderson, W.B., and Pastan, I., Advances in Cyclic Nucleo-
    tide Research, 5 (1975) 681.

5. Appleman, M.M., and Terasaki, W.L., Advances in Cyclic
    Nucleotide Research, 5 (1975) 153.

6. Appleman, M.M., Thompson, W.J., and Russell, T.R., Advances
    in Cyclic Nucleotide Research, 3 (1973) 65.

7. Arch. J.R.S., and Newsholme, E.A., Biochem. J., 158 (1976)
    603.

8. Bachrach, U., Biochem. Biophys. Res. Commun., 72 (1976)
    1008.

9. Balhorn, R., Bordwell, J., Sellers, L., Granner, D., and
    Chalkley, R., Biochem. Biophys. Res. Commun., 46 (1972)
    1326.

10. Bär, H.-P., and Hahn, P., Can. J. Biochem. Physiol., 49
    (1971) 85.

11. Bär, H.-P., and Henderson, J.F., Can. J. Biochem., 50 (1972)
    1003.

12. Berridge, M.J., Advances in Cyclic Nucleotide Research, 6
    (1975) 1.

13. Berridge, M.J., J. Cyclic Nucl. Res., 1 (1975) 305.

14. Birnbaumer, L., Pohl, S.L., and Rodbell, M., J. Biol. Chem.,
    246 (1971) 1857.

15. Birnbaumer, L., Pohl, S.L., Rodbell, M., and Sunby, F.,
    J. Biol. Chem., 247 (1972) 2038.

16. Bourne, H.R., Tomkins, G.M., and Dion, S., Science, 181
    (1973) 952.

17. Boyd, H., and Martin, T.J., Mol. Pharmacol., 12 (1976) 195.

18. Boyd, H., Louis, C.J., and Martin, T.J., Cancer Res., 34 (1974) 1720.

19. Bricker, L.A., and Levey, G.S., Biochem, Biophys. Res. Commun., 48 (1972) 362.

20. Brown, H.D., Chattopadhyay, S.K., Morris, H.P., and Pennington, S.N., Cancer Res., 30 (1970) 123.

21. Bucher, N.L.R. and Swaffield, M.N., Proc. Natl. Acad. Sci., 72 (1975) 1157.

22. Bürk, R.R., Nature, 219 (1968) 1271.

23. Butcher, R.W., and Sutherland, E.W., J. Biol. Chem., 237 (1962) 1244.

24. Butcher, F.R., Scott, D.F., Potter, V.R., and Morris, H.P., Cancer Res., 32 (1972) 2135.

25. Byus, C.V., Wicks, W.D., and Russell, D.H., J. Cyclic Nucleotide Res., 2 (1976) 241.

26. Byus, C.V., Costa, M., Sipes, I.G., Brodie, B.B., and Russell, D.H., Proc. Natl. Acad. Sci., 73 (1976) 1241.

27. Chasin, M., and Harris, D.N., Advances in Cyclic Nucleotide Research, 7 (1976) 225.

28. Chayoth, R., Epstein, S.M., and Field, J.B., Cancer Res., 33 (1973) 1970.

29. Cheung, W.Y., Bradham, L.S., Lynch, T.J., Lin, Y.M., and Tallant, E.A., Biochem. Biophys. Res. Commun., 66 (1975) 1055.

30. Chlapowski, F.J., Kelly, L.A., and Butcher, R.W., Advances in Cyclic Nucleotide Research, 6 (1975) 245.

31. Cho-Chung, Y.S., Cancer Res., 34 (1974) 3492.

32. Cho-Chung, Y.S., and Berghoffer, B., Biochem. Biophys. Res. Commun., 60 (1974) 528.

33. Cho-Chung, Y.S., and Clair, T., Biochem. Biophys. Res. Commun., 64 (1975) 768.

34. Cho-Chung, Y.S., and Clair, T., Nature, 265 (1977) 452.

35. Cho-Chung, Y.S., and Gullino, P.M., Science, 183 (1974) 87.

36. Christie, F., and Pawelek, J., Fed. Proc., 35 (1976) 1713.

37. Christoffersen, T., and Berg, T., Biochim. Biophys. Acta,
     381 (1975) 72.

38. Christoffersen, T., Bronstad, G.O., Walstad, P., and Øye,
     I., Biochim, Biophys. Acta, 372 (1974) 291.

39. Christoffersen, T., Morland, J., Osnes, J.B., and Eegjo, K.,
     Biochim. Biophys. Acta, 279 (1972) 363.

40. Christoffersen, T., Morland, J., Osnes, J.B., and Øye, I.,
     Biochim. Biophys. Acta, 313 (1973) 338.

41. Clark, J.F., Morris, H.P., and Weber, G., Cancer Res., 33
     (1973) 356.

42. Coffino, P., Bourne, H.R., Friedrich, U., Hochman, J.,
     Insel, P.A., Lemaire, I., Melmon, K.L., and Tomkins, G.M.,
     Rec. Progr. Horm. Res., 32 (1976) 669.

43. Craven, P.A., and DeRubertis, F.R., Biochim. Biophys.
     Acta, 497 (1977) 415.

44. Criss, W.E., and Morris, H.P., Biochem. Biophys. Res. Commun.,
     54 (1973) 380.

45. Criss, W.E., and Morris, H.P., Enzyme, 20 (1975) 65.

46. Criss, W.E., and Morris, H.P., Cancer Res., 36 (1976)
     1740.

47. Criss, W.E., and Murad, F., Cancer Res., 36 (1976) 1714.

48. Criss, W.E., Murad, F., and Kimura, H., J. Cyclic Nucl.
     Res., 2 (1976) 11.

49. Criss, W.E., Murad, F., Kimura, H., and Morris, H.P., Biochim.
     Biophys. Acta, 445 (1976) 500.

50. D'Armiento, M., Johnson, G.S., and Pastan, I., Proc. Natl.
     Acad. Sci., 69 (1972) 459.

51. DeCrombrugghe, B., Chen, B., Anderson, W.B., Gottesman, M.E.,
     Perlman, R.L., and Pastan, I., J. Biol. Chem. 246 (1971)
     7343.

52. DeRubertis, F.R., Chayoth, R., and Field, J.B., J. Clin.
     Invest., 57 (1976) 641.

53. DeRubertis, F.R., and Craven, P.A., Metabolism, 25 (1976) 1611.

54. DeRubertis, F.R., and Craven, P., J. Clin. Invest., 57 (1977) 435.

55. DeRubertis, F.R., and Craven, P., Cancer Res., 37 (1977) 15.

56. DeWys, W.D., Cancer Res., 32 (1972) 374.

57. Dolan, M.L., Coetzee, M.L., Spangler, M., and Ove, P., Cancer Res., 34 (1974) 3010.

58. Earp, H.S., Smith, D., Ong, S.H.-H., Steiner, A.L., Proc. Natl. Acad. Sci., 74 (1977) 946.

59. Emmelot, P., and Bos, C.J., Biochim. Biophys. Acta, 249 (1971) 285.

60. Farron-Furstenthal, F., Biochem. Biophys. Res. Commun., 67 (1975) 307.

61. Fausto, N., and Butcher, F.R., Biochim. Biophys. Acta, 428 (1976) 702.

62. Fisher, B., Szuch, P., and Fisher, E.R., Cancer Res., 31 (1971) 322.

63. Fishman, P.H., and Brady, R.O., Science, 194 (1976) 906.

64. Flores, J., Witkum, P., and Sharp, G.W.G., J. Clin. Invest., 57 (1976) 450.

65. Friedman, D.L., Physiol. Rev., 56 (1976) 652.

66. Friedman, D.L., Johnson, R.A., and Zeilig, C.E., Advances in Cyclic Nucleotide Research, 7 (1976) 69.

67. Gericke, D., and Chandra, P., Hoppe-Seyler's Z., Physiol. Chem., 350 (1969) 1469.

68. Goldberg, M.L., Burke, G.C., and Morris, H.P., Biochem. Biophys. Res. Commun., 62 (1975) 320.

69. Goldberg, N.D., Haddox, M.K., Nicol, S.E., Glass, D.E., Sanford, C.H., Kuehl, F.A. Jr., Estenson, R., Advances in Cyclic Nucleotide Research, 5 (1975) 307.

70. Goridis, C., and Reutter, W., Nature, 257 (1975) 698.

71. Goridis, C., Zwiller, J., and Reutter, W., Biochem. J., 164 (1977) 33.

72. Granner, D.K., Biochem. Biophys. Res. Commun., 46 (1972) 1516.

73. Granner, D.K., Arch. Biochem. Biophys., 165 (1974) 359.

74. Granner, D.K., Sellers, L., Lee, A., Butters, C., and Kutina, L., Arch. Biochem. Biophys., 169 (1975) 601.

75. Haddox, M.K., Furcht, L.T., Gentry, S.R., Moser, M.E., Stephenson, J.H., and Goldberg, N.D., Nature, 262 (1976) 146.

76. Hammes, G.G., and Rodbell, M., Proc., Natl. Acad. Sci., 73 (1976) 1189.

77. Hanoune, J., Lacombe, M.-L., and Pecker, F., J. Biol. Chem., 250 (1975) 4569.

78. Helson, L., Helson, D., Peterson, R.F., and Das, S.K., J. Natl. Cancer Inst., 57 (1976) 727.

79. Hepp, K.D., Edel, R., and Weiland, O., Eur. J. Biochem., 17 (1970) 171.

80. Hershko, A., Mamont, P., Shields, R., and Tomkins, G.M., Nature, 232 (1971) 206.

81. Hickie, R.A., Jan. S.-H. and Datta, A., Cancer Res., 35 (1975) 596.

82. Hickie, R.A., and Kalant, H., Cancer Res., 27 (1967) 1053.

83. Hickie, R.A., Thompson, W.J., Strada, S.J., Couture-Murillo, B., Morris, H.P., and Robison, G.A., Cancer Res., 37 (1977) (in press, October).

84. Hickie, R.A., Walker, C.M., and Croll, G.A., Biochem. Biophys. Res. Commun., 59 (1974) 167.

85. Hickie, R.A., Walker, C.M., and Datta, A., Cancer Res., 35 (1975) 601.

86. Ho, R.-J., Russell, R.T., Asakawa, T., and Sutherland, E.W., Proc. Natl. Acad. Sci., 72 (1975) 4739.

87. Hochman, J., Insel, P.A., Bourne, H.R., Coffino, P., and Tomkins, G., Proc. Natl. Acad. Sci. 72 (1975) 5051.

88. Hsu, H.H., Proc. Soc. Exp. Biol. Med., 149 (1975) 698.

89. Humes, J.L., and Strausser, H.R., Prostaglandins, 5
     (1974) 183.

90. Johnson, R.A., Pilkis, S.J., and Hamet, P., J. Biol.
     Chem., 250 (1975) 6599.

91. Johnson, R.A., Garbers, D.L., and Pilkis, S.J., J. Supramol.
     Struct., 4 (1976) 205.

92. Keller, R., Life Sci., 11 (1972) 485.

93. Kimura, H., Mittal, C.K., and Murad, F., J. Biol. Chem.,
     250 (1975) 8016.

94. Kimura, H., Mittal, C.K., and Murad, F., J. Biol. Chem.,
     251 (1976) 7769.

95. Kimura, H., and Murad, F., J. Biol. Chem., 250 (1975) 4810.

96. Kimura, H., and Murad, F., Proc. Natl. Acad. Sci., 72
     (1975) 1965.

97. Klein, I., Levey, G.S., Bricker, L.A., and Morris, H.P.,
     Endocrinology, 94 (1974) 279.

98. Koide, Y., Earp, S., Ong, S., and Steiner, A., Fed. Proc.,
     35 (1976) 347.

99. Kuo, J.F., Proc. Natl. Acad. Sci., 71 (1974) 4037.

100. Kuo, J.F., and Greengard, P., J. Biol. Chem., 245 (1970)
     2493.

101. Kuo, J.F., Krueger, B.K., Sanes, J.R., and Greengard, P.,
     Biochim. Biophys. Acta, 212 (1970) 79.

102. Kuo, J.F., Wyatt, G.R., and Greengard, P., J. Biol. Chem.,
     246 (1971) 7159.

103. Lacombe, M.L., Rene, E., Guellaen, G., and Hanoune, J.,
     Nature, 262 (1976) 70.

104. Langan, T.A., Advances in Cyclic Nucleotide Research, 3
     (1973) 99.

105. Lee, J.C.K., Am. J. Pathol., 65 (1971) 347.

106. Leffert, H., Alexander, N.M., Faloona, G., Rubalcava, B.,
     and Unger, R., Proc. Natl. Acad. Sci., 72 (1975) 4033.

107. Leffert, H.L., Koch, K.S., and Rubalcava, B., Cancer Res.,
     36 (1976) 4250.

108. Lefkowitz, R.J., Mukherjee, C., Limbird, L.E., Caron, M.G.,
     Williams, L.T., Alexander, W., Mickey, J.V., and Tate, R.,
     Rec. Progr. Horm. Res., 32 (1976) 597.

109. Letnansky, K., Cell Tissue Kinet., 8 (1975) 423.

110. Leray, F., Chambaut, A.-M., Hanoune, J., Biochem. Biophys.
     Res. Commun., 48 (1972) 1385.

111. Leray, F., Chambaut, A.-M., Perrenoud, M.-L., Hanoune, J.,
     Eur. J. Biochem., 38 (1973) 185.

112. Levey, G.S., Lehotay, D.D., Canterbury, J.M., Bricker, L.A.,
     and Meltz, G.J., J. Biol. Chem., 250 (1975) 5730.

113. Lin, M.C., Salomon, Y., Rendell, M., and Rodbell, M., J.
     Biol. Chem., 250 (1975) 4246.

114. Looney, W.B., Mayo, A.A., Allen, P.M., Morrow, J.Y., and
     Morris, H.P., Brit. J. Cancer, 27 (1973) 341.

115. Looney, W.B., Mayo, A.A., Kovacs, C.J., Hopkins, H.A.,
     Simon, R., and Morris, H.P., Life Sci., 18 (1976) 377.

116. Mackenzie, C.W. III, and Stellwagen, R.H., J. Biol. Chem.,
     249 (1974) 5755.

117. Mackenzie, C.W. III, and Stellwagen, R.H., J. Biol. Chem.,
     249 (1974) 5763.

118. Mackenzie, C.W. III, and Stellwagen, R.H., Arch. Biochem.
     Biophys., 179 (1977) 495.

119. MacManus, J.P., Braceland, B.M., Youdale, T., and Whit-
     field, J.F., J. Cell. Physiol., 82 (1973) 157.

120. MacManus, J.P., Franks, D.J., Youdale, T., and Braceland,
     B.M., Biochem., Biophys, Res. Commun., 49 (1972) 1201.

121. Maganiello, V., and Vaughan, M., Proc. Natl. Acad. Sci.,
     69 (1972) 269.

122. Matusik, R.J., and Hilf, R., J. Nat. Cancer Inst., 56
     (1976) 569.

123. Miller, Z., Lovelace, E., Gallo, M., and Pastan, I.,
     Science, 190 (1975) 1213.

124. Minton, J.P., Matthews, R.H., and Wisenbaugh, T.W., J.
     Natl. Cancer Inst., 57 (1976) 39.

125. Mittal, C.K., Kimura, H., and Murad, F., J. Cyclic Nuc.
     Res., 1 (1975) 261.

126. Miura, Y., and Fukui, N., Adv. Enz. Reg., 14 (1976) 393.

127. Miura, Y., Iwai, H., Sakata, R., Ohtsuka, H., Elhanan,
     E., Kubota, K., and Fukui, N., J. Biochem., 80 (1976) 291.

128. Morris, H.P., In: Handbuch der allgemeinen Pathologie,
     H.-W. Altmann et al., (eds.), Vol. 6, Part 7, Tumors III,
     p. 277, Springer-Verlag, New York, 1975.

129. Morris, H.P., and Meranze, D.R., In: Recent Results in
     Cancer Research: Special Topics in Carcinogensis, E.
     Grundmann (ed.), No. 44, p. 103, Springer-Verlag, New York,
     1974.

130. Morris, H.P., and Wagner, B.P., In: Methods in Cancer
     Research, H. Busch (ed.), Vol. 4, p. 125, Academic Press,
     New York, 1968.

131. Murad, F., Kimura, H., Hopkins, H.A., Looney, W.B., and
     Kovacs, C.J., Science, 190 (1975) 58.

132. Murray, A.W., Froscio, M., and Rogers, A., Biochem. Bio-
     phys. Res. Commun. 71 (1976) 1175.

133. Nambu, Z., and Terayama, H., J. Biochem., 80 (1976) 845.

134. Neethling, A.C., and Shanley, B.C., Lancet, 2 (1976) 578.

135. Nesbitt, J.A. III, Anderson, W.B., Miller, Z., Pastan, I.,
     Russell, T.R., and Gospodarowicz, D., J. Biol. Chem., 251
     (1976) 2344.

136. Nose, K., and Katsuta, H., Biochem, Biophys. Res. Commun.,
     64 (1975) 983.

137. Northup, S.J., Barthel, J.S., Brown, H.D., Chattopadhyay,
     S.K., and Morris, H.P., Mo. Med., 69 (1972) 934.

138. Novak, E., Drummond, G.I., Skala, J., and Hahn, P., Arch.
     Biochem. Biophys., 150 (1972) 511.

139. Okamura, N., and Terayama, H., Biochim. Biophys. Acta, 455 (1976) 297.

140. Otten, J., Johnson, G.S., and Pastan, I., Biochem. Biophys. Res. Commun., 44 (1971) 1192.

141. Paschkis, K.E., Cantarow, A., Stasney, J., and Hobbs, J. H., Cancer Res., I5 (1955) 579.

142. Pastan, I.H., Johnson, G.S., and Anderson, W.B., Ann. Rev. Biochem., 44 (1975) 491.

143. Pastan, I., and Perlman, R.L., Advances in Cyclic Nucleotide Research, 1 (1972) 11.

144. Pennington, S.N., Brown, H.D., Chattopadhyay, S., Conway, C., and Morris, H.P., Experentia, 26 (1970) 139.

145. Perkins, J.P., Advances in Cyclic Nucleotide Research, 3 (1973) 1.

146. Pickart, L., and Thaler, M.M., Nature, 243 (1973) 85.

147. Pickart, L., Thayer, L., and Thaler, M.M., Biochem. Biophys. Res. Commun., 54 (1973) 562.

148. Pliskin, M.E., Cancer Res., 36 (1976) 1659.

149. Pohl, S.L., Birnbaumer, L., and Rodbell, M., Science, 164 (1969) 566.

150. Pohl, S.L., Birnbaumer, L., and Rodbell, M., J. Biol. Chem. 246 (1971) 1849.

151. Pohl, S.L., Krans, H.M.J., Birnbaumer, L., and Rodbell, M., J. Biol. Chem., 247 (1972) 2295.

152. Potter, V.R., and Watanabe, M., In: Proceedings of the International Conference on Leukemia-Lymphoma, C.J.D. Zarafonetis (ed.), p. 33, Lea and Febiger, Philadelphia, 1968.

153. Pradhan, T.K., Criss, W.E., and Morris, H.P., Cancer Biochem. Biophys., 1 (1976) 239.

154. Prasad, K.N., and Sinha, P.K., Differentiation, 6 (1976) 59.

155. Prasad, K.N., Sinha, P.K., Sahu, S.K., and Brown, J.L., Cancer Res., 36 (1976) 2290.

156.   Rasmussen, H., Jensen, P., Lake, W., Friedmann, N., and
        Goodman, D.B.P., Advances in Cyclic Nucleotide Research,
        5 (1975) 375.

157.   Rebhun, L.I., Int. Rev. Cytol., 49 (1977) 1.

158.   Rendell, M., Salomon, Y., Lin, M.C., Rodbell, M., and
        Berman, M., J. Biol. Chem., 250 (1975) 4235.

159.   Rhoads, A.R., Morris, H.P., and West, W.L., Cancer Res.,
        32 (1972) 2651.

160.   Rhoads, A.R., Olowofoyeku, A.K., West, W.L., and Morris,
        H.P., Biochem. Pharmacol. 25 (1976) 97.

161.   Robison, G.A., Butcher, R.W., and Sutherland, E.W., Ann.
        N.Y. Acad. Sci., 139 (1967) 703.

162.   Rodbell, M., Birnbaumer, L., Pohl, S.L., and Krans, H.M.J.,
        J. Biol. Chem., 246 (1971) 1877.

163.   Rodbell, M., Birnbaumer, L., Pohl, S.L., and Sunby, F.,
        Proc. Natl. Acad. Sci., 68 (1971) 909.

164.   Rodbell, M., Krans, M.J., Pohl, S.L., and Birnbaumer, L.,
        J. Biol. Chem., 246 (1971) 1861.

165.   Rodbell, M., Krans, M.J., Pohl, S.L., and Birnbaumer, L.,
        J. Biol. Chem., 246 (1971) 1872.

166.   Rubalcava, B., and Rodbell, M., J. Biol. Chem., 248
        (1973) 3831.

167.   Russell, D.H., Life Sci., 13 (1973) 1635.

168.   Russell, T.R., Terasaki, W.L., and Appleman, M.M., J. Biol.
        Chem., 248 (1973) 1334.

169.   Ryan, W.L., and Heidrick, M.L., Advances in Cyclic Nucleo-
        tide Research 4 (1974) 81.

170.   Salomon, Y., Lin, M.C., Londos, C., Rendell, M., and
        Rodbell, J., J. Biol. Chem., 250 (1975) 4239.

171.   Seifert, W., J. Supramol. Struct. 4 (1976) 279.

172.   Seifert, W., and Rudland, P.S., Nature, 248 (1974) 148.

173.   Selkirk, J.K., Elwood, J.C., and Morris, H.P., Cancer
        Res., 31 (1971) 27.

174. Sharma, R.K., McLaughlin, C.A., and Pitot, H.C., Arch. Biochem. Biophys., 175 (1976) 221.

175. Sharma, R.K., McLaughlin, C.A., and Pitot, H.C., Eur. J. Biochem., 65 (1976) 577.

176. Sheppard, J.R., Proc. Natl. Acad. Sci., 68 (1971) 1316.

177. Sheppard, J.R., Nature, 236 (1972) 14.

178. Shikama, H., and Ui, M., Biochim. Biophys. Acta, 444 (1976) 461.

179. Shima, S., Kawashima, Y., Hirai, M., and Kouyama, H., Biochim. Biophys. Acta, 444 (1976) 571.

180. Short, J., Tsukada, K., Rudert, W.A., and Lieberman, I., J. Biol. Chem., 250 (1975) 3602.

181. Singer, A.L., Sherwin, R.P., Dunn, A.S., and Appleman, M.M., Cancer Res., 36 (1976) 60.

182. Smith, E.E., and Handler, A.H., Res. Commun. Chem. Pathol. Pharmacol., 5 (1973) 863.

183. Srivastava, A.K., and Stellwagen, R.H., Fed. Proc., 35 (1976) 1713.

184. Steinberg, R.A., O'Farrell, P.H., Friedrich, U., and Coffino, P., Cell, 10 (1977) 381.

185. Steiner, A.L., Ong, S.-H., and Wedner, H.J., Advances in Cyclic Nucleotide Research, 7 (1976) 115.

186. Strada, S.J., and Pledger, W.J., In: Cyclic Nucleotides in Disease, B. Weiss (ed.), p. 3, University Park Press, Baltimore, 1975.

187. Strada, S.J., and Thompson, W.J., In: Cyclic Nucleotides: Mechanism of Action, H. Cramer and J. Schultz (eds.), J. Wiley and Sons Ltd., Sussex, England, 1976.

188. Sudilovsky, O., and Gunter, R., Cancer Res., 35 (1975) 1069.

189. Sugden, P.H., and Corbin, J.D., Biochem. J., 159 (1976) 423.

190. Sulakhe, P.V., Sulakhe, S.J., Leung, N.L.-K., St. Louis, P.J., and Hickie, R.A., Biochem. J., 157 (1976) 705.

191. Sulakhe, S.J., and Hickie, R.A., Can. Fed. Proc. 20 (1977) 177.

192. Sulakhe, S.J., Leung, N.L.-K., and Sulakhe, P.V., Biochem. J., 157 (1976) 713.

193. Swislocki, N.I., and Tierney, J., Arch. Biochem. Biophys., 168 (1975) 455.

194. Swislocki, N.I., Tierney, J., and Essner, E.S., Arch. Biochem. Biophys., 174 (1976) 291.

195. Tashjian, A.H., Voelkel, E.F., Goldhaber, P., and Levine, L., Fed. Proc., 33 (1974) 81.

196. Thomas, E.W., Murad, F., Looney, W.B., and Morris, H.P., Biochim. Biophys. Acta, 297 (1973) 564.

197. Thompson, W.J., and Appleman, M.M. J. Biol. Chem., 246 (1971) 3145.

198. Thompson, W.J., and Appleman, M.M., N.Y. Acad. Sci., 185 (1971) 36.

199. Thompson, W.J., and Strada, S.J., In: Hormone Receptors: Peptide Hormones, B.W. O'Malley and L. Birnbaumer (eds.), Vol. II, Academic Press, New York, 1976.

200. Thrower, S., and Ord, M.G., Biochem. J., 144 (1974) 361.

201. Tomasi, V., Réthy, A., and Trevisani, A., Life Sci., 12 (1973) 145.

202. VanInwegen, R.G., Swafford, R.L., Strada, S.J., and Thompson, W.J., Arch. Biochem. Biophys., 178 (1977) 58.

203. VanWijk, R., Wicks, W.D., Bevers, M.M., and VanRijn, J., Cancer Res., 33 (1973) 1331.

204. Vinicor, F., Higdon, G., Clark, J.F., and Clark, C.M., J. Clin. Invest., 58 (1976) 571.

205. Voorhees, J.J., Ann. Rev. Med., 28 (1977) 467.

206. Voorhees, J.J., and Duell, E.A., Advances in Cyclic Nucleotide Research, 5 (1975) 735.

207.   Wang. J.H., Teo, T.S., Ho, H.C., and Stevens, F.C.,
       Advances in Cyclic Nucleotide Research, 5 (1975) 179.

208.   Watson, J., J. Exper. Med., 141 (1975) 97.

209.   Watson, J., J. Immunol., 117 (1976) 1656.

210.   Weber, G., In: The Role of Cyclic Nucleotides in
       Carcinogenesis, J. Schultz and H.G. Gratzner (eds.),
       Vol. 6, p. 57, Academic Press, New York, 1973.

211.   Weber, G., New Eng. J. Med., 296 (1977) 486.

212.   Weber, G., Trevisani, A., and Heinrich, P.C., Adv.
       Enz. Reg., 12 (1974) 11.

213.   Weiss, B., Advances in Cyclic Nucleotides Research, 5
       (1975) 195.

214.   Weiss, B., and Hait, W.N., Ann. Rev. Pharmacol. Toxicol.,
       17 (1977) 441.

215.   Whitfield, J.F., MacManus, J.P., Rixon, R.H., Boynton,
       A.L., Youdale, T., and Swierenga, S., In Vitro, 12 (1976) 1.

216.   Yanagi, S., and Potter, V.R., Life Sci., 20 (1977) 1509.

217.   Zeilig, C.E., and Goldberg, N.D., Proc. Natl. Acad. Sci.,
       74 (1977) 1052.

CYCLIC NUCLEOTIDE METABOLISM IN SOLID TUMOR TISSUES

Wayne E. Criss, Perpetua Muganda, Atul Sahai, and
Harold P. Morris

Department of Biochemistry
Howard University Cancer Research Center
Washington, D.C. 20060

SUMMARY

The examination of the regulation of the system of 3'-5' cyclic nucleotide monophosphates has only begun in cancer tissues. In human cancers, these studies are notably non-existent. However, in animal cancers, especially the Morris hepatomas, enough data has been gathered that, while risky, certain trends seem to begin to appear. Cyclic AMP is constant or lowered, while cyclic GMP is elevated in the fast growing hepatomas. Regulation of adenylate cyclase by protein hormones is reduced, while regulation by epinephrine may be increased. Binding of glucagon is decreased in the fast growing hepatomas. Guanylate cyclase, while being predominantly cytoplasmic in the normal liver, is predominantly membrane bound in the tumors. The liver enzyme is also readily stimulated by several chemical carcinogens. The cyclic GMP phosphodiesterases are decreased in these tumors; while the cAMP phosphodiesterases are increased. Although the cyclic nucleotide dependent protein kinases (histone as substrate) are altered in the hepatomas, observations of unique cyclic nucleotide binding proteins or cAMP independent protein kinases in cancer tissues may be of even greater significance for the development of or the maintenance of the neoplastic state of cells.

INTRODUCTION

The 3', 5' - cyclic forms of AMP and GMP, perhaps also CMP and UMP, are quite ubiquitous in nature and have been observed in extracellular fluids and tissues from both eukaryotes and prokaryotes. They seem to have a very general distribution in most mammalian cells where their concentrations can be altered with a wide variety of

polypeptide hormones, neurohormones, prostaglandins, and Ca^{2+}.
Levels of these cyclic nucleotides in extracellular fluids of man,
particularly in urine and plasma, have proved useful in diagnosing
some disorders and in studying the pathaphysiological states of
tissues (8, 10, 23, 36, 49, 66-67, 92-95, 139, 141, 159). Altered
levels of cyclic AMP and cyclic GMP have been observed in tissues
or in the urine of animals or patients with hyperparathyroidism
(67, 92, 95, 139), ectopic PTH-secreting tumors (67, 92), hepatomas
(36, 93, 141), renal adenomas and sarcomas (36), tumors associated
with the syndrome of inappropriate antidiuretic hormone secretion,
and Cushing's disease (159). The purpose of this manuscript is to
examine the cyclic nucleotide system in cancer, specifically in the
Morris hepatomas.

Preliminary to any such examination of cyclic nucleotide metabolism in cancer requires a brief statement of the current status
of the cyclic nucleotide components of this (or these) systems.
(Figure 1). Specific membrane receptors (for polypeptide hormones,
neurohormones, prostaglandins, drugs and several intracellular metabolites such as GTP and Ca) interact through the membrane structural
framework to effect the activity of adenylate cyclase and guanylate
cyclase. These cyclases convert ATP or GTP to cyclic AMP or cyclic
GMP, respectively. The cyclic nucleotides are hydrolized to their
corresponding non-cyclic nucleotide 5' - monophosphates by phosphodiesterases; or, the cyclic nucleotides interact with cyclic nucleotide binding proteins to allow activation of certain protein kinases.
The protein kinases phosphorylate a wide range of specific proteins.
Phosphorylation of these proteins results in the initiation or the
termination of specific intercellular biological functionings, from
membrane transport to genomic transcription. Extracellular substances (e.g. hormones) thus directly effect intracellular functioning. Many cancer cells have lost their capacity to respond to extracellular stimuli (e.g. hormones). And since the regulatability of
cyclic AMP and cyclic GMP involves this response capacity which
includes processes of cellular growth and differentiation, any modifications in the cyclic nucleotide system would directly effect the
cell's ability to grow and/or differentiate, including the cellular
state which we call cancer.

TISSUE CONCENTRATION OF CYCLIC NUCLEOTIDES

A number of recent studies have pointed to important roles for
3', 5' - cyclic AMP and 3', 5' - cyclic GMP in several experimental
cancer systems. Several labs have shown that addition of cyclic
AMP or its derivaties to cultured malignant cells will "seemingly"
restore these cells to "normal:"(60-63, 83, 151). Similarly, in
animals, solid and ascites tumor growth can be greatly reduced or
even inhibited if the animals are treated with certain derivatives
of the cyclic nucleotides (29, 30, 32).

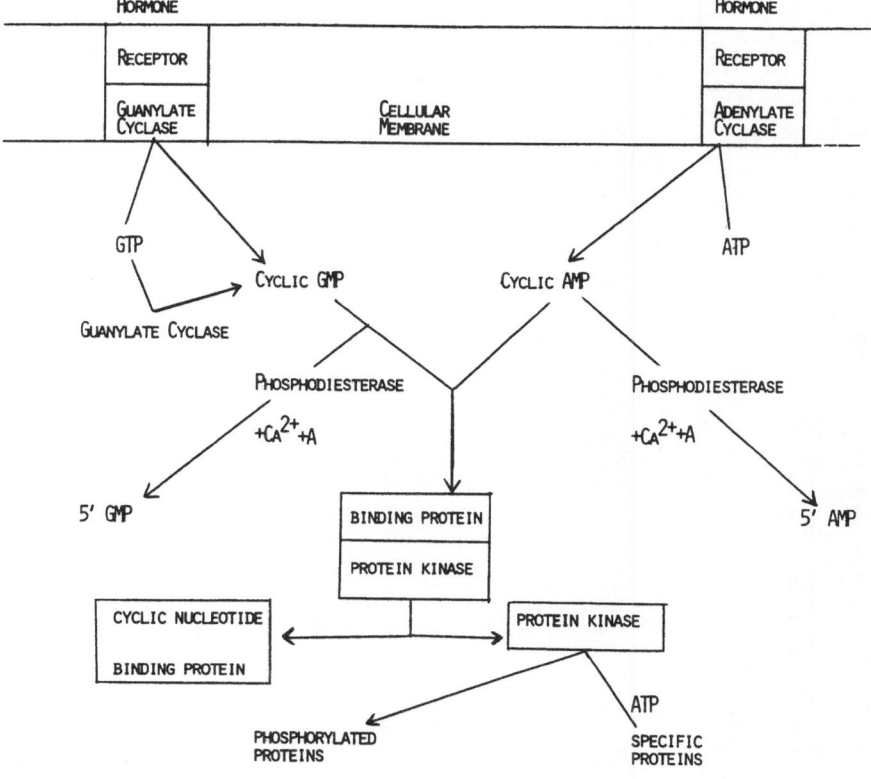

Figure 1
Cyclic nucleotide action in normal tissues.

It has been postulated that cyclic AMP and cyclic GMP may exert
a portion of their biological actions upon metabolic systems which
are in opposition (i.e. cellular differentiation versus cell division; see refs. 50-53, 76, 91, 116, 154, 157). Indeed the in vivo
cyclic GMP:cyclic AMP ratio has been observed to be increased in
numerous proliferating cell systems (See Tables 1 and 2). The levels
of both of these cyclic nucleotides are influenced by hormones and
numerous pharmacological agents in mammalian cells. Therefore,
regulation of the in vivo levels of the cyclic nucleotides may

Table One

In Situ Levels of Cyclic AMP and Cyclic GMP in Normal and Neoplastic Rat Tissues (Reprinted from Criss & Murad, Ref.37)

Tissue	pmoles/mg protein		Cyclic GMP	
	Cyclic AMP	Cyclic GMP	Cyclic AMP Ratio	
Normal Liver	3.50	0.11	0.03	0.04
Liver of Hepatoma Bearing Rats	3.50	0.09	0.03	
Normal Kidney Cortex	8.01	0.32	0.04	
Slow Growing Tumors				
Hepatoma 16	8.30	0.26	0.03	
Hepatoma 9633F	5.11	0.39	0.08	
Hepatoma 20	4.00	0.19	0.05	0.06
Hepatoma 21	6.30	0.50	0.08	
Hepatoma 9633	6.64	0.51	0.08	
Intermediate Growing Tumors				
Hepatoma 7800	11.00	0.56	0.05	
Hepatoma 9121	9.94	0.38	0.04	
Hepatoma 7316B	11.11	0.45	0.04	0.08
Kidney Sarcoma (MK2)	5.10	0.70	0.14	
Kidney Adenoma (MK3)	4.50	0.55	0.12	
Fast Growing Tumors				
Hepatoma 7288ctc	8.41	2.50	0.30	
Hepatoma 9618A2	5.10	0.99	0.19	
Hepatoma 5123tc	8.80	0.88	0.10	0.71
Hepatoma 3924A	9.86	22.40	2.27	

Table Two
Proliferating Systems with
Altered Cyclic Nucleotide Levels

System	Change Reported	Reference
Confluent Fibroblasts	Increased cAMP	91, 116, 123
Proliferating Fibroblasts	Increased cGMP	91, 116, 123
Proliferating Fibroblasts	Decreased cAMP	98
Viral Transformed Fibroblasts	No change in cGMP (resting/proliferation)	52, 91, 116
Renal Hypertrophy	Increased cGMP	118
Proliferating Epidermal Cells	Increased cGMP	154
Proliferating Lymphocytes	Increased cGMP	52
Regenerating Liver	Increased cGMP	89
Neonatal Kidney	Increased cGMP/cAMP Ratio	118
Immature Testis	Increased cGMP/cAMP Ratio	133
Primary Liver Tumors	Increased cGMP	43
Transplantable Liver Tumors	Increased cGMP	39, 50
Transplantable Kidney Tumors	Increased cGMP	37, 38
Adenocarcinoma of Human Colon	Increased cGMP/cAMP Ratio	42
Adenocarcinoma of Rat Colon	Decreased cAMP	79
Growing Cells of Plants	Have highest level of cGMP	56
Sporulation in Bacteria	Increased cGMP	131

occur through alterations of synthesis, hydrolysis, intracellular
binding, and cellular extrusion. Studies with the Morris hepatomas
(39, 50), proliferating cell systems of lymphocytes (50-52), epider-
mal tissues (76, 153 -154, 157), and fibroblasts (91, 116, 123)
support the concept that these two cyclic nucleotides do promote
opposing regulatory influences that may directly involve cellular
growth processes. It is obvious that these regulatory influences
are quite complex.

In addition to 3', 5' - cyclic AMP and 3', 5' - cyclic GMP,
other cyclic nucleotides have been identified. Cytidine 3', 5' -
monophosphate (cyclic CMP) has been observed in leukemia cells and
in the urine of leukemia patients (13). It has been postulated
to play a role in regulating the growth of these cells (15). The
same laboratory has also identified uridine 3', 5' - monophosphate
(cyclic UMP) in rat liver and in the urine of leukemia patients
(14). After future confirmation of their existence in several tissues and bodily fluids, the regulatory roles of these latter two
cyclic nucleotides and their relationship to the neoplastic state
will have to be elucidated.

ADENYLATE CYCLASE ACTIVITY AND ITS REGULATION BY HORMONES

Adenylate cyclase activity is associated with various membrane
structures of the cell, although there have been reports of "soluble"
adenylate cyclase activity in Yoshida ascites hepatoma cells (146)
and in rat testis (18). The membrane bound adenylate cyclase systems in most mammalian cells are modulated by biogenic amines, polypeptide hormones, guanine nucleotides, halides, the calcium ion, and
prostaglandins. Thus adenylate cyclase activity is highly regulatory
and must be considered an important aspect of the cell's regulatory
control mechanisms. It is probable that these adenylate cyclase
systems are composed of membrane elements which include specific
receptors for each of the above listed modulators, enzymatic catalytic units which are capable of converting ATP to cyclic AMP, and
some form of transducing elements which allow or disallow the interaction of the modulator-receptor complexes with the catalytic units
(45, 58, 99, 109, 111-112).

Several laboratories have examined the adenylate cyclase systems
in pre-neoplastic and neoplastic cells and tissues. Pre-neoplastic
or hyperplastic liver tissue from rats which have been fed 3'-methyl-
4-dimethylamino-azobenzene (16-17), ethionine (24), or acetylaminofluorene (25-27), showed modified responses to glucagon, epinephrine,
and prostaglandins. In general, it appears that glucagon responsiveness decreases and epinephrine responsiveness increases during the
course of neoplasia. SV40 transformed WI-38 cells has low basal
adenylate cyclase activities when compared to non-transformed WI-38,
but their adenylate cyclase was hyper-responsive to catecholamines,

adenosine, and prostaglandins (68); while sarcoma virus transformed cells showed decreased adenylate cyclase activity and were non-responsive to prostaglandin E_1(4). One study found that HeLa and hepatoma (HTC) cells had adenylate cyclases stimulatable by glucagon, epinephrine, or prostaglandins; while the cyclases from Chang's liver cells and fibroblast cell lines L929 and 3T3 responded well to catecholamines and prostaglandins (82). Adenylate cyclases from normal adrenal cells responded to ACTH by producing cortisone while the adrenocortical carcinoma 494 did not synthesize cortisone upon ACTH stimulation (20). Yet this same adrenocortical carcinoma con-tained an adenylate cyclase which had multiple hormone responsiveness, including ACTH (120). The sensitivity of the adenylate cyclase system to neurotransmitters and divalent ions, and the sensitivity of prostaglandin E_1 stimulated activity to GTP increased in malignant neuroblastoma cells which were induced to differentiate with cyclic AMP (105). Neoplastic thyroid nodules were reported to have increas-ed basal activity and showed hyper-responsiveness to thyroid stimulat-ing hormone (44, 48). We observed that liver tissue contained a mem-brane adenylate cyclase which was stimulated by glucagon, epinephrine, guanine nucleotides, fluoride, and prostaglandins; fast growing hep-atomas contained a membrane adenylate cyclase which was lower in basal activity and which was decreased or had no response to glucagon and modified responses to several prostaglandins (33-34, 102, Table 3). Thus, there would appear to be a wide variation in the ability of tumor adenylate cyclase systems to respond to various hormones and modulators. It is not known whether these modified character-istics reflect changes in the individual components of the hormonal-ly responsive membrane bound adenylate cyclase systems.

We observed the following trends in the fast growing Morris hep-atomas, in comparison to normal liver tissue: 1. increased levels of cGMP; 2. decreased stimulation by glucagon; 3. decreased binding by glucagon; 4. widely variable stimulation by prostaglandins; 5. fully intact responses to both fluoride and Gpp(NH)p; 6. decreased and altered activity of the basal catalytic unit; 7. altered com-ponent relationships within the membrane.

GUANYLATE CYCLASE ACTIVITY

Guanylate cyclase activity is distributed throughout all mamma-lian cells. It is associated with all membrane fractions and is also found to be soluble in the cytoplasm (57, 61, 71-74). The soluble and membrane bound (particulate) guanylate cyclases differ with re-spect to their activation and inhibition by Triton X-100, Ca^{2+}, ATP, mercurial reagents and by oxidation as with sodium azide; they also have different molecular weights (70-75, 136). The basal activities and subcellular distribution of both forms of guanylate cyclase are tissue specific. Ratios of particulate to soluble guanylate activity were altered in the liver during development and regeneration(37,88,89).

Table Three

Stimulation of Adenylate Cyclase and
Binding of Glucagon to Membranes from Liver and
Hepatoma Tissue
(Reprinted from Criss&Murad, Reference 37)

	Enzymatic Activity (nmoles/10 min/mg)					PGA_1	PGE_1	125 I-Glucagon Binding (pm/mg)
	basal	+Fl	+Epi	+Gluc	+Gpp(NH)p			
Normal Adult Liver	0.6	3.5	0.7	3.1	3.3	0.8	1.2	0.72
Slow Growing Hepatomas								
20	0.06	0.44	0.06	0.21	0.40	0.08	0.12	0.01
21	0.08	0.98	0.11	0.35	0.84	0.10	0.15	0.15
Intermediate Growing								
Hepatomas 9633F	0.3	2.0	0.3	0.4	0.6	0.4	0.05	0.06
Fast Growing Hepatomas								
3924A	0.1	2.8	0.1	0.2	2.3	0.1	0.02	0.01
7777	0.2	2.0	0.3	0.2	0.7	0.3	0.04	0.02
5124tc	0.5	4.9	0.6	1.2	2.3	0.3	0.05	0.04
9618A2	0.4	3.0	0.4	0.4	1.3	0.3	0.04	0.01

We recently separated and characterized the guanylate cyclase activities from Morris liver and kidney tumors and compared them with the guanylate cyclase activities from normal adult liver and kidney tissues (37-39. See Table 4). The total basal homogenate guanylate cyclase activities were lower in all tumors when compared to corresponding normal tissues. The soluble form of guanylate cyclase was predominant in the liver tissues, while the particulate form predominated in the tumor tissues. Comparisons of particulate enzymes from these normal and neoplastic tissues and comparison of soluble enzymes from these normal and neoplastic tissues indicated that the tumor guanylate cyclases were less able to utilize Mg^{2+} at low Mn^{2+} concentrations, were less stimulatable by Triton X-100, and apparently were not as stimulatable by azide (or nitrosamine) oxidation process. Ca^{2+} activation of the soluble enzymes and inhibition of the particulate enzymes, as well as the greater susceptibility of the soluble enzymes to be inhibited by ATP, was similar in guanylate cyclases from normal or neoplastic tissues. It is, therefore, possible that the observed elevated levels of cyclic GMP in these tumors may be related to the increased activity of the particulate form of guanylate cyclase. (Also recently observed in primary liver tumors - Ref. 43).

Subsequent studies in several research labs (43, 152, including our own lab, Ref 40 and Table 5) indicate that guanylate cyclase, or certain components of the cGMP system, are regulated by several chemical carcinogens such as nitrosamines (e.g., hydroxylamine, dibutylnitrosamine, dimethylnitrosourea, diethylnitrosamine and nitrosopiperidine) such that elevated levels of cGMP are observed when tissue extracts are incubated with these carcinogens. This could reflect the potential in vivo activation of guanylate cyclase by a variety of carcinogens.

Phosphodiesterases

Cyclic nucleotide phsophodiesterases occur in all biological systems which have cyclic nucleotides. Cyclic nucleotide phosphodiesterase activity is observed to be both membrane associated and soluble in most mammalian cells (3). It exists in multiple molecular forms which differ in substrate specificities (9, 64, 142-143), substrate affinities (101, 134, 143), heat and cation sensitivities (64, 96, 117) chromatographic and electrophoretic mobilities (107, 143), sensitivities to various inhibitors (2, 3, 130), subcellular location (110, 119, 142), and also possibly in physiological function (47, 122). There would appear to be two major forms of cyclic nucleotide phosphodiesterase activity in most tissues, high Km (10^{-4}M) and low KM (10^{-6}M) forms. Also both cyclic AMP and cyclic GMP phosphodiesterases exist in cells (2-3, 103, 122, 130). There may be interconversion of the high and low Km enzymes; and macromolecular activators and inhibitors of phosphodiesterase activity have been

Table Four

Subcellular Distribution of
Guanylate Cyclase Activities in Normal and Neoplastic Tissues
(Reprinted from Criss, Murad and Kimura, Ref 39)

| | Cyclic GMP Formed (nmoles/min/g tissue) | | Particulate: Soluble Ratio |
	Particulate	Soluble	
Normal Adult Liver	0.6	2.5	0.24
Normal Adult Kidney	0.9	1.8	0.50
Slow Growing Tumors			
Hepatoma 20	1.2	0.5	2.40
Hepatoma 21	1.8	0.9	2.00
Intermediate Growing Tumors			
Hepatoma 9633F	1.3	0.5	2.60
Kidney Sarcoma (MK2)	0.6	0.5	1.20
Kidney Adenoma (MK3)	0.7	0.7	1.00
Fast Growing Tumors			
Hepatoma 3924A	1.3	0.4	3.25
Hepatoma 9618A2	0.8	0.6	1.33

Table Five

In Vitro Activation of Liver Guanylate
Cyclase by Several Chemical Carcinogens*

Tissue Extracts	Cyclic GMP Formed (pmoles/min/mg protein)
Liver (soluble enzyme) - no additions to assay	32.1
+ 5 x 10^{-4}M azide	164.6
+ 2 x 10^{-3}M hydroxylamine	151.9
+ 2 x 10^{-3}M dibutylnitrosamine	128.6
+ 5 x 10^{-3}M nitrosopiperidine	187.2
+ 5 x 10^{-4}M diethylnitrosamine	211.9
+ 5 x 10^{-4}M methyl-nitro-nitrosguanidine	226.1

*Includes unpublished data from our laboratories.

-Experiments were performed with guanylate cyclase prepared
from the soluble portion of normal rat liver homogenates. Methods
have been previously published, Ref39.

described (5-6, 28, 65, 87, 140). In addition, the levels of phosphodiesterase activity are affected by hormones (6, 11, 144, 150).
Therefore, breakdown of cyclic AMP and cyclic GMP by mammalian cell
phosphodiesterase hydrolysis is accomplished by a complex and inter-
concerted set of mechanisms.

Phosphodiesterase activity has been examined in cultured astro-
cytoma cells (149-150),neuroblastoma cells (77, 103, 106, 149),
Krebs 2 ascites tumor cells (121), Mouse L cells (121), hyperplastic liver nodules (24), Novikoff and Morris hepatomas (31, 35,
59, 108, 121), and an adrenocortical carcinoma (124). Total cyclic
AMP phosphodiesterase activity in whole homogenates was decreased
in both hepatomas and in the adrenocortical carcinoma tissues when
compared with normal liver and adrenal tissues, respectively. In
hepatoma tissues we observed a large decrease in the high Km form
and a small increase in the low Km form of cyclic AMP phosphodiesterase. The normal adrenal and adrenal tumor contained only one
form of the enzyme which hydrolized cyclic AMP and cyclic GMP at
about the same rate.

In the fast growing Morris hepatomas, we recently observed decreased hydrolysis of cyclic AMP (Tables 6 and 7). We have found
the following trends in the fast growing Morris hepatomas, in comparison to normal liver tissue: 1. increased levels of cyclic AMP
(0.4 uM) phosphodiesterase activity; 2. decreased levels of cyclic
GMP (0.4 uM) phosphodiesterase activity; 3. increased responsiveness by the cyclic AMP enzyme to Ca^{2+} and the PDE activator; 4. increased total levels and an increased soluble:particulate ratio of
the phosphodiesterase activator. Also, one recent manuscript which
examined phosphodiesterase activity in normal and viral transformed
fibroblasts showed decreased capacity of the transformed cells to
hydrolize cyclic GMP (81). Therefore, it is quite likely that these
tumor cells may have increased capacity to hydrolize cyclic AMP and
decreased capacity to hydrolize cyclic GMP.

Cyclic Nucleotide Binding Proteins and Protein Kinases

A large number of physiological processes are modulated by the
enzymatic phosphorylation of proteins. Some of these phsophorylation
reactions require protein kinases that are activated by cyclic AMP
and/or cyclic GMP, and some are independent of cyclic nucleotide concentrations (19, 90, 97, 114, 137-138, 155). The postulated enzymatic model for the cyclic AMP dependent protein kinase is:

$$[R_2C_2 \quad + \quad 2 \quad cAMP \longrightarrow R_2(cAMP)_2 + 2C]$$

(inactive)   (active)

The native inactive enzyme is composed of two cyclic nucleotide

Table Six
Cyclic Nucleotide Phosphodiesterase
Activity in Normal Liver and in Hepatoma
Tissue* *

(Percent change)*

Tissue	Addition	0.4 uM cAMP		0.4 uM cGMP	
		sup	pellet	sup	pellet
Hepatoma 3924A	Ca+ Activator	+400	+620	+0	−40
Hepatoma 3924A	EGTA	+540	+670	−75	−10

Table Seven
Level of Phosphodiesterase Activator
Protein in Normal Liver and Hepatoma**

(Percent change)*

Tissue	sup	pellet	sup/pellet
Hepatoma 3924A	+430	−80	+500

*   Compared to normal rat liver as control.

**   Summarized from "Phosphodiesterase and Its Ca^{2+} Dependent
Modulator Protein in Morris Hepatoma Tissues" by K. Uenishi,
S. Kakiuchi, W. Criss, Y. Takai In: Second Cyclic AMP Con-
ference of Japan; soon to be translated and published in
English.

binding subunits (R) and two catalytic subunits (C). Cyclic AMP
causes disassociation of the binding subunits and catalytic subunits
by binding to the former subunits. The "free" catalytic subunits
then enzymatically catalyze the phosphorylation of substrate proteins. MgATP and a heat stable protein modulator (7, 46, 55, 155)
decrease the affinity of the catalytic subunits for the regulatory
subunits of the cyclic AMP dependent protein kinase. Activation
of the cyclic GMP dependent enzyme apparently (physiology) does not
require any disassociation of binding protein and catalytic subunit.
In all, proteins which are located in the plasma membranes, ribosomes,
cytoplasm, and chromosomes serve as substrate proteins for the
various protein kinase catalyzed phosphorylations (22, 69, 78, 80,
86, 115, 135, 137-138, 155-156, 197).

    The cyclic nucleotide binding proteins and the independent and
cyclic nucleotide dependent protein kinase systems have been examined
in normal and viral transformed thymic fibroblasts (147), normal and
malignant glicoma cells (1), neuroblastoma cells (104) Ehrlich ascites
tumor cells (113), HeLa cells (12), hepatoma cells (54, 85-95, 100),
Walker 256 carcinoma cells (132), adrenocortical carcinoma (125-126,
129), and Morris hepatomas (33, 41). The studies with Ehrlich ascites
tumor cells and HeLa tumor cells both show a complete loss of cyclic
AMP responsive protein kinase activities. Fractionation of cyclic
AMP binding activity and protein kinase activity from rat liver,
several Morris hepatomas, and a hepatoma cell line (HTC) revealed
that the tumors did not contain certain cyclic AMP responsive protein
kinase fractions which were found in the liver tissue. A part of
this deficiency was attributed to the absence of specific cyclic nucleotide binding proteins (84, 127-128). Purification and comparison
of the cyclic AMP responsive protein kinase from rat adrenal tissue
and from an adrenocortical carcinoma indicated that there was a decreased responsiveness to cyclic AMP and altered protein substrate
specificity in the tumor system (125, 129). We have recently observed that the cyclic GMP dependent protein kinase (histone as substrate) is reduced in Morris hepatomas (Table 8) and a unique polylysine stimulated, self phosphorylating protein kinase could be
isolated from the fast growing hepatomas (41, Table 9). The latter
protein kinase was independent of cyclic nucleotides. It is thus
quite possible that neoplastic tissues may have modified cyclic nucleotide binding proteins and protein kinase activities which could
lead to altered regulation of cellular functioning. However, much
information is necessary before these specific points of regulations
can be evaluated in cancer tissue.

INTERPRETATION

    Considering the numerous publications on the cyclic nucleotide
system in various tissues, it is surprising that there are relatively
few reports that have exmained the cyclic nucleotide systems in solid

<u>Table Eight</u>

<u>Cyclic Nucleotide Dependent Protein
Kinases in Normal and Neoplastic Tissues</u>*

	^{32}Pi incorporated/mg (cpm)
Normal Rat Liver	
cAMP Dependent	4,900
cGMP Dependent	2,800
Normal Rat Kidney	
cAMP Dependent	3,600
cGMP Dependent	2,150
Morris Hepatoma 3924A	
cAMP Dependent	5,100
cGMP Dependent	4,220
Morris Kidney Tumor-MK3	
cAMP Dependent	3,800
cGMP Dependent	3,100

*Includes unpublished data from our laboratories.
These studies will be published by Criss and Morris in Cancer Res.
Histone was used as substate in all assays.

Table Nine

Unique Polylysine Stimulated
Protein Kinase from Morris Hepatoma
3924A*

Substance (10µg)	^{32}Pi incorporated/mg (cpm)
None	800
Polylysine	7,900
Polyarginine	4,300
H_1 histone	8,900
H_{2A} histone	1,400
H_{2B} histone	2,000
H_3 histone	2,800
H_4 histone	2,400
Protamine	6,700
Spermine (3mM)	3,700
Spermidine (3mM)	1,400

*Includes data from our laboratories
These studies will soon be published by Criss, Takai, Kishimoto,
Inoue, Yamamato, and Nishizuka in Cancer Research.
No exogenous substrate was added to assay medium (See Ref 41).

tumors (see our recent review 37). Most of these reports are limited to a few select tumors in laboratory animals. From these reports it is difficult to delienate specific and consistent trends. However, some generalizations may be attempted. There does appear to be an increase in the ratio of cyclic GMP to cyclic AMP levels in several cancer tissues. Such changes in the in vivo levels of these two cyclic nucleotides could result from alterations in synthesis, hydrolysis, intracellular binding, or from cellular excretion. Synthesis of cyclic GMP may be reflective of an increase in membrane bound guanylate cyclase and/or an alteration of its properties and regulation. There is altered regulation of adenylate cyclase activity in tumors by various agents; the apparent trend is toward decreased activation of adenylate cyclase by the polypeptide hormones. Hydrolysis of cyclic nucleotides by the several phosphodiesterases and Ca-modulator indicates that these hydrolytic activities for cyclic GMP may be low in tumors while cyclic AMP is probably hydrolized at increased rates. It is also quite likely that neoplastic tissues have a unique "set" of cyclic nucleotide binding proteins and protein kinases which may directly influence numerous metabolic functions, from membrane transport to genomic expression. Obviously, much information is needed before one can begin to determine "essential" macromolecular lesions within the cyclic nucleotide systems of solid tumor tissues. Hopefully, the variability in the reported alterations of the cyclic nucleotide systems will prepare us for the even more complex analysis of data derived from human tumors, which to date is noticeably non-existent.

In summation, the solid tumors of the Morris hepatoma system have elevated levels of cyclic GMP which is a result of increased synthesis and decreased hydrolysis. Regulation of the synthesis of cyclic AMP is diminished and its hydrolysis is increased. The tumors contain unique cyclic nucleotide binding proteins and protein kinases (Fig 2).

ACKNOWLEDGEMENTS

This research was supported in part by grants NIH-CA11818 and 507-RR05361. WEC was the recipient of an Eleanor Roosevelt-American Cancer Society International Award and an NIH Research Career Development Award CA-70187.

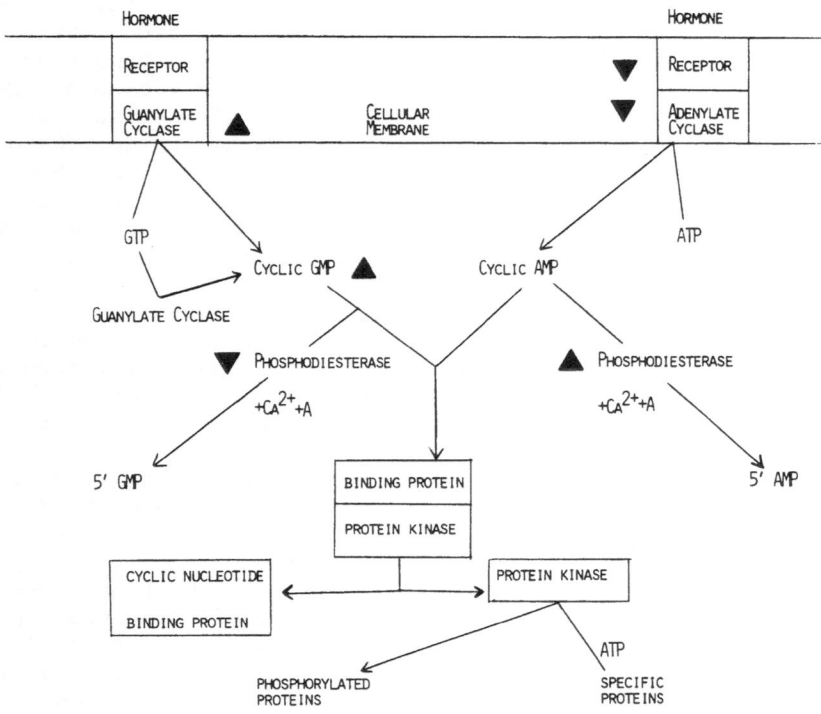

Figure 2
Cyclic nucleotide system in rapidly growing Morris hepatomas.

REFERENCES

1. Agren, C., and Ronquist, G. Acta Physiol. Scand. 92 (1974) 430.

2. Amer. M.S. Amer. J. Dig. Dis. 17 (1972) 945.

3. Amer. M.S., and Kreighbaum, W.E. J. Pharm. Sci. 64 (1975) 1.

4. Anderson, W.B., Gallo, M., and Pastan, I. J. Biol. Chem. 249 (1974) 7041.

5. Appleman, M.M., Thompson, W.J., and Russell, T.R. Adv. Cyclic Nucleo. Res. 3 (1973) 65.

6. Appleman, M.M., Thompson, W.J., and Russell, T.R. Adv. Cyclic Nucleo. Res. (1973) 99.

7. Ashby, C.D., and Walsh, D.A. J. Biol. Chem. 248 (1973) 1255.

8. Ball, J.H., Kaminsky, N.I., Hardman, J.G., Broadus. A.F., Sutherland, E.W., and Liddle, G.W. Man. J. Clin. Invest. 51 (1972) 2124.

9. Beavo, J.A., Hardman, J.G., and Sutherland, E.W. J. Biol. Chem. 245 (1970) 5649.

10. Bernstein, R.A., Linarelli, L., Facktor, M.A., Friday, G.A., Drash, A. and Fireman, P.J. Allergy Clin. Immunol. 49 (1972) 86.

11. Berridge, M.J. Adv. Cyclic Nucleo. Res. 6 (1975) 1.

12. Blanchard, J.M., DucampCn., and Jeanteur, Ph. Nature 253 (1975) 467.

13. Bloch, A. Biochem. Biophys. Res. Comm. 5 (1974) 659.

14. Bloch, A. Biochem. Biophys. Res. Comm. 64 (1975) 210.

15. Bloch, A. Dutschman, G., and Maue, R. Biochem. Biophys. Res. Comm. 59 (1974) 955.

16. Boyd, H., Louis, C.J., and Martin, T.J. Cancer Res. 34 (1974) 1720.

17. Boyd, H., and Martin, T.J. Molecular Pharm. 12 (1976) 195.

18. Braun, T., and Dods, R.F. Proc. Natl. Acad. Sci., USA 72 (1975) 1907.

19. Brostrom, C.O., Corbin, J.C., King, C.A., and Krebs, E.G. Proc. Natl. Acad. Sci. USA, 68 (1971) 2444.

20. Brush, J.S., Sutliff, L.S., and Sharma, R.K. Cancer Res. 34 (1974) 1495.

21. Burdon, R.H., and Pearce, C.A. Biochim. Biophys. Acta. 246 (1971) 561.

22. Chang, K-J, Marcus, N.A., and Cuatrecases, P. J. Biol. Chem. 249 (1974) 6854.

23. Chase, L.R., Melson, G.L., and Aurbach, G.D. J. Clin. Invest. 48 (1969) 1832.

24. Chayoth, R., Epstein, S.M., and Field, J.B. Cancer Res. 33 (1973) 1970.

25. Christoffersen, T., and Berg, T., Biochim. Biophys. Acta 381 (1975) 72.

26. Christoffersen, T., Moreland, J., Osnes, J.B., and Elgjo, K. Biochim. Biophys. Acta 279 (1972) 363.

27. Christoffersen, T., and Oye, I. Acta Endocrinologica, Suppl. 191, 77 (1974) 67.

28. Cheung, W.Y. J. Biol. Chem. 246 (1971) 2859.

29. Cho-chung, Y.S. Biochem. Biophys. Res. Comm. 60 (1974) 528.

30. Cho-Chung, Y.S. Cancer Res. 34 (1974) 3492.

31. Clark, J.F., Morris, H.P., and Weber, G. Cancer Res. 33 (1973) 356.

32. Cotton, F.A., Gillen, R.G., Gohil, R.N., Hazen, E.E., Kirchner, C.R., Nagvary, J., Rouse, J.P., Stanislowski, A.G., Stevens, J.D., and Tucker, P.W., Proc. Natl. Acad. Sci., U.S.A. 72 (1975) 1335.

33. Criss, W.E., and Morris, H.P. Biochem. Biphys. Res. Comm. 54 (1973) 380.

34. Criss, W.E., and Morris, H.P., Cancer Res. 36 (1976) 1740.

35. Criss, W.E., and Morris, H.P. Enzyme 20 (1975) 65.

36. Criss, W.E., and Murad, F. Cancer Res. 36 (1976) 1714.

37. Criss, W.E., and Murad, F. <u>Clinical Aspects of Cyclic Nu-
     cleotides</u>, ed. by L. Volicer, Spectrum Publications, N.Y.
     (1977) p. 350.

38. Criss, W.E., and Murad, F. J. Cyclic Nucleotide Res. 2 (1976)11.

39. Criss, W.E., Murad, F., and Kimura, H. Biochim. Biophys. Acta
     445 (1976) 500.

40. Criss, W.E., and Pradhan, T.K. Proc. Amer, Assoc. Cancer Res.
     18 (1977) 3.

41. Criss, W.E., Takai, Y., Kishimoto, A., Inoue, M., and
     Nishizuka, Y. Fed. Amer. Soc. Exptl. Biol. 36 (1977) 690.

42. DeRubertis, F.R., Chayoth, R., and Field, J.B. J. Clin.
     Invest. 57 (1976) 641.

43. DeRubertis, F.R., and Craven, P. Cancer Res. 37:15, 1977.

44. DeRubertis, F.R., Yamashita, K., Dekker, A., Larsen, P.R.,
     and Field, J.B. J. Clin. Invest. 51 (1972) 1109.

45. DeRubertis, F.R., Zenser, T.V., and Curnow, R.T. Endocrinol.
     95 (1974) 93.

46. Donnoley, T.E., Kuo, J.F., Reyes, P.L., Lui, Y.P., and Greengard,
     P. J. Biol. Chem. 248 (1973) 190.

47. Farber, D.B., and Lolley, R.N. J. Neurochem. 21 (1973) 817.

48. Field, J.B., Larsen, P.R., Yamashita, K., Mashiter, K., and
     Dekkar, A. J. Clin. Invest. 52 (1973) 1973.

49. Fichman, M., and Brooker, G. Clin. Res. 18 (1970) 121.

50. Goldberg, M.L., Burke, G.C., and Morris, H.P. Biochem. Biophys.
     Res. Comm. 62 (1975) 320.

51. Goldberg, N.D., Haddox, M.K., Estensen, R., White, J.G., Lopez,
     C., and Hadden, J.W. In: <u>Cyclic AMP, Cell Growth and the Immune
     Response</u>, W. Braun, L. Lichtenstein, and C. Parker (eds).
     Springer, Verlag, New York (1974) 247.

52. Goldberg, N.D., Haddox, M.K., Nicol, S.E., Glass, D.B., Sanford,
     A., Kuehl, F.A., and Estensen, R. Adv. in Cyclic Nucleotide Res.
     5 (1975) 307.

53. Goldberg, N.D., Haddox, M.K., Hartle, D.K., and Hadden, J.W. In: Pharmacology and the Future of Man, 5th Int. Congress of Pharmacology, Karger, Basel, 5 (1973) 146.

54. Granner, D.K. Biochem. Biophys. Res. Comm. 46 (1972) 1516.

55. Haddox, M.K., Newton, N.E., Hartle, D.K., and Goldberg, N.D. Biochem. Biophys. Res. Comm. 47 (1972) 653.

56. Haddox, M.K., Stephenson, J.H., and Goldbert, N.D. Fred. Proc. 33 (1974) 552.

57. Hardman, J.G., and Sutherland, E.W. J. Biol. Chem. 244 (1969) 6363.

58. Harwood, J.P., Low, H., and Rodbell, M.J. Biol. Chem. 248 (1973) 6239.

59. Hickie, R.A., Walker, C.M., and Datta, A. Cancer Res. 35 (1975) 601.

60. Hsie, A.W., and Puck, T. Proc. Natl. Acad. Sci., U.S.A. 68 (1971) 358.

61. Ishikawa, E.M., Ishikawa, S., Davis, J.W., and Sutherland, E.W., J. Biol. Chem. 244 (1969) 6371.

62. Johnson, G.S., Friedman, R.M., and Pastan, I. Proc. Natl. Acad. Sci., U.S.A. 68 (1971) 425.

63. Johnson, G.S., and Pastan, I., J. Natl. Cancer Inst. 48 (1972) 1377.

64. Kakiuchi, S. Pharmacology and Future of Man, 5 (1973) 192.

65. Kakiuchi, S., Yamazaki, R., Teshima, Y., Uenishi, K., and Miyamoto, E. Biochem. J. 146 (1975) 109.

66. Kanamori, T., Kuzuya, H., and Nagatsu, T. Dental Res. 53 (1974) 760.

67. Kaminsky, N.I., Broadus, A.E., Hardman, J.G., Jones, D.J., Ball, J.H., J. Clin. Invest. 49 (1970) 2387.

68. Kelly, L.A., Hall, M.S., and Butcher, R.W. J. Biol. Chem. 249 (1974) 5182.

69. Kemp, B.E., Bylund, D.B., Huang, T-S, and Krebs, E.G. Proc. Natl. Acad. Sci. U.S.A. 72 (1975) 3348.

70.   Kimura, H., and Murad, F. J. Biol. Chem. 249 (1974) 329.

71.   Kimura, H., and Murad, F. J. Biol. Chem. 249 (1974) 6910.

72.   Kimura, H., and Murad, F. J. Biol. Chem. 250 (1975) 4810.

73.   Kimura, H., Mittal, C.K., and Murad, F. J. Biol. Chem. 251
      (1976) 7769.

74.   Kimura, H., and Murad, F. Metabolism 24 (1975) 439.

75.   Kimura, H., and Murad, F. Proc. Natl. Acad. Sci. U.S.A. 72
      (1975) 1965.

76.   Kram, R., and Tomkins, G. Proc. Natl. Sci. U.S.A.70 (1973)1659.

77.   Kumar, S., Beckerm, G., and Prasad, K.N. Cancer Res. 35 (1975)
      82.

78.   Langan, T.A. Science 162 (1968) 597.

79.   Lawson, A.J., Stevens, R.H., Osborne, J.W., Smith, D.D., and
      Oberley, L.W. Proc. Fed. Amer. Soc. Exp. Biol.36 (1977) 47.

80.   Ljungstrom, O., Berglund, L., Hjelmquist, G., Humble, E., and
      Engstrom, L. Upsala J. Med. Sci. 79 (1974) 129.

81.   Lynch, T.J., Tallant, F.A., and Cheung, W.J. Biochem. Biophys.
      Res. Comm. 65 (1975) 1115.

82.   Makman, M.H. Proc. Natl. Acad. Sci. U.S.A. 68 (1971) 2127.

83.   Macintyre, E.H., Wintersgill, C.J., Perkins, J.P., and Vatter,
      A.E. J. Cell Sci. 11 (1972) 639.

84.   Mackenzie, C.W., and Stellwagen, R.H. J. Biol. Chem. 249 (1974)
      5755.

85.   Mackenzie, C.W., and Stellwagen, R.H. J. Biol. Chem. 249 (1974)
      5763.

86.   Matsumura, S., and Nishizuka, Y. J. Biochem. 76 (1974) 29.

87.   Miki, N., and Yoshida, H. Biocheim. Biophys. Acta. 268 (1972)
      166.

88.   Mittal, C.K., Kimura, H., and Murad, F. J. Cyclic Nucleotide
      Res. 1 (1975) 261.

89. Miura, Y., Iwai, H., Sakata, R., Ohtsuka, H., Ezra, E., Kubota, K., and Fukui, N. J. Biochem. 80 (1976) 291.

90. Miyamoto, E., Petzgold, G.L., Kuo, J.F., and Greengard, P. J. Biol. Chem. 248 (1973) 179.

91. Moens, W., Voaker, A., and Kram, R. Proc. Natl. Sci. U.S.A. 72 (1975) 1063.

92. Murad, F. Adv. Cyclic Nucleotide Res. 3 (1973) 355.

93. Murad, F., Kimura, H., Hopkins, H.A., Looney, W.B., and Kovacks, C.J. Science 190 (1975) 58.

94. Murad, F., Moss, W., Johnson, A.J., and Selden, R.F. J. Clin. Enc. Met. 40 (1975) 552.

95. Murad, F., and Pak, C.Y.C. N. Eng. J. Med. 286 (1972) 1387.

96. Murray, A.W., Spiszman, M., and Atkinson, D.E. Science 171 (1971) 496.

97. Nishiyama, K., Katakami, H., Yamamura, H., Takai, Y., Shimomura, R., and Nishizuka, Y. J. Biol. Chem. 250, 1297-1300, 1975.

98. Otten, J., Johnson, G.S., and Pastan, I. Biochem. Biophys. Res. Comm. 44 (1971) 1192.

99. Oka, H., Kaneko, T., Yamashita, K., Suzuki, S., and Oda, T. Endocrinol. Japan 20 (1973) 263.

100. Peterofsky,A., and Gzder, G. Proc. Natl. Acad. Sci. U.S.A. 68(1971) 2794.

101. Olson, M.O.J., Orrick, L.R., Jones, C., and Bush, H.J. Biol. Chem. 249 (1974) 2823.

102. Pradhan, T.K., Criss, W.E., and Morris, H.P. Cancer BioChemistry BioPhysics 1 (1976) 239.

103. Prasad, K.N., Fogleman, D., Gashler, M., Sinha, P.K., and Brown, J.L. Biochem. Biophys. Res. Comm. 68 (1976) 1248.

104. Prasad, K.N., Becker, G., and Tripathy, K. Proc. Soc. Exp. Biol. Med. 149 (1975) 757.

105. Prasad, K.N., Gilmer, K.N., Sahu., and Baker, G. Cancer Res 35 (1975) 77.

106. Prasad, K.N., and Kumar, S. Proc. Soc. Exptl. Biol. Med.
      142 (1973) 406.

107. Ramanathan, S., and Chou, S.C. Comp. Biochem. Physiol.
      46B (1973) 93.

108. Rhoads, A.R., Morris, H.P., and West, W.L. Cancer Res. 32
      (1972) 2651.

109. Robison, G.A., Butcher, R.W., and Sutherland, E.W.: In:
      Fundamental Concepts in Drug-Receptor Interactions, J.F.
      Danielli, J.F. Moram, and D.J. Triggle, (eds.), p. 59
      (Academic Press, N.Y.) 1968.

110. Robison, G.A., Butcher, R.W., and Sutherland, E.W. Cyclic
      AMP, Academic Press, New York, 1970.

111. Robison, G.A., Butcher, R.W., and Sutherland, E.W., Ann. N.Y.
      Acad. Sci. 139 (1967).

112. Rodbell, M., Lin, M.C., Salomon, Y., Londos, C., Harwood, J.P.,
       Martin, B.R., Rendell, M., and Berman, M. Acta Endocrinol.
      Suppl. 191 (1974) 11.

113. Ronquist, G., and Agren, G. Upsala, J. Med. Sci. 79 (1974) 138.

114. Rubin, C.S., Erlichman, J., and Rosen, O.M. J. Biol. Chem.
      247 (1972) 36.

115. Rubin, C.S., and Rosen, O.M. Biochem. Biophys. Res. Comm. 50
      (1973) 421.

116. Rudland, P.S., Seeley, M., and Seifert, W. Nature 251 (1974)
      417.

117. Rutten, W.J., Schoot, B.M., DePont, J.H.M., and Bonting, S.L.
      Biophys. Acta 315 (1973) 384.

118. Schlondorff, D., and Weber, H. Poc. Natl. Acad. Sci. U.S.A.
      73 (1976) 524.

119. Schmidt, S.Y., and Lolley, R.N. J. Cell Biol. 57 (1973) 117.

120. Schoor, I., Rathman, P., Saxena, B.B., and Ney, R.L. J. Biol.
      Chem. 246 (1971) 5806.

121. Schroder, J., and Plagemann, P.G.W. Cancer Res. 32 (1972)
      1082.

122. Schlutz, G., Hardman, J.G., Schultz, J., Davis, J.W., and Sutherland, E.W. Proc. Natl. Acad. Sci. U.S.A 70 (1973) 1721.

123. Seifert, W.E., and Rudland, P.S. Nature 248 (1974) 138.

124. Sharma, R.K. Cancer Res. 32 (1972) 1734.

125. Sharma, R.K. In: <u>Modified Cellular and Molecular Controls in Neoplasia</u>, (ed.) Wayne E. Criss, T. Ono, and J. Sabine, Raven Press, New York (1976) p.109.

126. Sharma, R.K., and Brush, J.S. Arch. Biochem. Biophys. 156 (1973) 560.

127. Sharma, R.K., McLaughlin, C.A., and Pitot, H.C., Arch. Biochem. Biophys. 175 (1976) 221.

128. Sharma, R.K., McLaughlin, C.A., and Pitot, H.C., Europ. J. Biochem. 65 (1976) 577.

129. Sharma, R.K., Shanker, G., and Ahmed, N.K., Cancer Res. 37 (1977) 472.

130. Sheppard, H., Wiggan, G., and Tsien, W.H. Adv. Cyclic Nucleo. Res. 2 (1971) 103.

131. Silverman, P.M., and Epstein, P.M. Proc. Natl. Acad. Sci. U.S.A. 72 (1975) 442.

132. Smith, D.L., Chen, C-C, Bruegger, B.B., Holtz, S.L., Halpern, R.M., and Smith, R.A. Biochemistry 13 (1974) 3780.

133. Spruill, W.A., Steiner, A.L., and Earp, H.S, Proc. Fed. Amer. Soc. Exp. Biol. 36 (1977) 347.

134. Song, S-Y, and Cheung, W.Y. Biochim. Biophys. Acta 242 (1971) 593-605.

135. Stein, G.S., Spelsberg, T.G., and Kleinsmith, L.J. Science 183 (1974) 817.

136. Steiner, A.L., Parker, C.W., and Kipnis, D.M., J. Biol. Chem. 247 (1972) 1106.

137. Takai, Y., Nishiyama, K., Yamamura, H., Nishizuka, Y. J. Biol. Chem. 250 (1975) 4690.

138. Takeda, M., Matsumura, S., and Nakaya, Y. J. Biochem. 75 (1974) 743.

139. Taylor, A.L., Davis, B.B., Pawlson, L.G., Josimovich, J.B., and Mintz, D.H. J. Clin. Endocrinol. Metab. 30 (1970) 316.

140. Teo, T.S., and Wang, J.H. J. Biol. Chem. 248 (1973) 5950.

141. Thomas, E.W., Murad, F., Looney, W.B., and Morris, H.P. Biochem. Biophys. Acta 297 (1973) 564.

142. Thompson, W.J., and Appleman, M.M. Biochemistry 10 (1971) 311.

143. Thompson, W.J., and Appleman, M.M. J. Biol. Chem. 246 (1971) 3145.

144. Thompson, W.J., Little, S.A., and Williams, R.H. Biochemistry 12 (1973) 1889.

145. Tisdale, M.J. Biochem. Biophys. Res. Comm. 62 (1975) 887.

146. Tomasi, V., Rthy, A., and Trevisani, A. Life Sciences 12 (1973) 145.

147. Troy, F.A., Vijay, I.K., and Kawakami, T.G. Biochem. Biophys. Res. Comm. 52 (1973) 150.

148. Ueda, T., Maeno, H., and Greengard, P. J. Biol. Chem. 248 (1973) 8295.

149. Uzunov, P., Shein, H.M., and Weiss, B. Neuropharm. 13 (1974) 337.

150. Uzunov, P., Shein, H.M., and Weiss, B. Science 180 (1973) 304.

151. Van Wijk, R., Wicks, W.D., and Clay, K. Cancer Res. 32 (1972) 1905.

152. Vesely, D.L., Rovere, L.E., and Levey, G.S., Cancer Res. 37 (1977) 28.

153. Voorhees, J., Stawiski, M., Kelsey, W., Smith, E., and Duell, E. In: The Role of Cyclic Nucleotides in Carcinogenesis,H.G. Gratzner (ed). (Academic Press, N.Y.) 1973, p. 325.

154. Voorhees, J., Stawiski, M., Duell, E.A., Haddox, M.K., and Goldberg, N.D. Life Sciences 13 (1973) 639.

155. Walsh, D.A., and Ashby, C.D. Rec. Prog. Horm. Res. 29 (1973) 329.

156. Walton, G.M., Gill, G.N., Abrass, I.B., and Garren, L.D., Proc

Natl. Acad. Sci. U.S.A. 68 (1971) 880.

157.   Watson, J. J. Med. 141 (1975) 97.

158.   Whitfield, J.F., Rixon, R.F., MacManus, J.P., and Balk, S.D.
       In Vitro 8 (1973) 257.

159.   Wray, H.L., Corrigan, D.F., Bruton, J., Schaaf, M., and Earle,
       J.M. Proceedings of the 57th Annual Meeting of the Endocrine
       Society (1975) p. 362.

TRANSFER RNA IN HEPATOMAS

E. Randerath, A.S. Gopalakrishnan and K. Randerath

Department of Pharmacology
Baylor College of Medicine
Houston, Texas 77030

SUMMARY

1. Altered column-chromatographic profiles of a number of hepatoma and other tumor aminoacyl-tRNAs have been observed, most frequently for tRNA^{Phe}, tRNA^{Asp}, tRNA^{Asn}, tRNA^{Tyr}, tRNA^{His}, and tRNA^{Ser}.

2. The chemical basis for the chromatographic alterations is still obscure, except that a tRNA^{Phe} in Morris hepatoma 7777, which is not present in liver, was reported to lack the hypermodified peroxy-Y base.

3. Base composition analysis by the tritium derivative method shows hepatoma tRNA to exhibit a number of relatively small, but statistically significant differences in the amounts of various constituents when compared with liver tRNA. No overall hypermethylation of the tRNA in hepatomas and other tumors has been observed. Hepatoma tRNA rather is slightly undermethylated and undermodified, as compared to liver tRNA.

4. Differences in the base composition between Morris hepatoma and liver mitochondrial tRNA are greater than those between hepatoma and liver cytoplasmic tRNA. Hepatoma mitochondrial tRNA was also found to be undermethylated and undermodified.

5. The activity of the tRNA methyltransferases is increased in hepatomas and other tumors.

6. Urinary excretion levels of modified nucleosides and bases originating from tRNA catabolism are elevated in tumor-bearing hosts.

517

The latter two changes may be due to increased tRNA turnover
in neoplasia. A mechanism has been proposed in the present article
by which the undermodification of tRNA in tumors may cause an increase in both tRNA methylase activity and tRNA turnover.

In view of the demonstrated regulatory functions of some modified nucleosides in tRNA and the stability of the tRNA modification
pattern during vertebrate evolution, the observed alterations of
tRNA modification in neoplasia must be regarded as highly significant
deviations from the norm. The observed tRNA alterations have been
discussed in the light of their role in dedifferentiation during
carcinogenesis and in the mechanism(s) underlying the metabolic advantages of neoplastic over normal cells.

We have emphasized in this article the necessity to further investigate in detail structure and function of tRNA and tRNA modifying
enzymes to enable a better understanding of the multiple roles of
tRNA in normal and cancer cells. Further studies of the effects of
drugs on tRNA structure and function appear also worthwhile.

1.   INTRODUCTION

During recent years the structures of macromolecules in cancer
cells have attracted increasing attention since it has been recognized that their investigation will be essential for defining the biochemical lesion(s) distinguishing cancer cells from normal cells. It
appears reasonable to assume that ultimately both prevention and
therapy of cancer will be improved by our knowledge of the structure
of macromolecules involved in DNA replication, transcription and
translation in mammalian cells.

Much attention has been focused on tRNA in cancer cells since
tRNA alterations very likely result in a derangement of cellular metabolism and regulatory processes because of the great structural complexity and the multitude of functions of tRNA. While initially the
major role of tRNA had been established as a carrier of amino acids
and an adaptor in the translation of the genetic code (for a review,
see 221), an increasing number of additional, nontranslational functions of tRNA has been uncovered during the past decade. Thus tRNA
has been shown to be involved in the suppression of nonsense, mis-
sense and frameshift mutations in bacterial systems (for a review,
see 102), feedback inhibition (11), feedback repression (184), and
peptidoglycan synthesis (for refs. see 102). It also serves as a
primer for initiation of DNA synthesis by the reverse transcriptase
of oncogenic RNA viruses (173). Regulatory functions of tRNA have
been much discussed in connection with the cancer problem. A role of
tRNA in the regulation of protein synthesis has been repeatedly suggested (23, 53, 54, 204, 220). In particular, the availability of
tRNAs may participate in the regulation of protein synthesis (3, 76,

110, 186) and there appears to be a relationship between the presence of certain tRNA species and cellular differentiation (38, 46, 97, 186). Thus it has been shown that specialized tRNA species are present in cells, in which a single protein is predominantly made, e.g., in reticulocytes (186), the posterior silk glands of silk worms (42, 46, 47), lactating mammary glands (38), and fibroblasts of healing wounds (97). Some of the nontranslational functions of tRNA mentioned above are also of a regulatory nature. The discovery that the lack of pseudouridine modification of tRNA^{His} in hisT mutants of S. typhimurium leads to a derepression of the histidine operon and also affects the regulation of the leucine, isoleucine and valine operons (27, 184) has shed some light on the possible regulatory role of modified nucleosides in tRNA. However, for the most part, the precise functions of the many tRNA modifications known to date (65, 125, 189) are still enigmatic. Ames and coworkers (28) have emphasized the idea that the increase in the frequency of modified bases in tRNA as one goes from mycoplasma to mammals may be related to the increasing importance of tRNA as a group of regulatory molecules during evolution.

Against this background, frequently observed alterations of tRNA in cancer are of special interest in the investigation of the causes of carcinogenesis and the maintenance of the neoplastic state. Numerous examples have been reported in the literature for alterations of the column-chromatographic profiles of aminoacylated tRNAs of neoplastic tissues when compared with those of normal control tissues (see Section 2a). These studies do not, however, define precisely the molecular or structural basis underlying the observed alterations. Direct methods are necessary to determine the molecular basis of the chromatographic changes. Base analysis, a step towards this goal, has shown tRNA from Morris hepatomas as well as from other tumors to differ significantly from tRNA of normal control tissue in the content of various nucleosides (See Sections 2c and 2d). At present, it is not known whether these alterations of tRNA in cancer are due to mutations or deletions of tRNA genes, mutations or deletions of genes coding for modifying enzymes, or the expression of oncofetal genes involving the appearance of additional tRNA species and/or additional modifying enzymes, or to a combination of these causes.

To answer these questions the isolation and nucleotide sequence analysis of various tRNA species from neoplastic and normal tissues is necessary. In the past, such a task could not be undertaken because of the lack of sequencing methods of sufficient sensitivity to allow one to work with small amounts of tissue ($< 1 - 2$ kg), the classical sequencing methods for nonradioactive RNA (73) requiring 50-100 kg of tissue. Only during the last 3-4 years, micromethods based on chemical or enzymatic "postlabelling" of RNA and RNA constituents have been developed, which are suited for nucleotide sequence analysis of tRNA species from normal and neoplastic mammalian tissues (See Section 2e). However, no primary structure of any tumor tRNA

species has been compared thus far with that of its normal counterpart. The nucleotide sequences of only three tumor tRNA species,
i.e., of tRNA$_f^{Met}$ (136, 137, 181), tRNA$_4^{Met}$ (134), and tRNA$_1^{Val}$ (135)
from mouse myeloma cells, have been determined. Since these cells
were grown in culture the tRNAs could be "prelabeled" with ^{32}P by
incubating the cells in the presence of ^{32}P-orthophosphate and nucleotide sequence analysis was then carried out by the procedures
described by Sanger et al.(172), (see also 21). This approach is,
however, not applicable to tumors growing in the intact organism,
because the high specific activity required for subsequent sequence
analysis cannot be achieved by in vivo labeling. The novel postlabeling methodology referred to above has opened up a new field for
investigation, and it may be expected that the fine details of tRNA
structure in neoplasia will be explored in the near future . The
availability of a well characterized spectrum of hepatomas derived
by Morris and coworkers (113, 116, 161), which differ in growth rate
and state of differentiation, provides a unique opportunity for comparative investigations on tRNA structure and function. Since the
cell of origin of these tumors is known to be the hepatocyte, normal
and regenerating liver can be readily used as control tissues. Such
studies may provide insights into the possible role that specific
tRNAs might play during tumor formation, cell growth, and differentiation. Furthermore, a wealth of biochemical and biological information
has been accumulated in these tumor model systems allowing one to correlate tRNA alterations with various biochemical and biological phenomena.

Since research on tRNA structure and function in neoplasia has
not yet progressed to a stage where definitive answers can be given
the following data and discussions must necessarily be of somewhat
preliminary nature.

A promising line of research has recently evolved from studies
in our laboratory on the effects of antimetabolites on tRNA in vivo.
Certain nucleoside analogs were found to inhibit specifically the
methylation and modification of the corresponding natural nucleosides
in tRNA, while there was little or no analog incorporation into tRNA.
This finding opens up the possibility to gain a better understanding
of the functions of tRNA modifications and may also be exploited thera·
peutically. A brief discussion of the effects of antimetabolites on
tRNA modification has therefore been included in this article (See
Section 2b).

2. CHANGES OF tRNAs IN HEPATOMAS

a. Column-Chromatographic Profiles of Aminoacyl-tRNAs

Column-chromatographic profiles are based on physicochemical
properties of the tRNA. tRNA isolated from a tumor, e.g., a hepatoma,

is charged with a specific (^{14}C)-amino acid (or (^{3}H)-amino acid), using a homologous or heterologous aminoacyl-tRNA synthetase preparation, and cochromatographed on a column with (^{3}H)-aminoacyl-tRNA (or (^{14}C)-aminoacyl-tRNA, respectively) prepared from normal control tissue (liver) in the same way. The profiles of (^{14}C)- and (^{3}H)-label in the column eluate are then recorded and a pattern of iso-accepting species (219) is obtained for each of the labeled aminoacyl-tRNAs. Various types of columns have been used in such studies e.g., methylated albumin kieselguht (MAK) columns (109) or reversed phase columns type 2 (RPC-2, (213) and type 5 (RPC-5) (82). Heterologous synthetase preparations are also being examined to make sure that differences in the profiles are not caused by synthetase differences.

Differences in the column-chromatographic profiles between amino-acyl-tRNA from tumor and normal tissue have been described for various amino acids in many tumors including a series of hepatomas, indicating that tumor tRNA populations differ from those of normal control tissue. Baliga et al. (7) compared the elution profiles from MAK-columns of 18 aminoacyl-tRNAs from Novikoff hepatoma cells with those from normal liver. The hepatoma was shown to contain new tRNA species for histidine, tyrosine, and asparagine; a shift in the elution profiles was observed for six other species isolated from tumor. Hayashi et al. (69) reported also on changed elution profiles of tyrosyl-tRNA from Novikoff ascites heaptoma as well as from other tumors. Ritter and Busch (165) reported on differences in the patterns of leucyl-tRNA between Novikoff hepatoma and rat liver, but found no differences in the valyl-tRNA patterns. Other tRNAs were not investiagted in this study.

Differences between normal and tumor tRNA elution profiles have been described for a series of Morris hepatomas (5, 57, 121, 192, 209) Volkers and Taylor (209) found Morris hepatoma 5123D, a tumor of in-intermediate growth rate and classified as intermediate between well and poorly differentiated, to contain two new seryl-tRNA species, one additional phenylalanyl-tRNA species, and to exhibit a slight change in the tyrosyl-tRNA profile, whereas two histidyl-tRNAs were missing when compared with tRNA from normal rat liver on RPC-2 columns. These authors pointed out that the observed alterations are tumor-specific and not growth-specific since the chromatographic patterns of aminoacyl-tRNAs prepared from regenerating rat liver overlapped those of the corresponding aminoacyl-tRNAs from normal liver. When the same aminoacyl-tRNAs were studied in the fast growing, poorly differentiated Morris hepatoma 3924A no changes in the profiles of seryl-tRNA and phenlalanyl-tRNA were observed, while the tyrosyl- and histidyl-tRNA profiles exhibited slight alterations. From these experiments it appears that there may be no definitive correlation between the changes in tRNA species and the malignancy of the tumor; the observed changes may rather represent individual features of each type of tumor.

An additional phenylalanyl-tRNA was also found in Morris hepatoma 5123C (54, 55), in Morris hepatoma 7777 (57, 121), and in
fetal rat liver (55). Since a new phenylalanine tRNA could not be
detected in regenerating rat liver (see above) the presence of the
additional species in the tumor cannot simply be growth-related.
The occurrence of the additional phenylalanine tRNA in fetal liver
might imply the presence in the hepatoma of a derepressed gene for
this species, which normally is active only in the embryonic stage.
The reappearance of embryonic tRNA species in malignant cells has
also been observed in Reuber hepatoma for tyrosine tRNA (217). In
this context, the analogy for instance to the carcinoembryonic antigen (CEA) of the human digestive system and the oncofetal antigen
(OFA) (2, 51, 52) is of interest. Gonano et al. (55) suggested
that the presence of embryonic tRNAs in the neoplastic cell may be
an epiphenomenon of the malignant transformation, but pointed out
the possibility that their function might be critical in maintaining
the cell in its typically dedifferentiated state. Although the hypothesis of the expression of oncofetal genes leading to the appearance
of additional tumor tRNA species appears reasonable, other mechanisms
could conceivably also underly the observed phenomena (see below).

Srinivasan et al. (192) compared tyrosyl-, histidyl-, aspara-
ginyl-, and phenylalanyl-tRNAs from a spectrum of Morris hepatomas
with the respective aminoacyl-tRNAs from normal liver on MAK columns.
The tyrosyl-, histidyl-, and asparaginyl-tRNAs from hepatoma 3924A
exhibited altered elution profiles similar to those found earlier in
Novikoff hepatoma (7). Hepatomas 9121, 9098, 3683F, and 5123C exhibited altered phenylalanyl-tRNA profiles. These results are summarized in Table 1 together with some properties of the tumors. As
the table shows, hepatomas 9121 and 9098, which are generally least
deviated from liver with respect to their karyotype, histology, growth
rate, and enzyme patterns, exhibit changes only in their phenylalanyl-
tRNA profiles; whereas new species of tyrosyl-, histidyl-, and asparaginyl-tRNAs are seen only in those hepatomas, which are generally representative of advanced states of malignancy, i.e., hepatoma 3924A
and Novikoff hepatoma. However, as the authors pointed out, the possibility that specific changes in tRNA may reflect the biochemical individuality of each tumor cannot be ruled out since hepatomas 3683F
and 5123C do not fit exactly into either category.

Other neoplasms and transformed cells, in which changes of the
aminoacyl-tRNA profiles were observed, include for instance Ehrlich
ascites tumor cells (69, 198, 199), mouse plasma cell tumors (18, 120,
218), mouse mammary tumors (118), SV-40-induced hamster tumors (19,
20, 43, 69), hamster cells transformed by adenovirus 7, SV40, or polyoma virus (44, 72, 199), white blood cells of patients with chronic
myeloid leukemia (138), human leukemic lymphoblasts (45), human mam-

Table One[a]

Rate of Growth, Karyotype, and the Occurrence of Alterations in Elution Profiles of Aminoacyl-tRNAs in Hepatomas

Hepatoma	Rate of Growth	Karyotype		New Species of tRNA			
		Ploidy	Structural Changes	Tyr	His	Asn	Phe
9121	Slow	Diploid	Min	-	-	-	+
9098	Slow	Diploid	Min	-	-	-	+
3683F	Rapid	Hypodiploid	28 Abn	-	-	-	+
5123C	Slow	Hypertetraploid	Min	-	-	+	+
3924A	Rapid	Hypotetraploid	10 Abn	+	+	+	-
Novikoff	Rapid	Hypotetraploid		+	+	+	-

a From ref. 192.

mary carcinoma (131) and a number of human carcinomas and adenocarcinomas (19).   Changes in aminoacyl-tRNA profiles have also been
observed during embryogenesis, differentiation, and hormonally
mediated development (for reviews, see 102, 195).   The relationship
of these changes to the alterations of tRNA in malignant cells is
not clear at this time and needs to be explored more fully in the
future.

Differences between tumors, including hepatomas, and normal
tissue have been described most frequently for phenylalanyl-, as-
partyl-, asparaginyl-, tyrosyl-, histidyl-, and seryl-tRNA profiles.
With the exception of a phenylalanyl-tRNA (see below), the structural
basis for the observed differences in the elution profiles is not
known.   These differences may reflect altered sequences or different
modification patterns of the tumor tRNAs or both.   It is of course
necessary in each case to exclude artifacts such as possible differences due to the origin of the synthetase preparation and/or
conformational changes or aggregation of the aminoacyl-tRNA.

Recently, suggestive evidence has been adduced for the basis of
such a structural difference involving the proxy-Y base in tRNA^{Phe}
(57).   tRNA^{Phe} of normal eukaryotic cells is known to contain a highly fluorescent and hydrophobic Y base, located next to the 3'-end of
the anticodon (141).   The Y compound is one of the most highly modified nucleic acid bases characterized so far, the others being Q and
its derivatives.   It consists of a tricyclic imidazo derivative of
guanine, to which is usually attached a 4-carbon side chain, mammalian tRNA^{Phe} in addition carrying a hydroxy peroxide group on the side
chain (12).   As mentioned above, several Morris hepatomas exhibit a
new, early eluting phenylalanyl-tRNA species when compared with rat
liver.   Grunberger et al. (57) showed that the additional species of
tRNA^{Phe} in Morris hepatoma 7777 differs from normal liver tRNA^{Phe} by
the absence of the peroxy-Y base.   This is illustrated by Figs 1 and
2.   In Fig 1 the profiles of phenylalanyl-tRNA from Morris hepatoma
7777 and normal rat liver on a RPC-5 column are shown, the hepatoma
tRNA giving two peaks, tRNA$_1$ and tRNA$_2$, and the liver tRNA one peak,
which overlaps hepatoma tRNA$_1$.   Fig 2 shows the profiles obtained
when acid-treated liver phenylalanyl-tRNA and untreated hepatoma tRNA
were cochromatographed.   As Thiebe and Zachau (201) have shown, mild
acid treatment will result in the excision of Y base from tRNA^{Phe}
without breaking the polynucleotide chain.   The acid treatment converted the liver tRNA almost quantitatively to an earlier eluting
species, tRNA$_{-Y}$, which lacked peroxy-Y but did not overlap completely
hepatoma tRNA$_1$ (Fig 2).   Isolation of the late eluting hepatoma tRNA$_2$
and analogous treatment gave the same result.   However, when the first
eluting hepatoma tRNA$_1$ was subjected to acid treatment its chromatographic position did not change.   Furthermore, the acid-treated early
eluting hepatoma tRNA$_1$ could still participate in poly(U)-directed
ribosomal binding, i.e., in codon recognition, as could untreated

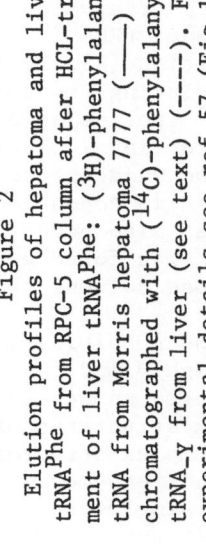

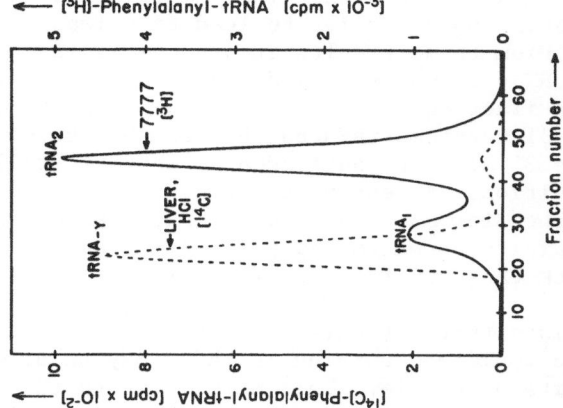

Figure 2

Elution profiles of hepatoma and liver tRNA^{Phe} from RPC-5 column after HCl-treatment of liver tRNA^{Phe}: (^{3}H)-phenylalanyl-tRNA from Morris hepatoma 7777 (———) co-chromatographed with (^{14}C)-phenylalanyl-tRNA$_{-y}$ from liver (see text) (----). For experimental details see ref 57, (Fig 1b).

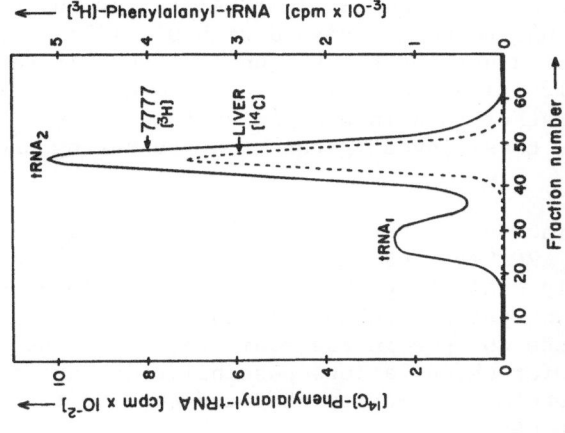

Figure 1

Elution profiles of hepatoma and liver tRNA^{Phe} from RPC-5 column: (^{3}H)-phenylalanyl-tRNA from Morris hepatoma 7777 (———) cochromatographed with (^{14}C0-phenylalanyl-tRNA from normal rat liver (----). For experimental details, see ref. 57. Figure redrawn schematically from Fig 1a of ref 57.

late eluting hepatoma $tRNA_2$ and untreated liver tRNA, whereas acid-treated late eluting hepatoma $tRNA_2$ and acid-treated liver tRNA no longer participated in codon recognition. The removal of Y base from yeast $tRNA^{Phe}$ had been shown earlier to lead to a loss of codon recognition (48, 201). From these results it was concluded that the early eluting hepatoma $tRNA_1$ is not simply derived from the normal $tRNA^{Phe}$ species as an artifact due to partial excision of the peroxy-Y base during isolation of hepatoma tRNA but has another base in the position adjacent to the 3' side its anticodon so that it still can function in codon recognition. Recently, a deficiency in peroxy-Y base has also been reported for mouse neuroblastomas, where 85% of $tRNA^{Phe}$ was found by affinity chromatography on anti-Y antibody-Sepharose columns to lack this modification (171).

The possibility exists that not only Y but also Q and Q*, the most highly modified nucleosides occurring in tRNA, may be affected by changed associated with neoplasia. This may be due to the very complex structures of these constituents of tRNA. The formation of such complex structures must be a multi-step process involving a number of enzymes and therefore may be more susceptible to changes than a single-step modification such as methylation. Q and Q* have recently been shown (78, 79) to be derivatives of 7-deazaguanosine containing a dihydroxy-cyclopentenyl-aminomethyl side chain, Q* compounds having in addition mannose and galactose respectively linked to the cyclopentene diol moiety. Q nucleoside has been found in $tRNA^{Tyr}$, $tRNA^{His}$, $tRNA^{Asn}$, and $tRNA^{Asp}$ from E. coli (68, 79) and Q or "Q-like" nucleoside in the same tRNAs from Drosophila (79, 214) and mammalian cells (80). Recently, the presence of Q and Q* in tRNA from a variety of eukaryotic organisms, including several mammalian tissues, was reported (77, 78), the Q* content being generally more abundant than that of Q. Furthermore, $tRNA^{Asp}$ from rabbit liver, rat liver, and rat ascites hepatoma was shown to contain a Q* nucleoside species having a mannose moiety, whereas in $tRNA^{Tyr}$ from the same sources galactose was found to be associated with Q* (127). The role of Q and its derivatives is not yet clearly understood. It has been suggested by White et al. (214) that Q may play a role in the regulatory function of tRNA rather than in protein synthesis since the amount of Q was found by these investigators to vary during the life cycle of Drosophila.

It may not be a coincidence that the tRNAs containing Q or Q*, i.e., $tRNA^{Tyr}$, $tRNA^{His}$, $tRNA^{Asp}$, and $tRNA^{Asn}$, belong to the category of tumor tRNAs frequently exhibiting changes in their column-chromatographic profiles when compared with normal and control tRNA (see above). This may indicate changes in the modification of the nucleoside in the Q position, for which various possibilities can be envisaged due to the structural complexity of Q and Q*. So far it has only been shown that rat ascites hepatoma cells have larger quantities of Q* than do normal cells (77, 78). In this context it is interest-

ing to note that mannose and galactose moieties occurring in Q*
are components specifying the properties of glycoprotein receptors
for lectins in cell membranes (101) and that the presence of the
same sugars in specific tRNAs containing Q* may reflect an important
regulatory role of these tRNAs in membrane function (127). The increase of Q* in rat ascites hepatoma could reflect increased synthesis of membrane glycoproteins. Alternatively, it might also be
casually related to changes in membrane glycoprotein structure and
function. Clearly, further research is desirable to elucidate the
possible role of tRNAs containing Q* in the synthesis of membrane
glycoproteins particularly in connection with neoplasia since
changes in membrane glycoproteins may be involved in loss of contact
inhibition of growth (see for instance 101).

It is not yet possible to decide whether the additional hepatoma
phenylalanyl-tRNA species represents the expression of a separate tRNA
gene, such as, for example, a fetal gene (as discussed above) in certain hepatomas or an immature form of $tRNA_2^{Phe}$ (Fig 1) resulting from
a failure to complete the synthesis of the Y base from its precursor
guanine molecule (100, 200). To answer these questions, it will be
necessary to determine and compare the primary structures of all
$tRNA^{Phe}$ species from Morris hepatoma 7777, other tumors having additional $tRNA^{Phe}$ species, and from normal adult and fetal rat liver.
It also appears desirable to study the Y modifying enzyme(s) in these
tissues. Complete sequence analysis of all these $tRNA^{Phe}$ species is
necessary for the following reasons:

1. In addition to the presence of a different nucleoside in the
Y position in the fast eluting tumor tRNA species, there may be dif-
ferences in other positions between the hepatoma and liver tRNAs
(Fig 1).

2. Fast eluting phenylalanyl-tRNA species need not necessarily
be the same for Morris hepatoma 7777 and other tumors or fetal rat
liver, even though they occupy the same position in the profile.

3. Similarly, the late eluting species from different tissues
may not have the same primary structure.

It cannot be assumed with certainty that the column-chromatographic methods used for establishing the profiles of isoaccepting tRNA
species are capable of discriminating between tRNAs of very similar
primary structure, e.g., two tRNAs differing in just one position of
the polynucleotide chain, especially if chromatography has been carried out only on one column. A chemically minor alteration nevertheless may have a profound effect on the biological properties of the
RNA possibly due to conformational changes.

It has been shown (for a review, see 162) that many of the nu-

cleosides in the invariant and semi-invariant positions of tRNA are
involved in tertiary interactions determining the three-dimensional
structure of the molecule. Conceivably, the very complex tertiary
structure of tRNA plays a major role in a large number of biological
functions, which require that many different protein molecules interact with tRNA in a highly specific manner. Thus, one might expect
changes of nucleosides particularly in these invariant or semi-
invariant positions to affect normal tRNA functions. In this regard
it is interesting to note that a number of nucleosides in the positions involved in establishing the three-dimensional structure are
methylated, i.e., 2-methylguanosine, N^2,N^2-dimethylguanosine, 2'-0-
methylguanosine, 7-methylguanosine, 5-methylcytidine, 5-methyluridine,
and 1-methyladenosine (for a review, see 162). Deficient methylation
in any of these positions (See Section 2c) might have similar consequences. Alterations of the primary structure of tRNA may be more
common than one would suspect on the basis of the chromatographic
profiles of aminoacyl-tRNAs. Only chemical analysis will be capable
of establishing the identity of molecules exhibiting the same chromatographic elution pattern. Such studies on the nucleotide sequence
of tumor tRNAs have been initiated recently in our laboratory (see
Section 2e) as well as by other groups since new methods have become
available, which, for the first time, make possible to undertake such
a task.

   b. <u>tRNA Methyltransferases and tRNA Methlation in vitro and in
       vivo</u>

   Since the discovery in the 1950s that nucleic acids contained
constituents other than the major two purine and three pyrimidine nucleotides (37, 103, 187, 216) more than 50 modified nucleosides have
been characterized in nucleic acids from various sources (1, 64, 65,
125, 126, 133, 159, 179). Most of these modified nucleosides occur
in tRNA where they may represent up to 23 per cent of the total nucleoside content in individual eukaryotic tRNA species. Although
there is a great variety of modifications, one major class, the methylated nucleosides, can be readily distinguished. This class accounts for 30 to 70 per cent of the modified nucleosides in various
tRNAs.

   In 1962 and 1963 Borek and coworkers demonstrated that the methylation of tRNA occurred posttranscriptionally (15, 40, 190), i.e.,
after completion of the polynucleotide chain rather than at the nucleotide precursor level, with S-adenosylmethionine serving as the
methyl donor (41). A number of specific tRNA methyltransferases were
subsequently described (74).

   The tRNA methyltransferases (or tRNA methylases) have attracted
great attention in cancer biochemistry ever since an increase of the
activity of these enzymes in tumors had been first reported (203).
Increases of the tRNA methylase activities have since been described

for many tumors (for reviews, see 14, 29, 87), including a series
of Morris hepatomas (178) (see also below). Such increases have
been found in all malignant neoplasms examined so far, but not in
benign ovarian tumors (176). tRNA methylase activities were also
reported to be increased during administration to animals of carcinogens (21a, 66, 67, 114, 194, 210, 215).

The tRNA methylases belong to the class of "key enzymes" as
described by Weber (for a review, see 211), i.e., enzymes involved
in the pattern of metabolic imbalance, which is linked with malignant transformation and/or progression in malignancy and which confers a biological advantage to the cancer cell over normal cells.
Therapeutically, the tRNA methylases are therefore of great interest
since the "key enzymes" in general are sensitive targets of anti-
cancer drugs (see also below).

The methylation of tRNA has attracted considerable interest
yet from another point of view: In 1963 Srinivasan and Borek (190)
hypothesized that methylating enzymes might constitute a naturally
occurring carcinogen. This hypothesis was based mainly on the observation by Magee and Farber (108) that alkylation in vivo of tRNA
by the carcinogen dimethylnitrosamine was more pronounced than that
of DNA and that the pattern of this alkylation was aberrant. The
reasoning leading to the hypermethylation hypothesis has been discussed (191). To prove whether this hypothesis is, at least in part,
valid it is necessary to demonstrate the general occurrence of aberrant methylation in tumor tRNA and perhaps in other tumor nucleic
acids. For recent detailed reviews on physiological and/or pathological alkylation of nucleic acids, see refs. 129 and 183, respectively.

The methylation of tRNA has been reviewed recently (123). Basically, there are two approaches to study the methylation of tRNA:

1. Investigation of the extent and pattern of tRNA methylation
in vivo in various organisms and tissues, and

2. Characterization of the tRNA methylases in vitro by studying
the incorporation of radioactive label from methyl-labeled S-adenosylmethionine into a heterologous tRNA substrate (see below).

The former has been a more difficult experimental task until recently because of the lack of sufficiently sensitive methods for structural analysis of nonradioactive RNA. Most studies described have
therefore dealt with the properties of the tRNA methylases in in vitro
assays. A large number of such studies have been carried out (for reviews, see 13, 16, 87, 123, 193). The tRNA methylases exhibit strict
specificity. Thus, methyl groups are incorporated only into a certain
limited number of positions in tRNA. As a rule, tRNA cannot be meth-

ylated by homologous enzymes since it has been fully methylated in
the cell. Further methylation can be achieved only on a heterologous tRNA substrate from an organism lower on the evolutionary scale
than that from which the methylase preparation originated since tRNA
from lower organisms is less methylated. The substrate most often
used in studies on mammalian tRNA methylases is E. coli tRNA. Although the physiological significance of in vitro assays with heterologous substrates may be questioned, nevertheless significant results have been obtained by in vitro experiments. However, when
such a heterologous substrate is used one cannot assume that extent
and pattern obtained by the in vitro methylation assay accurately reflect the degree and pattern of methylation in homologous tRNA in
vivo. An ideal substrate would be homologous unmethylated eukaryotic
pre-tRNA, but is has not been possible thus far to prepare such tRNA
in sufficient amounts. However, the recent discovery in our laboratory, that the administration to animals of certain nucleoside analogs caused undermethylation and undermodification of tRNA in specific
positions (see below) enables the use of such undermodified tRNA in
studies of the properties of methylases in homologous systems. tRNA
exhibiting in vitro methyl acceptor activity in a homologous assay
system can also be obtained from livers of rats treated with a mixture of the hepatocarcinogen ethionine and adenine (86, 139, 210).
As shown by base composition analysis in our laboratory (106), such
tRNA is methyl-deficient.

Another factor complicating the interpretation of in vitro assays with crude tRNA methylases is the dependence of the methylase
activities on the ionic environment (81, 99, 167), on polyamines
(63, 98, 99, 128), and on inhibitors (70, 83-85, 87).

The purification of tRNA methylases has proven quite laborious
and thus, no such enzyme has as yet been purified to homogeneity.
The difficulties encountered in the purification of the methylases
have been summarized (123). In mammalian organisms, work has concentrated mainly on tRNA methylases in rat liver, where adenosine-1
methylase and two different guanosine-N^2 methylases have been partially purified (8, 50, 90-93).

tRNA methylase activities in a series of Morris hepatomas have
been studied by Sheid et al. (178). These authors measured the extent of methylation of E. coli B tRNA by enzyme preparations from
Morris hepatomas 9633F, 8995, 7316B, 7800, 5123D, and 7777 as well as
from normal and host liver. The data obtained are summarized in
Table 2. Whereas enzyme activities of normal and host liver are very
similar, the methylase activities in the hepatomas were 1.4 -5 times
higher than in liver. As Table 2 shows, a direct positive correlation
between tRNA methylase activity and growth rate of the hepatoma was
found. Sheid et al. (178) also compared methylation patterns produced in the E. coli B substrate by methylase extracts from hepatomas

Table Two[a]

tRNA Methylase Activity in Some Morris Hepatomas and Normal Rat Liver

Specimen	Sex of animal	Generation used	Growth rate of tumors (cm 1 mo.)	Histological type[b]	Enzyme activity[c] $\mu\mu$moles (^{14}C)-CH$_3$ incorporated/mg tRNA (saturation level)		Ave. amount of protein used for saturation level (mg)
					Value	Ave.	
Liver (Normal)	M				130, 145, 170	148	20.0
Liver (tumor bearing)	M				130, 135, 155	140	18.6
Liver (normal)	F				95, 115, 130	113	20.2
Liver (tumor bearing)	F				100, 110, 120	110	18.6
Hepatoma 9633F	M	9	1.4	WD[d]	145, 195, 205	202	20.0
Hepatoma 8995	F	25	2.0	WD	225, 285	255	19.5
Hepatoma 7316B	F	41	2.5	WD	390, 435	413	18.6
Hepatoma 7800	F	48	2.6	WD-IWD and HD	350, 390, 405	382	21.8
Hepatoma 5123D	M	78	3.7	IWD and PD	505, 535, 615	551	24.4
Hepatoma 7777	M	57	5.0	PD	695, 715, 820	743	23.8

a From ref. 178.

b Characterized by Dr. David R. Meranze.

c Each value represents the tRNA methylase activity for an individual hepatoma in each particular series.

d Explanation of histological type: PD, poorly differentiated; WD; well-differentiated; HD, highly differentiated; IWD and HD, intermediate between well-differentiated and highly differentiated; IWD and PD, intermediate between well-differentiated and poorly differentiated.

methyl-deficient $\underline{E}$. $\underline{coli}$ as substrate, found the monkey hepatoma
tRNA methylases to produce increased levels of 7-methylguanine
N^2, N^2-dimethylguanine, and thymine, while the normal liver enzymes
yielded greater amounts of N^2-methylguanine. These differences
were, however not reflected in the base compositions of the homologous tRNAs. Base analysis may not be sensitive enough to detect
very small changes, i.e., if only a few species out of the total
tRNA population were altered in their patterns of methylation. Different distributions of nucleosides methylated in vitro have been reported for various tumor tRNA methylases (e.g. 62, 112, 124, 175).
On the other hand, there are reports on chemically induced rat kidney
and mouse colon tumors (130, 194) where no such changes in the tRNA
methylase properties were detected. All these results were obtained
with crude tRNA methylase preparations. Partially purified tRNA
methylases from normal and cancerous tissues appear to have identical
specificities (9, 90, 94). It thus appears that the specificity of
tRNA methylases may be altered in certain tumors but not in others.
One of the problems in assessing tRNA methylase specificities in in
vitro assays are the various factors discussed above, which may lead
to artifacts. Another difficulty stems from the use of heterologous
tRNA as the substrate. Ultimately, the question, whether there is
aberrant methylation of tumor tRNA, will be solved by nucleotide
sequence analysis of many tumor tRNA species.

An understanding of the mechanism underlying the elevated tRNA
methylase activities in tumors will require more detailed knowledge
about tRNA modification. This would probably also advance our understanding of the rather obscure functions of tRNA modifications. In
this context, recent results from studies in our laboratory on the
effects of nucleoside analogs in vivo on tRNA structure and modification are of interest. Thus, the antineoplastic agent 5-azacytidine
was found to be a potent specific inhibitor of the methylation of the
5-position of cytidine in mammalian tRNA in vivo under conditions
where this compound was not incorporated to a measurable extent into
tRNA (105). Similarly, fluorinated pyrimidines (e.g., 5-fluorouracil
and 5-fluorouridine), which are extensively used clinically in the
treatment of malignant disease, were found to cause a marked specific
reduction of 5-methyl-uridine, pseudouridine, and dihydrouridine but
not of 3-(3-amino-3-carboxypropyl)uridine in mammalian tRNA in vivo
under conditions where the amount of 5-fluorouridine incorporated was
too small to account for the decrease in these modified nucleosides
(107). These effects of tRNA modification were much more pronounced
in a 5-fluorouracil-responsive mammary tumor than in normal mammary
gland or liver (202). While the production of fraudulent nucleic
acids, following treatment with purine or pyrimidine analogs, has
usually been presumed to be the consequence of incorporation of analog
into RNA or DNA, these data suggest that major effects of antimetabolites on structure and function of mammalian nucleic acids may be
mediated by alterations of the patterns of modified nucleosides.

8895, 7316B, 5123D, and 7777 with those produced by liver enzyme.
These patterns were very similar for hepatomas and liver and thus
did not reflect specific increases of methylase activities in the
hepatomas. It was concluded therefore that the increase in tRNA
methylase activity in the hepatomas reflected an increase in overall
synthesis of RNA by the hepatomas rather than overmethylation of
heaptoma tRNA. This conclusion is in agreement with base composition data of tRNA from Morris hepatomas 5123D and 7777 determined
in our laboratory (see Section 2c), which showed that there was no
overall hypermethylation of hepatoma tRNA.

     Lakings et al. (95) studied the tRNA methylase activities and
compositions of homologous tRNAs in monkey hepatomas induced by N-
nitrosodiethylamine and in monkey liver as well as the urinary excretion levels of some tRNA catabolites in the same animals. tRNA
methylase activity and capacity, and also the urinary excretion
levels for selected tRNA degradation products were elevated for
the hepatoma-bearing monkeys when compared with the values for normal animals. Isolated tRNA from hepatoma and normal liver was hydrolized to the bases, which were analyzed by high-resolution liquid
chromatography. The base compositions of hepatoma and normal liver
tRNA were found to be similar (see also Section 2c). Thus, the increased tRNA methylase activity in the hepatoma was not paralleled
by hypermethylation of the hepatoma tRNA. The increased urinary excretion and higher methylase activity of the hepatoma-bearing monkeys
without an apparent increase in the methylated base content of the
hepatoma tRNA was interpreted to suggest increased tRNA turnover in
the hepatoma. Increased amounts in urine of several methylated bases
have also been reported in hepatoma patients, who excreted about 2
times the normal amounts (71). Other reports on elevated excretion
of modified purines and pyrimidines in tumor-bearing animals and
humans have been summarized (14). These observations together with
the lack of hypermethylation of bulk tumor tRNA support the idea
that in general increased tumor methylase activities are associated
with a higher tRNA turnover (biosynthesis and degradation). Unfortunately, virtually nothing is known about the mechanisms governing tRNA degradation in normal and neoplastic mammalian cells. It is
noteworthy that no increased tRNA methylase activity was found in regenerating liver (167, 77), whereas mammalian fetal tissues contained
a much higher tRNA methylase activity than did normal adult tissues
(70, 84, 164, 196). It is thus possible that the elevated methylase
activities in tumors may not be growth related, but may reflect the
expression of fetal properties.

     No clear answer has yet been provided to the question whether
the tumor tRNA methylases exhibit specificities different from the
normal methylases and thus may lead to aberrant methylation. While
Sheid et al. (178), for instance, did not observe changes in the in
vitro methylation patterns of heterologous tRNA produced by Morris
hepatoma and liver methylases (see above), Lakings et al. (95), using

Studies on the mechanism(s) of the drug-induced specific inhibition
of tRNA modifications are underway in our laboratory. Thus, the
modification reactions of tumor tRNA may provide specific targets
for drug therapy. Furthermore, the knowledge of the structure of
altered tumor tRNA species may enable the design of a rational therapeutic strategy, by which mainly the tumor tRNA is affected but not
its normal counterpart. In this context, it should be re-emphasized
that the tRNA methylases belong to the "key enzymes" (211) (see
above). Since these enzymes are connected with the metabolic imbalance characteristic of the neoplastic cell they may be singled out
as important sensitive targets for anticancer drugs. The studies
from our laboratory have shown the tRNA methylases indeed to be
specific targets for anticancer drugs.

    c. <u>Base Composition of Bulk tRNA</u>

    Base composition studies on bulk tRNA can provide answers to
the following questions:

    1. Do degrees of methylation and modification of tumor tRNA
differ from those of normal control tRNA, in particular, in view of
the factors discussed in the preceding section, is tumor tRNA hypermethylated?

    2. Does tumor tRNA contain methylated or modified nucleosides
not present in normal control tRNA or vice versa?

    3. Are there changes in the major nucleoside content in tumor
tRNA?

    4. How do changes in tumor tRNA base composition correlate with
changes observed in the column-chromatographic profiles of tumor tRNA
(See Section 2a)?

    Since the conventional spectrophotometric methods are not sensi-
tive enough for the analysis of modified constituents of tRNA in the
small amounts of material usually available from mammalian sources
the development of sensitive methods was necessary to analyze tRNA
base composition. Three methods have been used to analyze modified
and/or methylated constituents of tRNA from heaptomas and other
tumors:

    1. Biological labeling of the methylated nucleosides with radio-
active methionine,

    2. A chemical tritium derivative method, and

    3. High-resolution liquid chromatography.

In method 1, the tRNA lebeled <u>in vivo</u> is subjected to acid hydrolysis and the methylated bases are separated by a combination of column and paper chromatography (e.g., 75) or two-dimensional thin layer chromatography (119). This method allows one to analyze only the methylated bases but not the other modified bases. Another limitation is the possibility that, because of the higher turnover of tumor tRNA (see above), the control tRNA from normal tissue may not be labeled to the same degree as the tumor tRNA. To obtain meaningful results, this factor has to be corrected for. Method 2, which has been developed in our laboratory (146-149, 152, 153), is based on chemical "postlabeling" of nonradioactive RNA derivatives and thus does not involve in vivo labeling. The RNA is first degraded enzymatically to nucleosides, which are then converted to tritium-labeled nucleoside trialcohols by periodate oxidation and borotritide reduction. The nucleoside trialcohols are separated by two-dimensional thin layer-chromatography, detected by fluorography (142), eluted and counted. The base composition is calculated from the count rates of the nucleoside trialcohols. This method is suitable for assaying the four major the most methylated and modified bases in mammalian tRNA. A procedure for high-resolution liquid chromatography of methylated bases derived from tRNA by acid hydrolysis (method 3) has been described recently (96). Ten methylated bases and the four major constituents have been analyzed by this procedure. It requires, however, 100-200 times more tRNA than the tritium derivative method.

Using method 1, Inose et al. (75) compared the in vivo methylation patterns of cytoplasmic tRNA from four chemically induced rat ascites heaptomas with the pattern of cytoplasmic tRNA from normal rat liver. The content of methylated adenine was found to be in a narrow range of 13-14% of the total methylated components for all hepatomas and liver, while the total methylated guanine content was lower in the hepatomas than in liver. In view of the finding that the main methylated product in rat liver tRNA during administration of the carcinogen dimethylnitrosamine was 7-methylguanine (31, 174), it was of interest that the 7-methylguanine content of tRNA from the four hepatomas was below that of normal liver.

The major and modified base composition for 16 constituents of cytoplasmic tRNA from Morris hepatomas 7777 and 5123D and from rat liver was determined by the tritium derivative method in our laboratory (151). Figs 3 and 4 show fluorograms (142) of two-dimensional thin-layer chromatograms of chemically tritium-labeled nucleoside trialcohols obtained by digestion and labeling of cytoplasmic tRNA from Morris hepatoma 5123D (Fig 3) and host liver (Fig 4). The same spots are present on both maps and spot intensities are similar, indicating the absence of any additional unusual nucleosides in the hepatoma and an overall similarity of the base compositions. Fluorograms obtained from hepatoma 7777 and host liver tRNA (not shown) were also very similar to each other and to those depicted in Figs

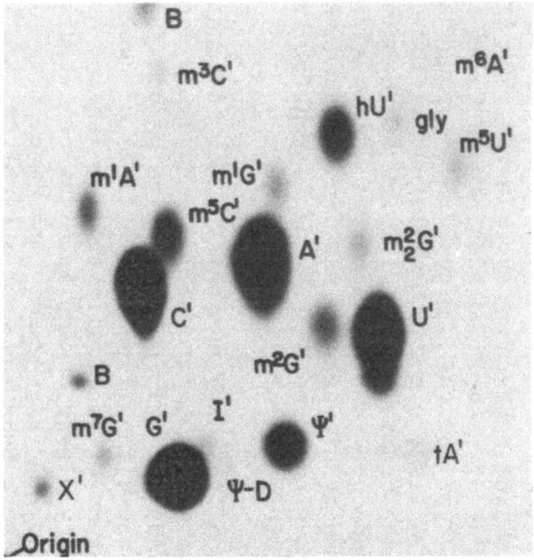

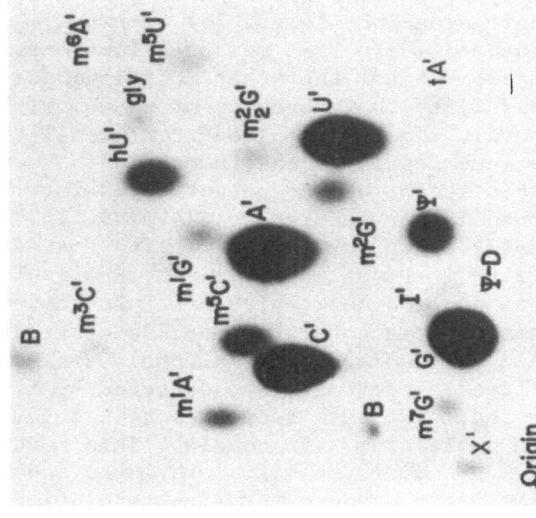

Figure 4

Fluorogram of tritium-labeled digest of host (5123D) liver tRNA. For explanations, consult legend of Fig 3. Figure taken from ref. 151.

Figure 3

Fluorogram of tritium-labeled nucleoside trialcohols obtained by digestion of hepatoma 5123D tRNA and chromatography on a cellulose thin layer. A', U', etc. nucleoside trialcohols of A, U, etc. For abbreviations of nucleosides, see footnote in text. B, background not derived from tRNA; gly, glycerol (153); Ψ-D, decomposition product derived from pseudouridine. For experimental details, see text and ref. 151. Figure taken from ref. 151.

3 and 4.

tRNA base composition data for host liver and Morris hepatomas
7777 and 5123D are listed in Tables 3 and 4, respectively, the left
part of the tables showing the total base composition and the right
part of the modified base composition. As shown by the data presented, tRNA base compositions are similar for all tissues investigated.
However, there are a number of statistically significant differences
between each hepatoma and host liver which have been indicated by encircled arrows. The base composition of tRNA from livers of normal
Buffalo rats, which was also investigated, was practically identical
with that of host liver. The total base composition of hepatoma 7777
tRNA, when compared with that of host liver tRNA (Table 3), exhibited
statistically significant differences in the four major and five modified constituents ranging from 2 to 10%, the greatest differences
being in the content of m^5U* (10%), m^3C (8%), and m^5C (7%). A comparison of the total base composition of hepatoma 5123D tRNA with
that of host liver tRNA (Table 4) showed differences in two major
and six modified constituents ranging from 1 to 16% the greatest differences being in the content of m^2_2G (13%) and X (16%). Differences
in the four major nucleosides between hepatomas and host liver were
very small (2 to 4%). The modified base composition was obtained by
excluding the major constituents from the calculations (Tables 3 and
4). This showed hepatoma 7777 tRNA (Table 3) to contain reduced
amounts of m^5U, Ψ, m^3C, m^5C but more hU and m^1_2G than liver, while hepatoma 5123D (Table 4) contained less hU and m^5C and more m^2_2G and X
than liver, differences ranging from 2 to 17%. The hepatoma tRNAs
showed no overall hypermodification or hypermethylation; their total
content in modified and methylated nucleosides was slightly reduced
as compared to liver tRNA. This can be seen from the data at the
bottom of Tables 3 and 4 where the degrees of modification (Σ modified
nucleosides/ Σ total nucleosides) and methylation (Σ modified nucleo-
sides/Σ total nucleosides) were compared for hepatoma and host liver
tRNA.

The data of Tables 3 and 4 pertain to cytoplasmic tRNA only,
which was isolated from a 100,000 g supernatant solution of a tissue
homogenate by precipitation at pH 5 and which constitutes about 50%
of total cellular tRNA. The base composition of most of the residual
cellular tRNA isolated from low-speed (15,000 x g) pellets (40-45%)
was also determined (151) (data not shown). A comparison of hepatoma
tRNA with liver tRNA isolated from low-speed pellets revealed the
following characteristics:

1. The pellet tRNA of the hepatomas was considerably more undermodified and undermethylated than the corresponding cytoplasmic tRNA.
The degrees of modification and methylation for hepatoma 7777 and
5123D pellet tRNA were both about 11 and 14% lower, respectively, than
those for pellet tRNA from liver.

Table Three[a]

Total and Modified Base Composition of Cytoplasmic tRNA from Morris Hepatoma 7777 and Host Liver

Nucleosides	Total base composition				Modified base composition			
	Hepatoma 7777 x̄ (%)[b]	Host Liver x̄ (%)	Hepatoma 7777 compared with host liver[c]	x̄ Hep.7777 / x̄ Host liv.	Hepatoma 7777 x̄ (%)	Host liver x̄ (%)	Hepatoma 7777 comp. w host liver	x̄Hep.7777 / x̄Host liver
Uridine	13.983	14.232	→	0.983				
Adenosine	16.618	17.377	→	0.956				
Cytidine	26.568	25.762	←	1.031				
Guanosine	28.460	27.860	→	1.022				
m^5U	0.515	0.572	→	0.900	3.587	3.868	→	0.927
hU	2.868	2.887	→	0.993	19.970	19.533	←→	1.022
ψ	3.455	3.605	→	0.958	24.017	24.410		0.984
m^1A[d]	1.260	1.303		0.967	8.767	8.830		0.993
I	0.330	0.325	→	1.015	2.302	2.205		1.044
m^3C[e]	0.315	0.343	→	0.918	2.202	2.340	→	0.941
m^5C	1.803	1.948	→	0.926	12.548	13.193	→	0.951
m^2G	0.582	0.572		1.017	4.055	3.870		1.048
m^2_2G	1.203	1.247		0.965	8.397	8.433		0.996
m^1G	0.842	0.780	→	1.079	5.855	5.275	←	1.110
m^7C[f]	0.803	0.787	→	1.020	5.603	5.328		1.052
X	0.388	0.403		0.963	2.700	2.705		0.998
Total	99.993	100.003			100.003	99.990		
Σ modif.nucl. / Σ total nucl.	0.1437	0.1477	→	0.973				
Σ methyl. nucl. / Σ total nucl.	0.0733	0.0755	→	0.971				

(See Footnotes under Table Five)

Table Four[a]

Total and Modified Base Composition of Cytoplasmic tRNA from Morris Hepatoma 5123D and Host Liver

Nucleosides	Total base composition				Modified base composition			
	Hepatoma 5123D x̄[b] (%)	Host Liver x̄ (%)	Hepatoma 5123D compared with host liver[c]	x̄Hep.5123D/x̄Host liv.	Hepatoma 5123D x̄ (%)	Host Liver x̄ (%)	Hep 5123D comp. with host liver	x̄Hep5123D/x̄Host liv.
Uridine	14.025	14.200	→	0.988				
Adenosine	16.928	17.093	←	0.990				
Cytidine	26.720	26.280		1.017				
Guanosine	27.908	27.675		1.008				
m^{5}U	0.585	0.615	→	0.951	4.053	4.165		0.973
hU	2.543	2.673	→	0.951	17.633	18.108		0.974
Ψ	3.525	3.595	→	0.981	24.483	24.390	→	1.004
m^{1}Ad	1.243	1.270	→	0.979	8.618	8.598		1.002
I	0.278	0.290		0.959	1.920	1.955		0.982
m^{3}Ce	0.308	0.330	→	0.933	2.133	2.220		0.961
m^{5}C	2.010	2.178	→	0.923	13.945	14.758	→←	0.945
m^{2}G	0.675	0.598	←	1.129	4.675	4.050	←	1.154
m$_2^2$G	1.265	1.265		1.000	8.773	8.575		1.023
m^{1}G	0.773	0.795		0.972	5.360	5.385		0.995
m^{7}Gf	0.735	0.735	←	1.000	5.103	4.980		1.025
X	0.478	0.413	→	1.157	3.310	2.823	←	1.173
Total	99.999	100.005			100.006	100.007		
Σ modif.nucl. / Σ total nucl.	0.1442	0.1475		0.978				
Σ methyl.nucl. / Σ total nucl.	0.0759	0.0778		0.976				

a Modified from ref. 151.

b x̄ = mean of 4 chromatographic analyses. For standard deviations consult ref. 151.

c--f See footnotes, Table 3.

2. In terms of total base composition, differences for individual modified nucleosides between the pellet tRNAs of the hepatomas and liver were generally somewhat greater than those between
corresponding cytoplasmic tRNAs. Some differences amounted to about
20 to 25%, e.g., m^3C in pellet tRNA of hepatoma 7777 was 24% lower
than in the corresponding liver preparation.

3. Pellet tRNAs and cytoplasmic tRNAs from hepatomas exhibited
similar trends. m_2^2G and X were elevated in hepatoma 5123D pellet
and cytoplasmic tRNA, while m^5U and m^3C were lower in hepatoma 7777
pellet and cytoplasmic tRNA.

Neither a comparison of the cytoplasmic tRNAs nor of the pellet
tRNAs between the two hepatomas provided evidence for a distinct correlation between altered modification and methylation patterns of
tRNA, growth rates and histological characteristics of these tumors
(see also Table 2, section 2b). The finding that hepatoma tRNAs were
slightly undermethylated is of particular interest with regard to the
report by Sheid et al. (178), who showed tRNA methylase activities to
be 3.7 and 5 times higher in Morris hepatomas 5123D and 7777, respectively, than in rat liver (Table 2, section 2b). Thus, increased tRNA
methylase activities are not necessarily accompanied by general hypermethylation of tRNA. Undermodification of tumor tRNA with regard to
several methylated or various methylated and modified constituents has
also been reported for human hepatomas (71a) and for thymic lymphoma-
bearing mice (205a), respectively.

The relatively small differences between hepatoma and liver tRNA
observed by us are consistent with differences in column-chromatographic profiles from various Morris hepatomas including hepatoma
5123D and rat liver (192, 209). tRNA from hepatoma 5123D was shown
to contain two new species of $tRNA^{Ser}$ and one new species of $tRNA^{Phe}$,
whereas two of the three $tRNA^{His}$ species found in Buffalo rat liver
could not be detected in the tumor (209). If one assumes that there
are about 60 tRNA species (45) in approximately equal amounts (chain
length, 80 nucleotides), a calculation shows that the insertion of one
additional modified base into one chain of the total tRNA population
would increase the base composition value of this particular base by
about 0.02% in terms of the total base composition or by about 0.15%
in terms of the modified base composition (see Tables 3 and 4). For
example, the increase in X and m_2^2G observed in hepatoma 5123D tRNA
(Table 4) would correspond to the addition of about 3 and 4 nucleosides, respectively, and the decrease in hU and m^5C to the deletion
of about 6 and 8 nucleosides, respectively. The values for hepatoma
7777 tRNA (Table 3) indicate similar changes. It thus appears possible that the differences in individual modified nucleosides observed by us may be the result of the presence of tumor-specific or
the absence of normal tRNAs in the hepatomas.

Regarding the question whether the heaptoma tRNAs exhibit aber-

rant methylation or modification, the increased amounts of m_2^2G and
X in hepatoma 5123D tRNA should be pointed out, which may possibly
be the result of aberrant modification. In this connection, the
report by Craddock (30) on increased activity of tRNA N^2-guanine di-
methylase in certain chemically induced rat liver and kidney tumors
should be noted. For a discussion of the possible mechanisms underlying the observed differences in tRNA base composition between the
hepatomas and liver, see also Section 3.

The data summarized here for the two Morris hepatomas are very
similar to data obtained earlier for tRNA from human brain and brain
tumors (143, 155), from avian leukemic cells and avian liver (158),
and from a variety of other normal and neoplastic mammalian tissues
(150). Our results did not confirm the substantial elevation of
various methylated bases reported by Viale and coworkers (132, 206,
208) for human brain tumor tRNA (e.g. an 80 fold increase in m^1G for
glioblastoma multiforme tRNA (207). They are not in agreement with
the hypermethylation reported earlier by Bergquist and Matthews (10)
for tRNA from certain mouse tumors. The values reported by these
authors may represent artifacts of preparation of the tRNAs (151).
As we have found (151), it is essential that the tRNA preparations
to be compared are not degraded and are free of contamination by
other RNAs and/or breakdown products of high molecular weight RNA.
Thus, purification of crude tRNA, e.g., by polyacrylamide gel electrophoresis or gel filtration, is essential to obtain meaningful results.

Recently, the methylated base content of tRNA from a caricongen-
induced monkey hepatoma has been compared with that of normal monkey
liver (95) by method 3 (see above). tRNA methylase activity in this
hepatoma and urinary excretion of tRNA catabolites by hepatoma-bearing
hosts were also determined (see also Section 2b). The base compositions for the hepatoma and normal liver were very similar (Table 5)
and there was no overall decrease in the methylated base content of
hepatoma tRNA, indicating that the latter is not hypermethylated in
spite of elevated methylase activity. These results are in agreement
with the results from our laboratory discussed above.

In summary, the questions posed at the beginning of this Section
may be answered as follows:

1. The degrees of methylation and modification of bulk tumor
tRNA do nor differ substantially from those of normal control tRNA.
Thus, tumor tRNA in general is not hypermethylated or hypermodified.
Recent work in several laboratories has indicated that the degree of
methylation and modification of tRNA from many tumors may be slightly
lower than that of normal tRNA. However, individual methylated or
modified tRNA constituents may be elevated in tumors, indicating the
presence of new tRNA species and/or possibly aberrant methylation or
modification.

Table Five[a]
Mole % Composition[b] of Monkey Liver and
Hepatoma tRNA

Compound	Liver[c]		Hepatoma[c]	
	Av.	S.E.	Av.	S.E.
m^3C	0.42	0.03	0.28	0.02
C_5	30.05	0.28	27.99	1.29
m^5C	1.91	0.11	1.57	0.07
m^1A	1.28	0.10	1.24	0.11
m^1G	0.70	0.05	0.49	0.04
m^5U[d]	1.38	0.11	5.67	2.16
U_7	19.33	0.53	21.46	1.45
m^7G	0.57	0.04	0.41	0.03
G_2	24.90	0.96	22.32	0.72
m^2A	0.37	0.02		
A	16.99	0.22	17.29	1.05
m^2G	1.44	0.09	1.18	0.13
m^1I	0.40	0.06	0.44	0.06
m_2^2G	0.51	0.04	0.49	0.05
ψ[e]	17.3	0.70	12.4	0.30

[a] From ref. 95.

[b] Mole % composition = (nmoles base/nmole total base) x 100.

[c] Average of 3 normal and 3 hepatoma tRNA pools. Each tRNA pool analyzed in duplicate.

[d] Possible DNA acontamination.

[e] Pseudouridine as (μmole/μmole uracil) x 100; determined in a separate assay.

From Table 3:

[a] Modified from ref. 151

[b] $\bar{x}$ = mean of 6 chromatographic analyses. For standard deviations, consult ref. 151.

[c] All statistically significant differences ($p \leqslant 0.05$) are indicated by encircled arrows. For p-values, consult ref. 151. Value for hepatoma > value for liver represented by ↑ . Value for hepatoma < value for liver represented by ↓ .

[d] The value for m^1A was obtained from the sum of the count rates of the (^3H)-trialcohols of m^1A and m^6A (147, 153).

[e] Corrected for 85% recovery (153).

[f] Corrected for 65% recovery (153).

From Table 4:

a Modified from ref. 151. b $\bar{x}$ = mean of 4 chromatographic analyses. For standard deviations see ref 151. c-f See footnotes, Table 3.

2.   No abnormal or additional methylated or modified nucleosides
were detected in tumor tRNA. All methylated and modified constituents found in tumor tRNA were also present in normal control tRNA.

3.   There appear to be slight changes in the major nucleoside
content in tumor tRNA, which may indicate the presence or absence
of some tRNA species or changes in the nucleotide sequence of species
normally present. The ratio of (G + C)/(A + U) is slightly elevated
in tumor tRNA.

4.   The magnitude of the changes found in tumor tRNA appears
to correlate well with the changes one would expect on the basis of
the absence or presence of a relatively small number of tRNA species,
in agreement with the chromatographic profiles of tumor tRNA.

d.   Base Composition of tRNA from Cellular Organelles

Only very few studies have been carried out on the base composition of tRNA in nuclei, nucleoli, and mitochondria, which will be
summarized here.

Nuclei and nucleoli have been shown to contain tRNAs capable of
accepting amino acids (115, 122) and also to synthesize proteins (22,
222). The base composition of 4S RNA preparations isolated from nuclei, nucleoli, ribosomes, and cell sap from Novikoff hepatoma ascites cells was investigated (160) by the tritium derivative method
described above (Section 2c). The data for 4S RNA from cell sap,
ribosomes, and nuclei were found to be very similar, whereas 4S RNA
from nucleoli contained considerably less dihydrouridine and 2-meth-
ylguanosine. Since nucleolar 4S RNA had been shown to have only 60%
of the amino acid acceptor activity as compared to nuclear or cytoplasmic 4S RNA (for refs. see 160) it appears possible that nucleolar
4S RNA contains a greater proportion of immature tRNA. Table 6 shows
a comparison of the base composition of nuclear 4S RNA from Novikoff
hepatoma ascites cells with that of nuclear 4S RNA from rat liver
(166). As can be seen, the base composition data were very similar.
However, there were statistically significant differences in two
major and five modified constituents and the degrees of modification
and methylation of the hepatoma nuclear 4S RNA appeared to be lower
than those of the liver nuclear 4S RNA.

It is now well recognized that mitochondria possess their own
specific transfer RNAs, which are coded for by mitochondrial DNA
and participate in mitochondrial protein synthesis (for reviews, see
4, 6, 17, 33). Mitochondria also appear to contain tRNA methyltransferases with specificities distinct from those of the cytoplasmic
enzymes (36, 88, 188). It is not known, however, whether the methylase activities in tumor mitochondria are increased. The base composition of mitochondrial tRNA from rat liver and Morris hepatoma

Table Six[a]
Total Base Composition of Nuclear tRNA from
Novikoff Hepatoma Ascites Cells and Rat
Liver

Nucleosides	Novikoff hepatoma		Rat liver		p[d]
	$\bar{x}$[b]	S[c]	$\bar{x}$	S	
Uridine	17.1	0.27	15.2	0.26	0.001
Adenosine	18.9	0.23	17.9	0.16	0.01
Cytidine	25.4	0.31	25.4	0.24	–
Guanosine	27.1	0.09	27.9	0.26	–
m^5U	0.5	0.03	0.6	0.03	0.05
hU	2.0	0.10	2.5	0.23	0.001
Ψ	3.0	0.11	3.5	0.09	0.01
m^1A	0.9	0.06	1.1	0.08	–
m^6A[e]	0.2	0.06	0.2	0.03	–
I	0.4	0.01	0.4	0.06	–
m^3C	0.2	0.04	0.2	0.03	–
m^5C	1.4	0.13	1.9	0.03	0.001
m_2^2G	0.5	0.04	0.5	0.05	–
$m^2{}_2G$	1.2	0.07	1.2	0.04	–
m^1G	0.7	0.05	0.8	0.02	–
m^7G	0.6	0.04	0.7	0.06	0.05

[a] Data of Ro-Choi (166).

[b] Mean of 9 chromatographic analyses.

[c] Standard deviation $|S| = \sqrt{[\Sigma\,(x - \bar{x})^2]/(N - 1)}$

[d] Probability values estimated on the basis of Student's t test.
$p \leq 0.05$, statistically significant.

[e] Trialcohol of m^6A originates from m^1A (147, 153).

5123D and 7777 was determined in our laboratory (25) by the tritium
derivative method (see Section 2c). Mitochondrial tRNA from these
sources, from cultured hamster cells (34, 35) and HeLa cells (5,
32) is characterized by some common features:

   1. Mitochondrial tRNA contains a rather high proportion of A*
and U, but less G and C, when compared with cytoplasmic tRNA.

   2. Mitochondrial tRNA is considerably less methylated than
cytoplasmic tRNA.

   3. Mitochondrial tRNA has a relatively high content of m^1A
and m^2G and a low content of m^5U (reported for rat liver, the two
hepatomas, and BHK cells).

   4. Mitochondrial tRNA resembles more its cytoplasmic counterpart than it does bacterial tRNA. This observation was unexpected
in view of the endosymbiont hypothesis, according to which mitochondria have evolved from domesticated bacteria (see 17).

   Regarding the high m^1A content of mitochondrial tRNA, it is interesting to note that a mitochondrial methylase preparation from
Phaseolus vulgaris was found to contain an additional adenosine-1
methylase activity with an unusual specificity (36).

   The investigation of the base composition of mitochondrial tRNA
from rat liver and from Morris hepatomas 5123D and 7777 was of particular interest since the data for the respective cytoplasmic tRNAs
were already available (see Section 2c). The two hepatoma mitochondrial tRNA preparations were found to exhibit relatively greater
alterations than the tumor cytoplasmic tRNAs when compared with their
normal counterparts. Both mitochondrial and cytoplasmic tRNA from
the two hepatomas were undermethylated and undermodified, but this
trend, which was only slightly apparent in the cytoplasmic tRNAs, was
much more pronounced in the mitochondrial tRNAs, particularly from the
more malignant, rapidly growing hepatoma 7777. Hepatoma 5123D mitochondrial tRNA contained 8%, hepatoma 7777 mitochondrial tRNA 17% less
methylated bases than liver mitochondrial tRNA. A comparison of the
base composition data for cytoplasmic and mitochondrial tRNA also
showed that the alterations of a specific base in the mitochondrial
tRNA of the two hepatomas usually was not paralleled by an analogous
alteration in the corresponding cytoplasmic tRNA. For example, the
relative amounts of m^1A, m^2G, and I were clearly elevated in the mitochondrial tRNAs of both hepatomas when compared with liver but none of
these bases was elevated to a statistically significant extent in cytoplasmic tRNA. Furthermore, the two hepatoma mitochondrial tRNAs
were found to have six alterations of the modified base composition in
common, i.e., an increase in m^1A, m^2G, and I, and a decrease in m^5U,
hU, and m^5C, while only one of these alterations, i.e., a decrease in

m^5C, was also found in the corresponding cytoplasmic tRNA.

The functional significance of these tRNA alterations in the hepatoma mitochondria is not clear at present. However, the mitochondrial tRNA alterations may be correlated with a number of other changes observed in mitochondria of Morris hepatomas. Mitochondria from various Morris hepatomas when compared with liver mitochondria were found to exhibit certain biochemical alterations, e.g., a decrease in monoamine oxidase and adenylate cyclase activity, a decrease in cytochromes a + a_3, b and c_1, a higher lability of the phosphorylative apparatus, alterations of membrane glycoproteins (for refs. see 25) and of phospholipids (117). Abnormalities of sedimentation properties, size, and shape of mitochondria from hepatomas and other tumors have also been reported (for ref. see 25). These biochemical and structural aberrations may conceivably be mediated by changes in the mitochondrial protein synthesizing system, in which altered mitochondrial tRNA may be involved. Moreover, if one assumes that mitochondrial tRNA modification serves some regulatory functions, the observed changes may also signify a loss of regulatory functions of tRNA in mitochondria and thus may mediate a derangement of biochemical processes in these organelles. Nucleotide sequence analysis of individual mitochondrial tRNA species should provide further insight into the nature and functional significance of tRNA alterations in tumor mitochondria.

e. Nucleotide Sequence Analysis of Individual tRNA Species

As pointed out in the preceding sections, a better understanding of the role of altered tRNA in neoplasia will be gained by sequence analysis of many individual tRNA species from normal and neoplastic cells. Only recently methods have become available to sequence the small amounts of individual tRNAs in tumors. Conventional sequencing methods based on UV spectrophotometry and/or biological isotope labeling were either impracticable because of the large amounts of biological material required or inadequate because of insufficient labeling of RNA in the intact mammalian organism. Work in our laboratory has therefore concentrated on the systematic development of highly sensitive isotope derivative ("postlabeling") methods suitable for sequencing small amounts of nonradioactive RNA. A number of possible sequencing schemes based on postlabeling have been discussed (149). Isotope label may either be introduced chemically into RNA fragments, e.g., (^3H)-label into 3'-terminal positions (140, 145, 146, 149, 156, 157, 185), or enzymatically, e.g., (^{32}P)-label into 5'-terminal (163, 182) or 3'-terminal (197) positions. Two highly sensitive tritium derivative methods, based on 3'-end labeling with tritium, have been developed in our laboratory (144, 156, 157, 185). These methods are several orders of magnitude more sensitive than classical spectrophotometric methods, requiring only a total of 20-25 A_{260} units of a tRNA species (about 1 mg; corresponding to about

1-2 kg tissue) to determine the entire nucleotide sequence. Two eukaryotic tRNA species have been sequenced by these procedures in our laboratory (154, 169). Thus, these methods are suitable for sequencing tumor and normal tRNA species from 1-2 kg of tissue. Recently two additional methods, based on the new principle of controlled endonuclease digestion of terminally labeled RNA, have been worked out in our laboratory, which require even less RNA (0.1 – 0.3 A_{260} unit of tRNA for sequencing all fragments in complete ribonuclease T_1 and A digests) (58-61). Thus, less than 100 g of tissue is needed for sequencing a tRNA by these methods. Related procedures have recently been developed independently in other laboratories (24, 104, 180). A distinct advantage of the post-labeling procedures developed in our laboratory is the feature of direct identification of each position in the polynucleotide chain. This is particularly important for oligonucleotides containing modified nucleosides and for large oligonucleotides from partial digests since such compounds may be difficult to characterize otherwise (21, 24).

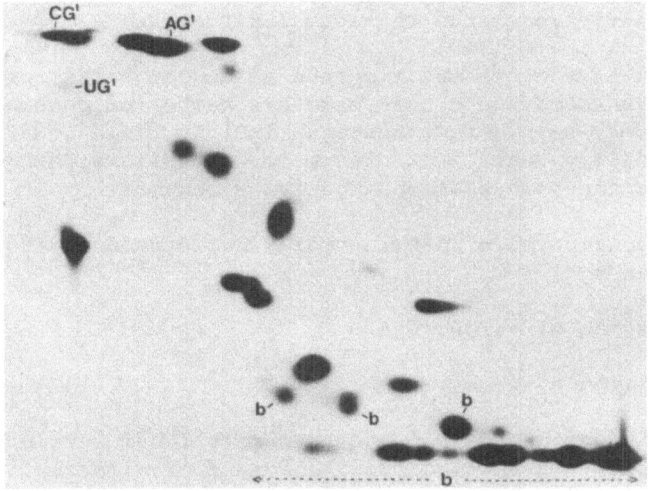

Figure 5
Fluorogram of a 3'-terminally tritium-labeled RNase T_1 digest of a tRNA^{Phe} from Morris hepatoma 5123D, isolated as described in the text (56). Two-dimensional chromatography (56) on a PEI-cellulose (141a) thin layer. CG', AG', UG', dinucleotide dialcohols, located by their coincidence with UV markers; b, background not derived from RNA.

Fig 5 illustrates a fingerprint of a Morris hepatoma tRNA^{Phe} digest currently being analyzed in our laboratory (56). This tRNA ^{Phe} species was isolated from Morris hepatomas 5123D by phenol extraction of total tRNA (168), followed by fractionation on a BD-cellulose column (49, 170), polyacrylamide gel electrophoresis of the ethanol fraction from the BD-cellulose column containing tRNA ^{Phe} acceptor activity (56), and extraction of the tRNA^{Phe} band from the gel (26). Fig 5 shows a fluorogram ($\underline{142}$) of a 3'-terminally (^{3}H)-labeled RNase T_1 digest of this tRNA^{Phe} species (60, 149). Sequencing work is in progress in our laboratory on this and other tRNAs from Morris hepatomas and normal liver to gain insight into the chemical basis of alterations in tumor tRNA.

3. DISCUSSION AND OUTLOOK

As has been shown in several laboratories (89, 149, 198), the pattern of modification and methylation of vertebrate tRNA has been preserved over a period of considerable evolutionary change. This stability indicates that the modifications of tRNA of vertebrates must have vital functions, which are however poorly understood at the present time. In recent years tRNA modifications have been increasingly implicated in nontranslational, regulatory functions of tRNA (see Introduction). The observed alterations of tumor tRNA and tRNA methylating enzymes have to be regarded therefore as highly significant deviations from the normal situation.

Although at the present time the molecular basis for these alterations is unknown, we can formulate a number of possible mechanisms, which may help direct research in this field toward specific goals. Basically, there are three major mechanisms that could cause qualitative changes in tRNA and modifying enzymes:

1. Transcription of new, normally not expressed (for example, oncofetal) genes,

2. Mutation of genes, and

3. Deletion of genes.

These changes at the DNA and transcriptional levels may affect tRNA indirectly (via the modifying enzymes) or directly.

Let us first consider the indirect effects.

1. Transcription of new genes for modifying enzymes may lead to increased levels of these enzymes. Unfortunately, the enzyme concentrations are difficult to determine and thus far only enzyme activities have been measured. The increased tRNA methylase activities in tumors could reflect the transcription of new genes or increased

transcription of normal tRNA methylase genes or both. The question whether tumor tRNA methylases exhibit new specificities has not yet been answered unambiguously (see Section 2b). Increased activities of the modifying and methylating enzymes may lead to aberrant modification and methylation of tRNA. Application of advanced techniques of tRNA analysis has however not demonstrated a general overmodification and overmethylation of tumor tRNA (see Section 2c). Increased activities of the modifying and methylating enzymes may lead to aberrant modification and methylation of tRNA. Application of advanced techniques of tRNA analysis has however not demonstrated a general overmodification and overmethylation of tumor tRNA (see Section 2c). In two Morris hepatomas investigated, there was overmodification only with respect to two constituents, while nine other nucleosides were found to be undermodified. The increase in the two nucleosides could possibly be the result of aberrant modification but could also be due to the presence of new tumor-specific tRNA species.

2. The mutation of genes coding for modifying enzymes may lead to alterations of enzyme structure and activity. It appears more likely that such altered enzymes would exhibit decreased activities leading to aberrant tRNA modification. The observed undermodification and undermethylation of tumor tRNA may be the result of such alterations at the enzyme level. Alternatively, it could also be the result of the presence of tRNAs having altered primary sequences (see below).

3. The deletion of genes for modifying enzymes would lead to deficient tRNA modification.

Let us now consider direct effects on tRNA caused by changes at the DNA and transcriptional level.

1. The transcription of new tRNA precursor genes will lead to the appearance of new tRNA species, provided the tRNA precursors are processed normally and the resulting tRNAs are metabolically stable. These species may be undermodified if certain modifying enzymes necessary for their complete modification are absent.

2. The mutation of genes may lead to altered sequences in the tRNA precursor, which may not be recognized by certain modifying enzymes. This may also lead to the appearance of undermodified tRNAs, if such tRNAs are sufficiently stable metabolically. Such a mechanism has actually been observed in $\underline{E}$. $\underline{coli}$ carrying phage T_4 mutants, which specify the production of undermodified phage tRNA^{Glu} and tRNA^{Ser}. It was shown (111) that single base mutations in the glutamine tRNA and the serine precursor tRNAs, respectively, led to absent or highly deficient modification of all modified nucleosides in the mutated tRNAs. Even single mutations apparently cause sufficient distortions of the three-dimensional structure of the mole-

cule so that it can no longer be recognized correctly by the
modifying enzymes, thus implying that these enzymes exhibit strict
stereospecificity.

    3. The deletion of tRNA genes would lead to a loss of tRNA
species.

    As may be inferred from this discussion, undermodification of
tumor tRNA is more likely to occur than overmodification. The increased tumor tRNA methylase activities as well as the increased
urinary excretion levels in tumor-bearing hosts, which have been
explained by a higher turnover of tumor tRNA, may well be direct
consequence of pre-tRNA or tRNA undermodification.

    The following hypothesis may explain how the increases in
both tRNA turnover and tRNA methylase activity in tumors may be
related to pre-tRNA or tRNA undermodification, which, in the context
of this hypothesis, is regarded as the primary tRNA lesion in tumor
cells, irrespective of whether it has its origin in faulty transcription of tRNA or tRNA methylase genes (see Discussion above).
Undermodified pre-tRNA or tRNA may be a better substrate for nuclease cleavage than normally modified pre-tRNA or tRNA, (Phospho-
diester bonds involving certain methylated and modified nucleosides
have been shown to be resistant to nuclease action, e.g., 205). This
decreased stability would lead to increased degradation of unmodified
tumor pre-tRNA or both precursor tRNA and modifying enzymes. Furthermore, the biosynthesis of the modifying enzymes might be regulated by
the intracellular concentrations of free modified nucleotides, nucleosides, and/or bases generated by tRNA degradation. Thus, increased levels of free modified tRNA constituents in tumors would
lead to increased synthesis of modifying enzymes.

    The observation that several carcinogens are capable of inducing
increased activities of tRNA methylases (Section 2b) may also be explained if one assumes that treatment with carcinogens leads to increased breakdown of tRNA but no systematic studies of this question
have been performed. In the special case of the hepatocarcinogen
ethionine, however, a decrease in tRNA methylation and a concomitant
increase in tRNA methylase activity have been demonstrated (Section
2b); it is possible that the increase in enzyme activity is mediated
by increased breakdown of labile undermethylated tRNA or pre-tRNA in
ethionine-treated cells. Unfortunately, very little is known about
tRNA metabolism during carcinogenesis. It is tempting to speculate
that alterations of tRNA metabolism, which are initiated at early
stages of carcinogenesis, are maintained during the preneoplastic
into the neoplastic phase and thus may play a crucial role in the
development and maintenance of the neoplastic state. As shown by
Farber (39), the pathogenesis of liver cancer proceeds in stages
from initiated preneoplastic cells to malignant neoplasia with an

interruption of differentiation in early new hepatocyte populations, both somatic mutation and altered differentiation probably playing important roles at different stages of this process. Since a new preneoplastic antigen (PN) was found to be present in preneoplastic cells and in primary hepatomas induced by a variety of different hepatocarcinogens, this author emphasizes that "common features of preneoplastic and neoplastic cell populations exist and should be looked for". It will be of great interest therefore to compare in detail tRNA and tRNA modifying enzymes in such early preneoplastic cell populations with those in neoplastic cells, particularly since changes of aminoacyl-tRNA profiles have been observed during embryogenesis and differentiation (Section 2a), which may imply that altered tRNA could be involved in the interruption of differentiation observed during the progression from initiated preneoplastic cells to primary hepatoma.

Another important characteristic of the cancer cell, in which tRNA may be implicated, is its metabolic advantage over normal cells. In this context, two aspects of possible tRNA involvement may be considered, i.e., 1. altered tRNA in tumor mitochondria and 2. the increased tumor tRNA methylases.

1. Studies on a spectrum of Morris hepatomas have demonstrated that the rate of glycolysis is directly proportional, while the respiratory rate is inversely proportional to the degree of cellular dedifferentiation (212). These metabolic changes are presumably a consequence of alterations of mitochondrial functions in tumor cells. It is well established that the ability of mitochondria to catalyze oxidative phosphorylation is directly linked to the structural integrity of the mitochondrial membranes, which depends on the structural integrity of the membrane proteins and other molecules. It appears possible that the mitochondrial tRNA alterations observed in Morris hepatomas (Section 2d) may be casually related to changes in both mitochondrial protein synthesis and regulatory processes, thus leading to defects in mitochondrial membrane structure and to the metabolic changes referred to above.

2. According to the molecular correlation concept formulated by Weber (see Section 2b), the tRNA methylases belong to the class of "key enzymes", As studies in a spectrum of Morris hepatomas have shown, these enzymes are involved in the pattern of metabolic imbalance, which is linked with malignant transformation and/or progression in malignancy because it confers a biological advantage of the cancer cell over normal cells.

This latter aspect is of particular interest in cancer chemotherapy since the "key enzymes" provide potential targets of anticancer drugs. Studies with anticancer drugs in our laboratory (Section 2b) have shown that the tRNA modifying enzymes are indeed specific targets for some antimetabolites.

It is apparent from the data presented in this article that our present knowledge of the role of tRNA and tRNA modification in neoplasia and carcinogenesis is rather limited. In order to better understand the role of altered tRNA and tRNA modifications in carcinogenesis and neoplasia, it is necessary to study the sequences and functional properties of tRNAs and to characterize the modifying enzymes in normal, preneoplastic, and neoplastic cells. Novel sensitive postlabeling methods have recently become available (Section 2e) which for the first time make it possible to sequence microgram amounts of tRNA. Several Morris hepatoma tRNAs have been isolated and are currently being sequenced ·in our laboratory. It will also be important to explore further the specific effects of nucleoside analogs and anticancer drugs on tRNA modification and function (Section 2b). It may be hoped that the knowledge of the structure of altered tumor tRNA species may enable the design of a rational therapeutic strategy, which would affect mainly structure and function of tumor-specific tRNA but not interfere with tRNA functions in normal cells.

ACKNOWLEDGEMENTS

Work in our laboratory referred to in this article has been supported by grants from the USPHS (CA-13591, CA-16840, CA-10893-P8) and an American Cancer Society Faculty Research Award PRA-108.

We wish to express our gratitude to Dr. Paul C. Zamecnik for encouragement and suggestions during our initial analytical work on tumor tRNAs.

* Abbreviations used are: m^5U, 5-methyluridine; m^3C, 3-methylcytidine; m^5C, 5-methylcytidine, m^1A, 1-methyladenosine, m^6A, 6-methyladenosine; m^1G, 1-methylguanosine; m^2G, 2-methylguanosine; m_2^2G, N^2, N^2-dimethylguanosine; m^7G, 7-methylguanosine; hU, dihydrouridine; Ψ, pseudouridine; I, inosine, X, 3-(3-amino-3-carboxypropyl)uridine; tA, N-[9-(β-D-ribofuranosyl)purin-6-yl-carbamoyl]threonine; U, uridine; C, cytidine; A, adenosine; G, guanosine.

REFERENCES

1. Adams, J.M. and Cory, S. Nature 255 (1975) 28.

2. Alexander, P. Nature 235 (1972) 137.

3. Anderson, W.F. and Gilbert, J. Biochem. Biophys. Res. Comm. 36 (1969) 456.

4. Ashwell, M. and Work, T.S. Ann. Rev. Biochem. 39 (1970) 251.

5. Attardi, B. and Attardi, G. J. Mol. Biol. 55 (1971) 231.

6. Attardi, G., Costantino, P., England, J., Lederman, M., Ojala, D. and Storrie, B. Acta Andocrinol. (Suppl). 180 (1973) 263.

7. Baliga, B.S., Borek, E., Weinstein, I.B. and Srinivasan, P.R. Proc. Natl. Acad. Sci. U.S.A. 62 (1969) 899.

8. Baguley, B.C. and Staehelin,M. Eur. J. Biochem. 6 (1968) 1.

9. Baguley, B.C. and Staehelin, M. Biochemistry 7 (1968) 45.

10. Bergquist, P.L. and Matthews, R.E.P. Biochem. J. 85 (1962) 305.

11. Blasi, F., Barton, R.W., Kovach, J.S. and Goldberger, R.F. J. Bacteriol. 106 (1971) 508.

12. Blobstein, S.H., Grunberger, D., Weinstein, I.B. and Nakanishi, K. Biochemistry 12 (1973) 188.

13. Borek, E., In: Exploitable Molecular Mechanisms and Neoplasia, The Williams and Wilkins Co., Baltimore (1969) 163.

14. Borek, E. and Kerr, S.J. Adv. Cancer Res. 15 (1972) 163.

15. Borek, E. and Srinivasan, P.R. In: Transmethyaltion and Methionine Biosynthesis, S.K. Shapiro and F. Schlenk (eds). Univ. of Chicago Press, Chicago (1965) 115.

16. Borek, E. and Srinivasan, P.R. Ann. Rev. Biochem. 35 (1966) 275.

17. Borst, P. Ann. Rev. Biochem. 41 (1972) 333.

18. Bridges, K.R. and Jones, G.H. Biochemistry 12 (1973) 1208.

19. Briscoe, W.T., Griffin, A.C., McBride, C. and Bowen, J.M. Cancer Res. 35 (1975) 2586.

20. Briscoe, W.T., Taylor, W., Griffin, A.C., Duff, R. and Rapp, F. Cancer Res. 32 (1972) 1753.

21. Brownlee, G.G., In: Laboratory Techniques in Biochemsitry and Molecular Biology, Determination of Sequences, T.S. Work and E. Work (eds), North Holland, Amsterdam/American Elsevier, New York (1972).

21a. Busby, W.F., Jr., Paglialunga, S., Newberne, P.M. and Wogan, G.N. Cancer Res. 36 (1976) 2013.

22. Busch, H. and Smetana, K. In: The Nucleolus, Academic Press, New York (1970).

23. Caskey, C.T. In: Prebiotic and Biochemical Evolution, A.P. Kimball and J. Oro (eds). North Holland, Amsterdam (1971) 153.

24. Chang, S.H., Brum, C.K., Silberklang, M., RajBahndary, U.L., Hecker, L.I. and Barnett, W.E. Cell 9 (1976) 717.

25. Chia, L.S.Y., Morris, H.P., Randerath, K. and Randerath, E. Biochim. Biophys. Acta 425 (1976) 49.

26. Chia, L.S.Y., Randerath, K. and Randerath, E. Anal. Biochem. 55 (1973) 102.

27. Cortese, R., Kammen, H.O., Spengler, S.J. and Ames, B.N. J. Biol. Chem. 249 (1974) 1103.

28. Cortese, R., Landsberg, R., Von der Haar, R.A., Umbarger, H.E. and Ames, B.N. Proc. Natl. Acad. Sci. U.S.A. 71 (1974) 1857.

29. Craddock, V.M., Nature 288 (1970) 1264.

30. Craddock, V.M., Biochim. Biophys. Acta 272 (1972) 288.

31. Craddock, V.M. and Magee, P.N. Biochem. J. 89 (1963) 32.

32. Davenport, L.W. and Dubin, D.T. Fed. Proc. 34 (1975) 612 (Abs).

33. Dawid, I.B. In: Mitochondria: Biogenesis and Bioenergetics; Biomembranes: Molecular Arrangements and Transport Mechanisms, S.G. Van den Bergh, P. Borst, L.L.M. Van Deenen, J.C. Riemersma E.C.Slater, and J.M. Tager (eds). North Holland, Amsterdam, 28 (1972) 35.

34. Dubin, D.T. and Friend, D.A. Biochim. Biophys. Acta 340 (1974) 269.

35. Dubin, D.T. and Montenecourt, B.S. J. Mol. Biol. 48 (1970) 279.

36. Dubois, E.G., Dirheimer, G. and Weil, J.H. Biochim. Biophys. Acta 374 (1974) 332.

37. Dunn, D.B. and Smith, J.D. Biochem. J. 60 (1955) XVII.

38. Elska, A., Matsuka, G. and Matiash, O. Biochim. Biophys. Acta 247 (1971) 430.

39. Farber, E. Arch. Pathol. 98 (1974) 145.

40. Fleissner, E. and Borek, E. Proc. Natl. Acad. Sci. U.S.A. 48 (1962) 1199.

41. Fleissner, E. and Borek, E. Biochemistry 2 (1963) 1093.

42. Fournier, A., Chavancy, G. and Garel, J.P. Biochem. Biophys. Res. Comm. 72 (1976) 1187.

43. Fujioka, S. and Gallo, R.C. Blood 38 (1971) 246.

44. Gallagher, R.E., Ting, R.C. and Gallo, R.C. Biochim. Biophys. Acta 272 (1972) 568.

45. Gallo, R.C. and Petska, S. J. Mol. Biol. 52 (1970) 246.

46. Garel, J.P., J. Theor. Biol. 43 (1974) 225.

47. Garel, J.P., Mandel, P., Chavancy, G. and Daillie, J. FEBS Lett. 7 (1970) 327.

48. Ghosh, K. and Ghosh, H.P. Biochem. Biophys. Res. Comm. 40 (1970) 135.

49. Gillam, I., Millward, S., Blew, S., von Tigerstrom, M., Wimmer, E. and Tener, G.M. Biochemistry 6 (1967) 3043.

50. Glick, J.M., Ross, S. and Leboy, P.S. Nucl. Acids. Res. 2 (1975) 1639.

51. Gold, P. Ann. Rev. Med. 22 (1971) 85.

52. Gold, P. and Freedman, S.O. J. Exp. Med. 121 (1965) 467.

53. Goldberger, R.F. Science 183 (1974) 810.

54. Gonano, F., Chiarugi, V.P., Pirro, G. and Marini, M. Biochemistry 10 (1971) 900.

55. Gonano, F., Pirro, G. and Silvetti, S. Nature New Biol. 242 (1973) 236.

56. Gopalakrishnan, A.S., Gupta, R.C., Randerath, E. and Randerath, K. Unpublished Experiments.

57. Grunberger, D., Weinstein, I.B. and Mushinski, J.F. Nature 253 (1975) 66.

58. Gupta, R.C. and Randerath, K. Nucl. Acids Res. 4 (1977) 1957.

59. Gupta, R.C. and Randerath, K. Submitted for Publication.

60. Gupta, R.C., Randerath, E. and Randerath, K. Nucl. Acids Res. 3 (1976) 2895.

61. Gupta, R.C., Randerath, E. and Randerath, K. Nucl. Acids Res. 3 (1976) 2915.

62. Hacker, B. and Mandel, L.R. Biochim. Biophys. Acta 190 (1969) 38.

63. Hacker, B. and McDermott, B.J. Physiol. Chem. Phys. 4 (1972) 41.

64. Hall, R.H. In: The Modified Nucleosides in Nucleic Acids, Columbia University Press, New York and London (1971).

65. Hall, R.H. and Dunn, D.B. In: Handbook of Biochemistry and Molecular Biology, Nucl. Acids, G.D. Fasman (ed). CRC Press, Cleveland 1 (1975) 216.

66. Hancock, R.L. Biochem. Biophys. Res. Comm. 31 (1968) 77.

67. Hancock, R.L. and Forrester, P.I. Cancer Res. 33 (1973) 1747.

68. Harada, F. and Nishimura, S. Biochemistry 11 (1972) 301.

69. Hayashi, M., Griffin, A.C., Duff, R. and Rapp, F. Cancer Res. 33 (1973) 902.

70. Heady, J.E. and Kerr, S.J. Cancer Res. 35 (1975) 640.

71. Ho, Y. and Lin, H.J. Cancer Res. 34 (1974) 986.

71a. Ho, Y. and Lin, H.J. Brit. J. Cancer 29 (1974) 324.

72. Holland, J.J., Taylor, M.W., Buck, C.A. Proc. Natl. Acad. Sci. U.S.A. 58 (1967) 2437.

73. Holley, R.W., Apgar, J., Everett, G.A., Madison, J.T., Marquisee,

M., Merrill, S.H., Penswick, J.R. and Zamir, A. Science 147 (1965) 1462.

74. Hurwitz, J., Gold, M. and Anders, M., J. Biol. Chem. 239 (1964) 3474.

75. Inose, M., Miyata, S. and Iwanami, Y. Biochim. Biophys. Acta 259 (1972) 96.

76. Itano, H.A. In: Abnormal Hemoglobins in Africa, Blackwell, Oxford (1965) p. 3.

77. Kasai, H., Kuchino, Y., Nihei, K. and Nishimura, S. Nucl. Acids Res. 2 (1975) 1931.

78. Kasai, H., Nakanishi, K., Macfarlane, R.D., Torgerson, D.F., Ohashi, Z., McCloskey, J.A., Gross, H.J. and Nishimura, S. J. Am. Chem. Soc. 98 (1976) 5044.

79. Kasai, H., Ohashi, Z., Harada, F., Nishimura, S., Oppenheimer, N.J., Crain, P.F., Liehr, J.G., von Minden, D.L. and McCloskey, J.A. Biochemistry 14 (1975) 4198.

80. Katze, J.R. Biochim. Biophys. Acta 383 (1975) 131.

81. Kaye, A.M. and Leboy, P.S. Biochim. Biophys. Acta 157 (1968) 289.

82. Kelmers, A.D. and Heatherly, D.E. Anal. Biochem. 44 (1971) 486.

83. Kerr, S.J. Biochemistry 9 (1970) 690.

84. Kerr, S.J. Proc. Natl. Acad. Sci. U.S.A. 68 (1971) 406.

85. Kerr, S.J. J. Biol. Chem. 247 (1972) 4248.

86. Kerr, S.J. Cancer Res. 35 (1975) 2969.

87. Kerr, S.J. and Borek, E. Adv. Enzymol. 36 (1972) 1.

88. Klagsbrun, M. J. Biol. Chem. 248 (1973) 2606.

89. Klagsbrun, M. J. Biol. Chem. 248 (1973) 2612.

90. Kraus, J. and Staehelin,M. Nucl. Acids Res. 1 (1974) 1455.

91. Kraus, J. and Staehelin, M. Nucl. Acids Res. 1 (1974) 1479.

92. Kuchino, Y. and Nishimura, S. Biochem. Biophys, Res. Comm. 40 (1970) 306.

93. Kuchino, Y. and Nishimura, S. Biochemistry 13 (1974) 3683.

94. Kuchino, Y., Endo, H. and Nishimura, S. Cancer Res. 32 (1972) 1243.

95. Lakings, D.B., Waalkes, T.P., Borek, E., Gehrke, C.W., Mrochek, J.E., Longmore, J. and Adamson, R.H. Cancer Res. 37 (1977) 285.

96. Lakings, D.B., Waalkes, T.P. and Mrochek, J.E. J. Chromatog. 116 (1976) 83.

97. Lanks, K.W. and Weinstein, I.B., Biochem. Biophys. Res. Comm. 40 (1970) 708.

98. Leboy, P.S. Biochemistry 9 (1970) 1577.

99. Leboy, P.S., FEBS Lett. 16 (1971) 117.

100. Li, H.J., Nakanishi, K., Grunberger, D. and Weinstein, I.B., Biochem. Biophys. Res. Comm. 55 (1973) 818.

101. Lis, H. and Sharon, N. Ann. Rev. Biochem. 42 (1973) 541.

102. Littauer, U.Z. and Inouye, H. Ann. Rev. Biochem. 42 (1973) 439.

103. Littlefield, J.W. and Dunn, D.B. Biochem. J. 70 (1958) 642.

104. Lockard, R.E. and RajBhandary, U.L. Cell 9 (1976) 747.

105. Lu, L.W., Chiang, G.H., Medina, D. and Randerath, K. Biochem. Biophys. Res. Comm. 68 (1976) 1094.

106. Lu, L.W., Chiang, G.H., and Randerath, K. Nucl. Acids Res. 3 (1976) 2243.

107. Lu, L.W., Chiang, G.H., Tseng, W.C. and Randerath, K. Biochem. Biophys. Res. Comm. 73 (1976) 1075.

108. Magee, P.N. and Farber, E. Biochem. J. 83 (1962) 114.

109. Mandell, J.D. and Hershey, A.D. Anal. Biochem. 1 (1960) 66.

110. Mauck, J.C. and Green, H. Cell 3 (1974) 171.

111. McClain, W.H. and Seidman, J.G. Nature 257 (1975) 106.

112. Mittelman, A., Hall, R.H., Yohn, D.S. and Grace, J.T. Cancer Res. 27 (1967) 1409.

113. Miyaji, H., Morris, H.P. and Wagner, B.P. Methods Cancer Res.
     H. Busch (ed). Academic Press, New York 4 (1968) 153.

114. Moore, B.G. and Smith, R.C. Can. J. Biochem. 47 (1969) 561.

115. Moriyama, Y., Hodnett, J.L., Prestayko, A.W. and Busch, H.
     J. Mol. Biol. 39 (1969) 335.

116. Morris, H.P. and Wagner, B.P. Methods Cancer Res. H. Busch
     (ed). Academic Press, New York 4 (1968) 125.

117. Morton, R., Cunningham, C., Jester, R., Waite, M., Miller, N.
     and Morris, H.P. Cancer Res. 36 (1976) 3246.

118. Mukerjee, H. and Goldfeder, A. Cancer Res. 36 (1976) 3330.

119. Munns, T.W., Podratz, K.C. and Katzman, P.A. Biochemistry
     13 (1974) 4409.

120. Mushinski, J.F. Biochemistry 10 (1971) 3917.

121. Mushinski, J.F. Nature 248 (1974) 332.

122. Nakamura, T., Prestayko, A.W. and Busch, H. J. Biol. Chem.
     243 (1968) 1368.

123. Nau, F. Biochimie 58 (1976) 629.

124. Nau, F., Garbit, F. and Dubert, J.M. Biochim. Biophys. Acta
     277 (1972) 80.

125. Nishimura, S. Prog. Nucl. Acid Res. Mol. Biol. 12 (1972) 49.

126. Nishimura, S. In: MTP International Review of Science, Bio-
     chemistry (Series One), Biochemistry of Nucleic Acids, K.
     Burton (ed). Butterworths, London/University Park Press,
     Baltimore 6 (1974) 289.

127. Okada, N., Shindo-Okada, N. and Nishimura, S. Nucl. Acids
     Res. 4 (1977) 415.

128. Pegg, A.E. Biochim. Biophys. Acta 232 (1971) 630.

129. Pegg, A.E. In: Advances in Cancer Research, G. Klein and S.
     Weinhouse (eds). Academic Press, New York (1977) in press.

130. Pegg, A.E. and Hawks, A.M., Biochem. J. 137 (1974) 229.

131. Penhoet, E.E. and Holland, J.J. J. Natl. Cancer Inst. 47 (1971)

1173.

132. Perria, L. and Viale, G.L. Acta Neurochir. 21 (1969) 257.

133. Perry, R.P. and Kelley, D.E. Cell 1 (1974) 37.

134. Piper, P.W. Eur. J. Biochem. 51 (1975) 283.

135. Piper, P.W. Eur. J. Biochem. 51 (1975) 295.

136. Piper, P.W. and Clark, B.F.C. Eur. J. Biochem. 45 (1974) 589.

137. Piper, P.W. and Clark, B.F.C. Nature 247 (1974) 516.

138. Rainer, H., Hocker, P., Stacher, A., Moser, K., Streit, I. and Deutsch, E. Neoplasma 21 (1974) 409.

139. Rajalakshmi, S. Proc. Am. Accos. Cancer Res. 14 (1973) 39.

140. RajBhandary, U.L. J. Biol. Chem. 243 (1968) 556.

141. RajBhandary, U.L. and Chang, S.H. J. Biol. Chem. 243 (1968) 598.

141a. Randerath, K., Angew. Chem. 74 (1962) 780, International Edition 1 (1962) 553.

142. Randerath, K. Anal. Biochem. 34 (1970) 188.

143. Randerath, K. Cancer Res. 31 (1971) 658.

144. Randerath, K. FEBS Lett. 33 (1973) 143.

145. Randerath, K. and Randerath, E. Experientia 24 (1968) 1192.

146. Randerath, K. and Randerath, E. Anal. Biochem. 28 (1969) 110.

147. Randerath, K. and Randerath, E. In: Proc. Nucl. Acid Res. G.L. Cantoni and D.R. Davies (eds). Harper and Row, New York, 2 (1971) 796.

148. Randerath, K. and Randerath, E. J. Chromatog. 82 (1973) 59.

149. Randerath, K. and Randerath, E. In: Methods in Cancer Res. H. Busch (ed). Academic Press, New York 9 (1973) 3.

150. Randerath, K. and Randerath, E. Unpublished Experiments.

151. Randerath, E., Chia, L.S.Y., Morris, H.P. and Randerath, K.

Cancer Res. 34 (1974) 643.

152. Randerath, E., Ten Broeke, J.W. and Randerath, K. FEBS Lett.
     2 (1968) 10.

153. Randerath, E., Yu, C.T. and Randerath, K. Anal. Biochem. 48
     (1972) 172.

154. Randerath, K., Chia, L.S.Y., Gupta, R.C., Randerath, E.,
     Hawkins, E.R., Brum, C.K. and Chang, S.H. Biochem. Biophys.
     Res. Comm. 63 (1975) 157.

155. Randerath, K., MacKinnon, S.K. and Randerath, E. FEBS Lett.
     15 (1971) 81.

156. Randerath, K., Randerath, E., Chia, L.S.Y., Gupta, R.C. and
     Sivarajan, M. Nucl. Acids Res. 1 (1974) 1121.

157. Randerath, K., Randerath, E., Gupta, R.C. and Chia, L.S.Y.
     FEBS Lett. 40 (1974) 187.

158. Randerath, K., Rosenthal, L.J. and Zamecnik, P.C. Proc. Natl.
     Acad. Sci. U.S.A. 68 (1971) 3233.

159. Reddy, R., R-Choi, T.S., Henning, D. and Busch, H. J. Biol.
     Chem. 249 (1974) 6486.

160. Reddy, R., Ro-Choi, T.S., Henning, D., Shibata, H., Choi, Y.C.
     and Busch, H. J. Biol. Chem. 247 (1972) 7245.

161. Reuber, M.R. Biol. Biochem. Eval. Malignancy Exp. Hepatomas
     Proc. U.S. Jap. Conf. 1 (1966) 43.

162. Rich, A. and RajBhandary, U.L. Ann. Rev. Biochem. 45 (1976)
     805.

163. Richardson, C.C. In: Proc. Nucl Acid Res. G.L. Cantoni and
     D.R. Davies (eds). Harper and Row, New York 2 (1971) 815.

164. Riddick, D.H. and Gallo, R.C. Cancer Res. 30 (1970) 2484.

165. Ritter, P.E. and Busch, H. Physiol. Chem. Physics 3 (1971)
     411.

166. Ro-Choi, T.S. Personal Communication.

167. Rodeh, R., Feldman, M. and Littauer, U.Z. Biochemistry 6
     (1967) 451.

168. Roe, B.A. Nucl. Acids Res. 2 (1975) 21.

169. Roe, B.A., Anandaraj, M.P.J.S., Chia, L.S.Y., Randerath, E., Gupta, R.C. and Randerath, K. Biochem. Biophys. Res. Comm. 66 (1975) 1097.

170. Rogg, H., Müller, P. and Staehelin, M. Eur. J. Biochem. 53 (1975) 115.

171. Salomon, R., Giveon, D., Kimhi, Y. and Littauer, U.Z. Biochemistry 15 (1976) 5258.

172. Sanger, F., Borwnlee, G.G. and Barrell, B.G. J. Mol. Biol. 13 (1965) 373.

173. Sawyer, R.C., Harada, F., Dahlberg, J.E. J. Virol. 13 (1974) 1302.

174. Shank, R.C. and Magee, P.N. Biochem. J. 100 (1966) 35.

175. Sharma, O.K., Biochim. Biophys. Acta 299 (1973) 415.

176. Sheid, B., Lu, T., Nelson, J.H., Jr. Cancer Res. 34 (1974) 2416.

177. Sheid, B. and Nelson, J.H., Jr. Biochim. Biophys. Acta 324 (1973) 69.

178. Sheid, B., Wilson, S.M. and Morris, H.P. Cancer Res. 31 (1971) 774.

179. Shibata, H., Ro-Choi, T.S., Reddy, R., Choi, Y.C., Henning, D. and Busch, H. J. Biol. Chem. 250 (1975) 3909.

180. Silberklang, M. Ph.D. Thesis, Massachusetts Institute of Technology (1976).

181. Simsek, M., RajBahndary, U.L., Boisnard, M. and Petrissant, G. Nature 247 (1974) 518.

182. Simsek, M., Ziegenmeyer, J., Heckman, J. and RajBhandary, U.L. Proc. Natl. Acad. Sci. U.S.A. 70 (1973) 1041.

183. Singer, B. Prog. Nucl. Acid Res. Mol. Biol. 15 (1975) 219.

184. Singer, C.E., Smith, G.R., Cortese, R. and Ames, B.N., Nature New Biol. 238 (1972) 72.

185. Sivarajan, M., Gupta, R.C., Chia, L.S.Y., Randerath, E. and Randerath, K. Nucl. Acids Res. 1 (1974) 1329.

186. Smith, D.W.E. Science 190 (1975) 529.

187. Smith, J.D. and Dunn, D.B. Biochem. J. 72 (1959) 294.

188. Smolar, N. and Svensson, I. Nucl. Acids Res. 1 (1974) 707.

189. Söll, D. Science 173 (1971) 293.

190. Srinivasan, P.R. and Borek, E. Proc. Natl. Acad. Sci. U.S.A
     49 (1963) 529.

191. Srinivasan, P.R. and Borek, E. Science 145 (1964) 548.

192. Srinivasan, D., Srinivasan, P.R., Grunberger, D., Weinstein,
     I.B. and Morris, H.P. Biochemistry 10 (1971) 1966.

193. Starr, J.L. and Sells, B.H. Physiol. Rev. 49 (1969) 623.

194. Stewart, B.W. and Pegg, A.E. Biochim. Biophys. Acta 281 (1972)
     416.

195. Sueoka, N. and Kano-Sueoka, T. Prog. Nucl. Acid Res. Mol.
     Biol. 10 (1970) 23.

196. Swiatek, K.R., Streeter, D.G. and Simon, L.N. Biochemistry
     10 (1971) 2563.

197. Szeto, K.S. and Söll, D. Nucl. Acids Res. 1 (1974) 171.

198. Taylor, M.W., Buck, C.A., Granger, G.A. and Holland, J.J. J.
     Mol. Biol. 33 (1968) 809.

199. Taylor, M.W., Granger, G.A., Buck, C.A. and Holland, J.J.
     Proc. Natl. Acad. Sci. U.S.A. 57 (1967) 1712.

200. Thiebe, R. and Poralla, K. FEBS Lett. 38 (1973) 27.

201. Thiebe, R. and Zachau, H.G. Eur. J. Biochem. 5 (1968) 546.

202. Tseng, W.C., Medina, D. and Randerath, K. (1977) Manuscript
     in Preparation.

203. Tsutsui, E., Srinivasan, P.R. and Borek, E. Proc. Natl. Acad.
     Sci. U.S.A. 56 (1966) 1003.

204. Turkington, R.W. J. Biol. Chem. 244 (1969) 5140.

205. Uchida, T. and Egami, F. In: Methods in Enzymology, L.
     Grossman and K. Moldave (eds). Academic Press, New York,
     12 (1967) 228.

205a. Uziel, M. and Smith, L.H. Fed. Proc. 15 (1976) 1675 (Abs).

206. Viale, G.L. Acta Neurochir. 21 (1969) 123.

207. Viale, G.L. Cancer Res. 31 (1971) 605.

208. Viale, G.L., Restelli, A.F. and Viale, E. Tumori 53 (1967) 533.

209. Volkers, S.A.S. and Taylor, M.W. Biochemistry 10 (1971) 488.

210. Wainfan, E., Moller, M.L., Maschio, F.A. and Balis, M.E. Cancer Res. 35 (1975) 2830.

211. Weber, G. New Eng. J. Med. 296 (1977) 486.

212. Weinhouse, S., Langan, J., Shatton, J.A. and Morris, H.P. In: Tumor Lipids, R. Wood (ed). Champaign III: American Oil Chemists' Society Press (1973) p. 14.

213. Weiss, J.F. and Kelmers, A.D. Biochemistry 6 (1967) 2507.

214. White, B.N., Tener, G.M., Holden, J. and Suzuki, D.T. J. Mol. Biol. 74 (1973) 635.

215. Wilkinson, R. and Pillinger, D.J. Intern. J. Cancer 8 (1971) 401.

216. Wyatt, G.R. Biochem. J. 48 (1951) 581.

217. Yang, W.K. Cancer Res. 31 (1971) 639.

218. Yang, W.K. and Novelli, G.D. Biochem. Biophys. Res. Comm. 31 (1968) 534.

219. Yang, W.K. and Novelli, G.D. In: Methods in Enzymology, S.P. Colowick and N.O. Kaplan (eds). Nucleic Acids and Protein Synthesis Part C K. Moldave and L. Grossman (eds). Academic Press, New York 20 (1971) p. 44.

220. Yang, W.K., Hollman, A., Martin, D.H., Hellman, K.B. and Novelli, G.D. Proc. Natl. Acad. Sci. U.S.A. 64 (1969) 1411.

221. Zamecnik, P.C. Cold Spring Harbor Symp. Quant. Biol. 34 (1969) 1.

222. Zimmerman, E.F., Hackney, J., Nelson, P. and Arias, I.M. Biochemistry 8 (1969) 2636.

THE SYNTHESIS AND SECRETION OF SERUM ALBUMIN IN MORRIS HEPATOMAS

5123tc AND 9121

Gerhard Schreiber, Jörg Urban, Heide Dryburgh and T.R.
Bradley

The Russel Grimwade School of Biochemistry
University of Melbourne (G.S., J.U., H.D.) and the
Peter MacCallum Cancer Institute, Melbourne (T.R.B.)
Victoria, Australia

SUMMARY

In vivo, Morris hepatomas 5123tc and 9121 do not secrete serum
proteins into the bloodstream. However, they synthesize albumin,
at a reduced rate, if compared with liver. The produced albumin accumulates, leading to an enlargement of the Golgi apparatus and the
appearance of intracellular vesicles. The proportion and the absolute amount of albumin found within the hepatoma cells is increased compared with liver.

As described recently for liver in vivo and for hepatocyte suspensions, albumin is synthesized also in hepatoma cells via a precursor protein.

Hepatoma cells in culture secrete albumin into the medium.
However, albumin accumulates in the cells with time in culture, indicating again a limited secretory capacity of the hepatoma cell.

INTRODUCTION

Serum albumin is the plasma protein which is present in largest
quantity in the bloodstream. Its physical and chemical characteristics are well established (for recent reviews see 1, 2). The complete amino acid sequence is known for man (3, 4) and bovine (5).
It is synthesized and secreted by the liver (6) and, in rats on a
20% protein diet, its synthesis rate amounts to 13% of total protein
synthesis (7). Thus, albumin synthesis is a specific function of the
liver and involves a major proportion of the protein synthesizing apparatus in this tissue. The following is a summary of our present

knowledge on the differences and similarities of albumin synthesis
and secretion in liver and the Morris hepatomas 5123tc and 9121,
in vivo and in cell suspension.

1. Lack of Secretion of Serum Protein by Transplanted Hepatomas in vivo

The secretion of serum protein into the bloodstream has been
investigated for the hepatomas Morris 9121 and Reuber H35 in ACI
rats and for the Morris hepatoma 5123tc in Buffalo rats (8).   In
these studies, hepatomas had been transplanted subcutaneously at 4
different sites on the abdomen and the thorax.   At the time, the
experiment animals were eviscerated under ether anesthesia and a
mixture of ^{14}C-labeled L-leucine, L-histidine and L-lysine was
given intraperitoneally.   Animals awoke from anesthesia 5-20 min
after the operations and were kept alive with i.p. injections of
glucose at 30 min intervals.   Two control groups were used: normal,
tumor-free, eviscerated rats and normal, intact rats.

Absorption and utilization of the administered radioactive
amino acids were studied by measuring non-protein radioactivity in
serum, and expired $^{14}CO_2$, respectively.   Expired $^{14}CO_2$/min/100 g
rat was lower in normal eviscerated rats than in normal intact rats.
It was, however, restored to values equal to those measured in intact rats, if the eviscerated rats were carrying hepatomas, suggesting that the tumor tissue contributed to the oxidation of the radioactive amino acids.   At times later than 1 hour after injection of
radioactive amino acids, the hepatomas in the eviscerated rats had
incorporated a larger amount of radioactivity into protein than the
liver of normal intact animals.   However, only a very small amount
of radioactivity could be detected in serum protein in blood from
hepatoma-bearing, eviscerated rats.   An example for this relationship if given in Fig 1.   The specific radioactivity of serum protein
in blood from eviscerated tumor-bearing animals was always lower
than in blood from normal, eviscerated rats.   These results indicated
that in eviscerated rats the Morris hepatomas 5123tc and 9121, and
the Reuber hepatoma H35 synthesized protein but did not secrete protein into the bloodstream.

2. Albumin Synthesis in Hepatomas

The failure of hepatomas to secrete protein into the bloodstream
as described in Section 1 can be explained in various ways.   For example, either the secretory mechanism or the synthesis of serum proteins could be affected.   The synthesis of the major plasma protein,
albumin, was therefore studied in Morris hepatomas 5123tc (9) and
9121 (10).   L-[1-^{14}C]leucine was injected into the caval vein of hepatoma-bearing animals, and hepatomas and livers were removed 12 to
14 min later.   This was well within the lag time (cf. Fig 1, curve

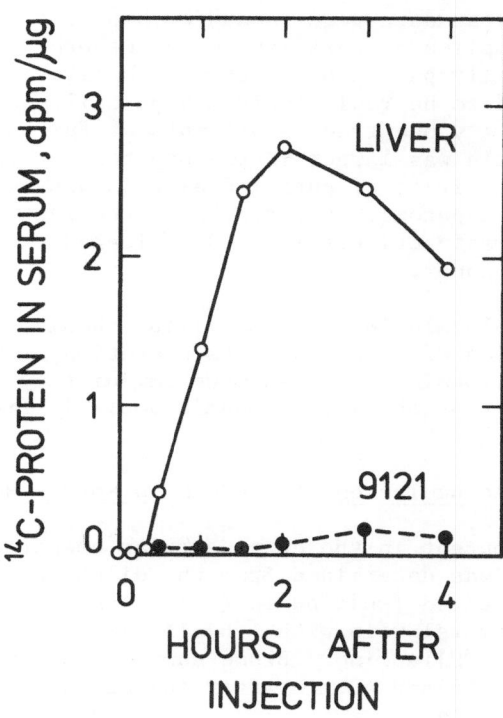

Figure 1
Absence of secretion of serum protein into the bloodstream by Morris hepatoma 9121 in vivo. The specific radioactivity of serum protein is given for various time intervals after intraperitoneal application of radioactive amino acids to normal (O——O, liver) and to eviscerated animals bearing hepatomas (●----●, 9121). Each animal received 7.89 µCi of a mixture of equal portions of uniformly ^{14}C-labeled L-leucine, 220-240 Ci/mole, L-histidine, 240 Ci/mole, and L-lysine, 180 Ci/mole, per 100 g body weight. Modified from (8).

for normal animals) between intravenous injection of radioactive
amino acid and appearance of radioactive protein in the bloodstream.
Therefore, no radioactive albumin synthesized in the liver could
have been secreted into the blood and transported to the hepatoma,
thus contaminating hepatoma albumin. Albumin was purified from the
homogenized livers and from the hepatomas by the procedure summarized in Table 1, which gives the values obtained for liver and hepatoma 5123tc. Similar data were found for hepatoma 9121 (10). A
rather long and complicated purification procedure was required to
obtain radiochemically pure albumin from both liver and hepatomas.
Albumin was assumed to be radiochemically pure if no change in its
specific radioactivity occurred in attempts at further purification.
The amount of albumin was larger in the hepatomas than in liver.
The specific radioactivity of purified albumin was very much higher
for liver than for hepatoma. Nevertheless, the fact that albumin
from hepatoma was radioactively labeled indicated that it had been
synthesized in the tumor.

Synthesis of albumin in hepatoma tissue should result in intracellular accumulation of albumin if its secretion is blocked, unless
newly synthesized albumin is broken down immediately. The next section deals with the intracellular albumin pools in liver and hepatomas.

3.   Intracellular Accumulation of Albumin in Morris Hepatoma 9121

The albumin content in the extravascular compartments of hepatoma 9121 and liver was determined from the dilution in these tissues
of intraveously injected [^{3}H]albumin (11). Tumor-bearing rats were
injected via the femoral vein with [^{3}H]albumin prepared from donor
rats injected with [^{3}H]leucine. Blood samples, hepatomas, and livers
were removed at 10, 25 and 40 min after injection. The values obtained for vascular and extravascular albumin did not differ significantly for the various time points (Table 2). Thus, the distribution
of [^{3}H]albumin had not changed between 10 to 40 min after injection,
suggesting that it was homogenously distributed in compartments accessible to albumin from the bloodstream within 10 min. Average
vascular albumin content per g of tissue wet weight was 2.1 $\pm$ 0.1 mg
(mean $\pm$ S.E.) in host liver and 1.4 $\pm$ 0.1 mg in hepatoma. The average
albumin content per gram of tissue wet weight was considerably larger
in the extravascular compartment of hepatoma 9121 (3.5 $\pm$ 0.1 mg) than
in that of host liver (1.0 $\pm$ 0.1 mg). The values were independent of
the tumor size. Tumors weighed between 3.6 and 10.1 g.

The biochemical observations could be correlated (11) with some
morphological characteristics of subcellular structures involved in
the synthesis and secretion of proteins. The fine structure of hepatoma cells differed most strikingly from that of hepatocytes by the
accumulation of vesicles at the cell periphery (Fig 2). Numerous

Table One

Purification of Albumin from Livers and Hepatomas 5123tc from 20 Rats
After Injection of L-[1-14C]leucine, 51 C/mole, 16 uC/100 g
Body Weight (Modified from (9))

Purification Step	Total Protein (mg)	Albumin in Total Protein (%)	Specific Radio-activity in protein (dpm/mg)
LIVER:			
Homogenate	45 800	1.9	3 440
Postmitochondrial supernatant	37 000	2.0	3 460
Partial heat denaturation (10 min at + 69°)	4 610	7.9	2 430
Precipitation with 10% tricholoacetic acid, extraction with acid ethanol, fractionation with ammonium sulfate	342	25	6 210
Molecular sieve chromatography on Sephadex G100	80.5	28	11 200
Ion-exchange chromatography on DEAE-cellulose	19.5	81	12 300
Preparative electrophoresis on poly-acrylamide gel at pH 10.3	6.1	88	9 550
Preparative electrophoresis on poly-acrylamide gel at pH 2.7	1.8	92	6 880
Charcoal treatment	0.4	108	6 050 (Cont'd)

(Continued)

Table One

Purification Step	Total Protein (mg)	Albumin in Total Protein (%)	Specific Radioactivity in Protein (dpm/mg)
HEPATOMA:			
Homogenate	52 200	4.3	2 500
Postmitochondrial supernatant	29 500	7.2	2 800
Partial heat denaturation (10 min at + 69°)	3 520	41	2 140
Precipitation with 10% trichloroacetic acid, extraction with acid ethanol, fractionation with ammonium.sulfate	476	74	2 550
Molecular sieve chromatography on Sephadex G100	297	115	2 200
First ion-exchange chromatography on DEAE-cellulose	117	96	687
Second ion-exchange chromatography on DEAE-cellulose	65.7	101	541
Preparative electrophoresis on polyacrylamide gel at pH 10.3	33.8	99	485
Preparative electrophoresis on polyacrylamide gel at pH 2.7	10.0	89	404
Charcoal Treatment	3.3	108	515

Table Two

Vascular and Extravascular Albumin Content of Morris Hepatoma 9121 and Host Liver

| Time after injection of [3H]albumin (min) | Albumin/g tissue wet wt in | | | |
| | Liver | | Hepatoma | |
	Vascular (mg)	Extravascular (mg)	Vascular (mg)	Extravascular (mg)
10	1.8 ± 0.1	1.0 ± 0.1	1.5 ± 0.1	3.9 ± 0.1
25	2.2 ± 0.1	1.0 ± 0.1	1.3 ± 0.1	3.5 ± 0.1
40	2.3 ± 0.1	0.9 ± 0.1	1.5 ± 0.1	3.0 ± 0.2

The vascular albumin content was obtained from multiplication of total tissue albumin by the specific radioactivity of albumin from tissue divided by the specific radioactivity of albumin from serum. Subtraction of the obtained value from total tissue albumin gives the extravascular albumin. Values are given as the mean ± S.E. of 6 liver or 12 hepatomas. Modified from (11).

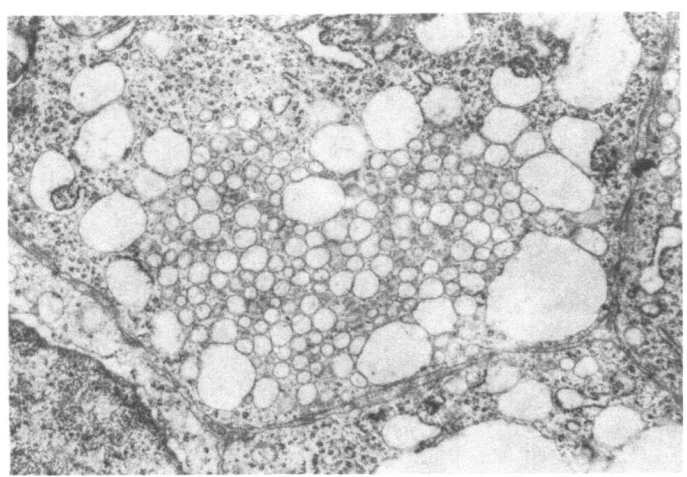

Figure 2
Electron micrograph of a thin tissue section from Morris hepatoma 9121. Four adjacent cells. Smooth-surfaced vesicles of two
size classes are densely accumulated in the cell periphery. Fixation with glutaraldehyde followed by OsO_4. Staining with uranyl
acetate and lead citrate. x 17 000. From (11).

Golgi complexes with many associated secretory vesicles were seen
in the hepatoma cells. The rough endoplasmic reticulum was less
frequent than in liver and predominantly formed slender and isolated cisternae. Free polysomes were more frequent than bound ones.

4. Protein Secretion in Cell Suspensions from Morris Hepatomas
   9121 and 5123tc.

With the introduction of continuous, recirculating perfusion
(12) of rat liver with a mixture of collagenase and hyaluronidase
(13), it became possible to prepare hepatocyte suspensions with a
high yield of viable cells. Under conditions optimized for protein
synthesis (14), such liver cell suspensions synthesize (15) and
secrete albumin (16). Attempts to utilize this technique for the
Morris hepatomas were unsuccessful because it was not possible to
establish continuous recirculating perfusion (17). However, in contrast to observations with adult rat liver, shaking of the minced
hepatoma in a solution containing collagenase and hyaluronidase resulted in cell suspensions of qualities obtained with continuous recirculating perfusion (17, 18; Fig 3). The hepatoma cells in sus-

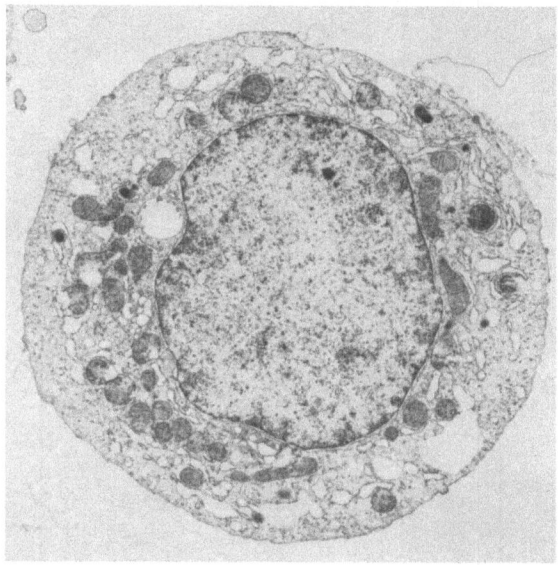

Figure 3
        Electron micrograph of a single cell from a Morris hepatoma
5123tc cell suspension incubated for 30 min at 37°. In general,
cell organelles are well preserved. The mitochondria have an
orthodox appearance. x 6000 (reduced 18% for reproduction). From (18).

pension transferred protein from the intracellular compartment into
the medium, with a lag time (Fig 4) similar to that observed for
protein secretion by regenerating liver (19). This was in contrast
to the lack of protein secretion described for hepatomas in vivo in
Section 1.

5. Involvement of a Precursor Protein in the Biosynthesis and Secretion of Albumin

        During many studies by other authors, albumin had been isolat-
ed by immunoprecipitation with anti-albumin without analyzing for
radiochemical purity. Therefore, values obtained for radioactivity
in albumin precipitated with anti-albumin were compared for each
step of the purification procedure described in Table 1 with the
value obtained by multiplying the specific radioactivity of radiochemically pure albumin with the amount of albumin present after
each purification step. The results for isolation from liver homogenate are given in Table 3. Invariably, immunoprecipitation gave
higher values for radioactivity in albumin than expected on the
basis of albumin concentration and specific radioactivity of pure

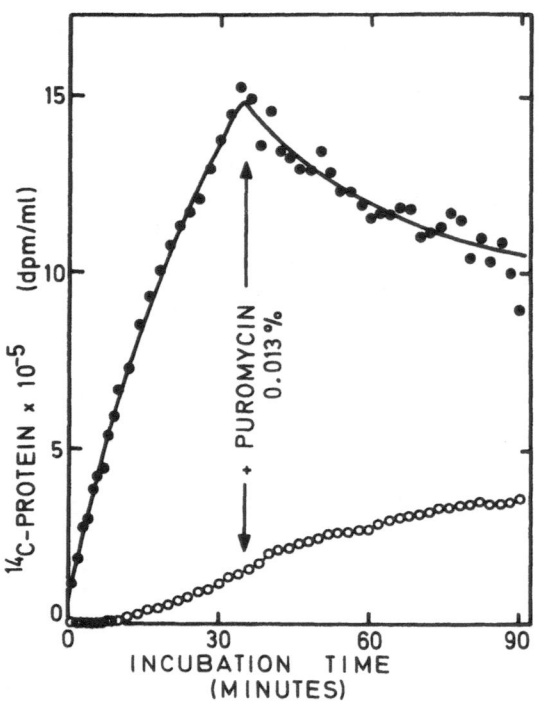

Figure 4
Incorporation of L-[1-^{14}C]leucine (59 Ci/mole) into intracellular (●) and extracellular (O) protein of cell suspensions from
Morris hepatoma 5123tc. After 35 min, addition of 133 μg of
puromycin per ml of incubation medium. From (18).

albumin. This held true also for Morris hepatoma 5123tc, but not
for tissues known not to be involved in albumin synthesis (20).
These observations suggested the presence of albumin-like protein(s)
in tissues which synthesize albumin. Anti-albumin precipitates both
albumin and albumin-like protein. However, shortly after injection
of radioactive amino acids, only the latter is labeled. From liver,
and albumin-like protein was isolated which differed from albumin by

Table Three

Radioactivity in Albumin at Consecutive Steps of a Purification from Liver

Purification Step	Radioactivity in albumin		Ratio A/B
	A. Immunoprecipitation (dpm/ml)	B. Albumin concentration x specific radioactivity of albumin at the end of purification procedure (dpm/ml)	
Homogenate	43 400	8 620	5.0
Postmitochondrial supernatant	20 100	7 320	2.7
Precipitation with 10% trichloroacetic acid and extraction with acid ethanol	9 640	3 490	2.8
Ammonium sulfate fractionation	142 000	49 300	2.9
Chromatography on Sephadex G100	11 900	4 790	2.5
Chromatography on DEAE-cellulose	40 800	20 200	2.0
Preparative electrophoresis on polyacrylamide gel at pH 10.3	3 550	2 360	1.5

At each purification step, radioactivity in albumin was determined (A) by precipitation with anti-albumin and (B) by multiplying the respective albumin concentration with the value for the specific radioactivity of albumin obtained at the end of the purification procedure. Modified from (10).

an oligopeptide extension at the N-terminus (21, 22) and which
was a precursor protein in the synthesis of albumin (7, 23, 24).

After the discovery of the participation of a precursor protein in the synthesis and secretion of albumin (for review, see
25), which is converted into albumin in the smooth endoplasmic re-
ticulum/Golgi apparatus region (26, 27), it seemed appropriate to
re-investigate albumin metabolism in hepatomas, a suitable system
being cell suspensions. In a pulse-chase experiment hepatoma
5123tc cells were labeled with L-[1-^{14}C]leucine for 25 min, exposed
thereafter to an 830-fold excess of non-radioactive L-leucine and
incubated for a further 30 min (28). Samples were removed at the
beginning, the middle and the end of the chase period. Albumin and
an albumin-like protein were purified from the samples. The observed changes in their specific radioactivities (Fig 5) clearly
indicated that the latter was a precursor of albumin. An albumin-
like protein was also found in hepatoma 5123tc _in_ _vivo_ (28).

The proportion of radioactive albumin plus albumin precursor
to radioactive total protein was lower (1.2%) than the value of 7%
obtained for liver cell suspension (24). _In_ _vivo_, the synthesis of
albumin plus precursor amounted to 13% of total protein synthesis in
liver (7) compared with 1.8% for hepatoma 5123tc (28).

6. Relationship Between Albumin Secretion, Cell Density and Growth
   Rate in Cell Cultures of Morris Hepatoma 5123tc

Cell suspensions from Morris hepatoma 5123tc were used to establish continuous monolayer cultures consisting of hepatoma cells as
shown by repeated transplantation to rats. On inoculation of the
hepatoma cells into flasks at low cell density, an initial phase of
slow growth was followed by rapid proliferation which then decreased
(Fig 6) as the cultures approached formation of a complete monolayer.
The rate of synthesis and secretion of albumin was high in the initial
resting stage, slowed down during the phase of rapid growth and increased again when the cells approached the second resting phase (Fig
7). Intracellular albumin concentration increased considerably with
time in culture (Table 4).

7. Interpretation

The secretory pathways of albumin in liver and in Morris hepatomas 5123tc and 9121 have common basic features. As in liver albumin
is synthesized in hepatoma via a precursor protein. However, no
albumin is secreted by the hepatomas into the bloodstream. Furthermore, the synthesis rate of albumin and its precursor protein is
greatly reduced in the hepatomas as compared to liver. A similarly
reduced rate of albumin synthesis has been reported also for Morris
hepatomas 7800 and 7777 (29). The failure to secrete the newly syn-

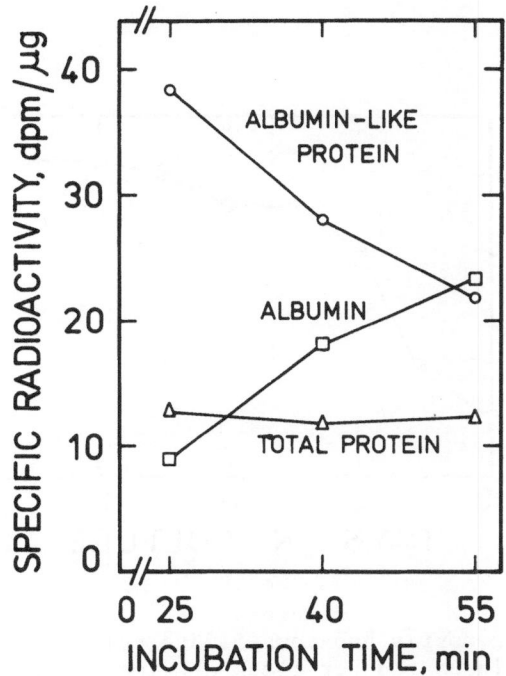

Figure 5
Specific radioactivity of albumin-like protein, albumin, and
total protein from Morris hepatoma 5123tc cells incubated with L-
[1-^{14}C]leucine followed by a chase with nonradioactive leucine.
From (28).

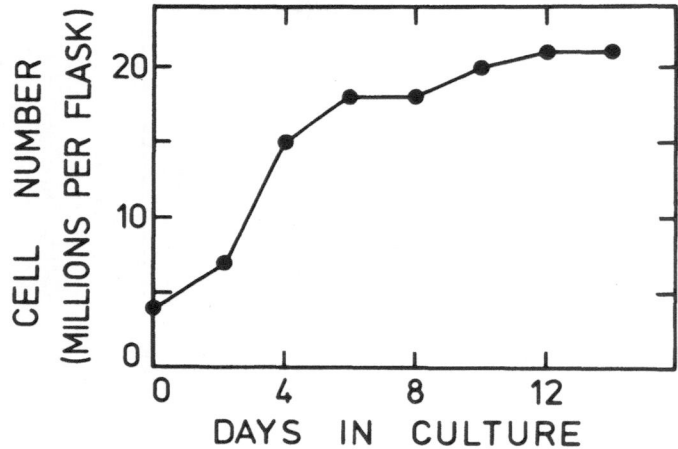

Figure 6
Growth curve of Morris hepatoma 5123tc cells in culture.
4×10^6 cells were incubated per flask at time zero. Culture medium
(Ham's F10 plus 10% fetal calf serum) was changed every two days.
Two flasks were used for each cell count.

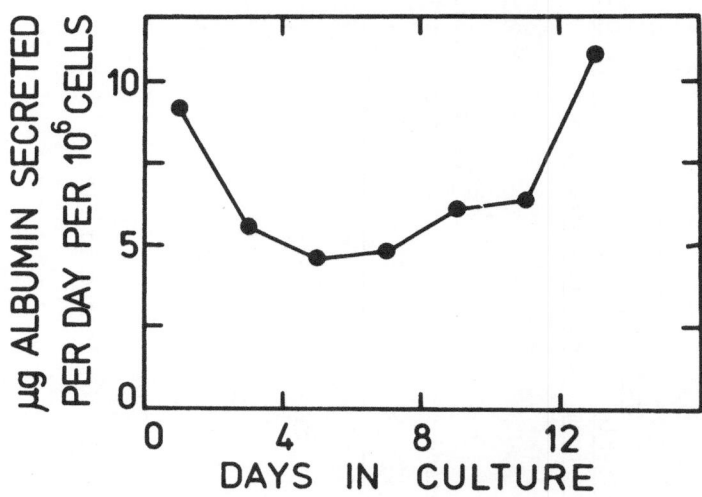

Figure 7
Rate of albumin secretion in the cell culture described in
Fig 6.

thesized albumin apparently leads to its accumulation in the hepatoma cell in vivo.

Synthesis and secretion of albumin has been observed in cell
cultures originating from hepatomas Morris 5123tc (this paper) and
7795 (30, 31) and from Reuber H35 (32-34). However, despite per-
sisting secretion, albumin accumulated in the cells of Morris hepatoma 5123tc with time in culture.

Table Four

Intracellular anti-albumin-precipitable Protein and Cell Concentration in Cell
Cultures from Morris Hepatoma 5123tc

Time in Culture	Cell Concentration	Intracellular anti-albumin-precipitable protein
(days)	(Cells/μl)	(μg/10^9 cells)
0	200	95
14	1 160	244

Conditions for cell culturing are described in the legend to Fig 6.

REFERENCES

1. Peters, T.,Jr. In: The Plasma Proteins, F.W. Putnam (ed).
    Academic Press Inc., New York 1 (1975) 133.

2. Peters, T.,Jr. Clinical Chem. 23 (1977) 5.

3. Beherns, P.Q., Spiekerman, A.M. and Brown, J.R. Fed Proc.
    34 (1975) 591.

4. Meloun, B., Moravek, L. and Kostka, V. Fed. Eur. Biochem. Soc.
    Ltters 58 (1975) 134.

5. Brown, J.R. Fed. Proc. 34 (1975) 591.

6. Miller, L.L., Bly, C.G., Watson, M.L. and Bale, W.F. J. of
    Exptl. Med. 94 (1951) 431.

7. Urban, J., Chelladurai, M., Millership, A. and Schreiber, G.
    Eur. J. Biochem. 67 (1976) 477.

8. Schreiber, G., Boutwell, R.K., Potter, V.R. and Morris, H.P.
    Cancer Res. 26 (1966) 2357.

9. Schreiber, G., Rotermund, H.M., Maeno, H., Weigand, K. and
    Lesch, R. Eur. J. Biochem. 10 (1969) 355.

10. Rotermund, H.M., Schreiber, G., Maeno, H., Weinssen, U. and
    Weigand, K. Cancer Res. 30 (1970) 2139.

11. Urban, J., Kartenbeck, J., Zimber, P., Timko, J., Lesch, R. and
    Schreiber, G. Cancer Res. 32 (1972) 1971.

12. Berry, M.N. and Friend, D.S. J. Cell Biol. 43 (1969) 506.

13. Howard, R.B., Christensen, A.K., Gibbs, F.A. and Pesch, L.A.
    J. Cell Biol. 35 (1967) 675.

14. Schreiber, G. and Schreiber, M. Sub-Cellular Biochem. 2 (1973)
    307.

15. Weigand, K., Muller, M., Urban, J. and Schreiber, G., Exp. Cell
    Res. 67 (1971) 27.

16. Weigand, K. and Otto, I. Fed. Eur. Biochem. Soc. Ltters 46 (1974)
    127.

17. Muller, M., Schreiber, M., Kartenbeck, J. and Schreiber, G. Cancer
    Res. 32 (1972) 2568.

18. Schreiber, M., Schreiber, G. and Kartenbeck, J. Cancer Res.
    34 (1974) 2143.

19. Schreiber, G., Urban, J., Zahringer, J., Reutter, W. and
    Frosch, U. The J. Biol. Chem. 246 (1971) 4531.

20. Urban, J., Zimber, P. and Schreiber, G., Analytical Biochem.
    58 (1974) 102.

21. Urban, J., Inglis, A.S., Edwards, K. and Schreiber, G.
    Biochem. Biophys. Res. Comm. 61 (1974) 494.

22. Russell, J.H. and Geller, D.M. J. Biol. Chem. 250 (1975) 3409.

23. Urban, J. and Schreiber, G. Biochem. Biophys. Res. Comm. 64
    (1975) 778.

24. Edwards, K., Schreiber, G., Dryburgh, H., Urban, J. and Inglis,
    A.S. Eur. J. Biochem. 63 (1976) 303.

25. Schreiber, G., Urban, J., Edwards, K., Dryburgh, H. and Inglis,
    A.S. Adv. in Enzyme Reg. 14 (1976) 163.

26. Edwards, K., Fleischer, B., Dryburgh, H., Fleischer, S. and
    Schreiber, G. Biochem. Biophys. Res. Comm. 72 (1976) 310.

27. Ikehara, Y., Oda, K. and Kato, K. Biochem. Biophys. Res. Comm.
    72 (1976) 319.

28. Edwards, K., Schreiber, G., Dryburgh, H., Millership, A. and
    Urban, J. Cancer Res. 36 (1976) 3113.

29. Ove, P., Coetzee, M.L., Chen, J. and Morris, H.P. Cancer Res.
    32 (1972) 2510.

30. Richardson, U.I., Tashjian, A.H., Jr. and Levine, L. J. of Cell
    Biol. 40 (1969) 236.

31. Hegna, I. and Prydz, H. Exptl. Cell Res. 77 (1973) 25.

32. Ohanian, S.H., Taubman, S.B. and Thorbecke, G.J. J. Natl. Cancer
    Inst. 43 (1969) 397.

33. Deschatrette, J. and Weiss, M.C. Biochimie, 56 (1974) 1603.

34. Peterson, J.A. Proc. Natl. Acad. Sci. U.S.A. 71 (1974) 2062.

LOSS OF REGULATION OF LIPID METABOLISM IN MORRIS HEPATOMAS: A POTENTIAL ROLE FOR CYTOPLASMIC BINDING PROTEINS

S. Mishkin* and M.L. Halperin

Department of Medicine, Royal Victoria Hospital and
McGill University Clinic, Montreal, Quebec: and
Department of Medicine, University of Toronto, Toronto,
Ontario

GENERAL HYPOTHESIS

It is well established that fatty acid and cholesterol synthesis are not inhibited in Morris hepatomas during the fasting
state in contradistinction to normal liver. The constitutive enzymes of these pathways in hepatomas appear to be normal. We observed that the tumor content of the feedback inhibitor of lipogenesis, long chain fatty acyl CoA and its cytoplasmic binding protein, Z protein, were both low and did not increase significantly
during fasting. We proposed that the basic defect could be defective net production of Z protein. Preliminary data suggest that
there is also a decrease in cholesterol affinity for its cytosolic
binding protein in Morris hepatomas. This raises the intriguing
possibility that the common denominator for these metabolic defects
in hepatomas resides in the abnormal metabolism of a family of cytosolic binding proteins.

INTRODUCTION

The chemically induced group of Morris hepatomas provide a most
interesting pathological model to study the mechanisms involved in
the regulation of tumor intermediary metabolism. In addition to a
variety of documented aberrations in lipid metabolism (1) these tumors manifest abnormalities in the integration of glucose and fatty
acid metabolism (2) An example of this group of abnormalities is the
observation by Weinhouse and coworkers of a reciprocal relationship
between the rates of glucose and fatty acid oxidation in hepatomas
with differing degrees of differentiation (3). Those well differentiated hepatomas which grew slowly had reduced capability for glucose

583

phosphorylation readily oxidized fatty acids, whereas the more
rapidly growing poorly differentiated tumors which had very rapid
rates of glycolysis but failed to oxidize fatty acids at appreciable rates. According to the molecular correlation concept of
Weber these abnormalities are classified as "progression - linked
alterations" (4). The conceptual framework for this hypothesis is
that "The operation of ordered and correlated expressions of morphological, biological and metabolic behavior in the neoplastic cell is
apparently linked with the expression of their malignancy and growth
rate". It would appear that this concept is correlative rather than
etiologic and pertains to the tumor cell after neoplastic transformation has taken place. The minimal deviation concept of Potter (5)
proposes that "there is some critical biochemical distinction common
to all hepatomas in contrast to nonneoplastic hepatic tissue". These
changes termed "transformation - linked alterations" are all-or-none
aberrations which may be considered as enzymatic markers of the malignant transformation (6). Much evidence has been accumulated for the
presence of two such "transformation - linked alterations" in the
lipid metabolism of hepatomas, namely the deletion of the feedback
control of cholesterol synthesis and the absent nutritional regulation
of fatty acid synthesis or lipogenesis. Normally the feeding of a
high cholesterol diet causes a prompt decrease in hepatic cholesterol
synthesis while fasting inhibits and refeeding of a fat-free diet after fasting leads to a great increase in fatty acid synthesis (7,8)[1].

A number of intriguing parallels exist between the physiologic
and pathologic aspects of cholesterol and fatty acid metabolism -
First while the respective rates of cholesterol and fatty acid synthesis differ significantly amongst tumor species, the regulation of
these processes is uniformly deleted irrespective of hepatoma growth
rate or degree of differentiation (10). Furthermore, the aberration
in the feedback regulation of cholesterol.synthesis has been extended
to all hepatomas of man, rodents and fish studied to date as well as
premalignant livers many months before hepatomas develop (11,12).
The second group of parallel observations are that the in vitro properties of regulatory enzymes isolated from hepatomas are not different from those of normal liver tissue; these include β - hydroxyl -
β methylglutaryl coenzyme A reductase (HMG CoA reductase) (13) and
microsomal methyl sterol demethylase (14) with regard to cholesterol
synthesis and acetyl CoA carboxylase and fatty acid synthetase in connection with fatty acid synthesis (15,16).

If the enzymatic machinery for the lipid biosynthetic pathways
appears to be intact what then is the mechanism for the deletion of
regulatory control? It has been postulated that the defective control
of fatty acid synthesis involves the regulation of enzyme production,
rather than short term modulation of enzyme activity (16,17). We are
not aware of any experimental data to support this hypothesis. In addition, the defective control of fatty acid synthesis in hepatomas is

not related to the absence of portal blood flow, since median lobe autografts that are devoid of portal blood flow behave like normal liver with respect to the nutritional control of lipogenesis (18). The recent demonstration in Morris hepatoma 7777 that the tumor content of palmitoyl - CoA was much lower than in hepatocytes and did not rise appreciably during the fasting state, has raised a number of interesting possibilities (19). In addition to the apparent role of palmitoyl CoA in the regulation of fatty acid synthesis (20, 21), palmitoyl CoA may be involved in the integration of glucose and fatty acid production (22). These observations prompted us to explore the possibility that the presumed physiological cytoplasmic binding protein for palmitoyl CoA, Z protein, might be altered in hepatomas. To date we have shown that the concentration of Z is reduced compared to control and host livers in 9 Morris hepatomas of different degrees of differentiation as well as one human hepatoma (23,24,25).

In parallel with fatty acid metabolism, a distinct set of cytoplasmic binding proteins termed sterol carrier proteins have been implicated in cholesterol synthesis (26,27). It is intriguing to note that preliminary evidence indicates that abnormalities exist in the sterol carrier proteins in the supernatant fractions obtained from Morris hepatoma 7777 (28) and Morris hepatoma 7787[2]. These observations raise the possibility that aberrations in the concentration and/or function of cytoplasmic binding proteins may provide the key to the abnormal regulation of cholesterol biosynthesis and fatty acid synthesis in hepatomas.

Although abnormal rates of lipoprotein synthesis have been documented in Morris hepatomas (29,30), the possible mechanisms of these oberrations will not be discussed in this review.

Z PROTEIN: STUDIES IN NORMAL LIVER

Z is a low M.W. protein (M.W.~12,000 daltons) present in the particulate-free supernatant fractions of liver, kidney, intestinal mucosa, adipose tissue, skeletal, cardiac and smooth muscle. Z is not present in serum nor erythrocytes (31,32). It was originally discovered in the cytosol of hepatocytes and was believed to be important for the cellular uptake and cytoplasmic binding of bilirubin and sulphobromophthalein (3,33). The observation that Z protein had affinity for long chain fatty acids (31) suggested that Z may regulate the cellular uptake of these substances. However, in vivo experiments with flavaspidic acid have cast doubt on the hypothesis that Z protein is a major determinant of the cellular uptake of long chain fatty acids (34). More recent observations indicated that the in vitro affinity of Z for the long chain acyl CoA exceeded that for long chain fatty acids (35) as well as other ligands studied. These results suggested that the possibility that the physiologic role for Z protein might be to bind chain fatty acyl CoA and thereby regulate fatty acid metabolism by a direct effect on various enzymatic reactions or by controlling the cytoplasmic concentration of free palmitoyl CoA.[3]

We have shown that partially purified Z protein was superior to albumin in stimulating the esterification of sn-glycerol-3-phosphate in the presence of palmitoyl CoA and rat liver microsomes (37). More recently it has been reported that Z stimulated the acylation of diacylglycerols to triacylglycerols in an assay system containing microsomes of rat liver and intestinal mucosa (38). These latter findings have been confirmed and extended to show that the stimulatory effect of Z is observed in a "palmitoyl - CoA containing system" (39). The explanation for these latter observations is currently under study. A protein does not appear to stimulate the activation of long chain fatty acids to their CoA derivatives. Whereas crude liver supernatant does stimulate the activation of long chain acyl - CoA synthetase, Z protein is without effect (40)[4]. Conclusions to the contrary are based on indirect evidence using flavaspidic acid, a competitive inhibitor of fatty acid binding to Z protein (41,42).

It should be noted that a number of liver supernatant proteins currently under study may in fact be identical to Z protein; these include the azocarcinogen metabolite binding protein (43), a thyroxine binding protein (31), a cortisol metabolite binding protein (44), a binding protein for cholecystographic agents (45), a hexachlorophene binding protein (46), a binding protein for penicilin analogues (47) and a protein which stimulates microsomal N-demethylation (48).

Z PROTEIN: STUDIES IN MORRIS HEPATOMAS

The Morris group of hepatomas provided an interesting experimental model to test the hypothesis that Z might be a regulator of fatty acid metabolism because long chain acyl CoA levels are low in one of these tumors (49). Furthermore, the nutritional regulation of lipogenesis, which may be mediated by palmitoyl CoA (20,21,50), is defective in all rodent hepatomas studied to date (51-57).[4]

We therefore set out to measure the contents of long chain acyl CoA and Z protein in Morris hepatomas with varying degrees of differentiation. We wished to determine whether there was a correlation between the quantity of Z, the in vitro binding of [^{14}C]palmitoyl CoA to Z, the long chain fatty acyl CoA levels and the degree of differentiation of the tumors.

EXPERIMENTAL PROCEDURE

Preparation of Liver and Hepatoma Supernatant Fractions

Buffalo and ACI strain rats were maintained on Purina Lab-chow diet with water containing 5% sucrose ad lib. Morris hepatomas were implanted in their hind limbs. The hepatomas and host livers were harvested when the tumors were 1-2 cm in diameter. Control liver denotes tissue obtained from animals of each strain free of implanted tumor. Livers were removed, rinsed and perfused with isotonic saline and homogenized to yield a 33% homogenate (Wt/V.). In the case of tumor tissue no perfusion could be carried out, instead capsular and necrotic tissue were carefully removed before the tissue was finely minced, rinsed in saline, blotted dry, weighed and homogenized in 0.45% saline to yield a 33% homogenate (Wt/V.).

Supernatant fractions were prepared by centrifugation of the homogenates at 110,000 x g for 90 minutes at 2° in a Model L Spinco ultracentrifuge. In some cases the homogenates were spun for 200,000 x g for 120 minutes to more completely spin down subcellular particulate matter. In other cases, Trasylol (50 units/ml) when added to liver and hepatoma 9108 homogenate to inhibit tissue proteolysis (58) did not alter the in vitro binding of [14C]palmitoyl CoA nor the concentrations of long chain acyl CoA or Z protein. The supernatant fractions once prepared were either used immediately or frozen and stored at -20°. Protein concentration was determined in these and other samples using Lowry method (59) with albumin as standard.

In order to assess the degree of serum contamination of liver and hepatoma supernatant, [131I]-albumin was administered intraveously to rats bearing hepatomas 7800 and 9121. The animals were sacrificed 10 minutes later and aliquots of serum, liver and hepatoma supernatant were analyzed for [131I]. While no serum contamination of liver supernatant was detected, the maximum contamination of hepatoma supernatant corresponded to 25λ of serum/ml of supernatant. This degree of serum contamination could not account for the results to be described. This was confirmed by the analysis of liver supernatant to which 25 and 250λ serum/ml had been added.

Sephadex Chromatography of Liver and Hepatoma Supernatant

Five ml aliquots of supernatant, equivalent to 2 g of liver or hepatoma tissue, were chromatographed on Sephadex G-100 columns (2.5 x 43 cm) as previously described (35).

The binding affinity of normal and hepatoma Z for [14C]palmitoyl CoA was determined by adding 4 nmoles of [14C]palmitoyl CoA to partially purified Z protein and chromatographing the mixture on Sephadex G-50 (1.6 x 14 cm). DPM and protein content (59) were determined for the binding zone and the specific activity was calculated. Methods for the identification, purification and quantitation of Z protein as well as the measurement of acid insoluble CoA have been described in other publications (25,35,60).

RESULTS

In Vitro Binding of [14C]Palmitoyl CoA to Liver Supernatant Proteins

The binding of [14C]palmitoyl CoA (4 nmoles) to liver supernatant proteins obtained from rats with or without tumor implantation in the hind limb was similar. In each case, palmitoyl CoA
radioactivity was localized to three regions labelled I, II and Z
(Fig 1), whose protein composition on 10% SDS PAGE[5] is depicted in
Fig 2. Region I corresponds to the void volume of the column and
contains lipoproteins and particulate matter, capable of binding
[14C]palmitoyl CoA. This particulate matter is released from intracellular organelles during homogenization[6]. Region II contains a
mixture of proteins with a M.W. range of 40,000 - 70,000 daltons.
The binding of [14C]palmitoyl CoA in this region is principally due
to albumin because this binding zone is absent after precipitation
of albumin with antibodies to rat albumin. In order to confirm
that the binding of [14C]palmitoyl CoA in the Z region is accounted
for entirely by Z protein, Z region proteins were electrophoresed on
alkaline gels after the addition of [14C]palmitoyl CoA. The gels
were stained, and individual 1.5 mm slices counted in scintillation
medium. Palmitoyl CoA radioactivity was found in those slices corresponding to the three bands present after electrophoresis of purified Z protein. Alkaline electrophoresis was repeated and protein
present in each of the three bands was eluted from 10 unstained gels
using 15 mM TRIS acetate (pH 7.6). The eluted protein fractions
were chromatographed using 10% SDS PAGE and in each case a single
band correpsonding to Z appeared. In addition, each protein fraction
gave a line of identity when reacted against mono-specific anti Z IgG
(courtesy of Drs. I.M. Arias and J. Fleischner). These results are
similar to those of Ketterer et al. (61) who showed that Z protein
separated into three components with isoelectric focusing.

In Vitro Binding of [14C]Palmitoyl CoA to Hepatoma Supernatant Proteins

The binding pattern of [14C]palmitoyl CoA to hepatoma supernatant proteins was very similar in each hepatoma studied (Figs 1 and
3). In all hepatomas, the binding to proteins in Region I and II was
increased significantly compared to Control or host liver, while it
was markedly reduced in the "Z region". In order to rule out the possibility that the increased binding of trace amounts of [14C]palmitoyl
CoA (4 nmoles) in regions I and II was responsible for the reduced
binding in the "Z region", increasing amounts of cold palmitoyl CoA
(up to 2.0 mmoles) were added to 5 ml of hepatoma supernatant prior to
Sephadex chromatography. In no instance was there any increased binding of [14C]palmitoyl CoA in the "Z region". In order to determine
whether the reduction in binding of [14C]palmitoyl CoA to the "Z

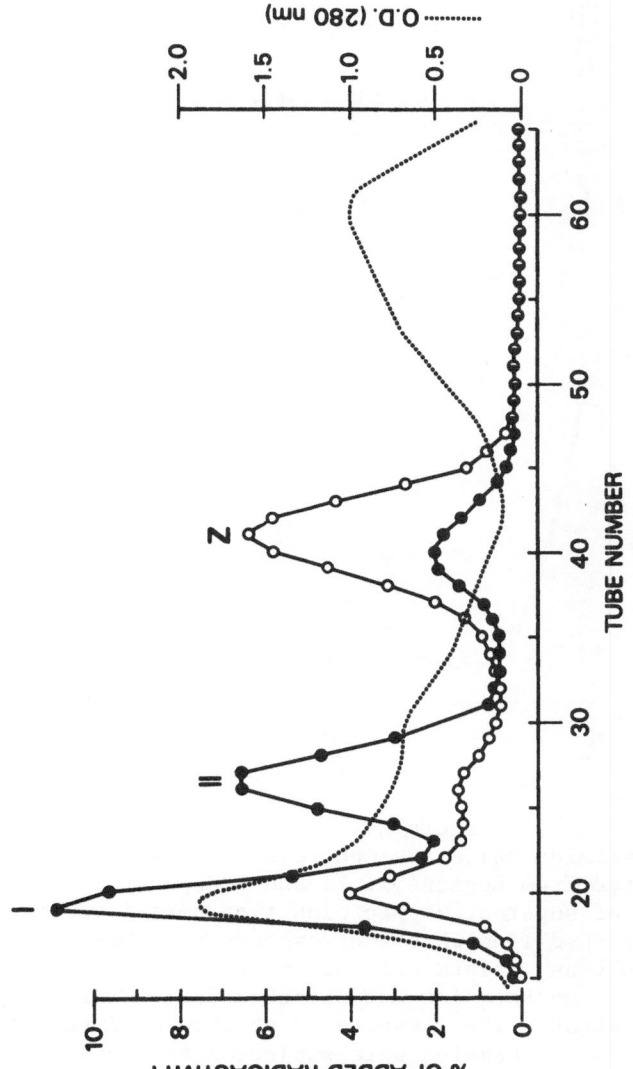

Figure 1

The binding pattern of $[^{14}C]$palmitoyl CoA to supernatant proteins of host liver (●——●) and hepatoma 7777 (○——○) after separation according to M.W. by Sephadex G-100 chromatography. Region I represents high M.W. (>100,000) proteins which appear in the void volume of the column, Region II represents proteins of M.W. 40-70,000 and the Z region contains Z protein, M.W. ~12,200. Four nmoles of $[^{14}C]$palmitoyl CoA dissolved in 50 μl of sodium acetate buffer were added to a 5 ml aliquot of supernatant representing 2 g of tissues.

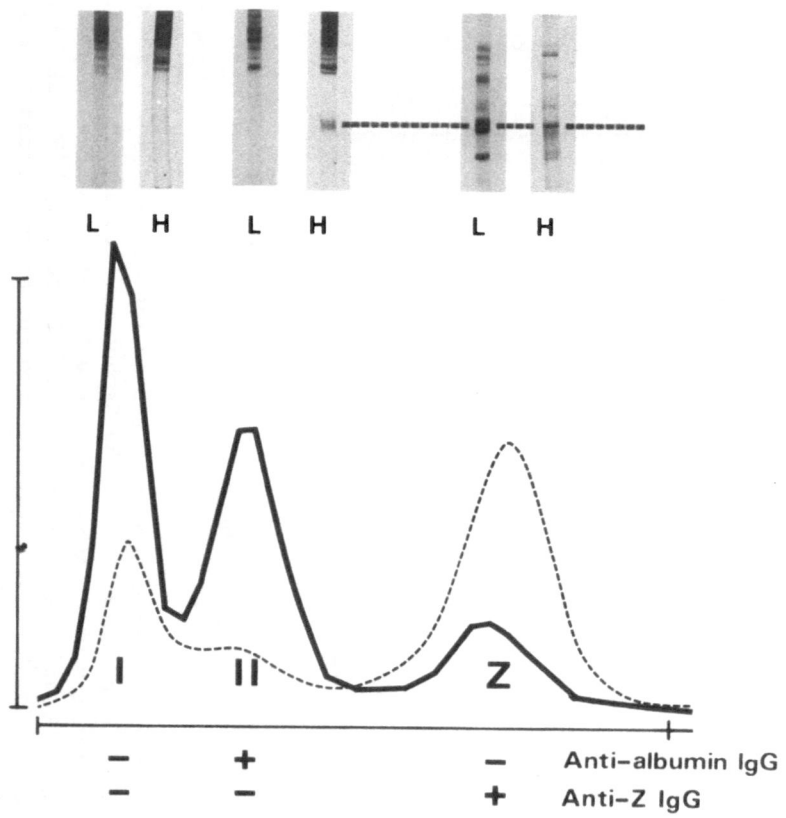

Figure 2

10% SDS polyacrylamide gel electrophoresis patterns of proteins pooled and concentrated from Regions I, II and Z separated by Sephadex G-100 chromatography of supernatant proteins from host liver (L) and hepatoma (H). The hatched line which corresponds to a M.W. of approximately 12,000 daltons, points out the location of Z protein in the Z region as well as another low M.W. protein derived from Region II of hepatoma supernatant. The presence or absence of lines of identity when the above protein samples were subjected to Ouchterlony immunodiffusion against anti-rat albumin IgG abd anti-rat Z IgG is indicated by + or − respectively. Beneath the gels is a schematic representation of the binding pattern of [14C]palmitoyl CoA to the proteins of Regions I, and II and Z in host liver (----) and hepatoma (——) supernatant as shown in Figure 1.

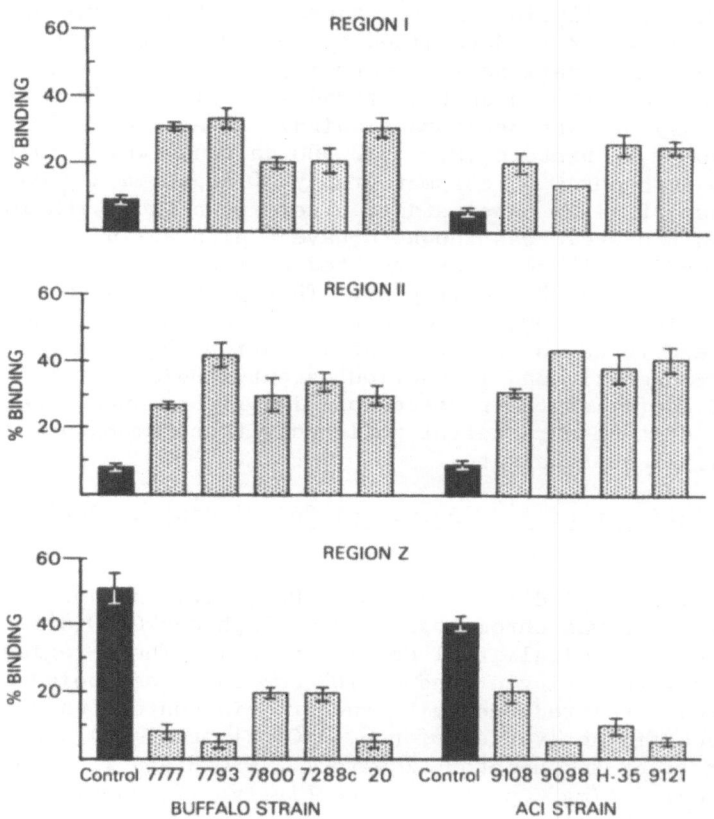

Figure 3
The percentage of exogenous [^{14}C]palmitoyl CoA recovered in the three binding regions separated from liver and hepatoma supernatant as depicted in Figure 1. The solid bars represent control and host livers from Buffalo and ACI rats respectively and the hatched bars represent the values obtained for supernatant proteins separated from various implanted hepatomas.

region" of hepatomas was due to competitive displacement by endogenous long chain acyl CoA, Z protein from liver and hepatoma 7800
supernatant was assayed for acid-insoluble CoA: no acid-insoluble
CoA could be detected on either normal or hepatoma Z. (Approximately 50 nmoles of Z protein were used). The lower limit of sensitivity of the CoASH assay was 20 pmoles.

The M.W. distribution and concentration of hepatoma proteins
in Region I, II and Z as determined by 10% SDS PAGE differed from
that for proteins separated from normal liver supernatant (Fig 2).
The most notable differences were found in Region II (M.W. 40,000 -
70,000 daltons) of each hepatoma studied. In each case SDS PAGE
yielded a low M.W. protein (M.W. 12,500 daltons) which could be
isolated by Sephadex G-50 chromatography of hepatoma Region II but
not from that of liver supernatant, after incubation with 10% SDS
(Fig 4). This protein was shown to have a high affinity for [14C]
palmitoyl CoA (Fig 4) and cross reacted with anti-rat albumin IgG
but not with anti-rat Z IgG (Fig 5). This protein may be derived
from albumin (M.W. 68,000), a potent binder of palmitoyl-CoA (34)
which has been found to be increased in various hepatomas (35,36).
Immunoelectrophoretic and immunoflourescent studies[7] with anti-rat
albumin IgG confirmed the presence of significant quantities of
albumin in hepatoma supernatant while only trace amounts were found
in normal liver supernatant.

Specific Activity of [14C]Palmitoyl CoA Binding to Purified Z Protein

Z protein purified from hepatoma 7800, 9121 and corresponding
liver supernatant was chromatographed on Sephadex G-50 after preincubation with [14C]palmitoyl CoA (4 nmoles). The Z region so obtained which gave a single band on 10% SDS PAGE was pooled and concentrated and total radioactivity and protein content was measured.
The mean specific activities of the [14C]palmitoyl CoA: Z protein
complex for liver and hepatoma Z were 1.2 ± 0.8 and 1.3 ± 0.6 nmoles
[14C]palmitoyl CoA/mg Z protein respectively. It should be noted as
well that the M.W. of hepatoma Z protein, (by 10% SDS PAGE), was 1.2,
185 ± 157 daltons, a value similar to that of normal Z ($12,173 \pm 59$
daltons). These results suggest that the physical properties of hepatoma and normal Z are similar.

Acid-Insoluble CoA Content of Liver and Hepatoma Tissues

Livers and hepatomas were frozen immediately between clamps
precooled in liquid nitrogen. The tissues were weighed and ground
in ice-cold perchloric acid. The acid insoluble CoA content was
significantly lower in all hepatomas than in corresponding host liver
tissue (Table 1).

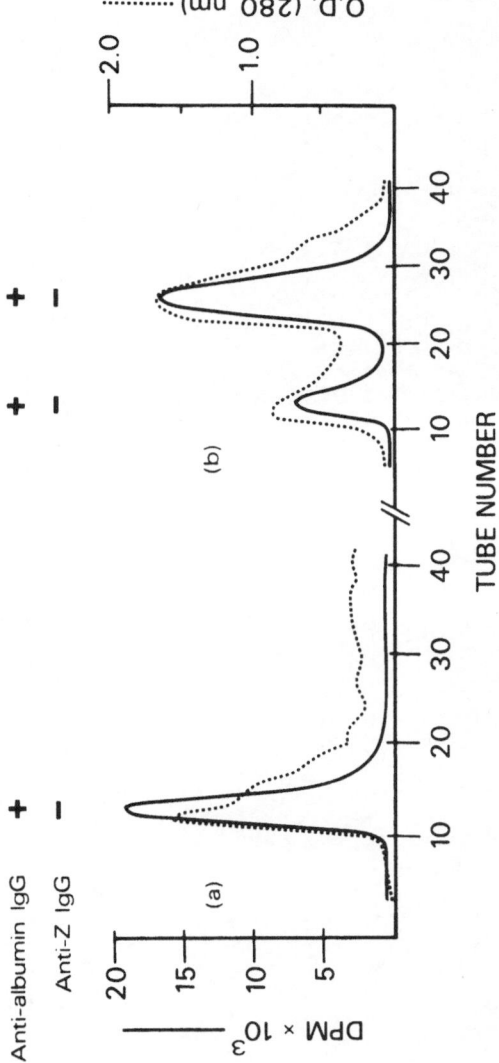

Figure 4

The binding pattern of exogenous [¹⁴]palmitoyl CoA to hepatoma 9121 supernatant proteins pooled and concentrated from Region II (see Fig 1) and further separated by Sephadex G-50 chromatography a) represents the binding pattern of untreated Region II proteins and b) represents the binding pattern after incubation with 0.1 ml 10% SDS (2 hours at 4°C). In each case, 4nmoles of [¹⁴C]palmitoyl CoA was added to 2.0 ml of Region II proteins (7.8 mg/ml). The hatched line (–––) represents 280 mu optical density reading. The presence or absence of lines of identity when proteins harvested from each binding zone are reacted against anti-rat albumin IgG and anti-rat Z IgG on Ouchterlony immuno-diffusion are depicted by + or – respectively (See Fig 5).

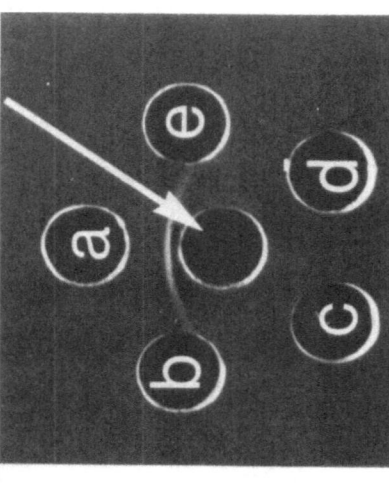

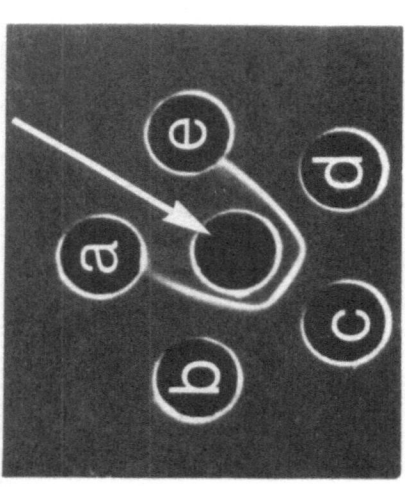

Figure 5

Ouchterlony immunodiffusion of 15 anti-rat albumin IgG and II anti-rat Z IgG against: a) normal of hepatoma Z protein, b) Region II proteins separated from hepatoma 9121 supernatant, c) proteins in void volume after Sephadex G-50 chromatography of the above Region II hepatoma proteins with or without prior incubation with 10% SDS (as described in Figure 4), d) proteins in low M.W. binding zone obtained after exposure of Region II hepatoma supernatant proteins to 10% SDS (see Figure 4), e) 0.5 N sodium chloride.

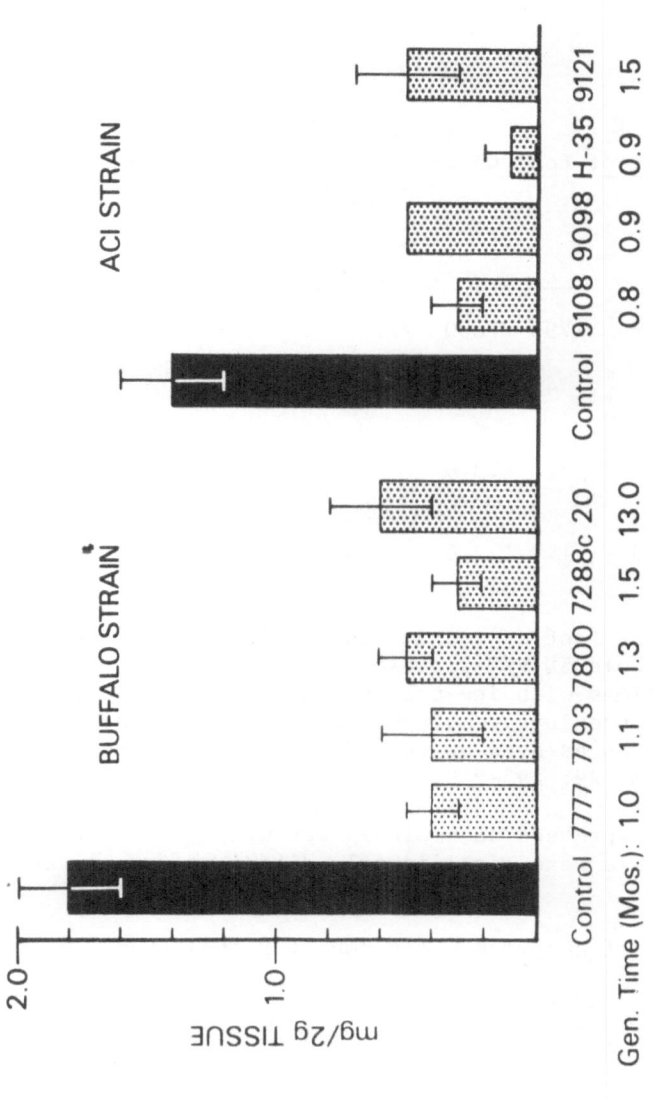

Figure 6

The concentration of Z protein in the Z regions from control and host liver supernatants (solid bars) and various hepatoma supernatants (hatched bars). See text for methods used to quantitate Z protein. Data are derived from Table II.

Table One
Content of Long Chain Acyl CoA in Liver and
Hepatoma[a]

	Liver	Morris Hepatoma Type						
		7793	7800	7288c	20	9108	9098	9121
# of specimens	20	4	9	4	2	4	4	4
long chain[b] acyl CoA	32.0	8.2	13.8	3.3	8.1	10.7	8.5	12.7
S.E.M.[c]	2.9	1.0	2.0	0.4		0.6	0.9	1.1

a - The tissues were fast frozen in liquid nitrogen, weighed and
ground in ice-cold 5% V/V perchloric acid. The precipitate
was washed 3 times with ice-cold perchloric acid and the CoA
content in the precipitate was determined after alkaline hydrolysis. CoASH was assayed as described by Allred and Guy (1969)
Analyt. Biochem. 29: 293-299.

b - Mean values - expressed as nmoles/g wet weight. The concentrations in hepatoma were significantly different from liver
($p < 0.01$).

c - Standard error of the mean - not done for less than 3 determinations.

Concentration of Z Protein in the Supernatant Fractions of
Liver and Hepatoma

The concentrations of protein in the Z region of liver and
hepatoma supernatant are shown in Table 2 and Figure 6. While
the concentration of Z protein in the supernatant fractions of
control and host liver were not statistically different, the concentration of Z as well as the in vitro binding of [14C]palmitoyl
CoA to the Z region were markedly reduced in all hepatomas studied
(p < 0.01).

INTERPRETATION

In this review we have discussed two examples of abnormal
regulation of hepatoma lipid metabolism which appear to be "transformation - linked" (i.e., abnormalities common to all hepatomas).
The abnormalities discussed are the loss of the negative feedback
regulation of cholesterol biosynthesis and the nutritional regulation of fatty acid synthesis which have been documented in all hepatomas studied to date irrespective of growth rate or degree of
histological differentiation (2,10,11). The etiology of these abnormalities is unknown as the key regulatory enzymes are not only
present in both liver and hepatomas, but possess identical physical
properties in vitro (13-16). We have observed that there is a reduced level of both Z protein and acid insoluble CoA in nine Morris
hepatomas with varying degrees of differentiation. The binding of
[14C]palmitoyl-CoA to cytoplasmic proteins was consequently different in these hepatomas, being significantly less in the Z region.

There are major implications resulting from this study which
may help to clarify the altered regulation of tumor metabolism.
Palmitoyl CoA is a potent reversible regulator of a variety of enzymatic reactions (8,20,21,50,56,57,62-67). It has been postulated
that increased hepatic levels of long chain fatty acyl CoA and/or
increased rates of oxidation of fatty acids during fasting will inhibit lipogenesis (56,57,62-67). Since long chain acyl CoA levels
are uniformly reduced in hepatomas studied and are unaffected by
nutritional state where examined (49,46,47) suggests a possible mechanism for the altered regulation of lipogenesis observed in these
hepatomas. The role for Z protein in these mechanisms is uncertain.
We and others hypothesized that by virtue of its high affinity for
long chain fatty acyl CoA, Z protein controls the intracytoplasmic
concentration of free palmitoyl CoA (35,64). We suggested that Z
may also serve as a cofactor in the enzymatic transformations of
fatty acids and their CoA derivatives (5). To date, there is evidence
that Z protein stimulates a number of steps in fatty acid esterification (37,38,39) and oxidation[8]. There is as yet no data on the direct effect of Z protein on lipogenesis.

We have alluded to preliminary studies of the properties of

Table Two
Concentration of Z Protein and Percent Binding
of [^{14}C]Palmitoyl CoA to Z Region of
Supernatant Fractions

	Z Concentration Mg per 2 g tissue	[^{14}C]Palmitoyl CoA Binding to "Z Region"	
BUFFALO STRAIN			
Control[a]	1.7 + 0.2[b]	51.0 + 4.3	(21)[c]
7777	0.4 + 0.1	7.6 + 2.2	(4)
7793	0.4 + 0.2	4.9 + 1.8	(3)
7800	0.5 + 0.1	19.5 + 1.5	(4)
7288c	0.3 + 0.1	19.5 + 2.0	(3)
20	0.6 + 0.2	5.1 + 2.1	(3)
ACI STRAIN			
Control	1.4 + 0.2	40.4 + 1.9	(10)
9108	0.4 + 0.1	20.2 + 3.5	(4)
9098	0.5	4.6	(2)
H-35	0.1 + 0.1	9.4 + 2.4	(3)
9121	0.5 + 0.2	5.2 + 0.8	(4)

a. Refers to combined data from control and host livers which were
   not significantly different.

b. Mean + S.E.M. numbers without S.E.M. represent the mean of two
   determinations on samples from different animals. These individual values did not differ by more than 15%.

c. Number of animals tested.

sterol carrier proteins in Morris hepatomas (28)[9] and must await
further studies to clarify their possible role in the regulatory
defect of cholesterol synthesis in these tumors. It is of interest
to note that in 1973 Horton et al. (71) theorized that the "loss in
the control of cholesterol synthesis in hepatomas is due to a defect in the binding and storage of cholesterol within the cell".
In addition to those already described a number of other observations
await explanation. Preliminary studies in our laboratory have indicated that the cytoplasmic binding of I^{125} triiodothyronine (T_3)
and I^{131} thyroxin (T_4) which is very low in the normal liver, is
markedly increased (200-500%) in Morris hepatomas as well as in one
human hepatoma (24,68). These findings are of interest in view of
the documented relationship between thyroid status and fatty acid
metabolism (69,70). The observation that hepatic lipoprotein synthesis in rats bearing transplanted Morris heaptomas 7777 differs
from that of control livers (29,30) is an example of how a transplanted hepatoma will influence the systemic metabolism of the host
animal. As the mechanisms for this effect is unknown, we would
wonder whether these effects may be caused by dearrangements of thyroid and/or other hormonal status.

     To date the major interest in the binding properties of hepatoma
tissue were based on the assumption that the presence of specific
binding proteins reduced the susceptibility of the liver to aminoazo
dyes, polycyclic aromatic hydrocarbon, and aromatic amines which induced carcinogenesis. The "deletion hypothesis" advanced by Miller
and Miller (72) to explain azo dye carcinogenesis in liver proposed
that neoplasms are characterized by the inability of their proteins
to bind these carcinogens. In recent years a variety of soluble proteins have been identified in rat liver, mouse liver, skin, and lung
which combine relatively specifically with aminoazo dye and polycyclic
aromatic hydrocarbon carcinogens. These include the "slow h_2 - 5S
protein" characterized in rat liver (73), the "h-protein" of mouse
liver, skin and lung (74), and the two azo dye binding carcinogens described by Ketterer et al in rat liver (75). The larger of these proteins, ligandin (or y protein) is a dimer with a molecular weight of
approximately 45,000 binds a wide range of cellular metabolites including hematin, bilirubin, glucuronic acid, steroid metabolites and
various drugs (76) and appears to be a major glutathione S-transferase
of rat liver cytosol (77). The second azo dye binding described by
Ketterer et al appears to be identical with Z protein. Thus the intriguing possibility exists that a number cytoplasmic binding proteins
which form an integral part of the regulation of normal metabolic
function may be closely linked to the ethiology of carcinogenesis.
The key question is whether the observed changes in these cytoplasmic
binding proteins are primary or are secondary changes resulting from
other primary defects of hepatoma metabolism.

FOOTNOTES

* Scholar of the Medical Research Council of Canada, to whom requests for reprints should be addressed: c/o Division of Gastroenterology, Royal Victoria Hospital, 687 Pine Avenue, W.,
Montreal, Quebec H3A 1A1.

This work was supported by grants #MA 5474 and MT 3363 from the
Medical Research Council of Canada. This article is dedicated
to the memory of the late Mr. Moe Yalovsky.

1 It should be noted that the nutritional control of acyl coenzyme
  A desaturase is retained in at least two Morris hepatomas - 5123C
  and 7777 (9). Thus the desaturation of saturated fatty acids is
  depressed in a normal manner by fasting in hepatomas which have
  lost the ability to inhibit lipogenesis under the same nutritional
  conditions.

2 Mishkin, S. and Scallen, T.J., unpublished observations.

3 It is of interest in this regard that taking into account the concentration of Z in liver cytosol ($\sim$ 200 nmoles/gm) and its affinity
  for palmitoyl CoA (0.5-1.0 nmole palmitoyl CoA per nmole of Z protein) the amount of Z protein is adequate to bind all long chain
  fatty acyl CoA present in the liver under normal conditions ($\sim$ 50
  nmoles/gm) (36).

4 This observation may not be common to all tumors as has been suggested (54), In Ehrlich ascites tumor cells fatty acid biosynthesis
  responds rapidly to added free fatty acids in the same manner as
  non malignant cells (17).

5 The abbreviation used is: PAGE, polyacrylamide gel electrophoresis.

6 Murthy, P.V.N. and Mishkin, S., unpublished observations.

7 Huan, S.N. and Mishkin, S. unpublished observations.

8 Halperin, M.L. and Mishkin, S., unpublished observations.

9 Scallen, T.J. and Mishkin, S., unpublished observations.

REFERENCES

1. Goldfarb, S. and Pitot, H.C. Front. of Gatroint. Res. 2 (1976) 194.

2. Morris, H.P. Adv. in Cancer Res. 9 (1965) 227.

3. Bloch-Frankenthal, B., Langan, J., Morris, H.P. and Weinhouse, J. Cancer Res. 25 (1965) 732.

4. Weber, G., In: The Molecular Biology of Cancer, H. Busch (ed). Academic Press, New York (1974) 487.

5. Potter, V.R. Cancer Res. 21 (1963) 1331.

6. Weber, G. New England Journal of Med. 296 (1977) 486.

7. Allman, D.W., Hibard, D.D. and Gibson, D.M. J. of Lipid Res. 6 (1965) 63.

8. Lane, M.D., Moss, J., Ryder, E. and Stoll, E. Adv. Enzyme Regul. 9 (1971) 237.

9. Lee, T., Stephern, S.N. and Snyder, F. Cancer Res. 34 (1974) 3270.

10. Morris, H.P. In: Biological and Biochemical Characteristics of Transplantable Hepatomas, Springer-Verlag, Berlin, Heidelberg, New York (1975) 313.

11. Siperstein, M.D. and L.J., Luby, In: Fish in Research, Neuhaus and Halver (eds), Academic Press, New York (1969) 87.

12. Bricker, L.A., Morris, H.P. and Siperstein, M.D. J. of Clin. Invest. 51 (1972) 206.

13. Brown, M.S., Goldstein, J.L. and Siperstein, M.D. Fed. Proc. 32 (1973) 2168.

14. Williams, M.T., Gaylor, J.L. and Morris, H.P. Cancer Res. 36 (1976) 291.

15. Sabine, J.R. and Chaikoff, I.L. Australian J. Exptl. Biol. Med. Sci. 45 (1967) 541.

16. Majerus, P.W., Jacob, S.R., Smith, M.B. and Morris, H.P. The J. of Biol. Chem. 243 (1968) 3588.

17. McGee, R. and Spector, A.A. Cancer Res. 34 (1974) 3355.

18. Bartley, H.C. and Abraham, S. Biochim. Biophys. Acta 260 (1972) 169.

19. Halperin, M.L., Taylor, W.M., Cheema-Dhadli, S., Morris, H.P. and Fritz, I.B. Eur. J. of Biochem. 50 (1974) 517.

20. Fritz, I.B. and Lee, L. Endocrin. 1 (1972) 579.

21. Volpe, J.J. and Vagelos, P.R. Ann. Rev. Biochem. 42 (1973) 21.

22. Fritz, I.B. and Halperin, M.L. Metabolic Inhibitors IV, Academic Press, New York & London (1973) 311.

23. Mishkin, S., Morris, H.P., Murthy, P.V.N. and Halperin, M.L. Gastroenterology 70 (1976) 988.

24. Mishkin, S., Murthy, P.V.N., Huang, S.N. and Halperin, M.L. Clin. Res. 24 (1976) 660A.

25. Mishkin, S., Morris, H.P., Murthy, P.V.N. and Halperin, M.L. J. of Biol. Chem. in press.

26. Dempsey, M.E. Ann. Rev. of Biochem. 43 (1974) 967.

27. Scallen, T.J., Seetharam, B., Srikantiah, M.V., Hansbury, E. and Lewis, M.K. Life Sciences 16 (1975) 853.

28. Longino, M.A., Gaylor, J.L. and Morris, H.P. Fed. Proc. 36 (1977) 779.

29. Narayan, K.A. and Morris, H.P. Int. J. of Cancer 5 (1970) 410.

30. Narayan, K.A. and Morris, H.P. FEBS Letters, 27 (1972) 311.

31. Levi, A.J., Gatmaitan, Z. and Arias, I.M., J. Clin. Invest. 48 (1969) 2156.

32. Mishkin, S., Stein, L., Gatmaitan, Z. and Arias, I.M. Biochem. Biophys. Res. Comm. 47 (1972) 997.

33. Mishkin, S., Stein, L., Gatmaitan, Z. and Arias, I.M. Gastroenterology 64 (1973) 154.

34. Mishkin, S., Stein, L., Fleischner, G., Gatmaitan, Z. and Arias, I.M. American J. of Physiol. 228 (1975) 1634.

35. Mishkin, S. and Turcotte, R., Biochem. Biophys. Res. Comm. 57 (1974) 918.

36. Tubbs, P.K. and Garland, P.B. Biochem. J. 93 (1964) 550.

37. Mishkin, S. and Turcotte, R. Biochem. Biophys. Res. Comm. 60 (1974) 376.

38. O'Doherty, P.J.A. and Kuskis, A. FEBS Letters, 60 (1975) 256.

39. Mishkin, S. and Roncari, D.A.K. Clin. Res. 24 (1976) 682A.

40. Suzue, G. and Marcel, Y.L. Canadian J. of Biochem. 53 (1975) 804.

41. Ockner, R.K. and Manning, J.A. J. of Clin. Invest. 53 (1974) 57a.

42. Wu-Rideout, M.Y.C., Elson, C. and Shargo, E. Biochem. Biophys. Res. Comm. 71 (1976) 809.

43. Ketterer, B., Ross-Mansell, P. and Whitehead, J.K. Biochem. J. 103 (1967) 316.

44. Morey, K.S. and Litwack, G. Biochemistry, 8 (1969) 4813.

45. Sokoloff, J., Berk, R.N., Lang, J.H. and Lasser, E.C. Radiology, 106 (1973) 519.

46. Warner, M. and Neim, A.H. Canadian J. of Physiol. and Pharm. 53 (1975) 493.

47. Kornguth, M.L., Monson, R.A. and Kunin, C.M. Arch. of Biochem. and Biophys. 174 (1976) 339.

48. Kotake, A. and Mannering, G.J. The Pharmacologist, 16 (1974) 216.

49. Halperin, M.L., Taylor, W.M., Cheema-Dhadli, S., Morris, H.P. and Fritz, I.B. Eur. J. Bicoehm. 50 (1974) 517.

50. Hsu, K.L. and Powell, G.L. Proc. Natl. Acad. Sci. U.S.A. 72 (1975) 4729.

51. Sabine, J.R., Abraham, S. and Chaikoff, I.L. Cancer Res. 27 (1967) 793.

52. Sabine, J.R., Abraham, S. and Morris, H.P. Cancer Res. 28 (1968) 46.

53. Elwood, J.C. and Morris, H.P. J. Lipid Res. 9 (1968) 337.

54. Majerus, P .W., Jacobs, R. and Smith, M.B. J. Biol. Chem. 243

(1968) 3588.

55. Zuckerman, N.J., Nardella, P., Morris, H.P. and Elwood, J.C. Natl. Cancer Inst. 44 (1970) 79.

56. Halperin, M.L., Cheema-Dhadli, S., Taylor, W.M. and Fritz, I. B. Adv. in Enzyme Regul. 13 (1975) 535.

57. Fritz, I.B., Cheema-Dhadli, S., Morris, H.P. and Halperin, M.L. Alfred Benzon Symp. on Hepatic Met., VI (1974) 645.

58. Moroz, C. and Hahn, Y. Proc. Natl. Acad. Sci. U.S.A. 70 (1973) 3716.

59. Lowry, O.H., Rosenbrough, N.J., Farr, A.L. and Randall, R.J. J. Biol. Chem. 193 (1951) 265.

60. Allred, J.B. and Guy, D.G. Analyt. Biochem. 29 (1969) 293.

61. Ketterer, B., Tipping, E. and Hackeney, J.F. Biochem. J. 155 (1976) 511.

62. Numa, S., Bortz, W.N. and Lynen, F. Adv. Enzyme Regul. 3 (1965) 407.

63. Goodridge, A.G. J. Biol. Chem. 247 (1972) 6946.

64. Halestrap, A.P. and Denton, R.M. Biochem. J. 142 (1974) 365.

65. Halperin, M.L., Robinson, B.H. and Fritz, I.B. Proc. Natl. Acad. Sci. (Wash) 69 (1972) 1003.

66. Cheema-Dhadli, S. and Halperin, M.L. Can. J. Biochem. 51 (1973) 1542.

67. Cheema-Dhadli, S. and Halperin, M.L. Can. J. Biochem. 54 (1976) 171.

68. Murthy, P.V.N., Morris, H.P. and Mishkin, S. Clin. Res. 24 (1976) 660A.

69. Roncari, D.A.K. and Murthy, V.K. J. of Biol. Chem. 250 (1975) 4134.

70. Kumar, S. and Dipak, K.D. Fed. Proc. 35 (1976) 746.

71. Horton, B.J., Horton, J.D. and Pitot, H.C. Cancer Res. 33 (1973) 1301.

72. Miller, E.C. and Miller, J.A. Cancer Res. 7 (1947) 468.

73. Sorof, S., Sani, B.P., Kish, V.M. and Meoche, H. Biochemistry 13 (1974) 2612.

74. Sarrif, A.M., Bertram, J.S., Kamarck, M. and Heidelberger, C. Cancer Res. 35 (1975) 816.

75. Ketterer, B. and Christodoulides, L., Chem-Biol. Interactions, 1 (1969) 173.

76. Arias, I.M., Fleischner, G., Kirch, R., Mishkin, S. and Gatmaitan, Z. In: Glutathione: Metabolism and Function, Arias and Jacoby (eds). Raven Press, New York 6 (1976) 175.

77. Habig, W., Pabst, M., Fleischner, G., Gatmaitan, Z., Arias, I.M. and Jacoby, W. Proc. Natl. Acad. Sci. U.S.A. 71 (1974) 3879.

VITAMIN B$_6$ EFFECTS ON THE GROWTH OF MORRIS HEPATOMAS AND THE

DEVELOPMENT OF ENZYMATIC ACTIVITY[1]

George P. Tryfiates

Department of Biochemistry
West Virginia University School of Medicine
Morgantown, West Virginia 26506

SUMMARY

Vitamin B$_6$ is not only required for normal growth and development, in general, but also for the growth of neoplasms. In attempts
to decipher the effects of the vitamin on tumor growth and metabolic
function, i.e., enzyme activity, studies were carried out in our
laboratory using Morris hepatomas of increasing degree of differentiation grown in animals fed ad libitum a pyridoxine free diet and
in pair-fed or ad libitum (controls) given the same diet supplemented
with pyridoxine[2]. The effects of the absence of pyridoxine from the
diet on (a) hepatoma growth, (b) enzyme activity, (c) enzyme induction and (d) enzyme expression in liver and hepatomas were investigated using, in addition to conventional and chromatographic procedures,
(a) immunoprecipitation in agar-gel and (b) in situ, 'on the gel',
histochemical staining for detection of resolved, enzymatically active protein bands. Further, the effects of progressive 'cofactor
depletion' (vitamin deficiency) and hepatoma growth on hormonal enzyme induction and vitamin B$_6$ were also investigated.

The growth of a spectrum of neoplasms was significantly impaired
in the absence of dietary PX. Moreover, treatment with dexopyridoxine
alone or in combination with other agents was effective in inhibiting
tumor growth. Our results with a number of Morris hepatoma lines are
in agreement with findings reported for other tumors. The growth of
eight transplantable hepatomas examined was significantly impaired in
the absence of PX. Generally, hepatomas from ad lib fed controls
were significantly heavier than those from the other groups. Hepatomas from pair-fed controls were 2x or even heavier than those from
depleted animals.

TAT and SD activity levels as well as their response to hormonal stimulation were significantly influenced by cofactor depletion. Expression of SD was highly facilitated by PX in normal liver and in three hepatomas examined but was repressed in the respective host livers. Host liver and hepatoma TAT activity levels, in practically all instances, were increased in the PX depleted state. Further, the magnitude and pattern of TAT response to hormonal administration were drastically affected by the absence of dietary PX. In this regard, PX depletion effected a TAT response to steroid stimulation which increased steadily and in a linear fashion (superinduction?) as duration of depletion increased in contrast to a controlled induction pattern seen in pair-fed control animals. TAT activity levels remained high during the period of depletion and after 40 days were approximately equal to the induced TAT level of the pair-fed controls. The presence of growing hepatoma No. 7777 completely altered the TAT hormonal induction pattern in both PX depleted and pair-fed controls. After 7 days of tumor growth, hormonal stimulation resulted in a 4-5 fold increase in TAT activity in both host liver and hepatoma of either PX depleted or pair-fed animals. However, after 14 and 21 days, host liver and tumor TAT was only minimally induced.

Rat liver, cytoplasmic TAT was highly purified ($>$ 3,000x) following its hormonal induction and subsequently resolved by electrophoresis on polyacrylamide gel into 4 protein bands. High-speed supernatants from liver and hepatoma No. 7777 were gel electrophoresed and resolved proteins tested in agar-gel for immunoreactivity by immunoprecipitation with TAT-specific rabbit antiserum prepared against the purified TAT preparation. Normal liver and hepatomas developed four immunoprecipitation bands while liver and hepatomas from depleted animals developed five and three bands, respectively. Gel electrophoresis of partially purified, uninduced, hepatic TAT and in situ, on the gel, detection of enzymatically active peaks by histochemical staining showed six peaks. In cofactor depleted animals the main TAT peak was bifurcated. Expression of hormonally induced TAT in normal liver resembled that of the uninduced, depleted animals. The presence of growing hepatomas altered the expression of this enzyme significantly. Only one, two and four peaks were detected in the host liver of animals bearing highly, well and poorly differentiated hepatomas, respectively. Similarly, only one, four and six peaks were, respectively detected in these hepatomas.

Liver cells incorporated twice as much PX* as hepatoma cells and maximal uptake occurred at 30 min and 6 hours, respectively. In the state of deficiency, normal liver cells retained the label through the seven-day period studied. Maximal synthesis of phosphorylated vitamin B_6 forms from labeled PX occurred sequencially, i.e., PX*$\rightarrow$ PX5P$\rightarrow$PXL5P$\rightarrow$PM5P. Albeit, this ordered sequence was not altered in the state of deficiency the reactions were highly accelerated. PM5P was retained, being continuously synthesized and increasing linearly

in proportion to the rate of PXL5P disappearance. Further, in
contrast to PX metabolism in normal liver, PM5P was also synthesized
and retained by the host liver of animals bearing hepatoma No. 7777.
PXL5P was, however, also maintained at a high level in this case.
On the other hand, hepatoma cells synthesized high amounts of PM5P
which was not retained but was further dephosphorylated to PM. The
latter observation concurs with normal hepatoma growth which, in the
vitamin depleted state, is significantly impaired and Pm5P is retained at least in the instance studied, i.e., animals without tumors
(this review paper concerns studies relating to PX, Morris hepatomas
and enzymatic activity known to the author prior to this Hepatoma
Symposium.)

INTRODUCTION

Vitamin B_6 refers to pyridoxine, pyridoxal and pyridoxamine.
The three vitamin forms are active biologically. They are present in
tissues as phosphate esters. The vitamin serves as the coenzyme of
many classes of enzymes with pyridoxal phosphate believed to be the
active coenzyme form. Among the enzymes requiring pyridoxal phosphate as coenzyme are transaminases, amino acid decarboxylases, race-
maces (i.e., D- or L-alanine), α , β-eliminases (i.e., serine), (phosphorylase), enzymes involved in tryptophan metabolism (i.e., trypto-
phanase), cystathionase and others. Vitamin B_6 is required for normal growth and development, in general. Its absence from the diet of
young rats results in the development of characteristic dermatitis affecting the paws and nose with swelling and edema. Certain tissues
are particularly sensitive to pyridoxine depletion. Impairment of
antibody response, anemia, atrophy of lymphoid tissue, functional
changes in the central nervous system and inhibition of tumor growth
have been seen in animals fed pyridoxine free diets.

Because pyridoxal $5'-PO_4$ is required by a variety of enzymes for
catalysis alterations in enzymatic activity levels have been seen in
the state of deficiency. Further, results of recent studies suggest
that the vitamin influences, in addition, the expression of gene product relating to its structure. In attempts to relate the effects of
pyridoxine to tumor growth and metabolic function, i.e., enzyme activity, studies in our laboratory have been concerned mainly with the influence of pyridoxine depletion on the growth of Morris transplantable
hepatomas and the development and expression of hormonally induced enzymes requiring pyridoxal $5'$-phosphate for catalysis. In addition,
possible aberrations in vitamin B_6 metabolism peculiar to hepatoma-
bearing animals and/or the deficient state as well as their relationship to enzyme inducibility were also investigated. In this paper,
examples from this work and relevant data from the literature are
presented and discussed in the light of possible application to limiting or controlling the growth of solid (or other) tumors biochemically
by such means as nutritional.

1. Inhibition of Tumor Growth

Investigators as early as 1943 demonstrated that the growth of sarcoma 180, two carcinomas and one fibrocarcinoma was impaired if rodents were fed semipurified diets lacking vitamin B_6 (1-2). Stoerk (3) reported that lymphosarcoma failed to grow in animals deprived of pyridoxine. Complete regression of sarcoma 180 was reported by Mihich and Nichol (4). The growth of six mouse tumors, i.e., adenocarcinoma 755, leukemia L1210 and L4946, Ehrlich carcinoma ascites clone 2, Ehrlich carcinoma solid, and plasma-cell tumor 70429 in addition to a rat lymphosarcoma, was also impaired in the absence of dietary vitamin B_6 (5). Further, antagonists of the vitamin such as 4-deoxypyridoxine (DOP) (6) exerted marked effects against experimental tumors (3, 7-12). The combination of DOP and 8-azaguanine was also found to be very effective in inhibiting tumor growth (9, 10). Whether absence of pyridoxine from the diet also affects the growth of transplantable Morris hepatomas was not investigated until recently. Studies in our laboratory have shown that the growth of several lines of Morris hepatomas was significantly impaired in the absence of dietary pyridoxine (13-17). The hepatomas examined included poorly differentiated lines (rapid growth), well differentiated (average growth) and one highly differentiated (slow growth; most liver-like hepatoma) lines. Since pyridoxine is needed for normal animal growth and development, in general, it is not surprising that the vitamin is also needed for growth of hepatomas and other tumors. Other vitamins, minerals and other dietary factors exert fundamental influence(s) on tumor growth, in general (18-29). Despite the lack of specificity there is merit in studying nutritional effects in detail on the theory that tumor cells might be more sensitive to deficiency than normal cells or that tumors might have unusual metabolites which could be blocked without much interference with normal cell function.

The results presented in Table 1 show the effect of the absence of dietary pyridoxine on the growth of the highly differentiated hepatoma No. 7794A. The growth of this very slowly growing tumor was minimal in animals fed the deficient diet and maximal in animals fed the sufficient diet ad libitum. Hepatomas grown in animals receiving the latter regimen were on the average 4x heavier than those on deficient animals. The average weight of hepatomas developed by pairfed controls depended on the time of inoculation of tumor cells. If inoculation was performed at the start of the experiment (time zero, t_0) there was no significant difference in average tumor weight between the deficient and paid-fed (control) animals. However, if the animals were fed the respective diets for 31 days and then inoculated with hepatoma cells, average tumor weights of 0.78, 2.40 and 2.80 grams were developed by the deficient, pair-fed and ad libitum fed control groups, respectively. This finding shows that control animals on a restricted food intake (pair-fed group) require a longer

Table One

Growth of Morris Hepatoma #7794A in the Absence and Presence of Vitamin B$_6$ and under ad libitum and Pair-Feeding Conditions

Group	# animals	Diet	Time of inoculation	Duration of tumor growth	Average wt(g) Body wt.	Liver weight	Tumor wt.	Body wt/ Tumor wt.rat	Ave. food consumed g/ rat per 24hr.
A	5	Vit.B$_6$(-) Ad libitum	t$_o$(50)*	47	94 ± 14.0	4.0 ± 0.2(5)+	0.73±0.2(4)+	129	8.1 ± 2
B	4	Vit.B$_6$(+) Pair-fed to A	t$_o$(50)	47	123 ± 5.8	2.5 ± 0.5(4)	0.91±0.1(8)	135	8.1 ± 2
C	4	Vit.B$_6$(+) Ad libitum	t$_o$(50)	49	278 ± 5.0	8.0 ± 0.4(4)	2.94±0.4(7)	95	17.0 ± 4
D@	4	Vit.B$_6$(-) Ad libitum	t$_{31}$(80)	48	154 ± 7.0	4.7 ± 0.5(4)	0.78±0.5(5)	198	8.4 ± 2
E	4	Vit.B$_6$(+) Pair-fed to D	t$_{31}$(106)	48	185 ± 1.0	4.8 ± 0.4(4)	2.40±0.5(8)	77	8.4 ± 2
F	4	Vit.B$_6$(+) Ad libitum	t$_{31}$(160)	48	348 ± 23.0	8.4 ± 0.6(3)	2.80±0.5(6)	124	19.1 ± 5

* Number in parenthesis is the average body weight of the group at the time of inoculation; t$_o$, t$_{31}$ indicate the number of days the animals (🐀) were fed the diets shown prior to inoculation with tumor cells.

+ Number in parenthesis is the number of livers averaged.

‡ Number in parenthesis is the number of tumors averaged. Numbers following the ± sign are the standard error of the mean in all cases.

@ After 31 days on the B$_6$(-) diet, pyridoxine was given for 3 days. Each animal consumed approximately 360 μg of pyridoxine during this period (ref. 16).

time period prior to inoculation with tumor cells to develop hepatomas of similar average weight as animals receiving the control
diet (vitamin B_6 plus) ad libitum. The requirement for a longer
feeding period may be necessary for the accumulation of vitamin B_6
by this very slowly growing hepatoma. It is interesting to note
that liver pyridoxal phosphate decreased steadily after ascites
hepatoma cells were inoculated into animals and that the coenzyme
content of the cancer cells increased as they proliferated (30).
Furthermore, hepatoma No. 7777 - a fast growing tumor - accumulated
as much as 5x pyridoxal 5'-PO_4 as host liver two weeks after inoculation at which time host liver was practically depleted of the cofactor (15). It was also reported that Buffalo strain pair-fed control animals continued to lose liver pyridoxal 5'-PO_4 up to 50 days
old. Afterwards, a minimal coenzyme level was maintained. At the
age of 50 days the liver cofactor content of the pair-fed animals
was less than 40% that found for 29 days old animals (31). These
observations indicate that during early development vitamin B_6 is
probably mobilized and utilized in essential metabolic processes.
It appears therefore, reasonable that the period of 31 days of
caloric restriction (pair-feeding) to be necessary for the animal to
satisfy its own needs for vitamin B_6 and for this very slowly growing
tumor to accumulate enough needed vitamin for its growth. Presumably,
accumulation of cofactor by hepatoma cells reflects the rate of multiplication. Therefore, well and poorly differentiated hepatomas
growing in pair-fed control animals should be expected to require a
shorter pre-inoculation time period for accumulation of needed vitamin B_6. Tables 2 and 3 show results obtained with the latter hepatoma lines. In these instances the pre-inoculation period was three
weeks. There is no doubt that lack of dietary pyridoxine impairs the
growth of the hepatomas. The possibility of considerable impairment
of metabolic function resulting from a 31 day depletion period should
not be overlooked (31, 32). Therefore, in the case of the slow growing hepatoma No. 7794A it is very probable that impairment in general
animal metabolism as a result of deficiency also contributes to the
retardation in the growth of this tumor (13). This would not, however, be the case for the other fast growing hepatoma lines since the
length of both pre-inoculation and tumor development periods taken
together is not unreasonable with regards to the welfare of the
animal.

2. Enzyme Activity and Induction

Since pyridoxal 5'-PO_4 is the coenzyme of many classes of enzymes
any alteration(s) in its availability would be expected to exert cor-
respondingly an influence in the activity levels of these enzymes.
Alterations in cofactor availability could also be involved in the
response of inducible pyridoxal 5'-PO_4-requiring enzymes to stimulation by an inducer. The activity levels of various enzymes have been
reported to be decreased during pyridoxine depletion, by deoxypy-

Table Two

Growth of Morris Hepatomas #7777, 5123A, 7316B, and 7800 without and with Vitamin B₆ under ad libitum and Pair-Feeding Conditions*

Group	Number of Animals	Diet+	Tumor Growth (days)	Average weights at death‡(g) Body	Liver	Tumor	Tumor wt/ Body weight	Average diet consumed (g/rat/24 hr)	P@
				#7777					
A	7	I	21	87 ± 6(7)	4.8 ± 0.3(7)	2.1 ± 0.6	0.024	9 ± 2	
B	8	II	21	96 ± 11(8)	4.7 ± 0.5(16)	4.7 ± 0.5(16)	.097	9 ± 2	< 0.001
C	8	III	21	161 ± 18(8)	7.4 ± 1.2(8)	7.7 ± 1.2(16)	.048	15 ± 3	< .001
D	8	IV	21	183 ± 14(8)	6.3 ± 0.8(8)	7.7 ± 0.6(16)	.042	17 ± 4	< .001
				#5123A					
A	6	I	28	86 ± 23(6)	5.2 ± 0.9(6)	1.1 ± 0.4(12)	.012	8 ± 2	
B	5	II	28	86 ± 9(5)	5.8 ± 1.2(5)	2.6 ± 1.0(10)	.030	8 ± 2	~ .001
C	5	III	28	129 ± 4(5)	5.5 ± 0.8(5)	2.7 ± 0.6(10)	.021	15 ± 2	< .001
D	6	IV	28	135 ± 19(6)	8.0 ± 0.7(6)	2.5 ± 0.7(12)	.018	16 ± 3	< .001
				#7316B					
A	7	I	30	84 ± 11(7)	4.6 ± 0.5(7)	1.2 ± 0.4(10)	.017	8 ± 2	
B	7	II	30	97 ± 9(7)	5.3 ± 1.8(7)	2.0 ± 0.4(10)	.021	8 ± 2	~ .001
C	7	III	30	178 ± 10(7)	6.8 ± 0.8(7)	3.3 ± 1.4(14)	.019	17 ± 4	< .001
D	8	IV	30	205 ± 12(8)	6.4 ± 1.0(8)	3.4 ± 1.3(14)	.018	18 ± 4	< .001
				#7800					
A	4	I	48	95 ± 12(4)	4.7 ± 0.7(4)	5.3 ± 0.2(8)	.056	9 ± 3	
C	7	III	48	172 ± 16(7)	7.5 ± 1.2(7)	7.6 ± 1.6(14)	.044	18 ± 5	< .001
D	6	IV	48	177 ± 16(6)	7.3 ± 2.0(6)	8.3 ± 1.8(10)	.047	18 ± 4	< .001

*± values are SD.

+ Group A received type I diet: vitamin B₆ deficient ad libitum. Group B received type II diet: B₆ deficient ad libitum, the B₆ supplemented at 21 days and pair-fed to group A. Group C received type III diet: B₆ deficient ad libitum, then changed at 21 days to B₆ supplemented until animals were killed. Group D received type IV diet: B₆ supplemented ad libitum throughout the experiment.

‡ Values in parenthesis are number of animal, liver, or tumor weights averaged. @ Determined by t test. All animals were (♀) inoculated with hepatoma cells after three weeks on the respective diets.

Table Three
Growth of Morris Hepatoma No. 7288tc and No.
7316A in Pyridoxine Depleted and Pair-
fed Buffalo (♀) rats

Group	Average Tumor Weight (g)	
	No. 7288tc	No. 7316A
Depleted	4.73 ± 0.7 (30)*	1.44 ± 0.2 (16)
Pair-fed	11.61 ± 1.5 (30)	3.75 ± 0.6 (16)

± values are SD. Numbers in parentheses are numbers of hepatomas averaged. The significance level was determined by the t-test and was $P < 0.001$ and $P \simeq 0.001$ for hepatomas #7288tc and #7316A, respectively. The number of animals in each group was 15 and 8 for No. 7288tc and No. 7316A hepatomas, respectively (Ref. 17).

ridoxine or by both (10, 11, 33-36). Brin and Thiele (37) found that the activity of two transaminase enzymes of different rat tissues increased with increasing the vitamin B$_6$ content of the diet and Milholland et al. (38) reported that the activity of tyrosine transaminase was decreased in vitamin B$_6$ deficiency. A similar finding was also reported from this laboratory in tests with male Wistar strain rats (39). On the other hand, a slight increase in the level of apotransaminase was observed by other investigators (40, 41). These workers used animals which were fed a vitamin B$_6$ deficient diet for over three months. In our laboratory we are unable to keep vitamin B$_6$ deficient animals alive for another 4-5 weeks on the deficient diet. The animals become deficient in 30-35 days, as has also been reported by others (42) and if left on the deficient diet for another 35 days they die soon afterwards. Perhaps the difference in results (10, 11, 30, 35-39) and (40, 41) are due to different lenghts of time of exposure of the animals to the vitamin B$_6$ deficient diet. In this regard, other variables such as animal strain and sex should also be considered as contributing factors. For example, we have observed that hepatic TAT activity levels of PX depleted and control Buffalo males are not very much dissimilar (13, 43) while Wistar PX depleted male rats have low TAT levels (32, 39). Albeit, PX depletion did not significantly decrease the TAT level of male Long-Evans rats (44). On the other hand, we have consistently found higher TAT levels in female PX depleted Buffalo rats than in the controls (14, 15, 17, 31). Greengard and Gordon reported (45) an increase in tyrosine transaminase activity upon injection of pyridoxine to adrenalectomized (or normal) rats which was prevented by puromycin but not by actinomycin D. However, Holten, Wicks and Kenney (46) reported later that actinomycin D does prevent the rise in transaminase activity elicited by either the administration of hydrocortisone or pyridoxine to adrenalectomized animals. Using vitamin B$_6$ deficient animals (about 50 days on the deficient diet) the rise in transaminase activity due to hydrocortisone or pyridoxine injection could not be prevented by either puromycin or actinomycin D but instead was further stimulated (39). The rise in enzymatic activity due to hydrocortisone administration was, however, inhibited by cycloheximide in normal animals (32). Enzymes which specifically degrade the apoprotein of pyridoxal phosphate-requiring enzymes have been isolated (47) and in one instance the activity of the inactivating enzyme was 20-fold greater in vitamin B$_6$ deficiency (48). The inactivating enzymes are predominantly found in the intestine and skeletal muscle but not in the heart liver or brain. They may function in the pyridoxine depleted state by reducing the level of certain apoenzymes in some tissues thus making pyridoxal 5'-PO$_4$ available for more important enzyme functions which require the coenzyme.

In attempts to shed light on tumor metabolism, in general, many investigators studied metabolic function in neoplastic tissues in

terms of alterations in enzyme activity levels. Several studies
(49-53) related the behavior of a number of enzymes including TAT,
in hepatocellular carcinomas. In certain Morris hepatomas TAT is
"derepressed", i.e., tumor TAT activity is several times greater
than that of host liver and does not respond to hydrocortisone
while host liver TAT does respond to the steroid. Further, after
adrenalectomy, the tumor enzyme levels returns to that of host liver
and acute administration of cortisone to adrenalectomized animals
returns the level of the tumor and host liver enzyme to that seen
in the tumor of the intact host.

In contrast to the behavior of tyrosine transaminase, another
extensively studied enzyme, tryptophan pyrrolase - which is hormonally inducible in normal rats - is present at low levels in rat hepatomas and, in general, does not respond to cortisone (49-53). More
recent studies by Potter and coworkers (54-59) have shown that the
activities of a number of enzymes oscillate in daily cycles in Morris
hepatomas and also in normal rat liver. Further, in some hepatomas
certain enzymes appear to be non-induced, in others derepressed and
some enzymes do not change in response to environmental change. The
activity of tyrosine transaminase varied greatly (in one hepatoma it
was almost zero) and depended both on the protein content of the diet
and feeding pattern peaking 6 hours after the start of the feeding
period. Under controlled feeding and lighting conditions the response of this liver enzyme to hormones given to adult rats was proportional to the protein content of the diet. Its response to hydrocortisone, glucagon and adrenalectomy, however, differed in the hepatomas studied, In normal animals fed ad libitum but under controlled illumination (8 p.m. to 8 a.m., darkness; 8 a.m. to 8 p.m., light)
the enzyme showed a daily cycle peaking soon after the onset of darkness. The activity rhythm persisted after adrenalectomy or hypophy-
sectomy (60).

3. Hormonal TAT Induction Patterns

Results of experiments carried in our laboratory strongly suggested that the expression of enzymatic activities (and/or their response to hormonal stimulation) is highly influenced by the availability of cofactor. In Morris hepatoma No. 7794A, for instance, TAT will
respond to hydrocortisone only if this tumor is grown in animals fed
a diet containing a high level of pyridoxine (13, 43). Lack of cofactor interfered also in the expression of serine dehydratase activity in tumors and normal liver (13, 43, 61). In normal liver and in
the host liver of animals bearing the highly differentiated hepatoma
No. 7794A both expression and hormonal induction in the host liver
was not demonstrated - a finding indicating interference by this hepatoma with the response of SD to steroid stimulation (13, 43). On
the other hand, expression of this enzyme in the well differentiated
Morris hepatoma Nos. 5123A, 7316B and 7800 was highly facilitated by

dietary PX but was significantly inhibited in the corresponding host livers (Fig 1). In this case, lack of PX facilitated SD expression in host liver (61). Moreover in regards to TAT, in practically all instances except for No. 7794A hepatoma (13, 43), host liver and hepatoma activity level were increased in the pyridoxine depleted state (14, 17). The influence of cofactor presence (and/or absence) on enzymatic activities and their response to hormonal stimulation prompted further studies regarding the effects of PX depletion and of progressive depletion on TAT hormonal induction in animals with and without hepatomas. TAT activity levels in PX depleted Wistar animals (male) were low. Hormonal TAT induction in these animals was characterized by (a) an early peak induction time (3.5-6 hours) when in vivo protein synthesis was normal; (b) a delayed incorporation of label into protein, including transaminase protein (8-10 hours); (c) an increased rate of protein synthesis; and (d) failure of cycloheximide to block the rise in enzymatic activity albeit it, at the same time, effectively inhibited in vivo protein synthesis. In contrast, hormonal induction of transaminase activity in control Wistar animals was characterized by: (a) the occurrence of peak induction at 6 hours, which was concurrent with peak in vivo protein synthesis, and antitransaminase-precipitable radioactivity, and (b) the effective inhibition by the antibiotic of both rise in activity and in vivo incorporated radioactivity into liver proteins, including transaminase (32). It was concluded that the rise in TAT activity (3.5-6 hours) in the absence of accelerated de novo synthesis of liver proteins was not due to the accumulation of apotransaminase brought about by a slower degradation rate but that it was probably due to activation of preformed enzyme following steroid stimulation (32).

The patterns of hormonally induced and noninduced hepatic tyrosine aminotransferase specific activity as affected by increasing age, progressive vitamin B$_6$ depletion, pair-feeding and repletion are shown in Figure 2a. The accompanying Figure 2b is a repeat of Figure 2a except that enzymatic activity was assayed in vitro (39) without the addition of cofactor pyridoxal phosphate. Tyrosine aminotransferase activity was maximal between 43-59 days of age at which time it began to decrease in the pair-fed and repleted animals reaching at 57 days a stationary value similar to that seen in animals less than 43 days old. The enzyme level of animals fed the pyridoxine free diet did not decrease at 57 days of age but remained high till sacrifice. Administration of hydrocortisone 4 hours prior to sacrifice resulted in increased TAT activity levels reaching a peak value at 50 days of age in pair-fed controls and continuing to increase in animals fed the vitamin deficient diet. The hormonal induction pattern in repleted animals appears to resemble that of animals fed the deficient diet since enzyme activity continued to increase with age till sacrifice. The level of cofactor saturated TAT in vivo appears to depend largely on the amount of total (available) apoenzyme provided enough coenzyme is also present. Approximately 50% of the total apoenzyme

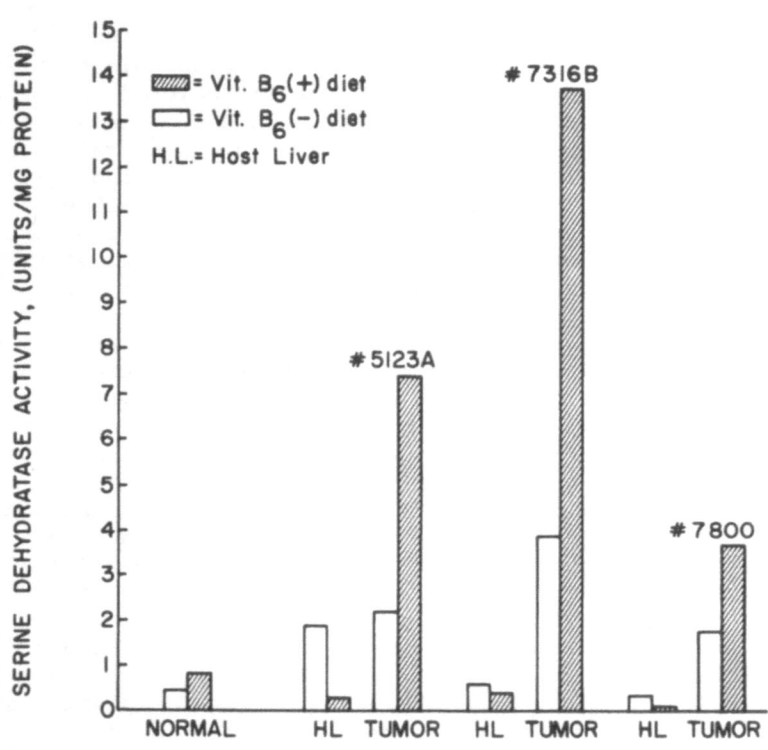

Figure 1

Serine dehydratase act. levels in normal, host liver, and Morris hepatomas Nos. 5123A, 7316B, and 7800 grown in animals fed vitamin B_6-deficient (-) and supplemented (+) diets. Animals per group: no tumors, 3; 5123A, 5(-), 6(+); 7316B, 6(-), 8(+); 7800, 4(-), 4(+); number of enzyme assays as number of animals (livers). Number of assayed tumors averaged: 5123A, 10(-), 12(+); 7316A, 10(-), 16(+); 7800, 8 each. Highest (activity level) $\pm$ SE observed was 0.4 for host liver of 5123A (-) group. All other averaged $\pm$ 0.15 SE.

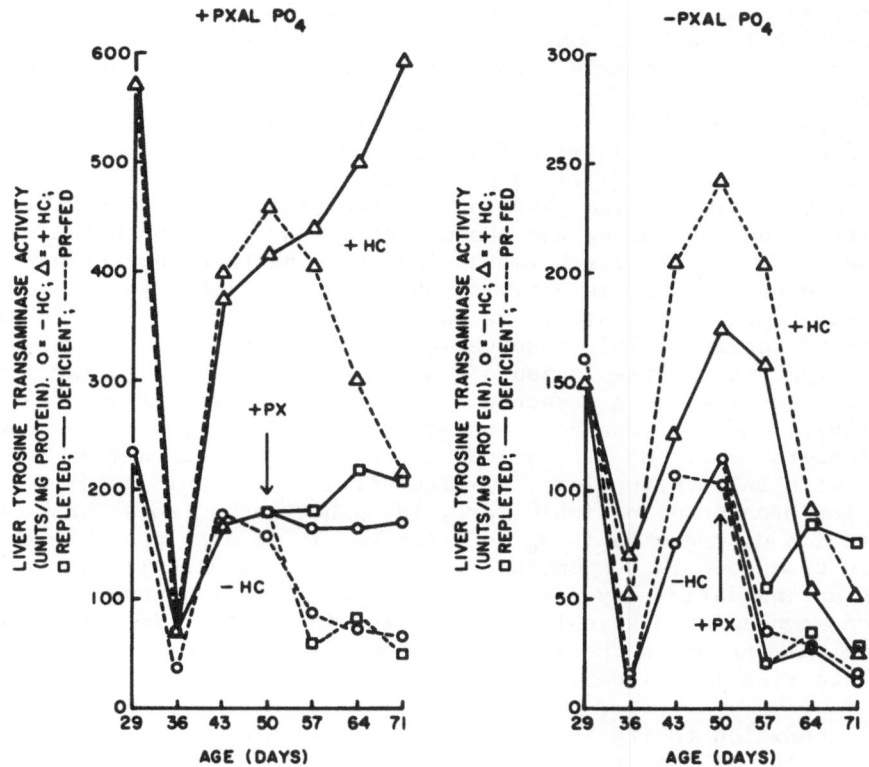

Figure 2a, 2b
     Hepatic TAT activity patterns before and after induction with
hydrocortisone during the post weanling period of animals fed the
vitamin deficient and control diets.   Left side: Figure 2a; Right
2B - Graph shows TAT activities assayed in the absence of coenzyme.
Each point in both figures represents the average from 4 separate
animals (4 separate assays).   Maximal standard deviation observed
was $\pm$ 20 TAT activity units.   The degree of cofactor saturated apoenzyme was arrived at as follows: (Act. in absence of cofactor/Act.
in presence of cofactor).

was found to be saturated with the coenzyme in pair-fed control
and repleted animals. In animals fed with vitamin B_6 deficient
diet the saturated enzyme level varied with progressive age and
degree of deficiency. The absence of dietary cofactor supply to
the animals resulted in continuously increasing levels of apoamino-
transferase protein in both hormonally induced and uninduced animals
(Figure 2a,2b). A high content of pyridoxal 5'-PO_4 was found in
weanling, pair-fed animals (6.5 μgm/gm liver) which decreased steadily reaching a constant level ($\approx$ 3 μgm/gm) after two weeks (43 days
old) on the diet. While repleted animals showed a similar pattern
the cofactor level of animals fed the PX depleted diet continued to
decrease till sacrifice (71 days of age) reaching a low level of less
than 1 μgm/gm liver. The results show the profound effects on TAT
activity brought about by the absence of dietary PX. Both the uninduced TAT level and its hormonal induction pattern were effected
(31). The peak in enzyme activity observed at 43-50 days of age in
pair-fed and repleted animals is only maintained in the absence of
dietary pyridoxine. This observation demonstrates the involvement of
the coenzyme in the regulation of TAT apoprotein levels in rat liver.
A similar conclusion was reached earlier and with male Wistar strain
rats (39). The maintenance of unreduced TAT activity could be due to
many factors, e.g. (a) alterations in the activity of enzymes concerned with TAT destruction; (b) alteration in TAT half-life; (c) removal (or breakdown) of inhibitors; (d) other mechanism(s) brought
into action during vitamin B_6 deficiency. It is also possible that
protein breakdown is responsible for the observed high TAT activity
levels during deficiency. Blood and liver amino acid levels were increased when animals were fed a high protein diet lacking PX (62).
Further, elevation in the level of amino acids has been reported to
stimulate rise in TAT activity (63, 64).

In addition to its involvement in the regulation of hepatic TAT
activity, lack of dietary pyridoxine effected a dramatic alteration in
the pattern of the hormonal induction of the enzyme. In pair-fed
animals, the observed maximal rise in TAT specific activity above the
uninduced level (i.e., at 50 days of age) was practically the same as
that seen in animals fed the deficient diet. Continued absence of
dietary pyridoxine resulted in further rise in TAT specific activity.
Whether the observed effects of cofactor deficiency on TAT activity
levels in vivo and on the hormonal enzyme induction pattern are direct
or are brought about via the mediation of other factors is not known.
It is well known that estrogen administration results in abnormal
tryptophan metabolism which is similar to that seen in the vitamin B_6
deficient state and which can be corrected by pyridoxine (65). It
has also been reported (66) that estrogen stimulates an increase in
the activity of certain enzymes including TAT. It is possible that
the maintenance of high TAT levels and the increased sustained TAT response to steroid stimulation seen during progressive vitamin B_6 depletion of female Buffalo rats reflect, in addition to cofactor ef-

fects, other operative processes mediated through endogenous levels
of sex hormones.

The presence of growing hepatoma No. 7777 drastically alters
the pattern of hormonal TAT induction in both host liver and the
hepatoma itself (15). Further, the effects of cofactor lack on the
induction process, in general, and in the TAT uninduced activity
level were abolished (31). The data show that: (a) pair-fed animals
developed heavier tumors (1.5-2 times), with tumor TAT activity
levels higher (two times) than those of host liver; (b) hormonal TAT
induction patterns in host liver and tumor were similar, with minimal
increase in activity occurring in the latter stages of tumor growth;
and (c) pyridoxal phosphate was depleted in host liver and was accumulated by the tumor during vitamin deficiency (15). Maximal TAT
induction in both host liver and hepatoma occurred when tumor growth
was minimal (1 week; 57 days old rats). As tumor growth increased
enzyme induction was minimized and the uninduced hepatoma TAT level
remained 2x that of the respective host liver (15) and was similar in
magnitude to that seen in normal liver (31). Figures 3 and 4 show
typical results. The presence of the growing hepatoma interfered
drastically with the vitamin and hormone functions seen in normal
animals.

4. Cofactor Effects on TAT Expression

The profound influence of the absence of dietary PX on enzymatic
activity levels in liver and hepatomas and on TAT hormonal induction
patterns prompted us to examine TAT expression by resolving the enzyme electrophoretically in polyacrylamide gel. Subsequently, a two
fold approach was utilized: 1) following gel electrophoresis of cytoplasmic high speed supernatants from liver and hepatomas, resolved
proteins on the gel were reacted immunochemically with aminotransferase (TAT)-specific antibody, i.e., anti-TAT, prepared against highly purified TAT (>3,000 fold). Reactive, resolved proteins were immunoprecipitated by imbedding the running gel in a precut trough made
on a glass plate coated with agar (67), and 2) following partial purification and resolution of TAT preparations on acrylamide, enzymatically active protein bands were identified in situ, on the gel, by staining histochemically and using L-tyrosine as substrate (68, 69).
Figure 5 shows the gel scan of the purified TAT preparation which was
used to prepare the antibody (67). This resolution pattern was repeatedly obtained. Figure 6 shows the immunoprecipitation lines developed with TAT-specific antiserum and reacting soluble liver protein
species following their separation by gel electrophoresis. Patterns
of cytosol proteins from pyridoxine deficient and control animals
after induction with hydrocortisone are shown. Five and four precipitation lines were developed by samples derived from the deficient
and control animals, respectively. Figure 7 shows precipitation patterns obtained with soluble Morris hepatoma No. 7777 protein species

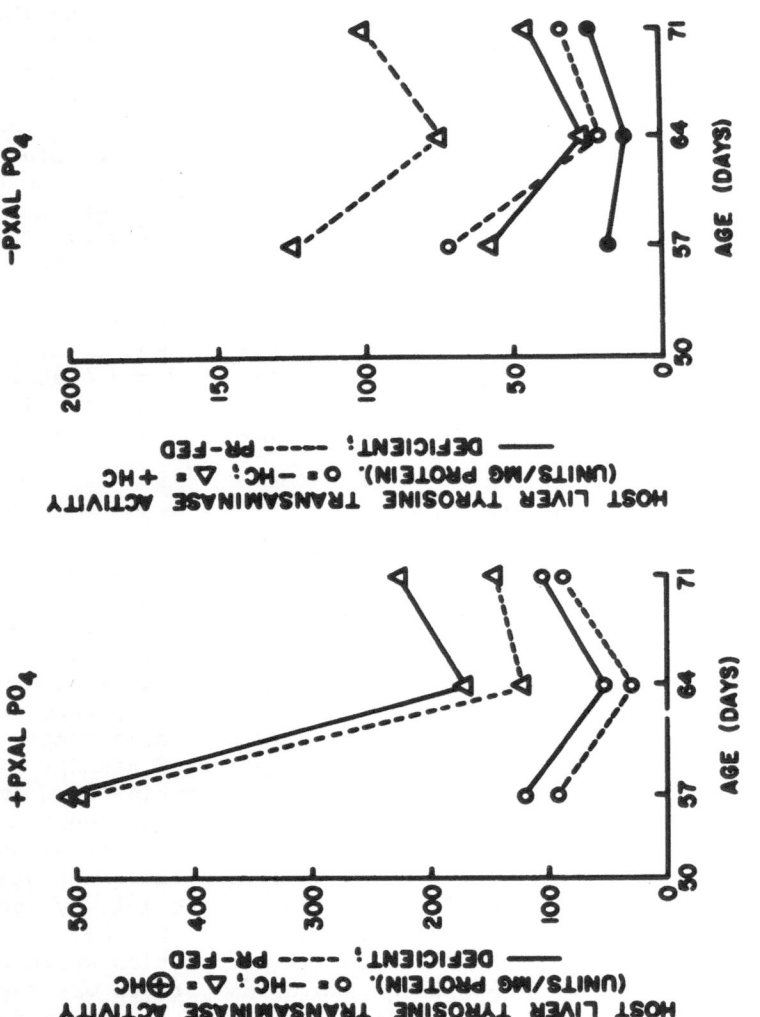

Figure 3

Host liver TAT activity patterns in host liver before and after induction with hydrocortisone
in BUF rats fed the pyridoxine-deficient and control (PR-fed) diets. Graph on right shows TAT
activities assayed in absence of cofactor (PXAL PO$_4$). HC = hydrocortisone. Each point represents
average of 4 determinations (4 animals). Maximum SD was $\pm$ 38 TAT activity units.

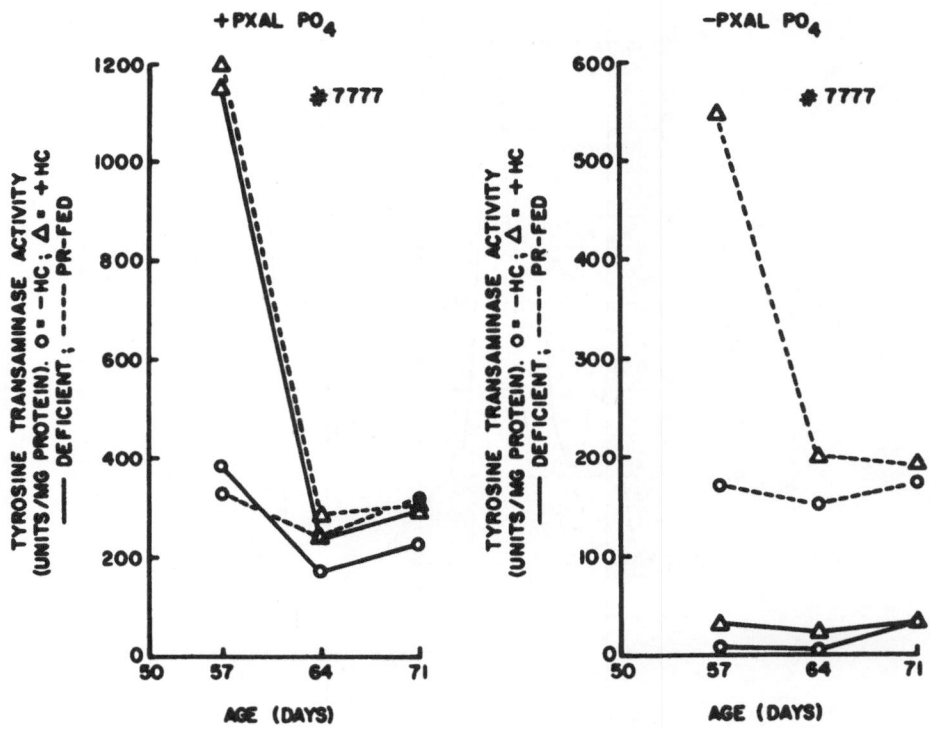

Figure 4

TAT activity patterns of Morris hepatoma No. 7777 before and after
induction with hydrocortisone. Other details as in Figure 3 except
that highest SD was ± 55 TAT activity units, observed after 1 weeks
tumor growth.

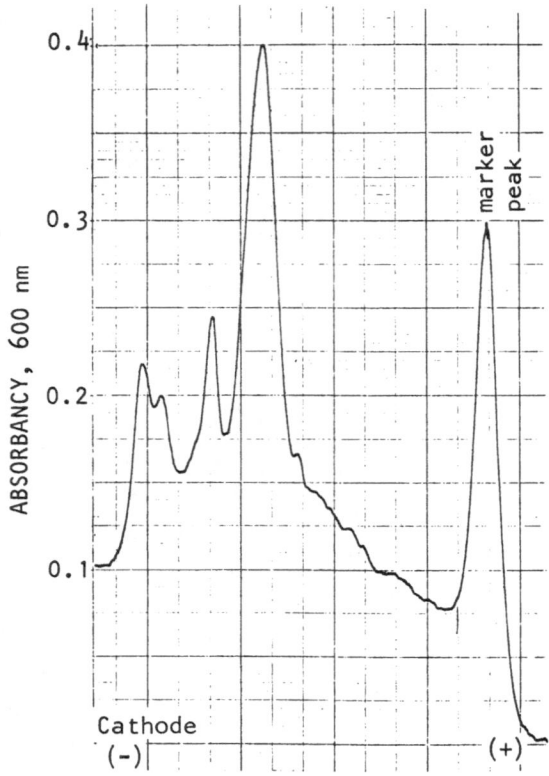

Figure 5
Gel electrophoretic pattern of highly purified soluble rat
liver TAT. Approximately 30 μg protein were electrophoresed. The
pattern was repeated several times.

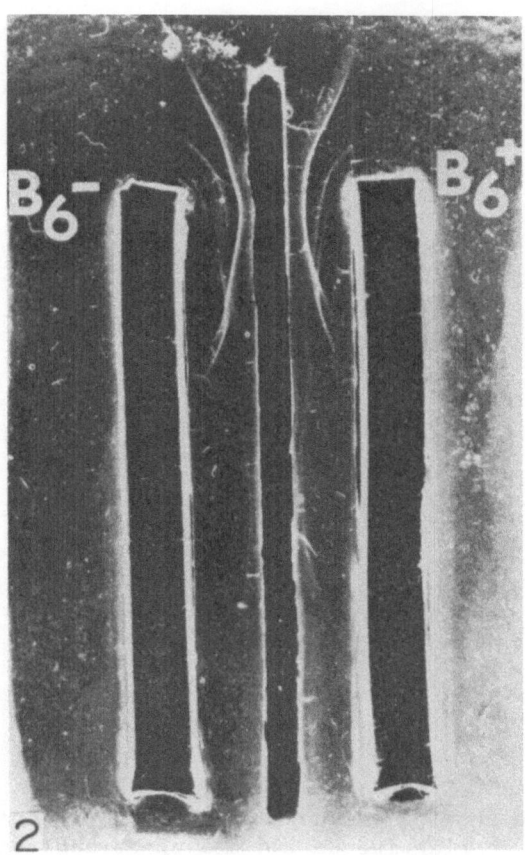

Figure 6
Photograph showing immunoprecipitation patterns developed with tyrosine aminotransferase-specific rabbit antiserum and gel electro-phoresed soluble, racting, liver protein species.

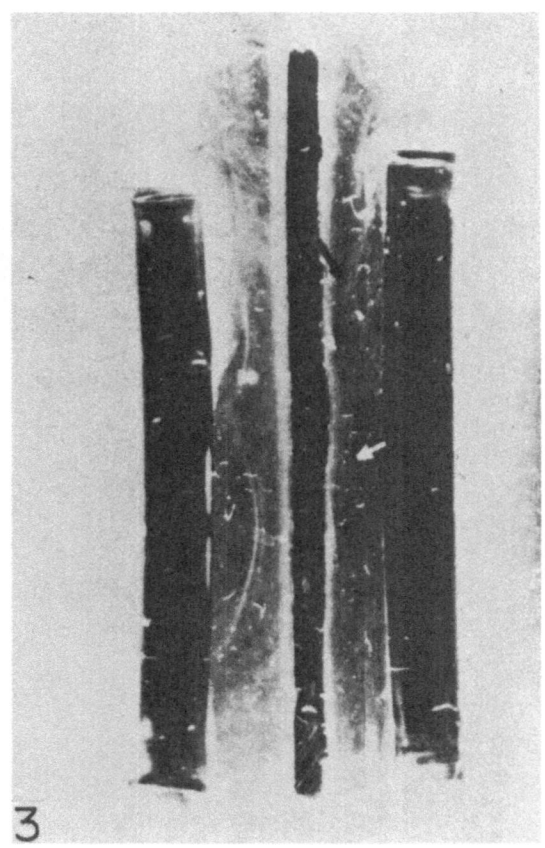

Figure 7
Photograph showing immunoprecipitation patterns developed with
TAT-specific rabbit antiserum and gel electrophoresed soluble, reacting, hepatoma proteins. Patterns on the left and right were
developed by tumors grown in deficient and control animals, respectively.

from pyridoxine deficient and control, hydrocortisone-treated animals. Three and four immunoprecipitation lines were developed by hepatoma samples from vitamin B_6 deficient and control (non-deficient, see arrows) animals, respectively. On the other hand, histochemical staining in situ, on the gel, of partially purified TAT preparations from control animals detected six enzymatically active species. Moreover, cofactor depletion effected further resolution of the enzyme into seven active forms as revealed by the bifurcation of the major active peak. Figures 8 and 9 show these results. Examination of TAT expression after induction with hydrocortisone using the same methodology showed seven active forms in normal liver. The presence of growing hepatomas altered significantly the expression of the enzyme. Only one, two and four activity peaks were detected in the host liver of animals with highly (most liver-like), well and poorly (least liver-like) differentiated hepatomas, respectively. Similarly, only one, four and six peaks were detected, respectively, in highly, well and poorly differentiated hepatomas (69).

The results shown in Fig 6 complement the gel scan of Fig 5. Cofactor depletion resulted in further TAT resolution. All five bands were immunoreactive with the anti-TAT antibody. In the pyridoxine depleted state, additional resolution of TAT was also seen by the histochemical staining method. The number of protein bands detected by this technique, however, was greater. Histochemical staining in situ is not a precise or particularly specific method. Staining may be effected by the presence of different proteins or other agents. Moreover, the method does not differentiate whether the observed bands are indeed TAT. Another aminotransferase could also have transaminated the L-tyrosine. Furthermore, cytoplasmic supernatants from different sources, i.e., liver, hepatoma, may contain different protein species which could interfere with histochemical staining, especially in quantitating enzymatic activity accurately. In spite of the foregoing, however, it should be pointed out that patterns peculiar to the hepatoma lines examined were seen using the histochemical method (69). In all instances, all samples were treated similarly to the last detail. The results with hepatomas were as follows:

(a) different hepatoma lines affect enzyme expression in host liver differently;

(b) enzyme expression varies in the different hepatoma lines;

(c) enzyme expression is facilitated (increased) in both host liver and hepatoma as the differentiation of hepatomas becomes less liver-like (69).

The results of an early study (70) suggested that TAT may exist

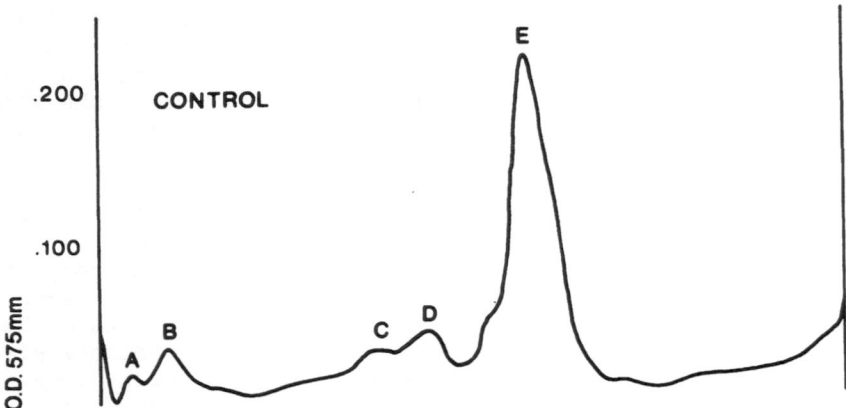

Figure 8
Polyacrylamide gel electrophoresis of partially purified hepatic
tyrosine aminotransferase from control animals. Each gel was loaded
with an amount of protein having 25 enzyme units. After electrophoresis enzyme activity was located histochemically and gel scans were
taken. The specific activity prior to purification (105,000 g; 1 h;
4°C) was 168 units/mg proteins. After the heat step, the specific
activity was 822 units/mg protein. The yield was 100%. For other
details (68).

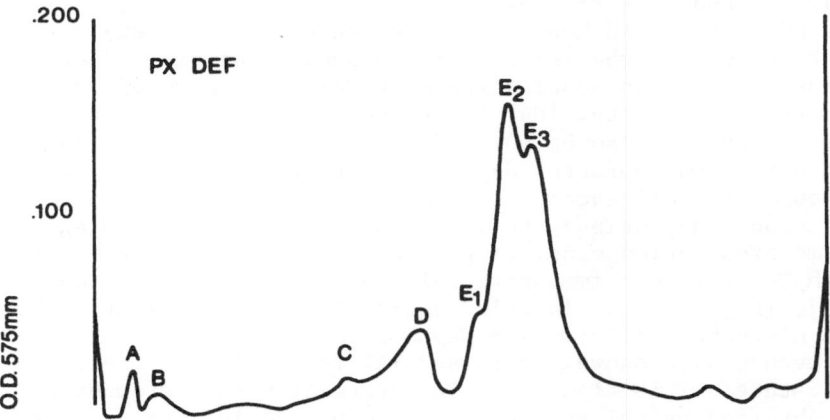

Figure 9

Polyacrylamide gel electrophoresis of partially purified tyrosine
aminotransferase from pyridoxine-deficient animals. All information
in figure 8 is also applicable in this figure except that pyridoxine-
deficient animals were used. The specific activity prior to purification (105,000 g; 1 h; 4°C) was 200 units/mg protein. After the
heat step, the specific activity was 980 units/mg protein. The
yield was 100%.

in multiple forms since several activity peaks were eluted upon
chromatographing on hydroxyapetite. Later, other studies (71-83)
showed that (a) the enzyme consisted of at least three or four
forms; (b) the proportion of each form can be affected by various
hormones or changes in the diet; (c) the forms are interconvertible
and may be due to post-translational modification, and (d) at least
one of the forms is in all likelihood another enzyme, probably aspartate aminotransferase. It has also been reported that the proportion of each enzyme form could be varied depending on the pH of
the medium during homogenization (84). More recently, a particulate
liver fraction component has been described which can interconvert
the TAT multiple forms and whose catalytic action is pH dependent
(85, 86). In contrast to other studies (73, 78, 79, 81), evidence
has been presented with hepatoma tissue culture cells (80) or rat
liver (82) that only the TAT form is induced by different hormones.
It is possible that hormonal effects on TAT forms may reflect effects on the liver factor (84, 85) responsible for their interconversion. It should also be pointed out that the increased TAT resolution during the cofactor depleted state (Figs 5, 6) may also reflect a cofactor influence on the same liver factor (84, 85).
Further, since the antibody to TAT (anti-TAT) was prepared against
the enzyme preparation consisting of all forms, it is not surprising
that each TAT form was immunoprecipitated after resolution on polyacrylamide (Figs 6, 7). In this regard, it should be stated that,
although histochemical staining may not be absolute, results obtained
by this method also showed increased TAT resolution in the PX-
depleted state. This finding is in agreement with aforementioned
results obtained by gel resolution - immuno precipitation. Our observations indicate that PX depletion and/or presence of growing hepatoma drastically effected both TAT hormonal induction and TAT multiple form expression in liver and the hepatoma itself. Cofactor effects on gene product expression presumably reflect cofactor-mediated
post-translational processes. To our knowledge evidence to the contrary has not been reported.

5. PX Depletion and Vitamin B_6 Metabolism

      Our observations regarding the effects of PX depletion are,
briefly, summarized below. Lack of dietary PX results in (a) inhibition of the growth of hepatomas; (b) alterations in enzymatic
activity levels; (c) alterations in enzyme expression; (d) increased
resolution of TAT; (e) facilitation of TAT inducibility by hydrocortisone; (f) alteration in the TAT induction pattern, and (g) increased pyridoxal 5'-PO_4 concentration by hepatoma cells even at the
face of depletion. Table 4 illustrates the last point (15). These
observations suggested to us that aberrations in vitamin B_6 metabolism in the depleted state may be related to enzyme inducibility and/
or expression and to the inhibition of tumor growth. Since these
processes are indeed influenced by cofactor presence or absence, any

Table Four
Pyridoxal 5'-PO$_4$ Content of Host Liver and Morris Hepatoma
No. 7777 in Pyridoxine Depleted and Pair-fed Buffalo
Rats

Group	ug Pyridoxal Phosphate/g Tissue[a]	
	Host Liver	Hepatoma #7777
Pyridoxine-Depleted, (ad lib).	1.47 ± 0.5	6.90 ± 2.0
Pyridoxine Supplemented, (pair-fed)	10.30 ± 2.3	9.35 ± 1.9

[a] In each case, the pyridoxal phosphate values from eight samples (i.e., eight host liver or eight tumors) were averaged; values are averages ± SD. Tumors were grown for two weeks.

aberration(s) in cofactor synthesis (function or utilization) would conceivably affect such processes.

The metabolic interconversions of tritiated pyridoxine in liver, carcass and brain have been studied by different laboratories (87-94). The results of time-course tests relating the appearance of labeled vitamin B$_6$ compounds following the injection of labeled pyridoxine to mice or rats showed the label to proceed mainly as follows: Pyridoxine* → Pyridoxine* 5'-P → Pyridoxal* 5'-P → Pyridoxamine* 5'-P. This ordered series of steps occurs at a slower rate in carcass (88). In this regard, it should be mentioned that the liver has been reported to be the principal, if not sole, organ responsible for the formation of plasma pyridoxal phosphate which is found principally bound to albumin (95, 96). The effects of vitamin B$_6$ depletion on the metabolic transformations of tritiated pyridoxine were studied in our laboratory (97). Although differences in pyridoxine metabolism were not observed with control animals (88, 89, 93, 94), pyridoxine metabolism affected significantly its own metabolism in rat liver. Liver cells incorporated significantly more labeled PX in the depleted state which was retained throughout the experimental period studied (97). Figure 10 shows the metabolic interconversions of tritiated pyridoxine in the liver of deficient animals. Lack of dietary pyridoxine caused rapid disappearance (conversion) of labeled

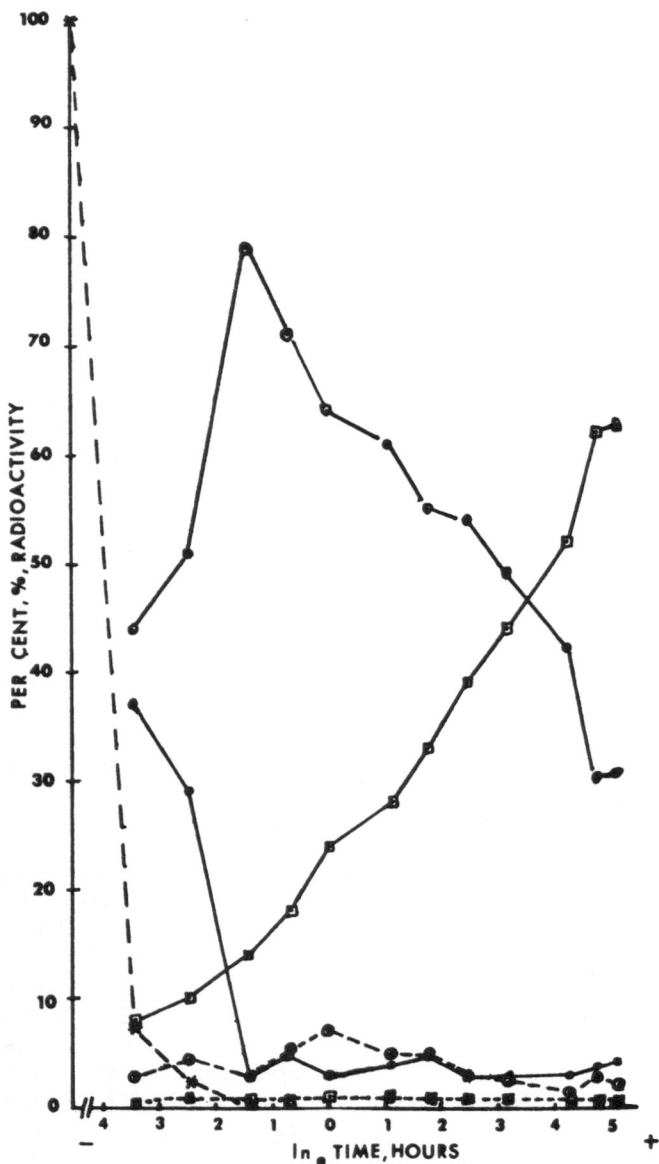

Figure 10

pyridoxine, rapid synthesis of pyridoxine 5'-P and practically
simultaneous synthesis of pyridoxal 5'-P. Synthesis of these two
phosphorylated vitamin derivatives was so fast that by 2 min pyridoxal 5'-P had reached a level of 44%, pyridoxine 5'-P dropped to a
minimal steady level (3%) by 15 min while, on the other hand, pyridoxal 5'-P rose proportionally at this time to a high of 79%. It
then began to drop in a linear fashion,reaching a constant level of
29% by 5 days. Synthesis of pyridoxamine 5'-P began early (8% at 2
min) increasing continually and practically in proportion to the rate
of disappearance of pyridoxal 5'-P. Some pyridoxal was also synthesized reaching a high level of 8% at 60 min and decreasing thereafter to low levels. Lack of dietary pyridoxine effected an accumulation and retention of pyridoxamine 5'-P which was not further metabolized.

The metabolic interconversions of tritiated pyridoxine in the
state of vitamin B$_6$ deficiency may be better understood in terms of
the following scheme (94, 98, 99):

Pyridoxine $\xrightarrow{1}$ pyridoxine 5'-P $\xrightarrow{2}$ pyridoxal 5'-P $\underset{4}{\overset{3}{\rightleftarrows}}$ pyridoxamine 5'-P

$$\downarrow 5$$

pyridoxal

The data presented demonstrate that synthesis of pyridoxal 5'-P
(reaction 2) from pyridoxine 5'-P via reaction 1 is of prime importance to the deficient animal. Both reactions 1 and 2 are very fast.
Reaction 3 (pyridoxamine 5'-phosphate oxidase) does not appear to occur in the deficient state (Fig 10), at least during the experimental

---

Figure 10

Metabolic interconversions of [6-^{3}H]-PX in the liver of vitamin
B$_6$-deficient Buffalo rats: Time-course of distribution of specific
radioactivity. Vitamin B$_6$ compounds were extracted from liver at
the indicated time intervals and chromatographically separated on
Dowex-[H$^+$] columns. Percent radioactivity of each separated peak
(compound) was calculated from the total cpm under the peak (fractions comprising each peak were pooled) and the total radioactivity
chromatographed. Recoveries of 97-99% were routinely obtained.
Samples of 10 ml were chromatographed. Symbols: x - - - -x, [^{3}H]
pyridoxine; ●——●, [^{3}H] pyridoxine 5'-P; ⊙————⊙ , [^{3}H] pyridoxal 5'-P; ⊡————⊡, [^{3}H] pyridoxamine 5'-P; ⊙ - - - - - -⊙, [^{3}H]
pyridoxal; ⊡------⊡,[^{3}H] pyridoxamine.

period studied. Conversion of pyridoxal 5'-P to pyridoxamine 5'-P
(reaction 4) occurs in practically linear fashion following maximal
(80%) synthesis of the former (Fig 10). An equilibrium between
these two vitamin B_6 forms was reached after 5 days with pyridoxamine
5'-P predominating in a ratio of 2:1.

Formation of pyridoxamine 5'-P presumably occurs via reaction
4 or by the reversability of reaction 3 which has yet to be demonstrated in vivo (94, 98, 99). The data strongly suggest that the
equilibrium of reaction 4 is well to the right, i.e. to the synthesis
of pyridoxamine 5'-P (fig 10). This reaction is known to occur with
the bound coenzymes during enzymatic transamination (100, 101). In
the state of vitamin B_6 deficiency the levels of L-amino acids in
blood and liver are increased while liver keto acid levels remain the
same (62, 102). Due to unbalanced metabolism in the direction of
amino acid catabolism the emergence of an acute need for increased
transamination is very likely. Increased transamination could conceivably occur with or without increased apoenzyme levels. Because
dietary pyridoxine is not supplied, the animal must regenerate pyridoxal 5'-P as rapidly as (enzyme bound) pyridoxamine 5'-P is formed
during enzymatic transamination that the process could continue. It
is possible that the regeneration of pyridoxal 5'-P from enzymatically bound pyridoxamine 5'-P is not as rapid. In that case, a higher
level of the latter coenzyme would be expected upon extraction of the
vitamin phosphorylated forms (both 'bound plus free') from liver homogenates (103, 104). The slow regeneration (or lack there-of) of pyridoxal 5'-P from (enzymatically bound) pyridoxamine 5'-P could be
causatively related with the observed inhibition of tumor growth in
the absence of dietary pyridoxine.

Results presented in Table 4 are not in disagreement with the
above statement. PXL5P content shown includes both "free plus bound"
coenzyme forms, i.e., total content. It is very probable that the
utilization of PXL5P by the hepatoma cells grown in Buffalo rats in
the absence of dietary PX is impaired. Moreover, impairment could involve vitamin binding. For the hepatoma cells to grow as well as in
the case when dietary PX is available enzymatic function should be
normal. Although the PXL5P content of hepatoma cells seen in the PX
depleted state may be high it is possible that only a fraction may be
utilizable by these cells in this state. That fraction should be regenerated from (enzymatically) bound PM5P. Otherwise, enzymes requiring the coenzyme for catalysis would be nonfunctional (inactive)
having PM5P bound to them. Cofactor regeneration is necessary to free
the enzymes from bound PM5P. It is, therefore, suggested that in the
case of this hepatoma the high PXL5P content seen in the depleted
state (Table 4) may be the result of (a) impaired enzyme-binding
(i.e., lack of binding; would result in 'free' PXL5P); (b) binding to
proteins other than enzymes (would result in 'bound' PXL5P but nonfunctional), and (c) enzyme binding, and, for reasons not known, non-

functional.

In other tests with hepatoma-bearing animals fed the PX supplemented diet high PXL5P and PM5P amounts were synthesized and retained by the host liver. In contrast, hepatoma cells synthesized a high amount of PM5P which was not retained but was dephosphorylated (105). This finding is in agreement with other results showing synthesis and retention of PM5P in the liver of depleted animals without hepatomas (97). PM5P was not retained but dephosphorylated to PM by hepatomas grown in the presence of dietary PX. Average hepatoma weight in this instance was 2x that of hepatomas grown in depleted animals. These results show that normal hepatoma growth (presence of dietary PX) is accompanied by nonretention of PM5P by the tumor. It would be interesting to learn whether PM5P dephosphorylation occurs also in hepatomas grown in PX depleted animals.

In attempts to decipher the mode of action of vitamin B_6 in the development of immune processes Axelrod et al. conducted several studies. Results of these have been reviewed (106, 107). Their observations were integrated into the conclusion that lack of vitamin B_6 impairs nucleic acid synthesis with consequent deleterious influence on protein production, cell division and/or repair. And moreover, that impairment in nucleic acid synthesis is due to the decreased production of C_1 fragments from serine which are needed for the biosynthesis of DNA and RNA. Serine hydroxymethyltransferase - a pyridoxal 5'-PO₄ requiring enzyme - catalyzes the transfer of the β - carbon of serine to tetrahydrofolate, the latter reaction product needed for deoxythymidylate synthesis. In this regard, it should be noted that Littman et al. (108) reported that the growth of sarcoma 180 was inhibited 50% in the absence of dietary pyridoxine. Furthermore, the vitamin stimulated the growth of this tumor, shortened the survival time of the mice, and further prevented the increase in the survival time of mice bearing this tumor that were treated with 5-fluorouacil. The latter inhibitor of DNA synthesis after conversion to 5-fluorodeoxyuridylic acid binds covalently to thymidylate synthetase thus immobilizing it (109). These observations suggest that our findings of hepatoma growth inhibition, altered expression of gene product and altered enzyme induction seen in the PX depleted state could also be directly related to aberrant nucleic acid and/or protein biosyntheses.

Studies in our laboratory and related literature reports regarding the effects of pyridoxine depletion (cofactor depletion) on the growth of Morris transplantable hepatomas, enzyme activity, expression and inducibility as well as on pyridoxine metabolism in liver and hepatomas were reviewed. In spite of the many and varied effects brought about by cofactor depletion it is felt that limiting dietary PX availability would be beneficial in efforts aimed at controlling tumor growth, particularly in cases of rapidly growing solid tumors. Effects, therapeutically favorable, would very likely result via a combination of antifolate therapy with (limited PX intake). To our knowledge such an approach has not been reported. Further, in spite of the lack of relatively nontoxic potent vitamin B_6 antimetabolites (110), it is felt that certain presently available such agents could effectively be employed provided methodological changes in treatment are concurrently made. In this regard, results of preliminary studies in this laboratory are much encouraging.

ACKNOWLEDGEMENTS

I would like to express sincere thanks to the following individuals for technical assistance, discussion and encouragement rendered during the course of these studies: Dr. Frank L, Saus, Mr. John K. Shuler, Nicholas (Hement) Senapati, M.D., Mr. Larry Larson, Mr. Thomas Puskar.

I especially owe deep appreciation and sincere thanks to Dr. Harold P. Morris who has continuously helped me with the hepatoma strains, editing, discussion and moral support throughout the course of these studies.

[1] Supported by General Reserach Support Award 5S01 RR05433-12(21) from the School of Medicine, by Research Award No. 2-210-1615(76) from the West Virginia University Medical Corporation and in part by USPHS grants CA13759 and CA10729.

[2] Abbreviations: [6-^{3}H]pyridoxine, 3-hydroxy-4,5-bis(hydroxymethyl)-2-methylpyridine; Pyridoxine, (PX); Pyridoxine 5'-phosphate, (PX5P); Pyridoxal, (PXL); Pyridoxal 5'-phosphate, (PXL5P); Tyrosine Aminotransferase (L-tyrosine:2-oxoglutarate aminotransferase, EC2.6.1.5) (TAT); Serine Dehydratase (L-serine hyrdo-lyase,deaminating EC4.2.1.13) (SD). TAT = tyrosine aminotransferase = tyrosine transaminase.

REFERENCES

1. Bischoff, F., Ingraham, L.P.and Rupp, J.J. Arch. Pathol. 35 (1943) 713.

2. Kline, B.E., Rusch, H.P., Baumann, C.A. and Lavik, P.S. Cancer Res. 3 (1943) 825.

3. Stoerk, H.C. J. Biol. Chem. 171 (1957) 437.

4. Mihich, E. and Nichol, C.A. Cancer Res. 19 (1959) 279.

5. Mihich, E., Rosen, F. and Nichol, C.A. Cancer Res. 19 (1959) 1244.

6. Ott, W.H. Proc. Soc. Exptl. Biol. Med. 61 (1946) 125.

7. Gellhorn, A. and Jones, L.O. Blood, 4 (1949) 60.

8. Weir, D.R. and Morningstar, W.A. Blood, 9 (1954) 173.

9. Shapiro, D.M. and Gellhorn, A. Cancer Res. 11 (1951) 35.

10. Shapiro, D.M., Shils, M.E. and Dietrich, L.S. Cancer Res. 13 (1953) 703.

11. Dietrich, L.S. and Shapiro, D.M. Proc. Soc. Exptl. Biol. Med. 84 (1953) 555.

12. Skipper, H.E., Thomson, J.R. and Schabel, F.M. Cancer Chemoth. Rep. 29 (1963) 63.

13. Tryfiates, G.P., Shuler, J.K., Hefner, M.H. and Morris, H.P. Eur. J. Cancer 10 (1974) 147.

14. Tryfiates, G.P. and Morris, H.P. J. Natl. Cancer Inst. 52 (1964) 1259.

15. Tryfiates, G.P., Saus, F.L. and Morris, H.P. J. Natl. Cancer Inst. 55 (1975) 839.

16. Tryfiates, G.P. and Morris, H.P. Eur. J. Cancer 12 (1976) 9.

17. Tryfiates, G.P. Oncology, in press.

18. Bollag, W. Chemotherapy 21 (1975) 236.

19. Gailani, S., Murphy, G., Kenny, G., Nussbaum, A. and Silvernail, P. Cancer Res. 33 (1973) 1071.

20. Rivlin, R.S. Cancer Res. 33 (1973) 1977.

21. Pamukcu, A.M., Yalciner, S., Price, J.M. and Bryon, G.F. Cancer Res. 30 (1970) 2671.

22. Raineri, R. and Weisburger, J.H. Ann. N.Y. Acad. Sci. 258 (1975) 181.

23. Schlegel, J.U. Ann. N.Y. Acad. Sci. 258 (1975) 432.

24. Rubin, D. and Levy, I.S. Pathol. Microbiol. 39 (1973) 446.

25. Han, J.R., Exon, J.H., Westwig, P.H. and Shanger, P.D. Clin. Toxicol. 6 (1973) 487.

26. Black, H.S. and Chan, J.T. J. Invest. Dermat. 65 (1975) 412.

27. Greenstein, J.P. In: Biochemistry of Cancer, Academic Press, New York (1954) 239.

28. Cancer Research 35 (No. 11), Part 2, Nov (1975).

29. Lasnitzki, I. and Goodman, D.S. Cancer Res. 34 (1971) 1564.

30. Ito, K., Nakahara, I. and Sakamoto, Y. Gann 55 (1964) 373.

31. Tryfiates, G.P. and Saus, F.L. Cancer Biochem. Biophys. 1 (1975) 63.

32. Puskar, T. and Tryfiates, G.P. J. Nut. 104 (1974) 1407.

33. Kuchinskas, E.J., Horvath, A. and duVigneaud, V. Arch. Biochem. Biophys. 68 (1957) 69.

34. Rosen, F. and Nichol, C.A. Adv. Enz. Reg. 2 (1964) 115.

35. Okada, M. and Ochi, A. Japanese J. Biochem. 70 (1967) 581.

36. Takami, M., Fujioka, M., Wada, H. and Taguchi, T. Proc. Soc. Exptl. Biol. Med. 129 (1968) 110.

37. Brin, M. and Thiele, V.F. J. Nut. 93 (1967) 213.

38. Milholland, R.J., Rosen, R. and Nichol, C.A. Ann. N.Y. Acad. Sci. 166 (1969) 126.

39. Tryfiates, G.P. Life Sciences 10 (1971) 1147.

40. Lin, E.C.C., Civen, M. and Knox, W.E. J. Biol. Chem. 233 (1958)

1183.

41. Greengard, O. Adv. Enz. Regulation 2 (1964) 277.

42. Bliss, C.I. and Gyorgy, P. In: Vitamin Methods, P. Gyorgy (ed). Academic Press, New York (1951) 214.

43. Tryfiates, G.P., Shuler, J.K. and Morris, H.P. Proc. Soc. Expt. Biol. Med. 145 (1964) 1363.

44. Yuwiler, A., Geller, E. and Eiduson, S. Biochim. Biophys. Acta 244 (1971) 557.

45. Greengard, O. and Gordon, M. J. Biol. Chem. 238 (1963) 3708.

46. Holten, D., Wicks, W.D. and Kenney, F.T. J. Biol. Chem. 242 (1967) 1053.

47. Katunuma, N. Curr. Top. Cell Reg. 7 (1973) 175.

48. Katunuma, N., Kominami, E. and Kominami, S. Biochem. Biophys. Res. Comm. 45 (1971) 70.

49. Pitot, H.C. and Morris, H.P. Cancer Res. 21 (1961) 1009.

50. Potter, V.R. In: The Molecular Basis of Neoplasia, University of Texas Press, M.D. Anderson Hospital and Tumor Institute, Austin, Texas (1961) 367.

51. Pitot, H.C. In: Symposium on Regulation of Enzyme Activity and Synthesis in Normal and Neoplastic Liver, G. Weber (ed). Pergamon Press, New York (1963) 309.

52. Pitot, H.C. Cancer Res. 23 (1963) 1474.

53. Pitot, H.C., Peraino, C., Morse, P.A. and Potter, V.R. In: Metabolic Control in Animal Cells, Natl. Cancer Inst. Monog. No. 13, USDH W.J. Rutter (ed),(1964) 229.

54. Potter, V.R., Gebert, R.A., Pitot, H.C., Peraino, C., Lamar, C. Jr., Lesher, S. and Morris, H.P. Cancer Res. 26 (1966) 1547.

55. Baril, E.F. and Potter, V.R. J. Nut. 95 (1968) 228.

56. Watanabe, M., Potter, V.R. and Pito, H.C. J. Nutr. 95 (1968) 107.

57. Potter, V.R., Watanabe, M., Pitot, H.C. and Morris, H.P. Cancer Res. 29 (1969) 55.

58. Watanabe, M., Potter, V.R. Reynolds, R.D., Pitot, H.C. and Morris, H.P. Cancer Res. 29 (1969) 1691.

59. Watanabe, M., Potter, V.R, Pitot, H.C. and Morris, H.P. Cancer Res. 29 (1969) 2085.

60. Wurtman, R.J. and Axelrod, J. Proc. Natl. Acad. Sci. U.S.A. 57 (1967) 1594.

61. Tryfiates, G.P. J. Natl. Cancer Inst. 54 (1975) 171.

62. Okada, M. and Suzuki, K. J. Nut. 104 (1974) 287.

63. Rosen, F. and Milholland, R.J. J. Biol. Chem. 243 (1968) 1900.

64. Rosen, F. and Milholland, R.J. In: Enzyme Synthesis and Degradation in Mammalian Systems, M. Rechcigl (ed). Univ. Park Press, Baltimore (1971) 77.

65. Rose, D.P., Strong, R., Adams, P.W. and Harding, P.E. Clin. Sci. 42 (1972) 465.

66. Braidman, I.P. and Rose, D.P. Endocrinology 89 (1971) 1250.

67. Tryfiates, G.P. and Saus, F.L. Eur. J. Cancer 12 (1976) 833.

68. Shuler, J.K. and Tryfiates, G.P. Enzyme, in press.

69. Shuler, J.K. and Tryfiates, G.P. Oncology, in press.

70. Kenney, F.T. J. Biol. Chem. 237 (1962) 1605.

71. Hayashi, S., Granner, D.K. and Tomkins, G.M. J. Biol. Chem. 244 (1967) 3998.

72. Valeriote, F.A., Auricchio, F., Tomkins, G.M. and Riley, W.D. J. Biol. Chem. 244 (1969) 3618.

73. Holt, P.G. and Oliver, I.T. FEBS Letters 5 (1969) 89.

74. Tryfiates, G.P. Biochim. Biophys. Acta 169 (1969) 779.

75. Auricchio, F., Valeriote, F.A., Tomkins, G.M. and Riley, W.D. Biochim. Biophys. Acta 221 (1970) 307.

76. Blake, R.L. and Broner, C. Biochim. Biophys. Res. Comm. 41 (1970) 1443.

77. Sadleir, J.W., Holt, P.G. and Oliver, I.T. FEBS Letters 6 (1970) 46.

78. Iwasaki, Y. and Pitot, H.C. Life Sciences 10 (1971) 1071.

79. Pitot, H.C. et al. Gann 13 (1972) 191.

80. Galehrter, T.D., Emannuel, J.R. and Spencer, C.H. J. Biol. Chem. 247 (1972) 6197.

81. Iwasaki, Y., Lamar, C., Danenberg, K. and Pitot, H.C. Eur. J. Biochem. 34 (1973) 347.

82. Johnson, R.W., Roberson, L.E. and Kenney, F.T. J. Biol. Chem. 248 (1973) 4521.

83. Spencer, C.J. and Gelehtrer, T.D. J. Biol. Chem. 249 (1974) 577.

84. Johnson, R.W. and Grossman, A. Biochem. Biophys. Res. Comm. 59 (1974) 520.

85. Smith, G.J., Pearce, P.H. and Oliver, I.T. Life Sciences 16 (1975) 437.

86. Rodriguez, J.M. and Pitot, H.C. Biochem. Biophys. Res. Comm. 65 (1975) 510.

87. Johansson, D., Lindstedt, S. and Register, U. Am. J. Phys. 210 (1966) 1086.

88. Johansson, S., Lindstedt, S. and Tiselius, H.G. Biochem. 7 (1968) 2327.

89. Colombini, C.E. and McCoy, E.E. Biochem. 9 (1970) 533.

90. Colombini, C.E. and McCoy, E.E. Anal. Biochem. 34 (1970) 451.

91. McCoy, E.E. and Colombini, C. J. Agr. Food Chem. 20 (1972) 494.

92. Tiselius, H.G. Clin. Chim. Acta 40 (1972) 319.

93. Tiselius, H.G. J. Neuroch. 20 (1973) 937.

94. Johansson, S., Lindstedt, S. and Tiselius, H.G. J. Biol. Chem. 249 (1974) 6040.

95. Lumeng, L., Brashear, R.E. and Li, T.K. J. Lab. Clin. Med. 84 (1974) 334.

96. _____ Nutr. Rev. 34 (1976) 40.

97. Tryfiates, G.P. and Saus, F.L. Biochim. Biophys. Acta 451 (1976) 333.

98. Snell, E.E. Vit. Horm. 22 (1964) 485.

99. Wada, H. and Snell, E.E. J. Biol. Chem. 236 (1961) 2089.

100. Jenkins, W.T. and Sizer, I.W. J. Amer. Chem. Soc. 79 (1957) 2655.

101. Snell, E.E. Vit. Horm. 16 (1958) 77.

102. Hawkins, W.W., MacFarland, M.L. and McHenry, E.W. J. Biol. Chem. 166 (1946) 223.

103. Novogrodsky, A. and Meister, A. Biochim. Biophys. Acta 81 (1964) 608.

104. Novogrodsky, A. and Meister, A. J. Biol. Chem. 239 (1964) 879.

105. Tryfiates, G.P., Saus, F.L. and Morris, H.P. manuscript in preparation.

106. Axelrod, A.E. Amer. J. Clin. Nutr. 24 (1971) 265.

107. Axelrod, A.E. and Trakatellis, A.C. Vit. Horm. 22 (1964) 591.

108. Littman, M.L., Taguchi, T. and Shimizu, Y. Proc. Soc. Exptl. Biol. Med. 113 (1963) 667.

109. Kornberg, A. In: DNA Synthesis, W.H. Freeman, San Francisco (1974) 45.

110. Rosen, F., Mihich, E. and Nichol, C.A. Vit. Horm. 22 (1964) 609.

IRON AND COPPER METABOLISM IN CANCER, AS EXEMPLIFIED BY CHANGES IN
FERRITIN AND CERULOPLASMIN IN RATS WITH TRANSPLANTABLE TUMORS

Maria C. Linder

Division of Biochemistry, Department of Chemistry
California State University, Fullerton
Fullerton, California 92634

INTRODUCTION

Iron and copper are crucial to the metabolism of all eukaryotic
cells and are often linked in their functions (17). Both elements
are associated with electron transport and in mammals are required
for the formation of hemoglobin in erythropoisis. Iron and copper
are stored in the liver of the fetus during the first part of gestation for utilization during the first part of life when the diet
(milk) contains little of these elements.

In the adult, normal man and animals, two-thirds of the iron in
the body is in the form of circulating hemoglobin. Thus the first
consequence of iron deficiency is a reduction in red cell number. A
similar anemia may be induced by copper deficiency, and this had been
variously explained on the basis that copper is required (a) for the
pathway of porphyrin biosynthesis (4), (b) is part of red cell proteins, particularly superoxide dismutase (4), and (c) in the form of
ceruloplasmin is necessary for the flux of iron from storage sites to
the marrow for incorporation into hemoglobin (17). Aside from hemoglobin, the other major forms of iron are muscle myoglobin (about 10%)
concerned with oxygen diffusion, and the iron storage protein,
ferritin, which along with its less well-defined partner, hemosiderin,
account for about 20% of body iron in the normal adult (17). In
contrast, iron containing enzymes (mostly heme enzymes) while equally
important contribute less than 1% to the body iron burden.

In the case of copper, a much larger percentage of body content
is associated with enzymes, including the circulating α_2-glycoprotein,
ceruloplasmin, intracellular superoxide dismutase and mitochondrial

643

cytochrome oxidase. Except in the fetus and neonate, copper is not stored to any great extent, and this lack of storage may be related to its relative ease of absorption from the diet and capacity for excretion through the bile. In contrast, the availability of dietary iron is low, averaging 10% as compared with 30% of more for copper, and the ability to excrete iron (also via the bile) is very limited. Indeed, much less than 0.1% of the total in the body enters and leaves daily, whereas about 1% of copper is exchanged (17).

In the face of limited uptake and excretion, the changing needs of the organism for iron are accomodated by a large and adaptive capacity for iron storage, primarily in ferritin. Ferritin is ideally suited for storing iron in that a single molecule may contain up to 5000 atoms of the element. The iron is sequestered as a crystalline ferric salt within a shell of protein subunits, thus rendering it harmless. If iron flows into a cell in increased amounts (as from increased breakdown of red cells), the capacity for iron storage is enhanced through stimulation by iron of ferritin subunit production (3, 15). The concentration of ferritin iron within a cell is therefore a hallmark of its availability for iron-dependent functions, both within the same cell, and generally also for other parts of the body.

When we embarked on a study of iron and ferritin in transplantable rat tumors it was unclear what we would find, both about the need for iron storage in these cells and the relative importance of iron for tumor metabolism. As will be described, our evidence suggests that iron storage and utilization are indeed important aspects of tumor cell metabolism.

Our interest in copper metabolism was aroused by reports that serum copper concentrations were elevated in cancer patients, and also the implication that serum ceruloplasmin was involved in allowing a flow of iron from liver storage sites into the blood (22, 24). We thus extended our studies of iron metabolism in cancer to include studies of copper and ceruloplasmin, with the hope that this would lead to a greater understanding of the functions and interactions of both elements in the disease. As with iron, we found that there are marked changes in the way this element is utilized and changes in the way it is distributed with the organism when cancer is present.

CHARACTERISTICS OF TRANSPLANTABLE USED IN THESE STUDIES

Transplantable rat tumors were selected to provide a range of growth rates and degrees of histological differentiation, as well as cell origins (Table 1). In this regard, the most useful group is the series of hepatomas developed by Dr. Harold P. Morris, who also established a number of differentiated renal tumors (Table 1). Two Dunning mammary tumors, one undifferentiated the other differentiated, were included to serve as a second non-hepatic tissue tumor source. This seemed particularly important in our examination of ceruloplasmin, since hepatocytes are the main source of this circulating plasma protein.

Rate constants for growth and weight doubling times of the tumors (Table 1) were determined by measuring three tumor diameters through the skin at various times after implantation (for subcutaneous tumors) and/or killing groups of rats at different times to obtain tumor weights. As Knox, Friedell and I had shown in earlier work (7), this provides a quantitative means of grading tumor growth which may then be used to assess parameters (such as enzyme activities) potentially associated with the growth process. As may be seen, the tumors used covered more than 10-fold range of tumor doubling times. We also measured the number of cell nuclei per g in order to place other measurements on a "per cell" basis. Bearing in mind that normal rat liver contains close to 2×10^8 nuclei per g (8), it may be deduced that the hepatomas and other tumors all contained cells with a much smaller mean size than hepatocytes (Table 1). Beginning with our studies of ceruloplasmin, we also began recording the hemotacrits of the tumor bearing rats (Table 1). Whereas the hematocrit of normal animals averaged 51%, many, but not all, of the implanted tumors had the effect of reducing red cell number. It has been found that this occurs at least in part through an increase in the fragility (and hemolysis) of the red cells, perhaps from damage during the passage of these cells through the tortuous circulation of the tumor (5). Normally, however, such hemolysis would be compensated for by the increased red cell synthesis, if iron and the other factors needed for production were in adequate supply. Our experience suggests that lack of iron availability is not part of the explanation for decreased hematocrits in tumor bearing rats since even with injection of excess iron a fall in hematocrit may be observed (Linder, unpublished observations).

IRON METABOLISM AND FERRITIN IN TUMORS

Iron and Ferritin Content of Transplantable Tumors in Comparison with Normal Tissues

Table 2 summarizes results obtained for assays of the iron and ferritin contents of rat tumors derived from threee different normal tissues. It is immediately apparent that the total iron content of the tumors varied greatly, not just from one type of tumor to another but even for a given tumor line in different generations. We have found that this is not the case for normal tissues such as liver and kidney. The latter give predictable values depending on the age, sex and diet of the animals (17). For liver tumors iron concentrations tended to be lower than in normal liver, and the same trend was apparent for kidney tumors compared with normal kidney; in the case

Table One

Origin, Growth Rate and Histology of Transplantable Rat Tumors Used in our Studies

Tumor Line	Tissue Origin	Histology Differentiation and Character of Carcinoma	No. of Nuclei (10^8/g)	Growth Rate Rate Constant (b ± Sb)	Doubling Time (days)	Rat Hematocrit
3683F	hepatic	Undifferentiated	3.44 ± 0.19(6)	0.593, 0.200	0.5, 1.5	34 ± 9 (13)
5A	mammary	Undifferentiated	1.72, 1.49 (2)	0.212 ± 0.039	1.4	51 ± 3(4)*
3924A	hepatic	Poorly or Undifferentiated	3.2 ± 0.5(8)	0.069 ± 0.011	4.4	
7777	hepatic	Well differentiated, trabecular	4.9 ± 0.6(12)	0.045 ± 0.005	6.6	42 ± 8(8)
5123tc	hepatic	Well differentiated, trabecular	5.3 ± 0.4(4)	0.043 ± 0.006	7.0	39 ± 9(8)
7A	mammary	Differentiated squamous cell carcinoma	3.6 ± 0.6(9)	0.038, 0.027	8.1-11.1	46 ± 4(15)
7793	hepatic	Well differentiated, trabecular	3.0 ± 0.5(8)	0.031 ± 0.006	9.8	
7800	hepatic	Highly or well differentiated, trabecular	2.16 ± 0.17(6)	0.025, 0.016	12.3, 19.3	53 ± 4(22)
MK-3	renal	Highly or well differentiated, tubular	4.30 ± 0.34(10)	0.012 ± 0.004	24.7	—
MK-1	renal	Highly or well differentiated, tubular	3.0 ± 0.25(3)		>12	—

* decreased with tumors larger than 10 g

Tumors were implanted intramuscularly except for 3683F which was intraperitoneal, and 5A and 7A which were subcutaneous. Histological information was taken from Linder et al.(13) for the hepatomas, Knox et al.(7) for the mammary tumors, and Morris et al.(21) for the renal tumors. Growth rates, based on tumor weights at two times after implantation, are given as the rate constant (b) ± S.E. (Sb) for the regression of log tumor weight against time (in days), or as weight doubling time calculated therefrom. The concentration of nuclei per g on non-necrotic tissue is given as mean ± SD with the number of tumors assayed in paranthesis. Similarly, hematocrit values (mean ± SD) are summarized for rats with tumors weighing 2-8 g. The normal hematocrit of Fischer, ACI and Buffalo rats is 51 ± 3 (53).

Table Two
Iron and Ferritin Contents of Transplantable
Rat Tumors and their Tissues of Origin

| Tissue | Untreated Rats | | | Iron-Treated Rats |
	Total Iron (µg/g)	Heme Iron (µg/g)	Ferritin Iron(µg/g)	Ferritin Iron (µg/g)
Hepatoma 3683F (9)	43	29	9	108*
(3 different (4)	53	24	10	
generations) (7)	103	51	23	
Hepatoma 7800 (5)	268	88	16	60*
Normal Liver, Adult(12)	237	58	121	2150*
Neonatal Liver (13)	305	67	167	351*
Renal Tumor MK-3 (5)	95	16	11	47*
Renal Tumor MK-1 (5)	93	69	15	73*
Normal Kidney, Adult(4)	123	33	19	66*
Mammary tumor 5A(2)	324	31	4	25*
Normal mammary gland (3)	31	1	10	–

Tumors were obtained from female rats when they were 2-6 g in size and the grossly viable fraction was assayed for its total content of iron, for heme iron, and ^{d}for ferritin iron (15). Normal tissues were taken from mature female Fischer rats, or in the case of neonatal liver from newborn animals of both sexes 1-3 days after birth. Mammary gland tissue was taken from the dams of these newborn animals at the same time. Some of the rats were treated with iron by giving 3 injections of iron dextran (20 mg Fe/rat at 2 day intervals) beginning one week before killing. In the case of newborn animals treatment was with 5 mg iron (iron dextran) 48 hours before death. The results are mean values for the number of rats indicated. For the determination, standard deviations were not more than 25% of the mean, and generally less.

* Significant increase over control ($p < 0.001$) due to iron treatment.

of single mammary tumor examined and normal lactating mammary gland
the reverse was found. There was a substantial but again variable
amount of heme iron present in tumor tissue homogenates. This may
be attributed to residual blood within the tissue and is not unexpected, as some tumors are more hemorrhagic than others even when
gross hemorrhage has been trimmed away (as was here the case).

In normal liver about 60% of the non-heme iron present is found
in the form of ferritin, with a somewhat smaller proportion as
ferritin in kidney and mammary gland (Table 2). In the tumors, a
large but variable percentage of the total was not accounted for by
ferritin and hemoglobin. This suggests the presence especially in
tumors of either hemosiderin (probably a degraded form of ferritin)
and/or as yet uncharacterized iron-containing components which may
be important for tumor metabolism. It is tempting to speculate
that the iron-containing, glucose-labeled components of tumor cells
grown in tissue culture and identified by Robbins et al. (26) as
associated with tumor cell proliferation accounts for some, or all,
of the "missing" iron in these cells. However, there was no correlation between the growth rate or histological differentiation of the
various tumors (Table 1) and their content of unidentified iron which
would support this concept.

Table 2 also indicates that administration of iron to rats by
injection (as iron dextran) markedly increased the ferritin iron
content of the tumors, as in the case with normal tissues. The
adaptive capacity of cells to store (and detoxify) iron in ferritin
thus persists in tumor of all kinds and is independent of their
degree of anaplasia or rate of growth. This is illustrated even more
clearly in Fig 1, which displays in quantitative terms the relationship between growth rate (or anaplasia) of hepatomas and their ferritin content, before and after injection of a large dose of iron.
Whereas hepatomas store decreasing amounts of ferritin iron as they
grow faster, there is no diminution in the capacity to store iron in
ferritin if it becomes available, as from injection. This is in line
with other observations (19) that the various hepatomas are able to
absorb about the same amounts of iron when infused intravenously as
$^{59}FeCl_3$.

Fig 1 also shows that whereas in untreated rats the concentration
of ferritin iron in tumors declined with their increasing rate of
growth, the concentration of ferritin protein (as determined immunologically) did not follow suit. Instead, it was quite similar in the
highly differentiated and completely undifferentiated hepatomas. The
ratio of iron to protein (or iron saturation) of the ferritins from
the different hepatomas thus decreased markedly with increasing tumor
growth rate and anaplasia. Indeed, the ratio values correlated inversely, in a linear manner, with the growth rate constants of the
range of hepatomas examined, giving a highly significant correlation

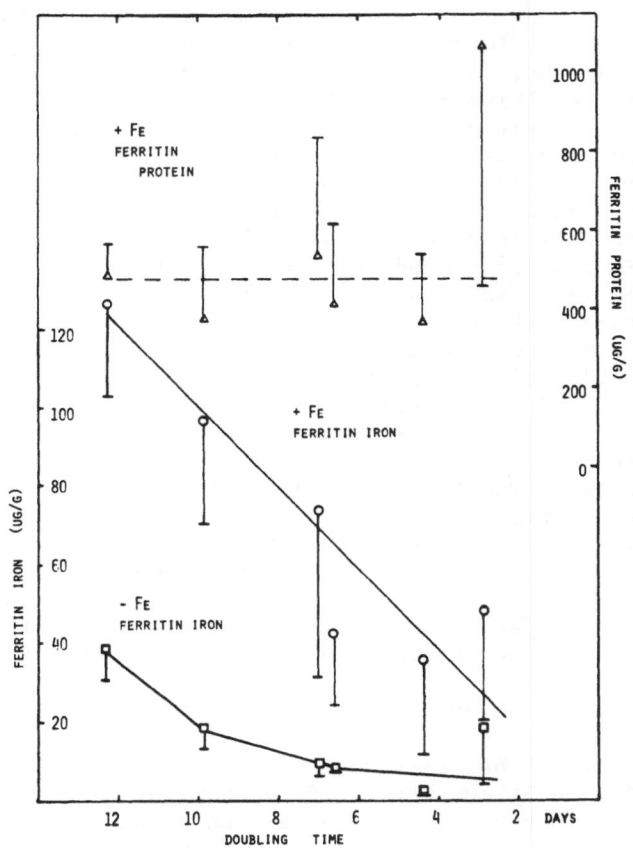

Figure 1
Relation of tumor ferritin content to growth rate. The mean
ferritin iron or ferritin protein content (μg/g) of hepatic tumors
obtained from untreated or iron injected rats, is plotted against
the growth rate (weight doubling time, in days) of individual tumor
lines. The bars represent one standard deviation of the mean, for
groups of 5 rats. From the slowest growing (to the left) to the
fastest growing, the 6 hepatoma lines examined were Morris 7800, 7793,
5123tc, 7777, 3924A, 3683F, and 383F. The data are from Linder et al.
(19).

(= -0.94 to -0.96; 4 D.F., p 0.01) for these parameters (19).
The presence of ferritin with a low iron content is in itself
apparently "abnormal", in that it has been our experience over
many years that normal rat tissues contain ferritin with high iron:
protein ratios (0.25 or more) (16). Several explanations for this
difference between the ferritins of normal and malignant tissues
are possible among them (a) that iron is rapidly utilized by proliferating cells resulting in less iron storage; (b) that the rate
of degradation of ferritin protein does not in the case of the
tumors keep pace with its rate of synthesis, particularly as the
rate of cell division increases; and (c) that the influx of iron
into tumor cells which normally occurs results in an over-stimulation
of ferritin synthesis (as compared with the normal), so that more
ferritin protein than is needed is produced. There is suggestive
evidence for the first and last points. Robbins et al.(26) have
been able to prevent DNA synthesis in HeLa cells by iron deprivation,
implicating iron in the process of cell division. Moreover, we have
found that induction of cell proliferation in normal liver by partial
hepatectomy results in a decrease in the amount of iron stored as
ferritin, and a fall in the ferritin iron:protein ratio from 0.24 to
0.13 (19). With regard to the possibility of over-stimulation of
ferritin synthesis in tumor cells, injection of a large dose of iron
increases the total iron and ferritin iron content of the tumors
Table 2, Fig 1), but the increase in ferritin protein concentration
is in proportion to the increase in ferritin iron, leaving the ratio
of iron:protein in the ferritin almost unchanged (19). The clear
persistence of the capacity for ferritin synthesis with increasing
tumor anaplasia, and the apparent enhanced sensitivity of ferritin
protein synthesis to iron influx would seem to underscore the importance of iron metabolism in cancer cells.

The picture which has emerged from our study of rat tumors is in
large part confirmed by our more limited examination of human neo-
plams (Table 3). Tumors tended to have less total iron than their
corresponding tissues of origin. A large proportion of the total
iron could not be accounted for by known components, such as ferritin
(and heme; not shown). Also, except in the case of the single sample
of stomach examined (consisting in part of rapidly proliferating
normal tissue), the ferritin from normal tissues had a much higher
iron saturation than that of the tumors, again pointing to a link
between iron saturation and cell proliferation. In collaboration
with the New England Deaconess Hospital we are currently examining
more carefully the correlation between these parameters in the human
using graded epidermoid lung carcinomas.

Structure of Ferritins from Normal and Malignant Tissues

Already in the mid-sixties Richter and his group reported that
the ferritins isolated from human or rat tumor cells had a different

Table Three
Iron and Ferritin Contents of Normal
and Malignant Human Tissues

Tissue Origin	Total Iron (μg/g)	Ferritin	
		Ferritin Fe (μg/g)	Ratio Fe: Protein
TUMORS:			
Breast	72	7	0.021
	34	7	0.017
Colon	82	18	0.095
	26	9	0.046
Kidney	17	7	0.080
Lung	50	35	0.065
	64	10	0.034
Rectum	40	11	0.048
Stomach	42	−	0.056
	52	13	0.045
NORMAL TISSUES:			
Kidney	86	13	0.078
Liver	347	98	0.093
Lung	335	61	0.128
Spleen	422	86	0.226
Stomach	119	17	0.066

Frozen samples of human tumors obtained at surgery and normal tissues obtained at autopsy from non-cancer patients were kindly provided by Dr. Ann Crosson at the Department of Pathology, New England Deaconess Hospital, Boston. These were homogenized and assayed for total iron and ferritin by the same procedures used previously for rat tissues. The results shown are for individual samples assayed in duplicate or triplicate.

rate of migration in qualitative gel electrophoresis than ferritins
of normal tissues from the same species (25). We soon were able to
confirm that this was the case for ferritins from a large variety of
rat tumor sources in comparison with normal rat liver ferritin (14,
19), using measurements of migration (R_f) relative to tracking dye
in disc gel electrophoresis. Of additional interest to us, however,
was the observations that normal rat tissues, as exemplified by liver,
kidney, heart and fetal liver, also contained electrophoretically
distinguishable species of ferritin, and that the tumor ferritin
appeared to correspond in migration to that of adult kidney or neonatal liver (14). [In previous studies with glutaminase, a similar
relation between tissue distribution of isozymes had emerged (8)].
Consequently, we ventured the hypothesis that during malignant transformation of normal cells, a change in gene expression occurs such
that a fetal, or kidney, cistron for ferritin is expressed, and
depending on the cell type involved the expression of other cistrons
for ferritin protein is lost. From this it would follow that a
partcular type of ferritin would be indicative of malignancy, at
least in certain cell types like hepatocytes.

To pursue this hypothesis, we isolated larger quantities of
ferritins from normal and malignant rat tissues and examined their
structure. It soon became apparent that ferritin structure and its
gene expression were more complex than had been envisaged, and that
our hypothesis was too simple to explain the structural differences
observed. In brief, ferritins from adult and neonatal rat liver,
kidney, heart,Morris hepatomas 3683 and 7800, and Morris renal tumor
MK-3 were analyzed by a variety of methods, including determination
of amino acid composition, mapping of tryptic peptides, analysis of
available sulfhydryl groups, and subunit composition after dissociation with sodium dodecyl sulfate. Except in the case of neonatal
ferritin from iron injected rats and adult liver ferritin, there were
significant and reproducible differences among all the ferritins
examined including differences between the ferritins from the different kinds of tumors (13). This was evident especially from amino
acid and peptide composition. Thus, although ferritins from the
different tumors, kidney and neonatal liver could not be distinguished
by electrophoresis (at least at one gel concentration), they differed
markedly in total amino acid composition and also gave different
peptide maps (Fig 2). Nevertheless, the two hepatoma and renal tumor
ferritins were the most similar (Fig 2), the next most similar being
neonatal liver ferritin and then kidney ferritin. Adult liver ferritin was most unlike the others, and judging from the number of
peptide spots, it was also the most complex (Fig 2).

Further studies using quantitative polyacrylamide gel electrophoresis over a range of acrylamide concentrations (28) revealed that
Morris 3683 hepatoma ferritin was of the same size as liver and kidney
ferritins (about 450,000 daltons) and that upon dissociation with SDS
contained primarily subunits of 19,000 daltons, in the line with other

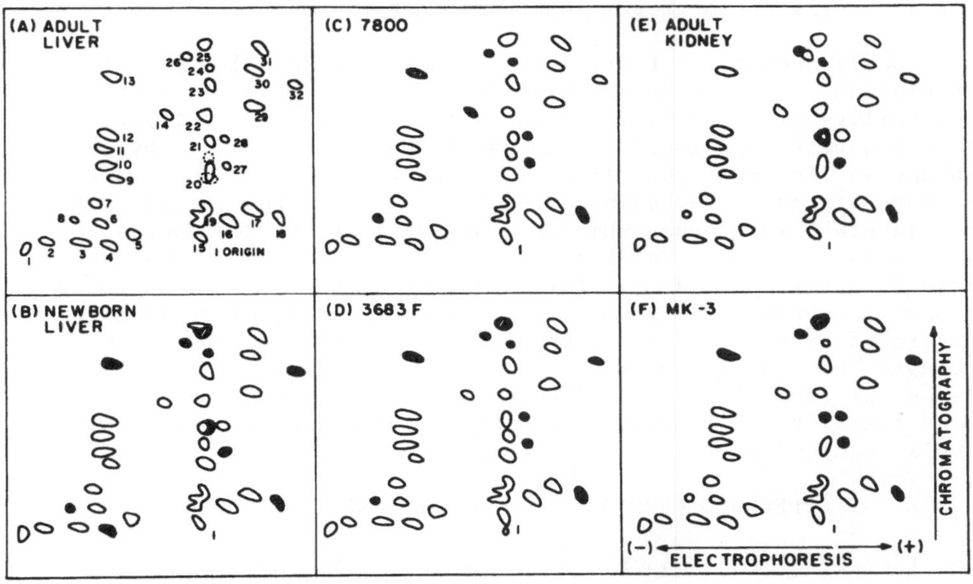

Figure 2

Peptide maps obtained on thin layer plates from tryptic digests of pure apoferritins isolated from normal and malignant rat tissues. The open spots are those found in a particular ferritin, while the hatched spots are those present in adult liver ferritin but missing from the ferritin in question. Numbers refer to Morris tumors (Table 1). Reprinted, with permission, from Linder et al. (13).

654 M. C. LINDER

ferritins (13). In the case of normal tissue ferritins considerable amounts of smaller subunits (11,000 - 14,000 daltons) were also found, but our more recent experiments suggest that most or all of these are attributable to limited proteolytic "nicking" of subunits during purification of the undissociated molecule (20). Therefore, despite considerable effort on the part of several laboratories using other techniques for dissociation and also isoelectric focusing, it is still unclear just how many genetic cistrons (and thus peptide chains or subunits types) in the rat (or any other species) contribute to the structural differences found in tumor ferritins or ferritins from other tissues (1).

Small amounts of ferritin are found extracellularly in the circulation. Serum ferritin concentrations are related to the availability of ferritin iron stores in liver and other tissues, but are often very much increased in cancer patients with no obvious changes in iron storage. Increases are also observed in a variety of other diseases, including infection (18), and the question of most interest is whether this increase reflects tissue damage (as is assumed to be the case for certain plasma enzymes during hepatitis or after myocardial infarction), or rather some other aspect of iron metabolism in disease. Analysis of the isoelectric focusing pattern of serum ferritins from normal and cancer patients does not indicate that the increased ferritin necessarily originates from tumor tissue, or from liver (1). Thus considerable further work is required to identify the mechanism leading to increased serum ferritin levels in cancer.

COPPER AND CERULOPLASMIN METABOLISM IN CANCER

Elevation of Plasma Copper and Ceruloplasmin in Cancer

A major portion of the copper in the body is found in the plasma, where 90% of it is part of the α_2-glycoprotein, ceruloplasmin. The remaining portion bound to amino acids and albumin is the fraction most readily available to tissues. Ceruloplasmin is made primarily or exclusively in the liver and has a number of possible functions. It is built like an enzyme, and in reactivity resembles the lacquer plant enzyme, laccase (29), with the capacity to oxidase a number of natural and synthestic substrates. P-phenylene diamine is the most common (synthetic) substrate used for its assay. Ceruloplasmin also catalyzes the oxidation of ferrus to ferric iron. This had lead to the concept that when iron is released from ferritin (in the ferrous form), oxidation by ceruloplasmin is an obligatory step preceding its attachment to transferrin (which binds ferric iron) and transfer to other parts of the body. Support for this has come from observations that copper deficiency results in a reduction of iron release from liver stores, and that infusion of ceruloplasmin rapidly reverses this process (22, 24). As regards other functions, ceruloplasmin may serve as a mechanism for ridding the liver of excess copper: liver copper concentrations are remarkably constant even when there are large variations in dietary copper intake (10). It may also serve as a special transport function, delivering copper to cytochrome oxidase (6) and to tissues such as the heart which are rich in respiratory enzymes (12).

It is now well established that elevations of plasma copper and ceruloplasmin concentrations occur in cancer in the human (11) as well as the rat (9). Table 4 provides a summary of studies on ceruloplasmin oxidase activities of plasma obtained from rats with and without transplantable tumors. The results are given in the order of decreasing growth rate of the tumor lines examined. In all the cases shown there was a significant but variable (50-300%) increase in ceruloplasmin oxidase in the tumor bearing rats, and this did not occur with either sham implantation or implantation of normal liver (Table 4) (9). More careful studies of the time course of increase in ceruloplasmin in the case of mammary tumor 5A indicated that significant elevations occurred when tumors weighed less than a g, but there was progressive increase with tumor size (9).

In an effort to understand the basis for the elevation of plasma ceruloplasmin, we measured the rates of ceruloplasmin synthesis in rats with and without tumors (Table 5). In the case of the three tumor lines tested, there was an enhanced rate of incorporation of ($3H$) leucine into ceruloplasmin (column B) in the tumor bearing animals. This was particularly significant when compared to rate of overall plasma protein synthesis (column A), as indicated by the ratio of counts in ceruloplasmin over those in plasma protein (third column). The enhancement of total plasma protein synthesis (along with ceruloplasmin synthesis) in the case of rats with Morris hepatoma 3683 may be explained on the basis that this tumor had a severe effect on hematocrit (Table 1). This would require a general increase in the rate of plasma protein synthesis to compensate for the increase in plasma volume which resulted (9).

In separate studies we examined the effects of copper administration on the rate of ceruloplasmin synthesis, using normal and copper deficient rats (12). An excerpt of our findings for normal rats is found in the last part of Table 5 for comparison with the effects of tumor bearing rats. As indicated by the results, rats fed a high copper diet maintained a greater than normal rate of ceruloplasmin synthesis, A more dramatic effect of copper on ceruloplasmin synthesis was seen in copper deficient rats, where a 5-fold increase in rate occurred by 8 hours after oral intubation (12).

The analogous effects of copper and tumors on the rate of ceruloplasmin synthesis suggested to us that tumors might be acting indirectly by enhancing the influx of copper from the diet. Our

Table Four
Ceruloplasmin Oxidase Activity of Plasma
from Rats with Transplantable
Tumors

Tumor Line Implanted	Tumor Weight (g)	Ceruloplasmin Oxidase Activity (10^2IU/ml)
Unimplanted Rats	-	21-25
Mammary Tumor 5A	1.6	42*
	4.1	36*
	11.7	78*
Hepatoma 3683	0.9	35*
	2.2	70*
Hepatoma 7777	1.6	26*
	4.7	29*
Hepatoma 5123tc	3.5	30*
	8.4	27*
Mammary Tumor 7A	2.4	48*
	4.5	61*
Hepatoma 7800	4.4	33*
	6.9	32*
Renal Tumor MK-2	4.2	28**
Implanted with Normal Liver	-	26
Sham-implantation	-	25

Mature, female rats were implanted with 1 mm cubes of tumor, or in the case of some controls, with a similar cube of normal liver. Sham-implanted rats were given saline by trocar at the implantation site, and other controls were not implanted. When tumors were various sizes, rats were heparinized, and killed by exsanguination. The blood obtained was separated into cells and plasma and the latter fraction assayed for ceruloplasmin oxidase activity, by following the linear rate of oxidation of p-phenylenediamine, at pH 5.4, 37°, in the presence of 10 mM EDTA (12). Results presented are mean values for assays of 4-10 rats (or much larger numbers of controls), and the order of the data is given in relation to the decreasing growth rate of the implanted tumors.

* $p < 0.01$ for difference from unimplanted rats

** $p < 0.05$ for difference from unimplanted rats

From Linder et al. (9).

Table Five

Increased Synthesis of Ceruloplasmin in Tumor Bearing
Rats and in Normal Rats Treated with Copper

| | Incorporation of (^{3}H) Leucine | | |
| | Specific Activity of | | Ratio |
	A Total plasma protein (10^{-3}dpm/mg)	B Ceruloplasmin (dpm/unit)	 10^3B/A
Mammary tumor 5A			
Control	6930	510	83
+Tumor	3380	750	222
% difference from control	-51*	+47	+170*
Mammary Tumor 7A			
Control	9040	305	51
+Tumor	6380	409	101
%difference from control	-29**	+34	+100
Hepatoma 3683			
Control	2180	400	18
+Tumor	3480	2870	104
%difference from control	+60*	+620*	+480*
Unimplanted rats			
Control	805	298	0.37
+Copper	937	434	0.46
%difference from control	+23*	+45*	+24*

* p<0.01 for difference ** p<0.05 for difference

     Rats bearing tumors weighing 0.5-3 g, and unimplanted controls,
were treated with (^{3}H) leucine (50 μCi:mammary tumors, or 25 μCi:
hepatomas and normal liver per 100 g body weight) 2-4 hours before
killing. Plasma was analyzed for incorporation of radiolabel into
total protein and ceruloplasmin. Similar experiments were done with
normal mature female rats maintained on normal and high copper diets
(5 and 300 μg/g, respectively) for more than a week. Except in the
case of the rats with hepatoma 3683, plasma protein concentrations
were unchanged by the presence of the tumor (with 3683 concentrations
were somewhat decreased), but ceruloplasmin levels were elevated
from 60-100% over the normal in the tumor bearing animals. They
remained unchanged in rats on the high copper diets. The results
are means for determinations on plasma from 9-10 rats, plasma from
2 rats being pooled for the ceruloplasmin isolation in most cases.
[From Linder et al. (9) (tumor bearing rats), and Linder et al. (10)
(copper treated rats).]

studies support this possibility. They show that at least in the case of the tumors examined (mammary tumors 5A), the capacity to absorb copper is increased 40-100% with tumor implantation (Table 6). $^{64}Cu(NO_3)_2$ was given by intragastric intubation to normal and tumor-bearing, fasted rats, and blood and tissues examined for radioactivity 2 hours later. Variations in the counts obtained for different experiments were due to the difference in the specific activity of the ^{64}Cu, which has a very short half life. The largest changes in copper uptake and distribution were evident in the plasma compartment. In all cases, and despite variations in tumor size, the plasma of tumor bearing rats contained 1-3 times as much radioactivity as that of normal controls. In contrast, and especially in the rat with larger tumors, there was a decreased amount of radioactivity in the liver, and some indication that this also occurred in the kidney. However, the decrease in liver and kidney radioactivity in no way offset the large increase in plasma radiocopper concentrations, as that overall, a 40-100% increase in total counts was obtained for the blood and organs examined. It was also evident that the tumor itself did not take up nearly as much of the newly absorbed copper as did liver and kidney. This may be due to its sequence in the circulation relative to the incoming radioactivity, since tumors were implanted subcutaneously in the flank, and liver and kidney would be expected to have a more direct access to the copper arriving from the gut.

More recently, we have tested absorption using everted gut sacs from normal and tumor bearing rats incubated with radiocopper in vitro (2). The results confirm that intestinal uptake of copper is enhanced in the rats with tumors and suggest that a change in the absorptive capacity of the intestinal mucosa is responsible. An indication of this is given by the data in the farthest column to the right of Table 6. It shows that while the mucosa of tumor bearing rats passed copper more rapidly into the circulation, less copper was retained by the mucosal cells, suggesting that a factor in the mucosa normally creates a "stumbling block" for entry of copper into the body. We are presently studying the possibility that a 10,000 dalton component, perhaps metallothionein, is present in reduced amounts in the mucosa of tumor bearing rats and that this allows a more rapid passage of the copper from the gut lumen into the blood.

The Copper Content of Rat Tumors

In an attempt to assess the importance of copper to tumor metabolism from another angle, we determined the total copper content of a variety of hepatic and mammary tumors, in comparison with normal liver (Table 7). Remarkably, the concentration of copper was almost constant among quite different tumors and very similar to the concentration in normal liver. On a per cell basis, copper content was much more variable but showed no trend relating to tumor growth rate

Table Six
Absorption of Copper by Tumor Bearing Rats
after Intragastric Intubation of ^{64}Cu(NO$_3$)$_2$

	Tumor Weight (g) Range	64Cu counts in plasma and tissues (dpm/g or ml)					
		PLASMA	LIVER	KIDNEY	HEART	TUMOR	INTESTINAL MUCOSA*
I. Unimplanted Rats (5)	–	53	499	579	44	–	
+Tumor (10)	2–14	164**	487	542	48	74	
II. Unimplanted Rats (5)	–	20	160	183	14	–	
+Tumor (5)	15–17	55**	115**	132**	14	22	
III. Unimplanted rats (3)	–	24	171	193	13	–	123
+Tumor (6)	13–24	41*	115*	158	13	19	49

* 30 min after intubation, 2 rats per group

** p<0.05-p<0.01 for difference from controls

    Rats with and without subcutaneous implants of mammary tumor
5A were fasted overnight and then intubated with ^{64}Cu (as Cu(NO$_3$)$_2$)
in about 0.05 M nitric acid, at doses from 26-93 ug/100 g body weight
(specific activity 1.08-3.85 μCi/ug), using an intragastric syringe.
Animals were killed 2 hours later and blood and tissues removed for
counting of radioactivity. The results given are means for determinations on 5-10 rats, as indicated. (From Cohen and Linder (2)).

Table Seven
Copper Contents of Hepatic and Mammary
Rat Tumors

Tissue	Total Copper Concentration (µg)	
	Per Gram Tissue	Per 10^8 Cells
Morris hepatomas		
7777	5.0 ± 0.9 (4)	1.02
5123tc	4.4 ± 0.5 (3)	0.83
7800	4.8 ± 0.7 (5)	2.09
9618A	3.9 ± 0.3 (3)	1.95
Mammary Tumor 5A	3.6 ± 0.9 (4)	2.24
Normal Liver Adult female*	4.9 ± 0.2 (5)	2.22

* From Linder et al. using published values for cell nuclei/g(19).

    Samples of apparently viable tumor tissue, and livers from
mature female Fischer rats, were assayed for their total content
of copper. Homogenates made with distilled-deionized water were
washed with a mixture of perchloric, sulfuric and nitric acids
prior to the copper determination (11). Results for copper concentration per g weight of tissue are given as mean ± SD, with the
number of samples assayed in parantheses. (From Moor and Linder,
unpublished).

or degree of anaplasia. A comparison of the values with those
obtained for other normal tissues of the rat indicate that tumors
have much higher concentrations of copper than almost all other
tissues (17).

Our Present Understanding of Copper Metabolism in Cancer

It is clear that we are just beginning the process of understanding the mechanisms underlying the changes in copper metabolism
and ceruloplasmin which occur in rats and humans with many kinds of
cancer. So far our findings show that the presence of a tumor results in an increased rate of synthesis of ceruloplasminm and that
this effect has some specificity, since it is not a general effect
on plasma protein synthesis. [It also is not a general effect on
the rate of synthesis of α_2-glycoproteins (9)]. One possible explanation stemming from our work is that tumors act by changing the
capacity of the intestinal mucosa to absorb copper, and that the
increased influx of copper, in turn, stimulates synthesis of ceruloplasmin. Unfortunately very little is known about the mechanism and
control of copper absorption to aid in our interpretation of these
results.

From a functional angle, it is possible to rationalize the
elevation of ceruloplasmin in cancer as a mechanism for delivering
copper to cytochrome oxidase, quantities of this enzyme being needed
for production of the respiratory apparatus of new cells. Hsieh
and Frieden (6) have recently shown that the copper in circulating
ceruloplasmin is much more readily transferred to cytochrome oxidase
in various tissues than is copper from the so-called "free" plasma
copper fraction (bound to albumin and amino acids). (The latter is
more readily available to other copper components within cells).
Complimenting this work we have acquired evidence that ceruloplasmin
as a whole is absorbed from the circulation by tissues such as heart
which are rich in respiratory enzymes (12).

One can also take quite the opposite view, and it may be argued
that the elevation in ceruloplasmin is part of the body's defense
against the presence of a tumor. In support of this idea, it is known
that copper can retard the growth of tumor cells in vitro (23, 27), or
inhibit their development in vivo (11), especially when given in combination with copper chelating agents. It is also known that ceruloplasmin may be elevated in infection (11) where other defense mechanisms are called into play. Still another possibility presents itself, and that is that ceruloplasmin is synthesized by the tumors
themselves. Indeed, we have found by immunological methods that extracts of tumor tissue contain ceruloplasmin antigen which cannot be
explained away on the basis of blood contamination. Also it has
already been mentioned that tissues may be absorbing ceruloplasmin
from the plasma (12). These divergent possibilities present a

challenge to those of us who are interested in iron and copper
metabolism as we continue our studies of the roles of these
elements in malignant disease.

REFERENCES

1. Aisen, P. and Brown, E.B. (eds). Proteins of Iron Metabolism,
    Grune and Stratton, New York (1977).

2. Cohen, D.I. and Linder, M.C. Cooper Absorption in Tumor Bearing
    Rats. Manuscript in preparation.

3. Drysdale, J.W. and Munro, H.N. J. Biol. Chem. 241 (1966) 3630.

4. Evans, G.W. Physiol. Rev. 53 (1973) 535.

5. Hevesy, G. and Lockner, D. Arkiv. Kemi. 19 (1961) 303.

6. Hsieh, H.S. and Frieden, E. Bioch. Biophys. Res. Comm. 67 (1975)
    1326.

7. Knox, W.E., Linder, M.C. and Friedell, G.H. Cancer Res. 30 (1970)
    283.

8. Knox, W.E., Linder-Horowitz, M. and Friedell, G.H. Cancer Res.
    29 (1969) 669.

9. Linder, M.C., Bryant, R.R., Lim, S., Scott, L.E., and Moor, J.R.
    Ceruloplasmin Elevation and Synthesis in Rats with Trasnplantable
    Tumors. Submitted for publication.

10. Linder, M.C., Houle, P.A., Isaacs, E., Moor, J.R. and Scott, L.E.
    Regulation of Ceruloplasmin by Copper in Normal and Copper-
    Deficient Rats. Submitted for publication.

11. Linder, M.C. and Moor, J.R. Plasma Ceruloplasmin and Copper in
    Pulmonary Cancer. In: Proceedings of the Third International
    Conference on Detection and Prevention of Cancer, New York,
    in press, (1977).

12. Linder, M.C. and Moor, J.R. Plasma Ceruloplasmin: Evidence for
    its Presence in and U take by Heart and Other Organs of the Rat.
    Bioch. Biophys. Acta. in press (1977).

13. Linder, M.C., Moor, J.R., Munro, H.N. and Morris, H.P. Biochem.
    Biophys. Acta 386 (1975) 409.

14. Linder, M.C., Moor, J.R., Munro, H.N. and Morris, H.P. In: Gann
    Monograph for Cancer Res. S. Weinhouse and T. Ono (eds). 13
    (1972) 299.

15. Linder, M.C., Moor, J.R., Scott, L.E. and Munro, H.N. Biochem.
    Biophys. Acta 297 (1973) 70.

16. Linder, M.C. and Munro, H.N. Analyt. Bioch. 48 (1972) 266.

17. Linder, M.C. and Munro, H.N. Enzyme 15 (1974) 111.

18. Linder, M.C. and Munro, H.N. Mechanism of Iron Absorption. Fed. Proc., in press, (1977).

19. Linder, M.C., Munro, H.N. and Morris, H.P. Cancer Res. 30 (1970) 2231.

20. Linder, M.C., Zahringer, J., Baliga, B.S., Drake, R.L., Barres, B., and Munro, H.N. In: Proteins of Iron Metabolism. P. Aisen and E.B. Brown (eds). Grune and Stratton, New York, in press (1977).

21. Morris, H.P., Wagner, B.P. and Meranze, D.R. Cancer Res. 30 (1970) 1362.

22. Osaki, S. and Johnson, D.A. J. Biol. Chem. 244 (1969) 5757.

23. Petering, H.G. and Vangiessen, G.J. In: The Biochemsitry of Copper. J. Peisach, P. Aisen and W.E. Blumberg (eds). Academic Press, New York (1966) p. 197.

24. Ragan, H.A., Nacht, S., Lee, G.R., Bishop, C.R. and Cartwright, G.E. Am. J. Physiol. 217 (1969) 1320.

25. Richter, G.W. Nature 207 (1965) 616.

26. Robbins, E. and Pederson, T. Proc. Natl. Acad. Sci. U.S.A 66 (1970) 1244.

27. Takamiya, K. Nature 185 (1960) 190.

28. Vulimiri, L., Catsimpoolas, N., Griffith, A., Linder, M.C. and Munro, H.N. Biochem. Biophys. Acta 412 (1975) 148.

29. Vanngard, T. In: Biological Spplications of ESR. H.M. Swartz, J.R. Bolton, and T. Borg (eds), Wiley-Interscience, New York, (1972) p. 411.

ABNORMAL DIETARY REGULATION OF GLUTAMINE SYNTHETASE IN

MORRIS HEPATOMAS

Thomas F. Deuel, Marjorie Louie, and Harold P. Morris

Department of Medicine
Jewish Hospital of St. Louis
St. Louis, Missouri 63310

INTRODUCTION

The series of Morris hepatomas offer unique opportunities to investigate the regulation of the cancer cell and how this regulation differs from that found in normal liver. One area of special interest concerns the failure of certain anabolic enzymes in hepatomas to change specific activity in response to dietary changes of the host animal in a manner similar to the enzyme in normal or host liver. Siperstein et al. (1, 2) showed that the biosynthesis of cholesterol was not suppressed in hepatomas from rats fed a cholesterol rich diet whereas a sharp reduction in cholesterol biosynthesis occurred in the liver of identically fed, tumor-free rats. Subsequently, Brown, Goldstein, and Siperstein (3) demonstrated that the synthesis of the rate limiting enzyme in cholesterol biosynthesis, β-hydroxy β-methylglutaryl coenzyme A reductase(HMG CoA reductase), was decreased in host liver when rats were subjected to the cholesterol rich diet; the synthesis of the enzyme in hepatomas did not change in response to an identical feeding schedule given to the host rat.

Majerus et al. (4) demonstrated an altered dietary regulation of the enzymes acetyl coenzyme A reductase and fatty acid synthetase in Morris hepatomas. When fasted animals were fed a fat free diet, both enzymes had increased activity in host and control rat livers; the enzyme activity in the Morris hepatomas was unaltered, These results and others, such as described by Pitot et al. (5), suggested the general hypothesis that critical anabolic enzymes in Morris hepatomas are not subject to the dietary regulation found in host liver and in control livers. To further test this hypothesis, we studied the

665

changes in the levels of the enzyme glutamine synthetase that occur
when the diet of the host rat is modified from a normal diet to a
nitrogen free diet, comparing results in control livers, host livers,
and hepatomas.

Glutamine synthetase was chosen for study because this enzyme
occupies a unique position in anabolic nitrogen metabolism by virtue
of the diverse metabolic end products that require either the amide
or the amino nitrogen of glutamine for biosynthesis. The amide
nitrogen of glutamine is preferentially utilized in the biosynthesis
of purines, pyrimidines, and pyridine nucleotides, in the biosynthesis
of complex carbohydrates, and in the biosynthesis of certain amino
acids. The amino nitrogen of glutamine is utilized in specific transamination reactions and glutamine itself is incorporated into protein
without further modification (6-13). In order to insure the continued
availability of glutamine for other diverse pathways, the enzyme synthesizing glutamine is a logical site for cellular regulation.

Glutamine synthetase has been isolated in pure form from many
different microorganisms and the purified enzyme has been studied in
detail. Complex regulatory mechanisms governing the overall activity
of the enzyme have been described. In Eschericia coli, a close correlation is found between the catalytic activity of glutamine synthetase and the state of nitrogen balance within the cell. The correlation of enzyme activity with cellular needs for nitrogen is mediated by the post-translational enzymatic adenylylation and deadenyl-
ylation of preformed glutamine synthetase, as elegantly worked out by
Stadtman et al (14). Bacillus licheniformis (15, 16) and Bacillus sub-
tilis glutamine synthetase (17-21) are also subject to complex regulation but the regulation is achieved through different mechanisms than
those encountered in E. coli.

The regulation of glutamine synthetase in animals has been less
intensively studied but detailed investigations are available with
glutamine synthetase from sheep brain and rat liver (22-25). The enzyme appears to play an important role in the intermediary metabolism
of mammals as suggested by the fact that glutamine, the product of the
reaction catalyzed by glutamine synthetase, is that amino acid found
in highest concentrations in the blood; high levels of glutamine are
also found in mammalian heart and brain. In the nervous system,
glumatine may play another important role because of its relationship
to λ-aminobutyric acid and glutamate, putative mediators of synaptic
transmission (26, 27). Apparent induction of glutamine synthetase in
response to glutamine deprivation or glucocorticoid administration has
been demonstrated in several different tissue or cell culture systems
(28-34). In neoplastic tissue, glutamine synthetase activity is lower
than that found in normal tissue (35). In order to study in greater
detail the regulation of glutamine synthetase in rat liver and Morris
hepatomas, we turned to the methods of Schimke (36) to determine the

turnover rates of glutamine synthetase structural protein in normal and neoplastic tissue and how these rates are modified when the nitrogen intake of the host rat was eliminated.

PURIFICATION AND PROPERTIES OF RAT LIVER GLUTAMINE SYNTHETASE

For these investigations, glutamine synthetase was required in highly purified form. Using techniques developed in our laboratory, methods similar to those developed by Meister et al. (22, 23), glutamine synthetase was purified 231 fold from rat liver, with a 31% recovery of enzyme activity. The enzyme appears to be essentially pure as judged by sedimentation velocity analysis, standard disc gel polyacrylamide electrophoresis, and electrophoresis in polyacrylamide gels in the presence of sodium dodecyl sulfate. A constant specific activity is found across the activity peak eluted during hydroxylapatite chromatography. Glutamine synthetase is associated with the microsomal particles when rat liver is fractionated in isotonic sucrose. The enzyme is released from the microsomal fraction, however, after incubation in physiological salt concentrations, suggesting that the in vivo synthesis of glutamine may occur when the enzyme is in the liver cytosol, unassociated with the membrane fraction. Divalent cations are required in the biosynthetic reaction and have a major effect on glutamine synthetase activity. The enzyme is more active in the presence of Mg^{2+} than in Mn^{2+}. The apparent K_m for glutamate depends upon the concentration of divalent cation in the assay. When 8 mM Mn^{2+} is used during assay, the apparent K_m is 0.3 mM. At 2 mM Mn^{2+}, the apparent K_m has risen to 5.0 mM. The enzyme is inhibited by several different metabolites, including alanine, histidine, and the product of the reaction, glutamine. No evidence of enzyme-bound adenylyl groups, as are found with E. coli glutamine synthetase, was found using ultra-violet absorption spectroscopy to analyze many different preparations of purified glutamine synthetase.

INDUCTION, PARTIAL PURIFICATION AND CHARACTERIZATION OF RABBIT ANTI-RAT LIVER GLUTAMINE SYNTHETASE SERA

With purified rat liver glutamine synthetase as antigen, rabbit anti-glutamine synthetase sera was obtained. The antisera was partially purified by ammonium sulfate precipitation and DEAE chromatography before use. The specificity of the antisera for the enzyme was analyzed using immunodiffusion and quantitative precipitin techniques. When antiserum is placed in the center well of immunodiffusion plates, the addition of partially purified and fully purified glutamine synthetase preparations to the surrounding wells resulted in single lines of precipitation. The precipitation of rat liver glutamine synthetase was evaluated quantitatively by adding increasing amounts of antiserum to fixed levels of enzyme. A progressive loss of activity in the supernatant was observed; this loss was directly proportional to the amounts of the antiserum added. Essentially all enzyme activity was

removed from the supernatant at appropriate levels of antisera.
These results were identical using highly purified or partially
purified rat liver extracts. The properties of the enzyme described above and the antiserum obtained were then used to compare
glutamine synthetase from rat liver with the enzyme from several
Morris hepatomas.

GLUTAMINE SYNTHETASE ACTIVITY IN EXTRACTS OF MORRIS HEPATOMAS

The transplantable Morris hepatomas 7777, 7800, 7749B, and 8999
were maintained in male Buffalo rats and crude extracts of the four
hepatomas from these rats were prepared for assay. The specific
activity of glutamine synthetase in the hepatomas ranged from 9% to
43% of the specific activity of the enzyme found in similarly prepared crude extracts of host liver. The enzyme specific activity
in crude extracts of liver from tumor bearing rats ranged from 90%
to 101% of the specific activity of glutamine synthetase in liver
extract from non-tumor bearing control rats. We found no apparent
correlation netween the specific activity of glutamine synthetase
and either the histological classification of the Morris hepatoma or
the growth rate of the individual tumors. Hepatomas 7777, 7794B, and
8999 had approximately equal enzyme specific activities even though
their histological classifications ranged from poorly to highly differentiated and their growth rates ranged from rapid to slow.

COMPARISON OF GLUTAMINE SYNTHETASE ACTIVITY IN HOST LIVER AND
HEPATOMA EXTRACTS FROM RATS ON A NORMAL DIET AND FROM RATS ON A
PROTEIN FREE DIET

We next studied the effect of eliminating dietary protein fed to
the host rat on the specific activity of glutamine synthetase in host
liver and in the four Morris hepatomas. In host liver extracts from
tumor bearing rats fed protein free diet for ten days, a drop in the
specific activity of glutamine synthetase was demonstrated to levels
ranging from 26% to 62% of the enzyme specific activity levels found
in similar liver extracts from rats fed a normal protein diet. Results from liver extracts from control, non-tumor bearing rats were
in all instances identical to results found in extracts ·of livers from
tumor bearing animals. In contrast, however, an increase in the specific activity of glutamine synthetase was found in extracts of hepatomas from rats on protein free diets, ranging from 131% to 260% of
the enzyme specific activities found in hepatoma extracts from rats
fed a normal protein diet. Thus, the specific activity of glutamine
synthetase in the hepatoma was increased under dietary conditions
which depressed enzyme specific activity in host and control livers.
Furthermore, when tumor bearing rats were refed a regular diet after
protein starvation, the specific activity of glutamine synthetase returned towards that activity found in tissues of animals on a normal
diet. Six days after initiation of refeeding, the specific activity

of glutamine synthetase in extracts of host livers from previously
protein starved rats had increased to 92% of the enzyme specific
activity in rats maintained on a normal protein diet. The enzyme
specific activity in hepatoma extracts from previously starved
rats had decreased to 84% of the enzyme level in rats previously fed
a normal-protein diet. These experiments demonstrate the specific
activity of glutamine synthetase in hepatomas was depressed under
dietary conditions which enhanced the specific activity in host
liver. Thus, the dietary regulation of glutamine synthetase in hepatomas differs both in direction and in amount from the regulation
of this enzyme in normal or host liver of tumor bearing rats.

COMPARISON OF PHYSICAL, KINETIC, AND IMMUNOLOGICAL PROPERTIES OF GLUTAMINE SYNTHETASE FROM CONTROL LIVER, HOST LIVER, AND MORRIS HEPATOMAS

We next wished to characterize further the nature of the changes
in glutamine synthetase specific activity that occurred when rats were
switched from a regular diet to a diet free of protein. Glutamine
synthetase from control liver, host liver, and hepatomas was partially purified for use in experiments to define different kinetic and
immunological properties of the enzymes. The goal in these experiments was to determine whether the enzymes from the different sources
behaved identically under differing conditions and thus was likely to
be the same structural enzyme. These studies also sought to determine
whether the changes in enzyme specific activity. in our experiments
reflected changes in the level of glutamine synthetase enzyme protein.
By precipitating the enzyme from crude extracts at pH 5.0 and resolu-
bilization of the precipitated enzyme in buffer, a four to nine fold
purification of glutamine synthetase was achieved with 90% or greater
recovery of enzyme activity in all cases.

Partially purified enzymes from hepatoma, host liver, and control
liver were heated at 50° and residual enzyme activity determined at
time intervals thereafter. In each instance, the $t_{1/2}$ of inactivation
was approximately nine minutes. Furthermore, glutamine synthetase
from both liver and hepatoma was completely protected from heat inactivation when the enzyme substrates glutamate, ammonia, and Mn ATP
were included in the buffer during heating. The kinetic properties of
the partially purified preparations were compared by measuring the
ratio of biosynthetic activity in the presence of 50 mM Mg^{2+} to its
activity in the presence of 2 mM Mn^{2+}, by comparing the inhibition of
the enzyme by alanine, histidine, and glutamine, and by comparing the
apparent K_m of the enzyme preparations for the substrate glutamate.
No differences between the three enzyme preparations were demonstrated.

Further comparative studies were performed by reacting the enzymes from different sources with the partially purified rabbit anti-
rat liver glutamine synthetase serum. Immunodiffusion pattern ob-

tained with extracts from control liver, host liver, and each of
the hepatomas in the surrounding wells and with partially purified
antisera in the center well showed reactions of identity and suggested that enzymes from all three sources were antigenically in-
distinguishable. Immunotitration analysis of the antiserum and
partially purified extracts of host liver, control liver, and hepatomas was performed also. All three enzyme preparations had the
same equivalence point in these experiments. Thus, no differences
between the enzyme from the three different sources were found in
comparing various physical, kinetic, and immunological criteria.
We concluded that the enzyme most likely was structurally identical
in all three tissues. True structural identity cannot be determined
with certainty in the absence of direct studies, however.

DETERMINATION OF THE DEGRADATIVE RATE OF GLUTAMINE SYNTHETASE IN HOST LIVER AND HEPATOMA FROM RATS ON A NORMAL DIET AND FROM RATS ON A PROTEIN FREE DIET

     Because the antibody precipitated equal amounts of enzyme from
each different preparation at all points studied, as judged by the
loss of enzyme activity in the supernatant after immunoprecipitation
of the enzyme antibody complex, it can be concluded that the changes
in enzyme specific activity in response to changes in host dietary
protein intake reflect changes in the enzyme levels in the respective
tissues. Furthermore, the differences in the activities and thus
levels of the enzyme in hepatoma tissue and the host liver as well as
the changes in activities when the host animals are converted from a
normal to a protein free diet can be concluded to reflect changes in
the steady-state turnover of glutamine synthetase. Experiments were
therefore done to determine directly the rate of degradation of
glutamine synthetase in hepatomas and host livers of rats on protein
free and normal protein diets. These experiments utilized the techniques described by Schimke (36). When rats were fed a normal diet,
the half-life of glutamine synthetase in host liver was determined to
be 5.2 days. When rats were fed a protein free diet, the half-life of
the enzyme was shortened to 3.0 days. The half-life of the enzyme in
hepatoma tissue from rats fed a normal diet was 1.4 days, but when
measured in hepatomas from rats fed a protein free diet, the half-life
had lenghtened to 3.8 days. These studies then demonstrated that the
rate of degradation of enzyme protein in both host liver and hepatomas
changes significantly when the diet of the host rats are changed from
a normal protein diet to a protein free diet. The directions of these
changes in the rates of degradation of enzyme protein are consistent
with the directions of the changes in the enzyme levels determined in
both tumor and host liver in response to the dietary changes.

DISCUSSION

The regulation of the turnover rates of glutamine synthetase

structural protein operates differently in hepatomas than it
operates in normal liver, serving to modify the enzyme levels of
glutamine synthetase in opposite ways when the hepatoma and host
liver are compared from host rats converted from a normal diet to
a protein free diet. Wu and Morris (37) were able to show that a
high protein diet reduced glutamine synthetase specific activity in
Morris hepatomas 8999 and 7800 but that a diet low in protein increased the enzyme specific activity in the hepatoma. Wu (38)
demonstrated also that the specific activity of glutamine synthetase
in the host liver was approximately the same whether the protein content in the diet was fixed at 5% or at 75%. The specific activity
of the enzyme significantly decreased however in the livers of rats
fed a protein free diet. No comparisons were made between the enzymes of the hepatoma and liver and the biochemical basis in the
change in the specific activity of glutamine synthetase was not established. The results that we have obtained show that glutamine
synthetase in hepatomas does respond to protein starvation. The
response, however, consistently is in a direction opposite to the
response of the enzyme in normal rat livers. Protein starvation depresses glutamine synthetase levels in host liver but results in
elevated enzyme levels in each of the four hepatomas that we have
studied. The observed differences in the levels of glutamine synthetase in liver and in hepatomas under the different conditions of
study correlate well with the changes in the degradative rates of
the enzyme as measured in these studies. For example, the increased
levels of glutamine synthetase in hepatomas of protein starved rats
is consistent with the observed decrease in the rate of degradation
of this enzyme in the hepatoma tissue. Conversely, the lowered levels
of the enzyme in the liver of the protein starved tumor bearing rats
correlates directly with the observed increase in the rate of degradation of liver enzyme.

It is unlikely that the enzyme in hepatomas is structurally different or modified in vivo from the enzyme in host or control liver
based on heat inactivation curves, kinetic parameters, and several
immunological properties of the respective enzymes. Additional experiments, including measurements of glutaminase activities and
measurements of the uptake of glutamine by isolated hepatoma and liver
cells would provide additional information on other mechanisms which
regulate the intracellular concentrations of glutamine and how these
mechanisms are modified in hepatoma and normal liver under different
physiological conditions.

The absent negative feedback control of glutamine synthetase in
the presence of protein starvation supports earlier theories of Potter
(39, 40) that a relationship exists between deranged feedback control
and malignant transformation. Which event is primary or secondary,
however, is not established. Rats with transplantable carcinomas
subjected to a six-day fast were observed by LePage (41) to have

increased tumor size when the liver, spleen, and kidneys of the
fasted animals were reduced in size. Labeled glycine was injected
into the rats immediately prior to fasting. The kidneys and the
liver lost radioactivity preferentially but the radioactivity continued to be incorporated in the tumors. Monroe (42) showed that
labeled glycine and phosphorus had a depressed uptake into the RNA
of livers of fasted rats as compared with the uptake of these
materials into liver RNA of control rats. In contrast, the uptake
of labelled glycine and phsophorus into the hepatoma RNA was not
lowered by fasting the host animals. Foster and Pardee (48) showed that the apparent rate of uptake and the V_{max} of uptake of λ-
aminobutyric acid and cycloleucine were increased in polyoma virus-
transformed 3T3 cells relative to the uptake in nontransformed 3T3
cells. More recently, Isselbacher (44) found that the uptake of
λ-aminobutyric acid, cycloleucine, and 2-deoxyglucose in polyoma
virus transformed baby hamster kidney cells and Simian virus 40-
transformed BALB/3 cells was increased 2.3-3.5 fold in comparison
with non-transformed cells. Thus these experiments as well as those
from our laboratory with the Morris hepatomas provide additional
biochemical evidence that hepatomas and other neoplasms have selective
advantage over normal tissues in fasted host animals. Specific regulatory mechanisms that serve to insure the overall metabolic har-
mony of normal cells in response to dietary stress do not operate
in the hepatoma cell. Further study of these altered regulatory
mechanisms may serve to provide specific targets for anti-tumor
therapy.

REFERENCES

1. Siperstein, M.D. and Fagan, V.M. Cancer Res. 24 (1964) 1108.

2. Siperstein, M.D., Fagan, V.M. and Morris, H.P. Cancer Res. 26 (1966) 7

3. Brown, M.S., Goldstein, J.L. and Siperstein, M.D. Fed. Proc. 32 (1973) 2168.

4. Majerus, P.W., Jacobs, R. and Smoth, M.D. J. Biol. Chem. 243 (1968) 3588.

5. Pitot, H.C., Potter, V.R. and Morris, H.P. Cancer Res. 21 (1961) 1001.

6. Buchanan, J.M. In: The Nucleic Acids, E. Chargaff and J.N. Davidson, (eds). Academic Press Inc. New York 3 (1960) 303.

7. Harlbert, R.B. and Chatroborty, K.P. Fed. Proc. 20 (1961) 361.

8. Picard, A. and Waime, J.M. Biochem. Biophys. Res. Comm. 15 (1961) 761.

9. Leloir, L.R. and Cardini, C.E. Biochim. Biophys. Acta 12 (1953) 15.

10. Shrinivasam, P.R. J. Am. Chem. Soc. 81 (1959) 1772.

11. Neidle, A. and Waelsch, H. J. Biol. Chem. 234 (1959) 586.

12. Meister, A. In: The Enzymes, P.D. Boywer and K. Myrback (eds). Academic Press Inc. New York 6 (1962) 193.

13. Cooper, A.J.L. and Meister, A. In: The Enzymes of Glutamine Metabolism, S. Prusiner and E.R. Stadtman (eds). Academic Press New York (1973) p. 77.

14. Stadtman, E.R. In: The Enzymes, P.D. Boyer (ed). Academic Press New York I (1970) 387.

15. Hubbard, J.S. and Stadtman, E.R. J. Bacteriol. 94 (1967) 1007.

16. Hubbard, J.S. and Stadtman, E.R. J. Bcateriol. 94 (1967) 1016.

17. Deuel, T.F., Ginsburg, A., Yeh, J., Shelton, E. and Stadtman, E.R. J. Biol. Chem. 245 (1970) 5195.

18. Deuel, T.F. and Stadtman, E.R. J. Biol. Chem. 245 (1970) 5206.

19. Deuel, T.F. J. Biol. Chem. 246 (1971) 599.

20. Deuel, T.F. and Turner, D.C. J. Biol. Chem. 247 (1972) 3039.

21. Deuel, T.F. and Prusiner, S. J. Biol. Chem. 249 (1974) 257.

22. Tate, S.S. and Meister, A. Proc. Natl. Acad. Sci. U.S.A. 68 (1971) 781.

23. Tate, S.S. and Meister, A. In: The Enzymes of Glutamine Metabolism, S. Prusiner and E.R. Stadtman (eds). Academic Press Inc, New York (1973) p. 77.

24. Deuel, T.F., Lerner, A. and Albrycht, D. In: The Enzymes of Glutamine Metabolism, S. Prusiner, S. and E.R. Stadtman (eds). Academic Press, New York (1973) p. 129.

25. Deuel, T.F., Lerner, A. and Albyrcht, D. Biochem. Biophys. Res. Comm. 48 (1972) 1419.

26. Johnson, J.L. Brain Res. 37 (1972) 1.

27. Bloom, F.E. Neurosciences Res. Prog. Bull. 10 (1972) 122.

28. DeMars, R. Biochim. Biophys. Acta 27 (1958) 453.

29. Paul, J. and Fottrell, P. Biochim. Biophys. Acta 67 (1963) 334.

30. Piddington, R. and Moscona, A.A. J. Cell Biol. 27 (1965) 247.

31. Piddington, R. and Moscona, A.A. Biochim. Biophys. Acta 141 (1965) 429.

32. Moscona, A.A. and Piddington, R. Biochim. Biophys. Acta 121 (1966) 409.

33. Reif-Lehner, L. J. Cell Biol. 51 (1971) 303.

34. Kulka, R.G., Tomkins, G.M. and Crook, R.B. J. Cell Biol. 54 (1972) 125.

35. Wu, C., Roberts, E.H. and Boon, J.M. Cancer Res. 25 (1965) 677.

36. Schimke, R.T. and Doyle, D. Ann. Rev. Biochem. 39 (1970) 929.

37. Wu, C. and Morris, H.P. Cancer Res. 30 (1970) 2675.

38. Wu, C. Arch. Biochem. Biophys. 106 (1964) 402.

39. Potter, V.R. Fed. Proc. 17 (1958) 691.

40. Potter, V.R. Cancer Res. 24 (1964) 1085.

41. LePage, G.A., Potter, V.R., Busch, H., Heidelberger, C. and Hurlbert, R.B. Cancer Res. 12 (1952) 153.

42. Munro, H.N. and Clark, C.M. Brit. J. Cancer 13 (1959) 324.

43. Foster, D.O. and Pardee, A.B. J. Biol. Chem. 244 (1969) 2675.

44. Isselbacher, K.J. Proc. Natl. Acad. Sci. U.S.A. 69 (1975) 585.

SOLID TUMOR MODELS FOR THE ASSESSMENT OF DIFFERENT TREATMENT
MODALITIES: VI: PERTURBATIONS IN THE KINETICS OF TUMOR AND HOST
ORGAN CELLULAR REGULATION DEMONSTRATED BY SINGLE AND COMBINED
EXPERIMENTAL THERAPY

W.B. Looney, H.A. Hopkins, and J.S. Trefil

Division of Radiobiology and Biophysics
University of Virginia
Charlottesville, Virginia 22901

INTRODUCTION

The Morris hepatomas, the large series of over fifty different
lines of transplantable rat hepatomas with multiple genetic, biochemical, metabolic and morphological changes, have been extensively
used in cancer research. A correlation between tumor cell kinetics
and tumor growth for this series of solid tumors was needed because
many studies used tumor growth rates as reference points. The parameters of cell cycle time, growth fraction and cell loss factor, in
addition to potential and actual volume doubling times, have been
determined in nine Morris hepatomas. These parameters of tumor cell
proliferation kinetics and tumor growth rates were determined in
selected rapid, intermediate and slow growing hepatomas. Information
obtained from these multiple parameter studies is necessary to quantitatively evaluate net tumor growth rates and provide baseline information regarding tumor growth classification. In fact, this additional
information on tumor cell kinetics of the different hepatoma lines
should be most helpful in the interpretation of the numerous studies
in cancer research utilizing these solid tumors. Most of the studies
using the different tumor lines use growth rates as the key reference
when differences are found between the tumor lines.

Solid tumors which comprise the majority of human cancer continue to challenge the best efforts of both the clinician and the ex-
perimentalist. At present no specific solid tumor or group of solid
tumors has provided all of the necessary information for clinical
utilization in therapuetic scheduling of different forms of cancer
treatment. The Morris hepatomas provide a diverse group of solid
tumors so that specific questions relating to cancer management can
be answered by selection of the appropriate tumor line. Well de-

fined and rapidly analyzable animal solid tumor models can yield
quantitative information concerning the time sequence of host toxicity to therapy and the kinetics of recovery of host and tumor. A
two-way translation of information between the animal model and
patient provides an approach for improved cancer management by the
rapid exchange of information between animal model and clinical
studies of solid tumors in man. The approach to the evaluation of
different treatment modalities has been multi-disciplinary. We
have examined the end points at four organizational levels; the
molecular, cellular, organ and animal levels in our studies of the
effects of therapy and the sequencing of therapy. The extensive
information and correlated parameters of therapeutic and toxic effects of therapy should assist the clinician in the overall management of patients with solid tumors.

The perturbations of tumor growth following experimental cancer
therapy provides information which may be utilized in the studies of
tumor regulation under both equilibrium and non-equilibrium conditions. The chemotherapuetic studies permit the evaluation of cellular
organ regulation as well as the interrelations of organ regulation to
tumor regulation.

KINETIC DESCRIPTION OF TUMOR LINES USED FOR THE ASSESSMENT OF SINGLE AND COMBINED MODALITY THERAPY

Nine tumor lines selected from rapid, intermediate and slow-
growing tumor lines are arranged in descending order of growth
rates in Table 1. Cell cycle phase times (Table 2) for these tumors
were estimated from percent labelled mitosis curves using an automated
analytical program. The model utilized assumes that the cell cycle is
composed of four distinct phases (G_1, S, G_2, M), and that the time
spent by a cell in a phase has a Gamma distribution. The mean and
standard deviation of these phase distributions are optimized by the
computer program to best fit the experimental percentage labelled
mitosis curve by the method of least squares. Estimates of the mean
time spent in each phase are shown in Table 2 for the tumor lines that
could be adequately analyzed.

Solid tumor models, each having the biological properties to
answer specific questions, have been selected from this series of
Morris hepatomas. Studies on the assessment of therapeutic response
to different modalities of treatment for these particular tumors can
provide guidelines for future attempts to improve the clinical management of solid tumors.

The most extensively used tumor line in these studies has been
hepatoma 3924A. Repeated cell kinetics and growth studies over the
past ten years have shown 3924A to be extremely stable and reproducible. It was induced originally in an ACI female rat by feeding N-2

Table One
Characteristics of Tumor Lines Studied

Hepatoma Line	Average of Tumor Generations Used*	Tumor Growth* cm/mo	Volume Doubling Time (Hours)	L.I.**	Histological Description*	Chromosome Number	Group***	Tumor Generation Used in this study	Animal Strain
7288ctc	50-59	10.0	56.2	31.3	Poorly Differentiated	43	III	79	BUFF
3924A	264-272	7.0	104.4	17.6	Poorly Differentiated	73	III	269	ACI
5123tc	71-77	5.0	120.7	16.9	Interm.between well and poorly Differentiated	47	II	99	BUFF
7316B	32-41	2.5	139.9	16.2	Interm.between highly diff. and well Differentiated	44	III	50	BUFF
7800	42-48	2.8	145.7	13.3	Well to highly Differentiated	42	I	57	BUFF
9121	20-29	3.5	191.0	23.0	Well Differentiated	42	I	36	ACI
9618A	1-5	0.7	243.6	6.3	Highly Differentiated	42	I	7	BUFF
9633	5-9	1.3	419.0	1.6	Interm.between well and highly Differentiated	42	I	12	BUFF
16	1-4	0.5	587.0	2.0	Interm.between well and highly Differentiated	42	I	7	BUFF

*Morris, H.P. and Meranze, D.R. In: Recent Results in Cancer Research, Vol.44, E. Grundmann (ed). Berling-Heidelberg-NewYork: Springer-Verlag, (1974) pp. 103-114. **L.I.- One hr. Thymidine Labeling Index. ***Norwell,P.C.,Morris,H.P. and Potter, V.R. Cancer Research, 27 (1967) 1565.

Table Two
Tumor Cell Kinetics and Growth Characterisctics

Hepatoma Lines	H-4-II-E	3924A	5123tc	7316B	9618A	16
Actual Doubling Time (Hrs).	49.2	104.4	120.7	139.9	243.6	587
Potential Doubling Time (Hrs).	34.8	42.0	33.5	48.5	72.5	300
Cell Loss Factor	0.29	0.60	0.72	0.65	0.70	0.42
Growth Fraction	100	65	100	100	78	100
L.I.	13.8	17.6	16.9	1 6.2	6.3	2.2
T_{g1}	30.5	14.0	28.1	43.0	45.5	316
T_s	6.0	9.3	7.1	9.8	5.7	8.4
T_{g2}	2.1	3.7	5.3	6.5	4.7	6.5
T_m	0.5	0.4	0.2	0.2	0.3	1.0
T_c	39.1	27.4	41.5	60.3	56.2	331.9

L.I. = 1 hour thymidine labeling index; tumor volume doubling time
in hours.

T_c = cell cycle time (hours); T_m = mitotic time; T_{g2} = gap 2; T_s =
DNA synthetic time; T_{g1} = gap 1.

fluorenyldiacetamide and is maintained in this host by transplantation at monthly intervals (27). It is a fast-growing, poorly differentiated tumor. The parenchymal tumor cells are hypotetraploid,
having 73 chromosomes, 10 of which are abnormal. The tumor contains
at least two populations of cells, one having a model DNA content
similar to that of diploid mammalian cells and the other having a
DNA content corresponding to that of tetraploid tumor cells. The
kinetics of cell proliferation and tumor growth are as follows:
the actual volume doubling time for 3924A is 96.3 hr, the potential
volume doubling time 42 hr. The cell cycle time is 27.4 hr. The
different phases of the cycle are: T_{G1}-14 hr; T_S-9.3 hr; T_{G2}-3.7 hr,
and T_M-0.4 hr. The 1 hr thymidine labelling index is 17.6, the
growth fraction 0.66, and the cell loss factor 0.61 (19).

The percentage composition for hepatoma 3924A remained constant
at 51% tumor, 18% necrotic, 26% connective and 5% blood for tumors
with volumes ranging from 70-350 mm^3. Over a range of tumor size
(0.2 - 12.0 g) the relative cell density of 3924A remains constant
5% of the cells being of parenchymal tumor type with the remainder
being associated with the connective tissue and vascular framework
of the hepatoma.

One major advantage of this tumor line is that it rarely metastasizes. This permits studies with the primary which are related to
the effects of treatment on the tumor without the deleterious effects
of metastases on the host. Wepsic, Nickel, and Alaimo (41) have demonstrated that 3924A has tumor specific antigens. Therefore, the
failure of the tumor to metastasize may be related to this antigenic
response of the host to the tumor.

Hepatome H-4-II-E, which metastasizes to the lungs and axillary
nodes, is carried in our laboratory both in vivo and in vitro. In
vivo H-4-II-E can be used to evaluate (a) the deleterious effects of
tumor on host, (b) the effect of ionizing radiation on the tumor, and
(c) the combined effects of chemotherapy on the tumor and its metastases. Destruction of the primary tumor can be accomplished by local
X-radiation or surgery. The role of the primary tumor on the rate of
growth of metastases could then be studied and attempts made at control
or eradication of the metastases by chemotherapy, or the sequential
use of the chemotherapeutic agents. In vivo, H-4-II-E has an actual
doubling time of 49.2 hr, a potential doubling time of 34.8 hr, and a
cell cycle time of 39.1 hr. T_{G1} is 30.5 hr, T_S 6.0 hr, T_{G2} 2.1 hr and
T_M 0.5 hr. The 1 hr thymidine labelling index is 13.8%, the growth
fraction 100%, and the cell loss factor 0.32 (19).

The effects of therapy are also being evaluated for the very
slow growing hepatoma 16 in order that greater generalization can be
made from results on slow, intermediate, and rapidly growing tumors.
The results from hepatoma 16 may also have more immediate clinical ap-

plication. Hepatoma 16 is a well differentiated tumor with a normal chromosome complement. The volume doubling time for 16 of 587
hr is greater than 10 times that of H-4-II-E (49 hr) and 5 times
greater than that of 3924A (104 hr).

ANALYSIS OF TUMOR GROWTH CURVES

The rate of change of tumor volume with time is one of the
basic measurements for the study of tumor growth. The analysis of
growth curves provides important theoretical and practical information for clinical and experimental oncology.

For an encapsulated tumor, weight would be the best measure of
tumor size since the density is approximately constant. However,
weight measurements of the tumor in vivo are impossible. Therefore,
an external measurement of the tumor mass becomes necessary. Three
methods have traditionally been used to determine tumor size. Each
method relies on external measurements of length, width, and height.
These are tumor volume (1/2 lwh) assuming a hemiellipsoid, surface
area (l x w), and the sum of length and width (l + w).

Although all three formulations can serve as indices of tumor
growth, l x w and l + w were found less meaningful, biologically,
then l x w x h. The measurement (l + w) most often does not double
during the time frame in which reliable measurements can be obtained.
The surface area (l x w) doubling time, if used to compute cell loss
rates, leads to erroneous results, because the surface area doubling
times are much larger than the volume doubling times. Fortunately,
the 1/2 lwh formulation overcomes both of these problems. The simple
exponential growth equation ln (1/2 lwh) = lnVo+B(t) accounts for the
greatest percentage of the total error of the growth of untreated hepatoma 3924A (18) (where Vo is some initial volume; t is time; lwh is
length, width, and height).

Although useful information can be obtained from simply averaging
the tumor response to a given treatment mode, a more comprehensive
picture of the effect of treatment on the tumor can be obtained by considering individual tumor responses. Using both types of analysis has
the advantage of presenting both an overview of the main effects of
treatment, via the averages, and a more detailed examination of the
mechanism by which these effects occur through the analysis of individual responses.

The basic problem of analysis is to extract useful information
about tumor behavior from fluctuating raw data. The rationale behind
the averaging technique is that if the measurement errors are random
(that is, if they give too large a value as often as they give too
small a value), then these errors should cancel out when averaging
over a large sample, leaving the average value as an estimate of the

"true" volume at a given time. In general, the averaging technique
will reveal the overall features of tumor response to a given treatment. However, the process of taking volume averages has a number
of drawbacks when it comes to extracting detailed information from
a set of experimental results, so that it is often necessary to go
beyond this technique in analysis.

The response of individual tumors to treatment is becoming increasingly important since information obtained about differences
in response has more relevance to the clinical management of patients.
The best representation of the data is needed. Therefore, a mathe-
matical function must be found whose parameters can be adjusted so
that the function, when graphed with the data, becomes the best fit
to the data. The functional form used most often is the polynomial
(37). The volume of a tumor as a function of time is represented by:

$$\ln (V/V_o) = a_o + a_1 t + a_2 t^2 + \ldots + a_N t^N$$

Where v is volume, V_o the volume at treatment, and the coefficients
$a_o \ldots a_N$ are the parameters which are adjusted for the fit. With
real data N up to 6 is needed to give good fits.

For a tumor in the exponential phase of growth when it is treated, any one of a number of responses can be seen in the growth curves after treatment (Fig 1). The most desirable result is complete
regression of the tumor. An example of this is labelled "I-A" in
Fig 1. The growth curve is characterized by a steadily decreasing
tumor volume, with no discernible regrowth.

The next most desirable result is typified by the curve reduction of tumor volume below the volume at treatment, but with a subsequent regrowth of the tumor. The term "definite local regression"
is utilized since the volume actually regresses from treatment volume,
but this happens only over a definite time interval.

The curve labelled "II" represents a "pseudo-local regression"
response, and is characterized by a lessening of the tumor volume
below its previous maximum. However, unlike class I-B responses,
these tumors never regress below the volume at the day of treatment.

Finally, there are tumors where the volume never decreases from
one time period to the next, but always exhibits growth. These are
class III responses, with the name "slowdown".

One example of a slowdown response would be a control tumor. No
regression is seen in these tumors, but a steadily changing growth
rate is evident as the tumor ages. For small doses associated with
the treatment, regular changes in growth rate may be observed as well.
In fact, the term "slowdown" is used to refer to those tumors whose

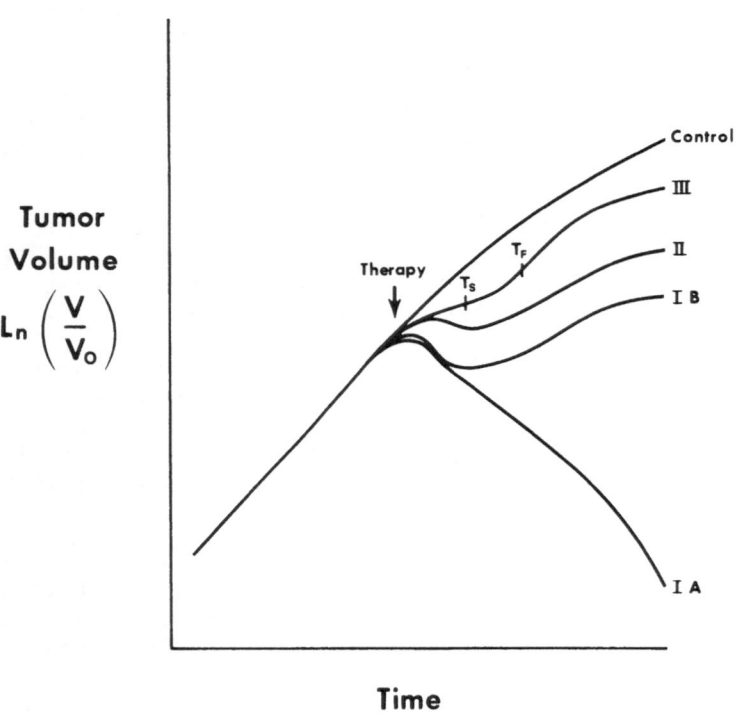

Figure 1

Three classifications of solid tumor response to treatment.

average growth after treatment falls below that of the controls, and the question of whether the growth rate at a specific time following treatment exceeds that of the controls is left open.

For ease of reference, the response classes for post-treatment growth curves are listed below:

Class	Names
I-A	Complete regression
I-B	Definite local regression
II	Pseudo-local regression
III	Slowdown

The actual response curves are a continuum, ranging from those tumors which treatment affects only slightly to those which are completely eliminated. The division of this continuum into the classes listed above is done primarily for reasons of convenience, and because the classes have some relevance in the design of treatment schedules.

THE TIME SEQUENCE OF EFFECTS OF 5-FLUOROURACIL AND ADRIAMYCIN ON CRITICAL HOST ORGANS OF NORMAL AND TUMOR-BEARING RATS

The successful use a chemotherapeutic agent in achieving tumor remission depends both on the cytotoxic effect of the drug on the tumor cell and on the ability of critical organs of the host to recover from these toxic effects.

Scheduling of cancer chemotherapeutic agents for optimal destruction of tumor cells must be within the constraints imposed by the vulnerable host tissues. The gastrointestinal epithelium and the bone marrow usually present the most life-threatening toxic reactions during cancer chemotherapy with cell cycle specific agents. However, the limiting factor in other forms of chemotherapy may be cumulative toxicity to such critical organs as the heart. Studies are in progress on the effects of 5-fluorouracil which is representative of the former type of host organ response and adriamycin which is representative of the latter type of response.

Since its synthesis by Heidelberger and associates (8), 5-fluorouracil (5-FU) has been widely used in the treatment of a number of cancers in man. It is perhaps the most important compound in the treatment of disseminated solid tumors (1), being of value in disseminated cancer of the breast, female genital cancer, and, in combination with radiation, head and neck and bronchogenic cancer. Furthermore, no commercially available drug other than 5-FU is useful, with any

degree of consistence or for a significant duration, in the most
common tumor type encountered, cancer of the gastrointestinal tract
and its appendages.

Early regimens with this drug produced severe toxicity and
some deaths in man (43). Adjustment downward of the dosage (2)
and experience in evaluating toxic symptoms have so reduced the
risk of death that the drug is now considered by some (3, 30) to
be safe for use as an adjuvant following resections for gastrointestinal, breast, or testicular cancers that are high risk for re-
currence.

Adriamycin was first isolated from a mutant strain of Strepto-
myces peucetius by DiMarco and associates (6). It is related structurally to daunomycin, an antibiotic produced by the parent strain
and also having anti-tumor activity, differing from daunomycin only
in the replacement of a hydrogen atom in the acetyl radical of the
aglycone moiety by a hydroxyl group (33). Adriamycin has been quite
successful in preliminary trials in treating patients with a wide
range of tumors. It is believed to act by intercalating or associat-
ing with DNA in a manner similar to that reported for daunomycin (44).
DNA replication and RNA transcription are blocked, with viability
being most affected for cells in the S phase of the cell cycle (11).
Blocks in G_2 (42) and in mitosis (12) have also been reported.

A. Effects of 5-FU on Bone Marrow and Peripheral White Blood Cell Concentrations

The total DNA content of the tibial marrow of rats with hepatoma
3924A following treatment with 150 mg/kg 5-FU is given in Fig 3.
Total DNA content of the tibial marrow as 92% of initial values at 1
hr after treatment and decreased to 11% of initial values 5 days after treatment. Incorporation of ^{3}H-deoxyuridine into marrow DNA was
13% of control during the first hour following 5-FU treatment and
continued to be depressed for 24 hr following treatment (Fig 2). Subsequently, a slow recovery of ^{3}H-deoxyuridine incorproation occurred,
lasting 4 days, and finally on the fifth day after treatment, rapid
recovery was initiated. An increase in total marrow DNA began 6 days
after treatment (Fig 2), in excellent agreement with the ^{3}H-deoxyuridi
incorpoation data. The major increase in bone marrow DNA took place
between 9 and 11 days after treatment. It should be noted in Fig 3
that ACI rats with tumors did not differ appreciably from rats without
tumors with respect to the magnitude and timing of the loss of tibial
marrow DNA after 5-FU treatment.

In Fig 2, the incorporation of ^{3}H-deoxyuridine into marrow DNA
(dpm/mg DNA) for the 5-FU treated rats was approximately twice that
of the non-treated rats at 8 days after drug treatment, then returned
to non-treated values over the subsequent 6 days. However, when the

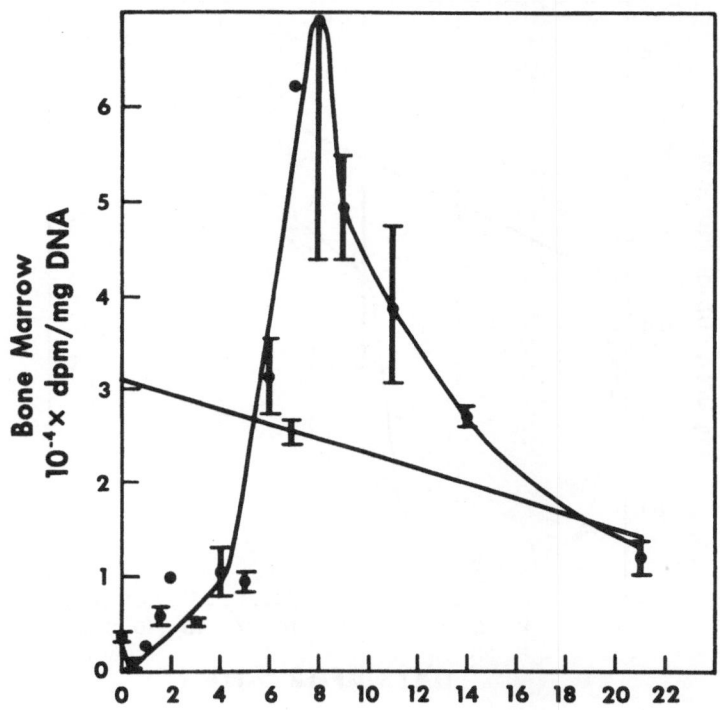

Figure 2
^{3}H–Deoxyuridine incorporation into tibial DNA of rats bearing
hepatoma 3924A, expressed as dpm/mg DNA.

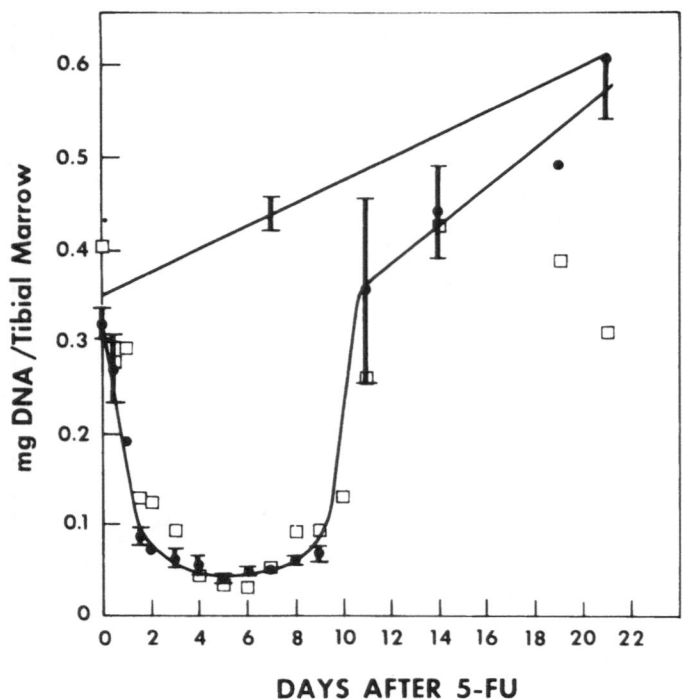

Figure 3
Total DNA content of the tibia marrow from normal and tumor
bearing rats.

data were expressed as dpm/tibia, incorporation of ^{3}H-deoxyuridine
into marrow DNA for the 5-FU treated rats was less than for control
rats during recovery and did not return to control levels until 11
days after treatment (Fig 4). Furthermore, there was no increase
in dpm/tibia from 1 to 4 days following drug treatment, suggesting
that the slow recovery of ^{3}H-deoxyuridine incorporation observed
during this time interval in Fig 1 could be attributed to the continued slow loss of DNA instead of to recovery of proliferative
potential.

White blood cell concentrations were determined in the peripheral blood of these animals. Relative to average initial levels
of 7200 WBC per mm^3 of blood, WBC concentrations were depressed for
9 days after treatment and corresponded to approximately 60% of
the initial levels. Recovery of white cell concentrations in the
blood occurred by day 11. Changes in peripheral white blood cell
concentrations obviously do not indicate the magnitude of the loss
of bone marrow, but do reflect the time interval of marrow depression.

B. Recovery of Host Bone Marrow Following Different Doses of
    5-FU

The times considered to be most sensitive to differences in
initiation of recovery of the various organs were chosen from the
time-course of recovery of host organs following 150 mg/kg 5-FU.
Doses of 0, 50, 100 and 150 mg/kg were compared at 1, 3, 6 and 9
days after injection; larger doses were not evaluated since animal
lethality precludes their therapeutic usefulness. The 3 doses of
5-FU tested were equally effective in inhibiting incorporation of
^{3}H-deoxyuridine at 24 hrs after administering the drug. Inhibition
of incorporation was greater than 90% for each dose and each host
organ at this time.

Recovery of bone marrow took place earlier following 50 mg/kg
5-FU than following 100 or 150 mg/kg 5-FU. This is indicated by the
larger average incorporation of ^{3}H-deoxyuridine into tibial DNA for
the 50 mg/kg dose at 3 days (71,700, 7,400 and 6,400 dpm/mg DNA for
50, 100 and 150 mg/kg 5-FU, respectively), and the larger average
DNA content per tibia for the 50 mg/kg dose at 6 days (0.29, 0.06 and
0.07 mg DNA/tibia for 50, 100 and 150 mg/kg 5-FU respectively).

C. Effects of Adriamycin on the Heart, Bone Marrow and
    Peripheral Blood

Changes in the total DNA content of the tibia after 10 mg/kg of
adriamycin are shown in Fig 5. This is an index of cell loss and cell
regeneration after adriamycin. The data suggests a compensating
"over shoot" during the second week. The magnitude of depression of
the cellular content of the tibia is much less than after 150 mg/kg

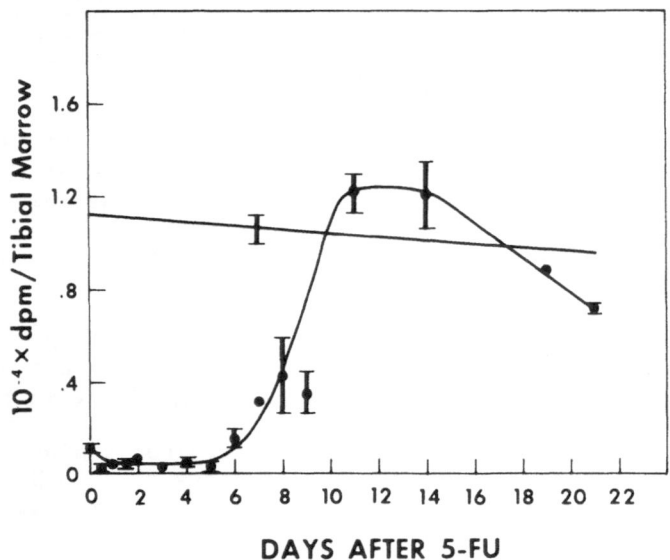

Figure 4
³H-Deoxyuridine incorporation into tibial DNA of rats bearing hepatoma
3924A, expressed as dpm/tibial marrow. ●, mean ± standard error for
3 rats with hepatomas given a single injection of 150 mg/kg 5-FU.
☐, mean for 3 ACI rats without hepatomas given 150 mg/kg 5-FU.
_____, linear regression line ± standard error of the overall mean
for data from rats with hepatomas given 0.9% NaCl.

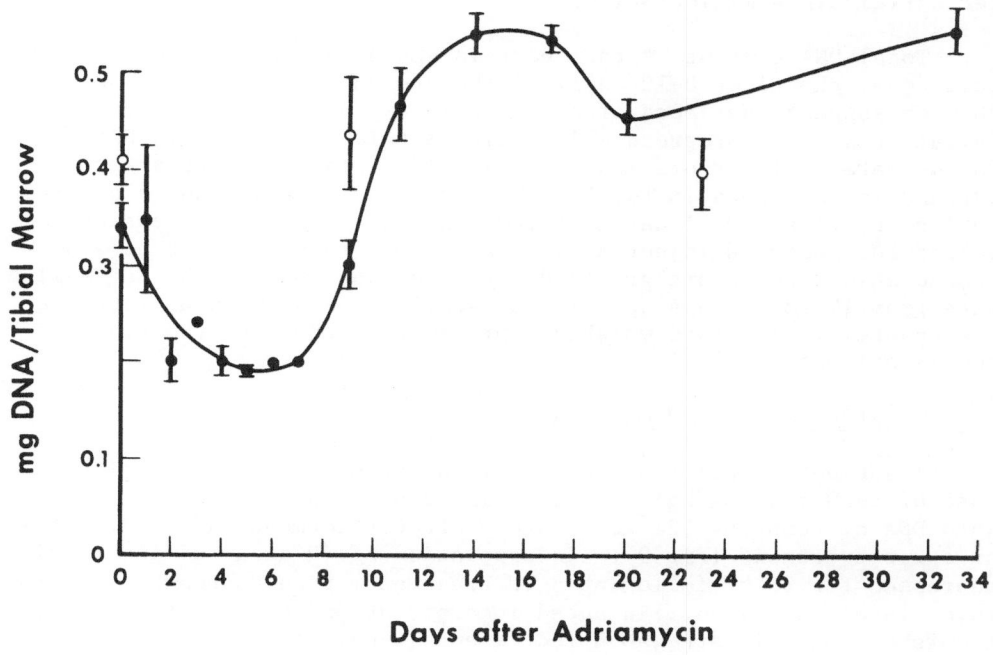

Figure 5
Effect of adriamycin (10mg/kg) on tibial bone marrow of ACI rats.
Total tibial bone marrow DNA of three rats. Control rats O; adria-
mycin treated rats , expressed as mean ± standard error.

5-FU; however, the time sequence of changes are similar since the recovery of both 5-FU and adriamycin occurs 10-11 days after treatment. The changes in the rate of ^{3}H-thymidine incorporation into bone marrow DNA are shown in Fig 6. The incorporation rates return to control values in 8 days compared to 16 days for 5-FU. Peripheral WBC concentrations were only marginally depressed by the adriamycin treatment during the period of bone marrow depression. Hemoglobin and hematocrit values indicated some hemoconcentration at 2-3 days; however, they were within normal limits over the 33 day period after adriamycin administration.

Total DNA content of the heart is shown in Fig 7. Fluctuations occur over the first 8-10 days. These are not significant; however, they do suggest that loss of heart cells may be occurring. Pathological studies in progress will evaluate this possibility. Changes in the rate of incorporation of ^{3}H-thymidine in the heart after adriamycin are shown in Fig 8. The most significant changes occur during the first 10-11 days, as for bone marrow. The decreasing values for controls injected with saline may be the result of continued animal and heart growth during the experiment. The decreasing rate from 12 to 33 days appears to parallel the decreasing rates in the controls. The rats weighed approximately 120 g at the start of the experiment.

D. Effects of 5-FU on Hepatoma 3924A

Treatment of rats bearing Morris hepatoma 3924A with a single dose of 5-FU (150 mg/kg) inhibited incorporation of ^{3}H-deoxyuridine into DNA of tumor by 92% immediately after treatment and by 97% at 12 hr after treatment (Fig 9). Incorporation of ^{3}H-deoxyruidine remained depressed for 36 hr following 5-FU treatment, then approached control tumor levels by day 4. Enhanced incorproration relative to that for tumors of control rats was noted 11 and 14 days after treatment but this did not exceed the incorporation for control tumors at the beginning of the experiment. In a separate experiment it was found that incorporation of ^{3}H-deoxyuridine into tumor DNA was also inhibited by more than 90% 24 hr after injection of 5-FU for doses of 50 or 100 mg/ kg. Tumor growth inhibition following 50, 100, 150, 200 and 250 mg/kg 5-FU resulted in tumor volumes which averaged 88, 67, 37, 35 and 50 percent, respectively, of those of non-treated rats 11 days after treatment.

E. Animal Survival Following a Second Injection of 5-FU

A second injection of 150 mg/kg 5-FU was given normal rats at various times after a first injection. Percentage survival for these rats is presented in Fig 8. Survival is clearly a function of the time which has elapsed since the previous injection. When the second injection was given 12 hrs after the first, 68% of the rats survived.

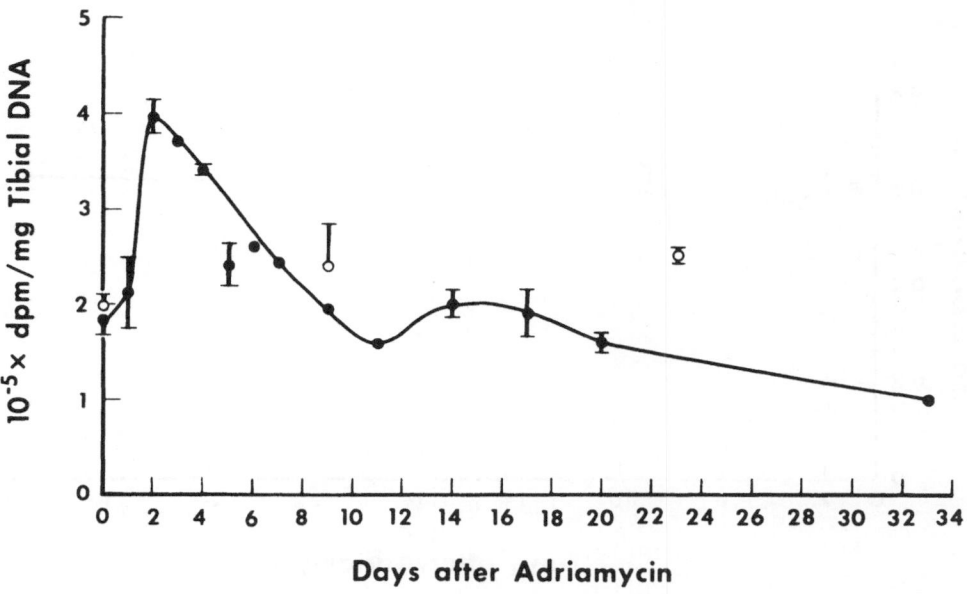

Figure 6

³H-thymidine incorporation into tibial DNA of normal rats and rats
given adriamycin (10 mg/kg) expressed as means ± standard errors for
three rats. Control rats 0; adriamycin treated rats .

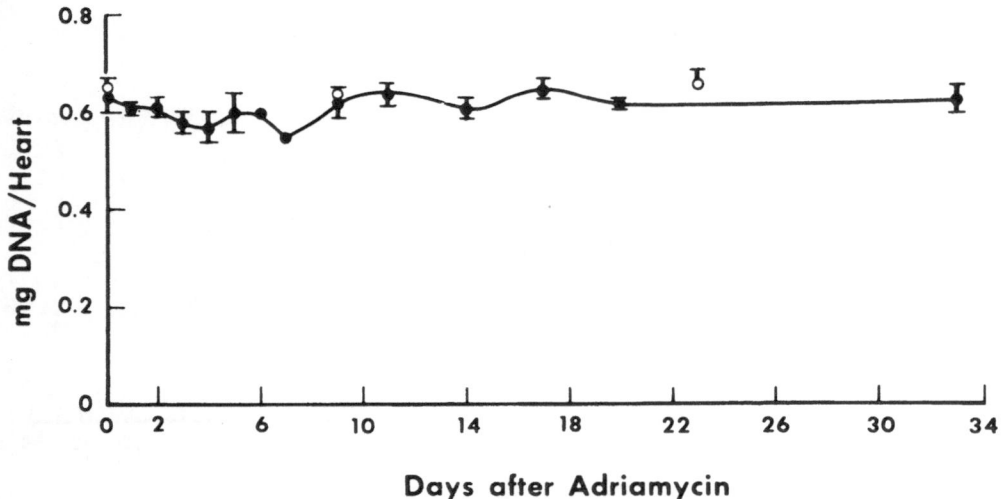

Figure 7
Effect of adriamycin (10 mg/kg) on the total DNA content of the
heart. Expressed as mg DNA/heart for three rats. Control rats 0;
adriamycin treated rats   .

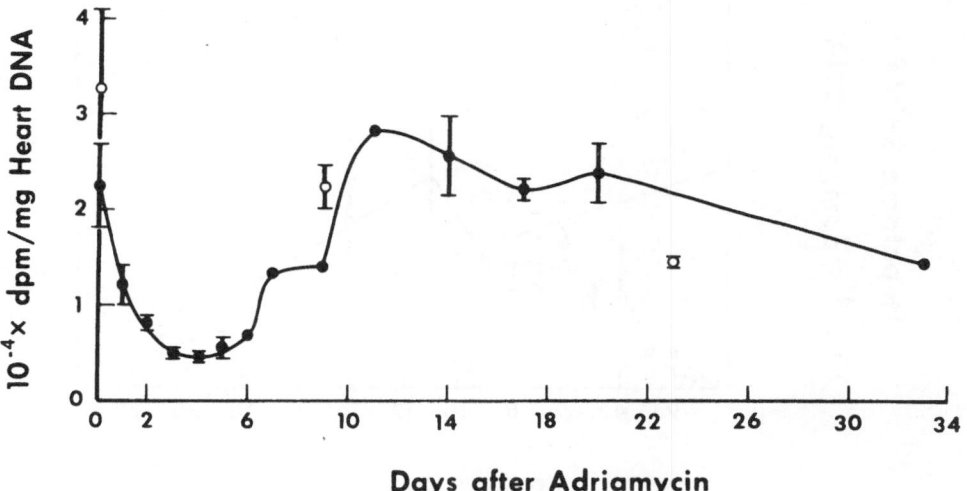

Figure 8

^{3}H-thymidine incorporation into heart DNA of normal rats and rats
given adriamycin (10 mg/kg) expressed dpm/mg heart DNA. The values
are expressed as means $\pm$ standard errors for three rats. Control
rats 0; adriamycin treated rats .

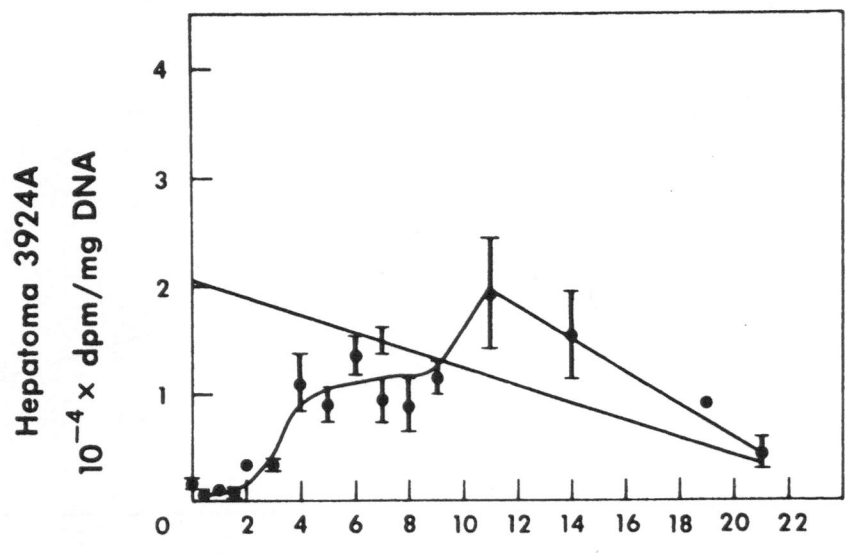

Days after 5 - FU

Figure 9

Effect of 5-FU on ^{3}H-deoxyuridine incorporation into DNA of
hepatoma 3924A. Each rat received 50 uCi (16 nmoles) deoxyuridine-
6-H[3] 1 hr prior to sacrifice. •, mean ± standard error for 3 rats
given a single injection of 150 mg/kg 5-FU, except 2 rats when no
standard error is indicated. _____, linear regression line ±
standard error of the overall mean for data from rats given 0.9%
NaCl.

At longer time intervals of 3-4 days between treatments, just
prior to rapid cell proliferation in bone marrow (Fig 10) and coinciding with rapid cell proliferation in intestinal mucosa, the
second injection resulted in the death of 100% of the rats tested.
Still longer intervals between injections were characterized by
progressively increasing animal survival. By 10-11 days following
the first injection when the DNA contents of both intestinal mucosa
and tibial marrow had returned to pre-treatment levels all the rats
survived the second 150 mg/kg injection of 5-FU.

EFFECTS OF INCREASING DOSES OF RADIOTHERAPY AND CHEMOTHERAPY (5-FU)
ON TUMOR GROWTH

For radiation studies, groups of 16 rats were given OR, 375R,
750R, 1500R, 2250R and 3750R of radiation locally to the tumor,
which was growing subcutaneously. Local tumor radiation was carried out with a 250kV, 30MA General Electric Maxitron 250 using
filters if 0.25 mm Cu and 1.0 mm Al. Prior to irradiation the
animals were anesthesized with ether and placed in a lead-shielded
box through which the tumor protruded. The midpoint of the tumor
was approximately 6 cm from the X-ray tube target and received the
calculated dose while the animal body received 0.5% of the dose delivered to the irradiated tumor. A plexiglass cover was placed
over the animal and the target cone lowered to prevent tumor displacement. The rats in the 5-fluorouracil studies were divided into
groups of 12 rats each. One group served as control and other
groups were given single intraperitoneal injection of 50, 100, 150
200 and 250 mg 5-FU/kg body weight (21).

There was a rapid decrease in tumor volume with increasing
radiation doses up to 1500R, the rate of decrease falling with
doses in excess of 1500R. At varying times after irradiation tumor
growth was reestablished and was comparable to the rate of growth
in the control groups (Fig 11). After 3750R, tumor regression occurred (Fig 12). The effects of different radiation doses on the
mean tumor volumes 30 days after tumor inoculation and 16 days after
irradiation are shown in Fig 13. The delay in days for each irradiated group to reach 40,000 mm^3 was compared to the number of days
required for the control group to reach 40,000 mm^3 (Fig 14).

Tumor response to increasing doses of radiation and 5-FU have
been summarized in Table 3 according to class of response.
Examination of the table reveals several important points:

i) As the radiation dose is increased from 375R to 3750R, the
predominant response goes from class III (slowdown) to class I-A
(complete regression). The "crossover" dose, at which a sizeable
percentage fall into each of the three classes, appears to be at
about 1500R.

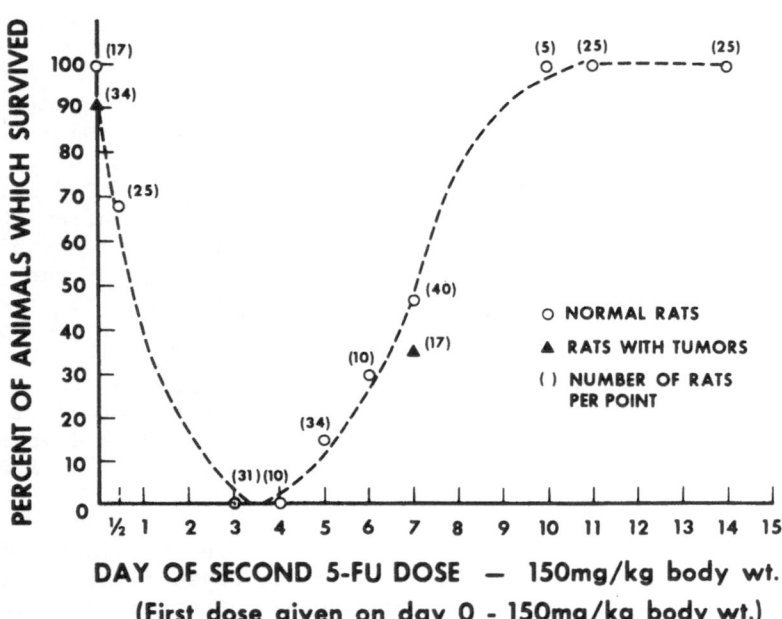

Figure 10
Survival of normal and hepatoma 3924A bearing ACI rats given
two injections of 5-FU. A second injection of 150 mg/kg 5-FU was
given at varying intervals of time after the first injection and
survival determined 19 days later. Data plotted at time 0 was obtained for rats given only a single injection of 150 mg/kg 5-FU.

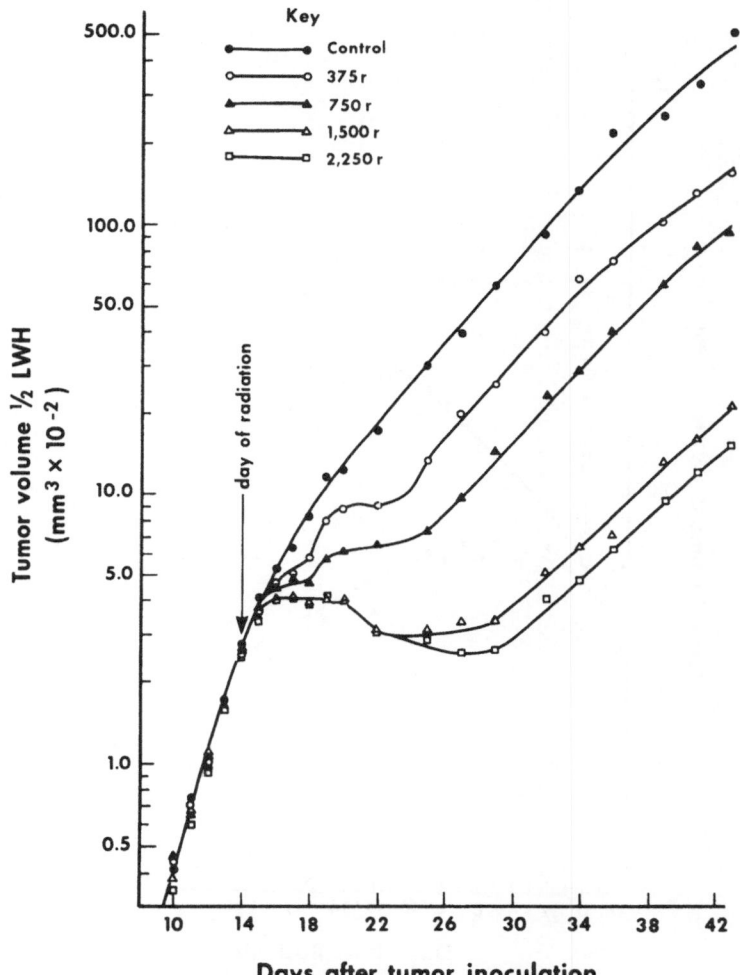

Figure 11
Growth curves for hepatoma 3924A after 375R, 750R, 1500R, and
2250R. Each symbol represents the average volume for 16 tumors.

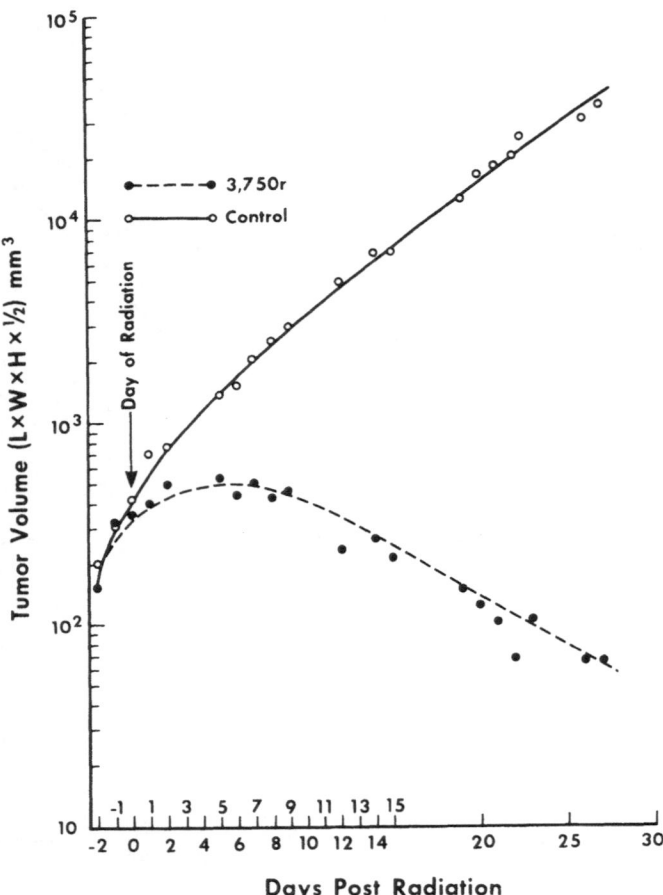

Figure 12
Growth curves for hepatoma 3924A after 3750R.

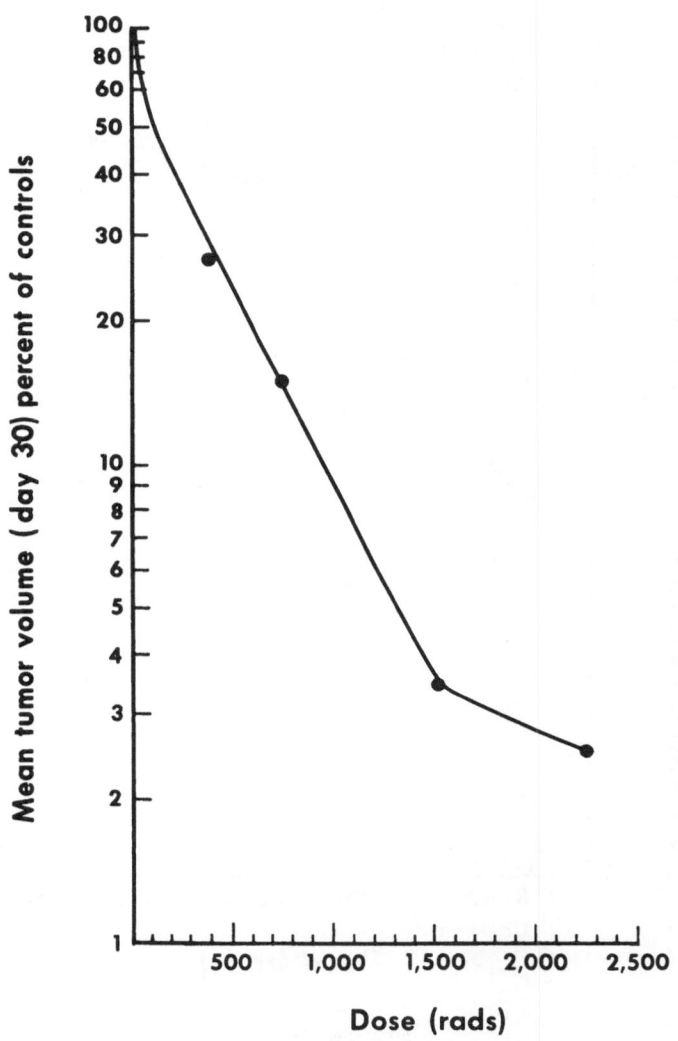

Figure 13
The mean tumor volumes in the irradiated and control groups
30 days after inoculation and 16 days after radiation.

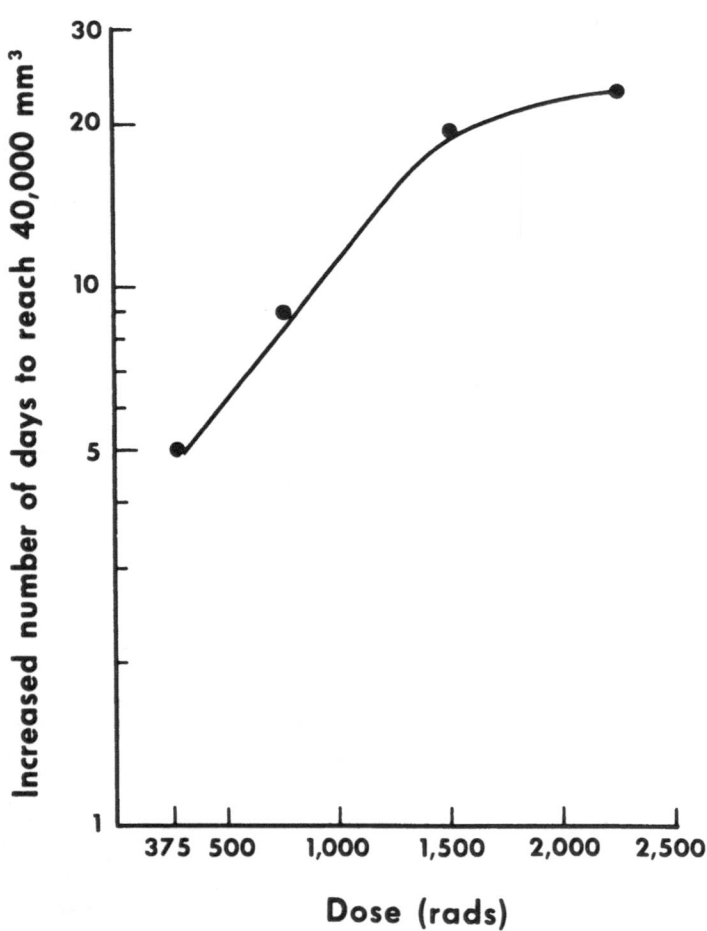

Figure 14
The time in days necessary for the mean tumor volumes in the
irradiated and control groups to reach 40,000 m³.

Table Three
Classification of Tumor Response to Treatment
(Percentage)

Class	Radiation R						5-FU (mg/kg)					
	0	375R	750R	1500R	2250R	3750R	0	50	100	150	200	250
IA Regression				.06		1.00						
IB Definite Local Regression				.38	.64					.13	.20	
II Pseudo Regression				.38	.21					.50	.40	.27
III Slowdown	.75	1.00	.93	.19	.14		.92	.91	.92	.38	.40	.71
Number of Animals	16	16	15	16	14	6	12	11	12	8	5	7

ii) Although it is possible to specify which type of reaction
is predominantly induced by each dose, for most doses there are a
wide variety of responses from individual tumors, so that it is impossible to predict how an individual tumor will respond to most
treatment modes.

iii) 5-FU shows a dose response similar to radiation for
doses less than 1500R. The response is predominantly class III
(slowdown), with some hint of the onset of class II at 200-250 mg/
kg. Unfortunately, the toxicity of the drug makes it impossible
to increase the dose beyond this level.

iv) The transition from one predominant reaction to another is
not smooth and gradual, but rather in the nature of a fairly sharp
plateau, beyond which doses may again be increased for a while without making major changes in response patterns.

Examining the details of the responses within each category
revealed interesting regularities in the data. The most striking
of these occurred in the slowdown type reaction.

The time for minimum tumor growth after radiation was approximately 6 days and for 5-FU 5 days. These times for minimum tumor
growth following either radiation or 5-FU were essentially independent of dose over the entire range of therapy for both treatment
modalities. The time for maximum tumor growth after radiation increased from day 18 for 375R to day 22 for 1500R. On the other
hand, the day of maximum growth after 5-FU was day 12 for the entire
dose range from 50 to 250 mg/kg.

The times, relative to the day of treatment (t=0), when the
tumor achieves minimum and maximum growth rates are shown in Fig 15.
In addition, the effect of dose on these two responses are presented.
The time it takes for the tumor to respond to small doses of 5-FU or
radiation seems to be independent of the dose itself, and to depend
only moderately on the treatment mode.

The magnitude of the treatment induced change in growth rate is
defined by a "treatment efficiency"

$$Q_{III} = 1 - \frac{b_{min}}{\langle b \rangle}$$

where b_{min} is the minimum value of the growth rate a particular tumor
assumes after treatment, and $\langle b \rangle$ is the average growth rate of the
controls at the time the growth rate minimum occurs. Q_{III} varies
smoothly from zero (when there is no difference between the treated
tumors and the controls) to one (when the growth rate goes to zero
and the response moves into class II). In a similar way, a parameter

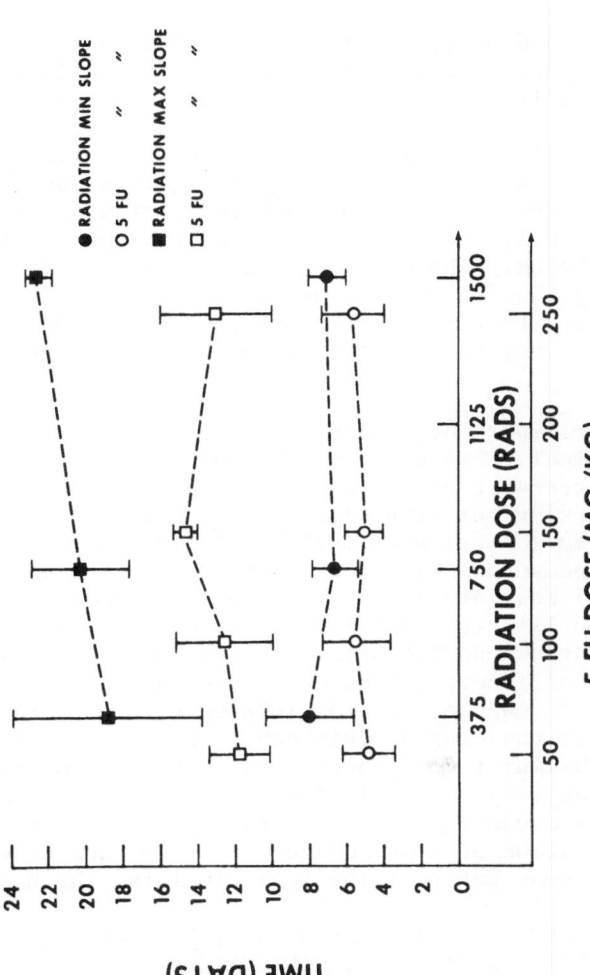

Figure 15

The times for minimum and maximum tumor volume change following treatment (t=0) as a function of dose. ●, radiation minimum slope, ○, 5-FU minimum slope; ■, radiation maximum slope;□ , 5-FU maximum slope.

which measures the maximum growth rate can be obtained from:

$$Q'_{III} = 1 - \frac{b_{max}}{\langle b \rangle}$$

where b_{max} is the value for the growth rate at its maximum.

In Fig 16, Q_{III} and Q'_{III} are plotted for both 5-FU and radiation. A consistent increase of both indices is seen with increasing doses of radiation until saturation (at the value one) is reached.

Quantitative regularities in the growth response following radiation demonstrated a continuous increase in efficiency of treatment for radiation. Progressive changes in growth response from III, slowdown, to I, regression, occurred through the radiation dose range 375R to 3750R. The efficiency of treatment for 5-FU with dose up to 150 mg/kg then remained constant for further increases in dose to 250 mg/kg. Factors such as increased 5-FU toxicity to the host may prevent increase in effectiveness of 5-FU for doses above 150 mg/kg.

One of the most important findings of the study in particular with regard to clinical relevance, was the observation of well defined times after treatment at which minimum and maximum tumor growth occur. These consistent perturbations of growth reflect the perturbations induced by radiation on cell birth and are a direct reflection of the response of cell proliferation kinetics to radiation. Recovery of critical host organs from the toxic effects of 5-FU is essentially complete 11 days following treatment as evidenced by (1) normal tibial marrow and intestinal mucosa DNA contents; (2) nearly normal rates of incorporation of ^{3}H-deoxyuridine into DNA of marrow and intestinal mucosa, and (3) 100% survival for rats given a second injection if the drug on this day. The convergence of these parameters (maximum tumor growth rate, maximum DNA synthesis in the tumor, and recovery of critical host organs) at 11 days after initial treatment is advantageous from a therapeutic standpoint since it permits administration of a second dose of 5-FU when effectiveness is maximal for the tumor but toxicity is minimal for the host.

THE EFFECTS OF A SINGLE DOSE OF IRRADIATION (1500R) ON THREE TUMORS
WITH MARKEDLY DIFFERENT GROWTH RATE, HISTOPATHOLOGIC AND CELL KINETIC
CHARACTERISTICS

Three hepatoma lines with widely differing growth rates, histopathologic and cell kinetic characteristics were selected for comparative studies of response to a single dose (1500R) of radiation. The volume doubling times of the heaptomas are: H-4-II-E - 49 hr; 3924A - 96 hr; and 16 - 587 hr; and the cell cycle times determined for the three tumor lines are 39.1 hr, 27.9 hr and 331.9 hr. respec-

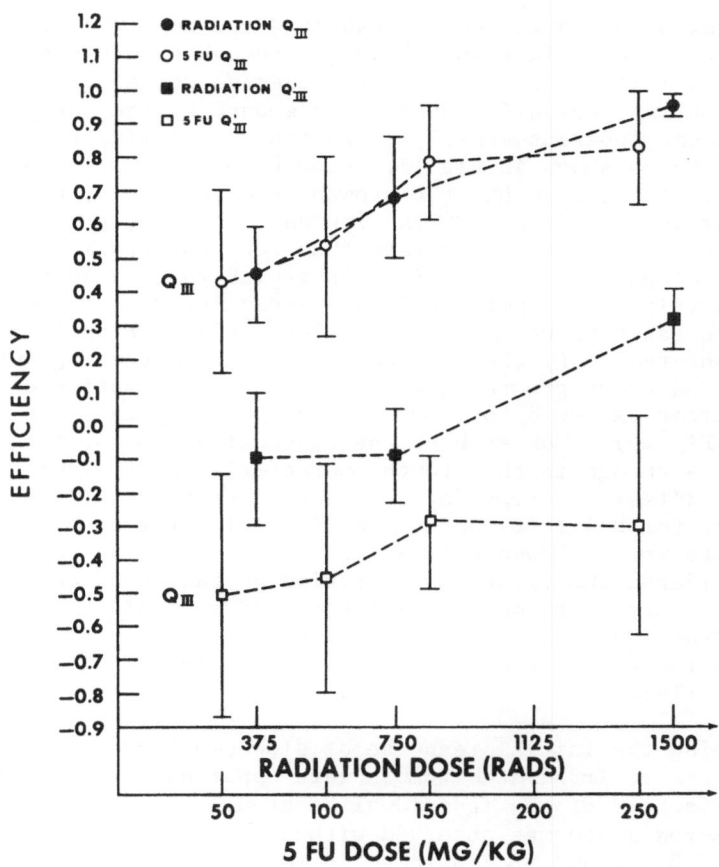

Figure 16
The minimum tumor volume change (Q_{III}) and the maximum tumor
volume change (Q'_{III}) efficiency indicated as a function of dose.
●, radiation Q_{III}: O, 5-FU Q_{III};■ ,radiation Q'_{III};□ , 5-FU Q'_{III}.

tively (See Tables 1 and 2). The response of all three tumors was
assayed by relative change in tumor volume. The response to a
single exposure of X-radiation is discussed from a multiparametrical
viewpoint in hopes of contributing additional insight into the
problems involved in attempting to better define the radiosensitivity
and radioresistance of solid tumors (14).

The growth curves for both irradiated and non-irradiated hepatomas are reproduced in Figs 17-19. Although growth rates similar
to those of non-irradiated tumors are observed for at least 24 hr
postradiation, obvious differences in response by the three tumors
to 1500R become apparent shortly thereafter. H-4-II-E tumors respond to 1500R as shown in Fig 17. Growth continues for 48 hr and
during the subsequent 24 hr, the growth rate is slowed, remaining
retarded for about 3 days. By the 7th day, however, growth is re-
sumed but at a somewhat slower rate than for non-irradiated tumors.
Hepatoma 3924A undergoes a slowdown in growth rate 24-48 hr after
irradiation (Fig 18). There follows a 4-day interval where essentially no growth takes place, and on days 7-8 a slight drop in mean tumor
volume is observed. By the 15th day, tumors commence regrowth at a
non-irradiated tumor growth rate. The first perturbation of hepatoma
16 growth after exposure to 1500R appears to commence on day 26 postradiation (Fig 19). For each of the respective tumors, the first indication of a change in the growth characteristics following 1500R
occurred at different times for the respective tumors (24 hr for
3924A, 48 hr for H-4-II-E, and 624 hr for 16). For each tumor, this
response involved a slowdown in growth. These initial perturbations
can be considered the first manifestation of radiation damage on the
tumor growth rate. It would appear that these initial radiation-in-
duced perturbations are linked to the cell cycle time (Table 4), the
response to 1500R occurring after 1.8 cell cycle times for all three
tumor lines (14).

Following the initial response of slowdown, however, subsequent
volume changes in irradiated tumors were apparently related to the
"cell loss factor" of the individual hepatoma. The most dramatic response to X-radiation was observed with 3924A (with the highest cell
loss factor, $\emptyset$ = 0.60), followed by 16 ($\emptyset$ = 0.42), and lastly by H-4-
II-E ($\emptyset$ = 0.32).

If there is a dose effect on the relationship between the cell
loss factor and the radiation response of solid tumors it must be an
indirect effect, mediated through the presence of a radioresistant
anoxic or hypoxic cell population. At least for the carcinomas, the
presence of an anoxic cell population has been related to both the
structural and vascular architecture of the tumors. Denekamp (5) has
suggested that the difference in radiation response between carcinomas
and slowly growing sarcomas may be related either to the vascular supply, the manner in which tumor cells die and are removed, or the amount

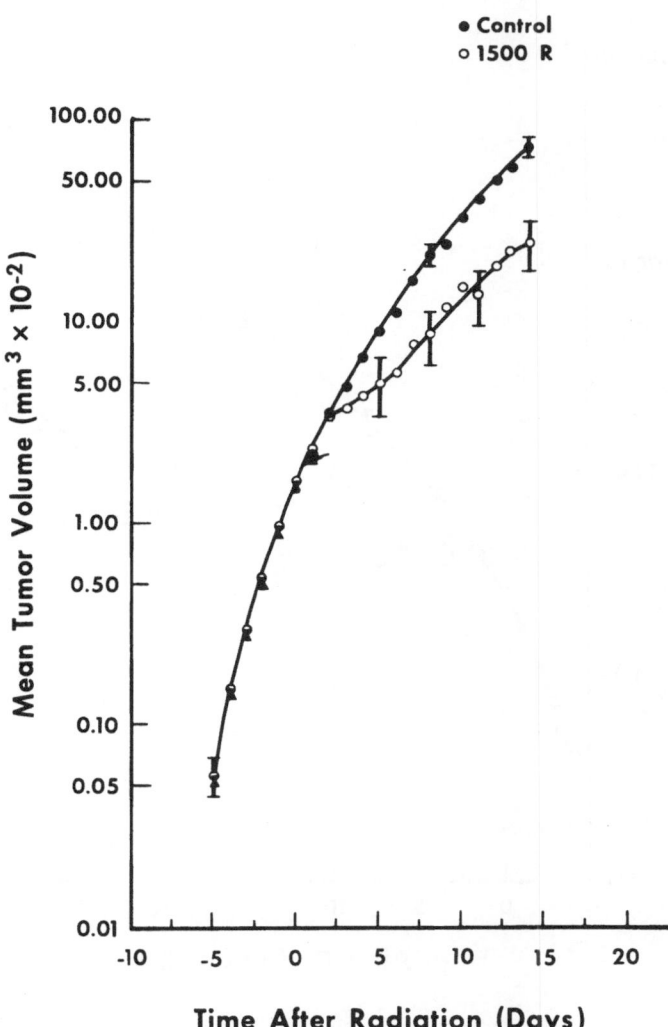

Figure 17
The effect of 1500R of local tumor radiation on the growth characteristics of hepatoma H-4-II-E. Each point represents the mean tumor volume of 12 tumors. Standard errors are given for different times for both control and irradiated tumors. Day 0 is the day of local tumor radiation.

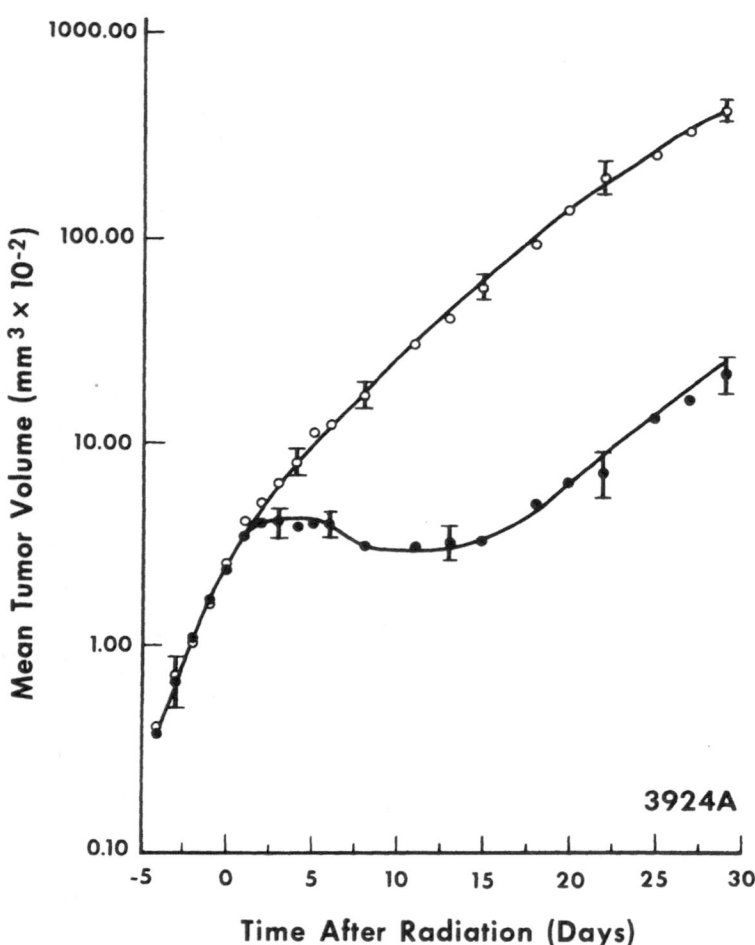

Figure 18
    The effect of 1500R of local tumor radiation on the growth
characteristics of hepatoma 3924A.   Each point represents the mean
tumor volume of 12 tumors.   Standard errors are given for different
times for both control and irradiated tumors.   Day 0 is the day of
local tumor radiation.

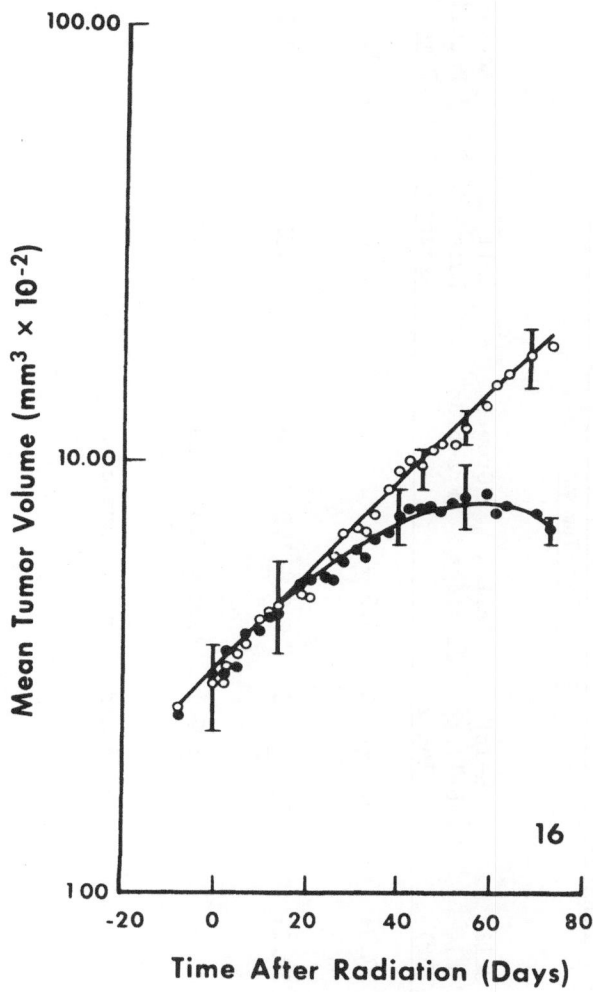

Figure 19
The effect of 1500R of local tumor radiation on the growth
characteristics of hepatoma 16. Each point represents the mean
tumor volume of 12 tumors. Standard errors are given for different
times for both control and irradiated tumors. Day 0 is the day of
local tumor radiation.

Table Four

Comparative Growth and Cell Proliferation Kinetics of

Three Rat Tumors

Tumor Line	Cell Cycle (hr)	^{3}H-TdR Labelling Index	Cell Density*	Growth Fraction	Cell Loss Factor	Actual Doubling Time (hr)
3924A	27.9+	16.3 $\pm$ 0.6	78.0 $\pm$ 4.1	65	0.60	96
H-4-II-E	39.1+	13.8 $\pm$ 0.5	49.5 $\pm$ 1.0	100	0.32	49.2
16	331.9+	2.2 $\pm$ 0.1	23.2 $\pm$ 0.3	100	0.42	587

* Cell number per unit microscope field of tumor parenchyma

+ 3924A, reference (23)
   H-4-II-E, reference (16)
   16, reference (20)

of edema resulting from radiation damage. The efficiency of dead
cell removal is probably related to the vascular architecture and
the position of dead cells relative to the surrounding blood ves-
sels. Hepatoma H-4-II-E is a highly vascularized tumor with a distinct microvasculature in addition to numerous sinosoids. One
would therefore expect that at a dose of 1500R, H-4-II-E would respond more rapidly than hepatoma 3924A where the vascularization is
less extensive and capillaries are difficult to distinguish in 4 μ
histological sections due to the extensive fibrous components of
the stroma. Furthermore both H-4-II-E and 3924A have similar
amounts of necrotic tissue (Table 5) suggesting that little distinction can be made between the efficiency of cell removal in
these two hepatomas.

    The question remains, therefore: Why does hepatoma H-4-II-E
respond less to a dose of 1500R X-ray than 3924A? The most obvious
differences between these two rapidly growing hepatomas, in addition
to the number of cells proliferating and the cell loss factor, are
the amounts of blood within the capillaries and sinusoids and the
connective tissue associated with the tumor mass (Table 5). The
concepts of "cell loss", and to a certain extent the rate of cell
proliferation, have already been discussed above. Radiosensitivity,
however, is generally described clinically in terms of the severity
of a radiation effect such as the reduction in size of a tumor. Inherent in the definition of radiosensitivity is the turnover rate of
cells (i.e., the rate of cell production and removal by lysis or
phagocytosis). From the data presented here, we have been unable to
confer sole responsibility for the radiation effect on either of
these measurable parameters of tumor growth. While there have been
reports of a correlation between tumor doubling time and ^{3}H-TdR
labeling indices with radiosensitivity, our data suggests that these
parameters, by themselves, are inadequate to categorize the radiosensitivity of solid tumors.

    In addition to vasculature, the hepatomas show diversity in
their relative interstitial and vascular connective tissue content
(Table 5). Changes in tumor volume require that both the parenchymal
and stromal tissues increase during growth and decrease during regression. It is possible then that tumors with high parenchymal cell
densities and connective tissue contents would require more efficient
cell removal and connective tissue resorption for shrinkage.
Thomlinson (36) suggests that a slower rate of removal of tumor tissue sterilized by radiation occurs when adjacent connective tissue
has been heavily irradiated. Collectively, then, the rate of cell
loss and the amount of interstitial connective tissue offer an explanation for the type of initial dose response observed with hepatomas 3924A and H-4-II-E.

    It is evident that many of the basic questions of solid tumor

Table Five

Comparative Histopathology of Three Rat Tumors

Relative Tissue

Constituents*

Tumor Line	Tumor	Necrotic	Connective	Blood
3924A	51.1 ± 1.5	17.6 ± 0.9	26.0 ± 2.3	5.2 ± 0.8
H-4-II-E	44.8 ± 1.9	10.5 ± 1.0	6.0 ± 0.5	38.5 ± 2.1
16	72.0 ± 1.9	4.4 ± 0.7	8.4 ± 0.8	8.1 ± 0.8

*Percent of total

radiosensitivity or radioresistance remain unanswered. Studies
such as these on different tumor lines with different morphological
cell kinetic and growth characteristics provide one of the more
promising approaches to gaining new insight into the radiosensitivity and radioresistance of solid tumors. Evaluation of changes in
cell cycle times, actual and potential volume doubling times, cell
loss factors and growth fractions provides a more comprehensible
evaluation of net tumor growth following therapy. These additional
parameters along with classical studies of morphological changes
following therapy should permit correlation of the dynamic changes
that occur in the tumor in relation to the pathological changes.
Further studies should provide the framework for updating our
traditional concepts of radiosensitivity and radioresistance primarily based on tumor morphology to more dynamic concepts based on the
multi-parametric evaluation of tumor response following therapy.

THE UTILIZATION OF THE TUMOR LINE H-4-II-E FOR IN VIVO AND IN
    VITRO EVALUATION OF SINGLE AND COMBINED MODALITY THERAPY

    Studies of the effects of radiation and chemotherapeutic agents
in tissue culture provides the means of elucidating the mechanism of
action of the chemotherapeutic agents and radiation under standard
and well defined conditions. Results of studies in vitro should be
most helpful in in vivo experiments designed to produce maximum cell
kill from the use of chemotherapy followed by radiotherapy and radiotherapy followed by chemotherapy. More importantly, transplanted
tumor lines, adapted to or selected for growth in cell culture allows
the survival (clonogenicity) of cells of solid tumors treated in vivo
to be assayed in vitro.

    The advent of assay systems which can quantitatively relate
treatment efficacy with cell survival (i.e., clonogenicity) is a
major requisite for understanding the long-term cellular response of
both normal and neoplastic tissue. Both in tissue culture and by the
transplantation of dispersed cellular systems, accurate quantitative
estimates of cell survival after irradiation and chemotherapy are possible. Recently, a number of solid tumor systems have been adapted
for in vitro assay of reproductive intergrity: the R-1 rhabdomysar-
coma (9), the EMT6 sarcoma (32), and the HLAC adenocarcinoma (35).
The H-4-II-E tumor cell system joins this small but expanding number
of diverse solid tumor models that can be used to quantitatively relate clonogenicity of the primary tumor to treatment efficacy (13, 19).

    The H-4-II-E cell line was derived from the Reuber H-35 hepatoma
(31) which was chemically induced in a male ACI rat following the
feeding of N-2-fluorenyldiacetamide. The primary culture (H-4) was
subcultured five times and passed through a male ACI rat giving rise
to a transplantable tumor ($H-35_{tc1}$) and a second cell culture (H-4-
II). This culture produced a second transplantable tumor ($H-35_{tc2}$)
when passed through female ACI rats. The H-4-II culture was sub-

cultured twice and "colony cloned" three times to give rise to the
cell line H-4-II-E which has been continuous culture since that
time (29). The H-4-II-E hepatoma, growing in the male ACI rat, results from subcutaneous injection of cultured H-4-II-E cells. The
H-4-II-E cells obtained from the hepatoma were passaged alternately
between culture and animal to select for optimal clonogenic characteristics, thus preventing adaptation to either the in vivo or the
in vitro environment exclusively.

H-4-II-E has a cell cycle time of 39.1 hr, an actual volume
doubling time of 49 hr, a growth fraction of 100% and a cell loss
factor of 0.32. The cell kinetics at the center and periphery of
the tumor are similar to the cell kinetics of a random evaluation
throughout the tumor (See Table 4) (19).

Cell cycle analysis by the percent labelled mitoses (PLM) method
was carried out on both exponential and plateau phase growth cultures.
From the data PLM curves were generated by computer analysis. In
each case, the cultures were supplied with fresh medium at the time
cell cycle experiments were initiated, but not during the experiment.
For exponential cultures, the maximum PLM was 100 with a second maximum at 61 percent. The cycle time (T_C) was calculated to be 17.7 hr,
compatible with a population-doubling time of 18.4 hr (Table 6) (13).

Notable characteristics of the PLM curve for plateau phase cells
are the failure of the first wave to reach 100% and the absence of a
well defined second wave. The projected T_C for plateau phase is approximately 128.4 hr, although the PLM curve suggests that G_1 is
probably highly variable in duration and that a certain population of
G_2 cells are retained in G_2 for long periods of time prior to passing
into mitoses. The greatest prolongation of phase occurs in G_1
although G_2 and S are also somewhat longer in plateau phase.

The progression of cells through the cell cycle in both exponential and plateau phase cultures was measured by continuous incubation
with labelled thymidine. For exponential phase cultures, approximately 27% of the cell population was in the S phase initially (33% L.I.
after 1 hr). The rate of entry of G_1 cells into S is seen to approach
7-8% per hr. Based on this rate of entry and the cell cycle phase
durations, all cycling cells should be labelled within 11 hr (T_{G2} +
T_M + T_{G1}) following the addition of labelled thymidine. Experimentally, all cells were labelled after 12 hr in ^{3}H-TdR indicating a growth
fraction of 100%; this value is in good agreement with a GF of 96.2
approximated from the T_C (13).

The results of the in vivo and in vitro survival curves following radiation demonstrate how this tumor line can be used to evaluate
the effects of different forms of treatment in tissue culture and in

Table Six
Kinetic Parameters for Exponential and
Plateau Phase Cultures Fed
Daily

	Exponential	Plateau
*T_{G1}	7.6 ± 4.2	114.0 ± 207.0
*T_{G2}	2.3 ± 0.8	6.1 ± 2.6
*T_S	6.8 ± 0.4	7.3 ± 0.7
*T_M	1.0	1.0
*T_C	17.7	128.4
Mitotic index (M.I.)	4.3	0.04
^{3}H-TdR L.I.	33.0	8.0
Population doubling time (PD)	18.4	-----
Maximum cell density (cells/20 cm^2 dish)	-----	2.5 x 10^7
Plating efficiency (PE)	53.1 ± 7.9	

* mean duration of cell cycle time phases given in hr ± S.D.
  Values for L.I., M.I. and PE are given in %.

the animal. The survival curve for exponentially growing cultures
of H-4-II-E cells irradiated in vitro under conditions of normal
aeration is shown Fig 20. The Do is 190R with an extrapolation
number of 1.6. Each point represents the mean value of 10 samples.
The survival curve for hepatoma H-4-II-E cells irradiated in situ
is shown in Figure 21. The Do is 240R with an extrapolation number
of 4. Each point represents the mean value $\pm$ S.E. of 3-9 air breathing animals (16).

The growth of hepatoma H-4-II-E is shown in Fig 22. The mean
latent period following injection of 1-2 X 10^6 cells into ACI male
rats is 8-10 days. Thereafter, tumor growth is rapid, resulting in
host mortality 37 days later. The radiation response of tumors remaining in situ after irradiation, as measured by the time course
variation in tumor volume, increased with dose. While high doses
(3750R) resulted in temporary eradication of the primary tumor, and
delayed host mortality, metastatic infiltration of the lung continued,
resulting in only marginal extension of host survival (Fig 22).
These observations, including the spontaneous pulmonary metastases
associated with this tumor, make the H-4-II-E tumor cell system well
adapted for experimental therapeutic investigations involving adjuvant or combined radiation-chemotherapeutic treatment.

The sequential utilization of radiotherapy with chemotherapy,
or the sequential utilization of two or more chemotherapeutic agents
is one of the more promising areas for the improvement of the treatment of cancer patients. The utilization of the second agent at a
time to block repair of cells potentially lethally damaged by the
first agent or at a time of maximum tumor cell synchronization by
the first agent needs further investigation. These are two examples
of how increased cell kill may be realized if the optimum times for
the sequential utilization of combined chemotherapy or radiotherapy
combined with chemotherapy are determined. The results of experiments with 5-FU and adriamycin are presented in the last two figures.

In the H-4-II-E cell line growing in vitro, 5-FU acts as a cell
cycle phase specific agent. Cell survival decreased to 53% of control for a concentration of 7 μg/ml and remained at this level when
the drug concentration was raised to 15 μg/ml (Fig 23). For other
cell lines (24), this drug is cycle phase non-specific. Cell kill
following adriamycin is consistent with first order kinetics, as
observed by others with other cell lines.

Combinations of 6 μg/ml 5-FU and 2.5 μg/ml ardiamycin, concentrations which singly gave cell survivals of 66% after 1 hr exposure,
were tested in the in vitro system (Fig 24). When both drugs were
simultaneously, survival was not different than seen for either drug
alone. However, when adriamycin was given 8 hr after 5-FU, survival
decreased to 48% of control. Longer intervals between the two drugs

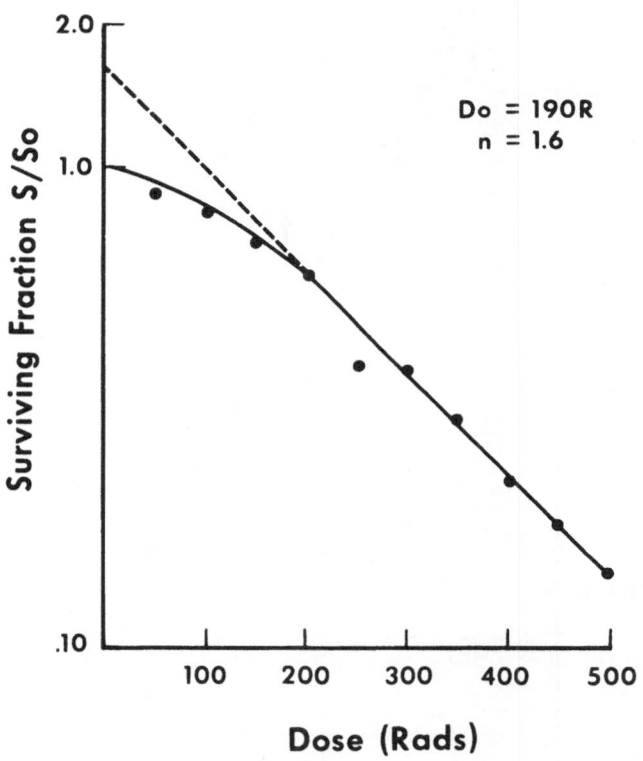

Figure 20
Survival curve for exponentially growing cultures of H-4-II-E
cells irradiated in vitro under conditions of normal aeration. Each
point represents the mean value of 10 samples.

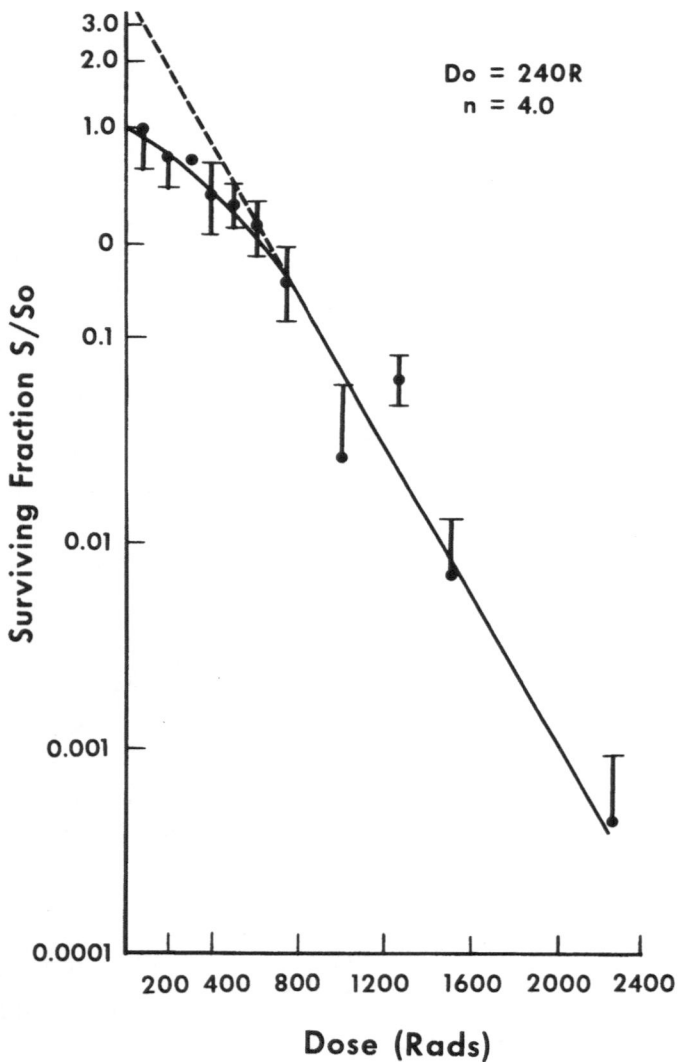

Figure 21
Survival curve for hepatoma H-4-II-E cells irradiated in situ.
Each point represents the mean value ± S.E. of 3-9 air breathing
animals.

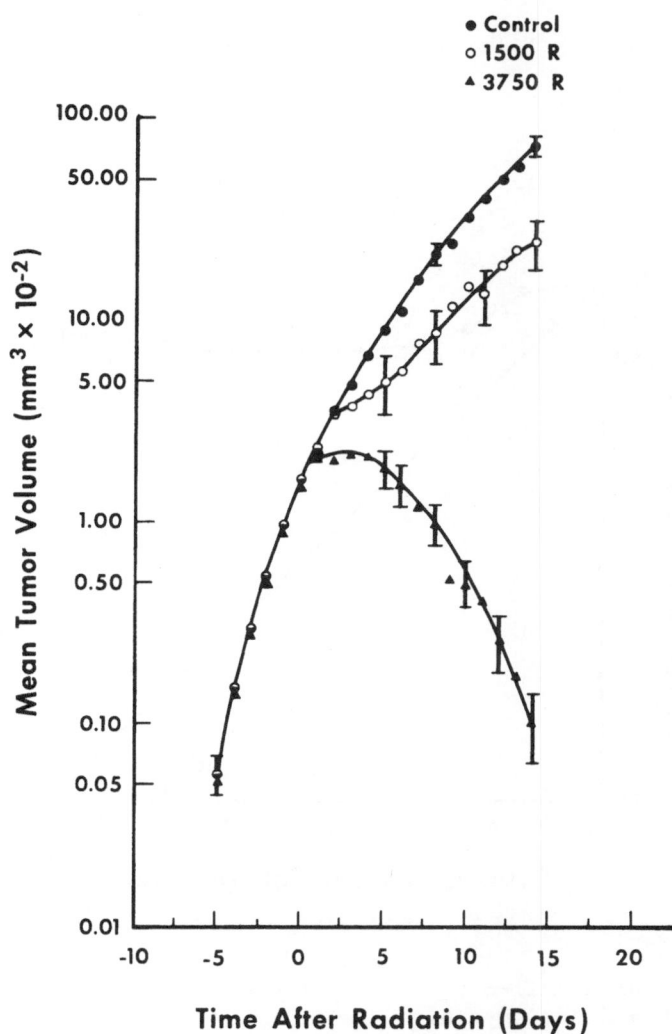

Figure 22
The effect of 1500R and 3750R of local tumor radiation on the growth characteristics of H-4-II-E. There was no significant effect of 375R on tumor growth. The curves are the mean values of groups of 12 animals for both the control and radiated tumors. Standard errors are given at different times after local tumor radiation on Day 0.

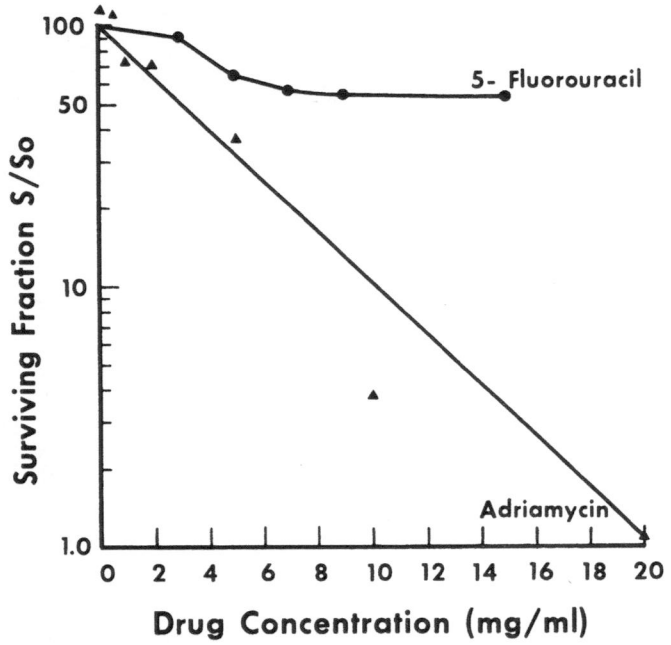

Figure 23
Survival of H-4-II-E cells <u>in</u> <u>vitro</u> after increasing concentrations of 5-FU and adriamycin.

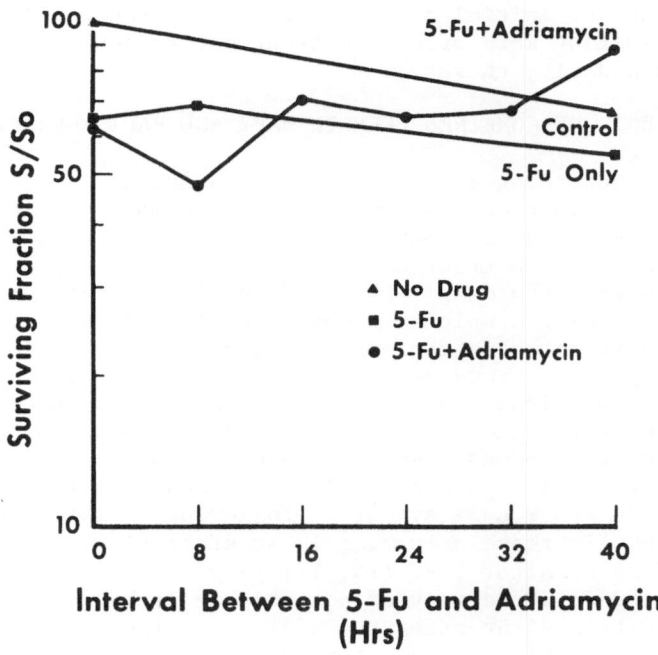

Figure 24
Survival of H-4-II-E cells _in vitro_ in which 2.5 µg/ml of
adriamycin was added at increasingly longer time intervals after
the addition of 6 ug/ml of 5-FU. The survival of 5-FU alone (6 µg/
ml) as well as control cultures are included for comparison with
the combined 5-FU and adriamycin treated cultures.

permitted recovery of cell survival. Bhuyan has obtained increased cell kill for L1210 by using low, non-toxic, synchronizing doses
of 5-FU for 8 hr, followed by adriamycin (4).

     Tumor cell lines such as the H-4-II-E, capable of growth
both in vitro and in vivo, offer increased opportunity for finding
more effective schedules for the clinical utilization of both combined chemotherapy as well as radiotherapy combined with chemotherapy. Those combinations and schedules resulting in increased
cell kill in culture can be immediately tested in the animal for
efficacy in tumor volume reduction and animal toxicity. These results represent our initial attempts to utilize the H-4-II-E cell
line for elucidating more effective treatment schedules for sequential combined modality therapy.

THE EFFECTS OF COMBINED CHEMOTHERAPY AND RADIOTHERAPY

     There is increasing evidence that human neoplasms are more
responsive to combination therapy. One of the more promising areas
for improving the clinical management of solid tumors is the proper
sequence of one or more treatment modalities. A synergistic effect
has been noted when the drug 5-FU is given 20 hr before or 10 hr
after radiation using a spleen colony assay (39) (Fig 25). These
observations have not been thoroughly evaluated in experimental
solid tumors. However, one possible explanation for this synergistic
effect is that the first agent produces a partial synchrony, increasing the number of cells in the more sensitive stages of the
cell cycle when the second agent is given, Results from studies with
the solid tumor model hepatoma 3924A have shown that there is a 2-3
fold increase in tumor cell synchrony following radiation or 5-FU
with the maximum increase occurring 12 hr after single exposure to
radiation and 24 hr after 5-FU (15, 17) (Fig 26). Twentyman (38) has
shown that a 100-fold recovery of potentially lethally damaged EMT6
cells occurs within 24 hr after the administration of cyclophosphamide (Fig 27). This suggests that radiation could prevent the repair of the damaged cells if given within 24 hr after cyclophosphamide. The results of all these studies suggest combined chemotherapy and radiotherapy could be more effectively utilized clinically if the optimum time for giving one modality after the other could
be better elucidated.

     Comparison was made of the tumor response to radiation alone,
5-FU alone, and 5-FU given 12 hr after local tumor irradiation in
this solid tumor model. Three different doses of radiation and three
different doses of 5-FU were given to determine the relationship
between these two different groups of treated tumors and also by computer fitting of individual growth curves and tabulating the percentage of tumors exhibiting three types of response (20) as a function
of 5-FU and radiation. A comparison of these two treatment modalities

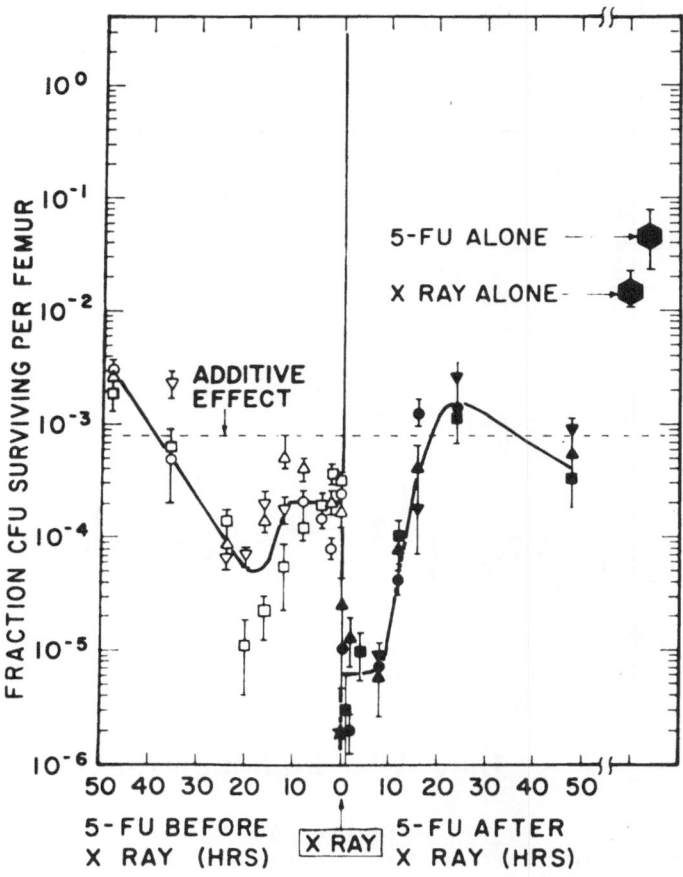

Figure 25

Survival of leukemic CFU after administration of 5-FU, radiation, or both agents. The time scale on the abscissa represents
the time interval between administration of these agents. Open
symbols represent 5-FU given before radiation; closed symbols represent drug given after radiation. Different symbols represent
different experiments. Limits shown are one standard error of
the mean.

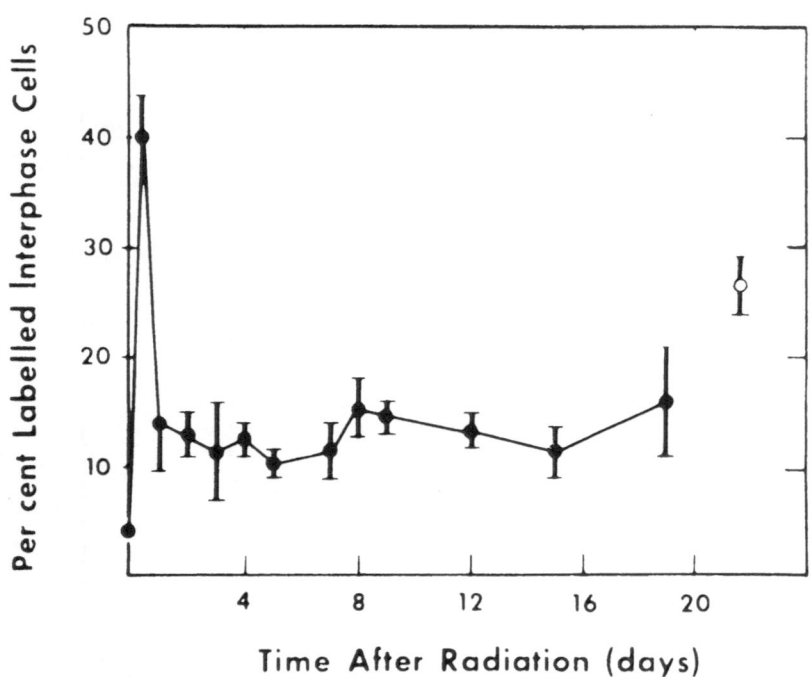

Figure 26

The effect of 3750R of X-ray on the S phase population of hepatoma 3924A. Each closed circle represents the mean percent labelled interphase cells ± the standard error of the mean in three irradiated tumors. The open circle represents the control unirradiated mean percent labelled interphase cells ± the standard error of the mean. The control value has been calculated from 40 tumors.

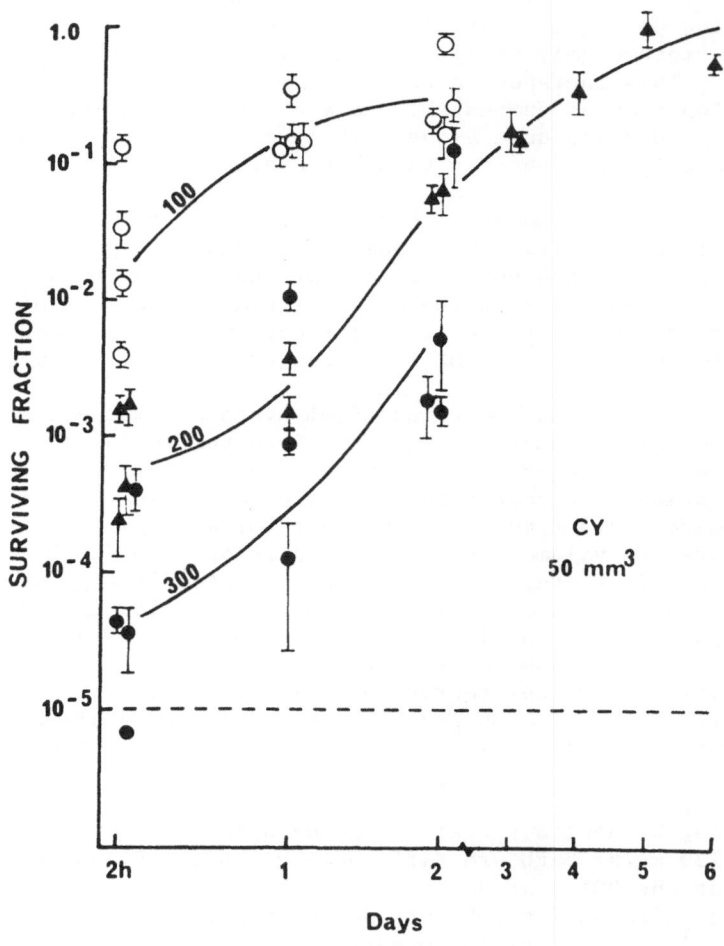

Figure 27
Change in surviving fraction of cells from solid tumors with
time between CY administration and preparation of cell suspension.
Tumors treated at a volume of 50 mm³. O, 100 mg/kg CY; ▲, 200 mg/
kg CY; ●, 300 mg/kg CY. Horizontal dotted line shows lower limit
of measurement in this assay system. Each point represents the
mean value of surviving fraction for groups of 4 mice within the
same experiment. Error bars show the standard error of the mean.
The scale of the abscissa is broken.

has uncovered specific responses to radiation and 5-FU which were masked in the analysis using only mean tumor volumes as the evaluating index. The results indicate that a series of combined 5-FU and radiation doses given at 11-day intervals should, in principle, result in progressively smaller tumor volumes until the tumor is eradicated. This therapeutic protocol would essentially transform the situation from an untreatable to a treatable one inasmuch as neither the radiation dose alone (375-1500R) nor the 5-FU dose alone (50-250 mg/kg) controls tumor growth.

Figure 28 shows the average volume relative to initial volume at time of treatment (V_0) for a number of treatment groups. Representative errors are shown on each of the curves; these errors are $\pm$ one standard error of the mean which are about 15% of the volume over the entire range for all treatments. The standard deviations are approximately 50% for these groups of 11 animals.

Analysis of the data obtained from average tumor volume changes of the different treatment group has given the following results. The response to 150 mg/kg 5-FU shows on the average, that the tumor is growing steadily except between days 4 and 10 where it is constant at approximately 2.5 times the treatment volume (V_0). For the 1500R dose, the average volume continues to increase from day 0 to $2 V_0$ at day 3; then it regresses to $1.5V_0$ and eventually regrows to $2V_0$ at day 11. The combined modality curve (1500R + 150 mg/kg) is essentially parallel to the 1500R curve but lower by a factor of approximately 2/3. Because of this the response does not attain $2V_0$ until day 16, with actual regression below V_0 occurring at day 8. Thus the effect of the combined treatment is to maintain the tumor at a smaller volume for a longer period of time than either 1500R or 150 mg/kg alone.

Applying Student's t-test to the data in Fig 28, the curves for 1500R and 150 mg/kg 5-FU are different on a point-by-point basis to day eight at the 90% confidence level. In addition, the two curves overall are different at 90% confidence from the day of treatment to day 20. It is also possible to perform an analysis of variance on the average tumor volumes for all doses (groups A-I) to see if the reduction in volume for the combined treatment is more than the simple sum of the two treatments taken individually. Our results indicate that at the 90% confidence level, the combined treatment effect is simply additive at eight days (where the volume reduction is maximal). There is some evidence for a marginally significant synergistic effect at 16 days. However, the difference between 1500R alone and 1500R plus 5-FU is not great at this point.

The data in Fig 29 are representative of both the raw data and the fitted functions. The errors shown are representative standard deviations of the spread in the volume measurements on a single tumor.

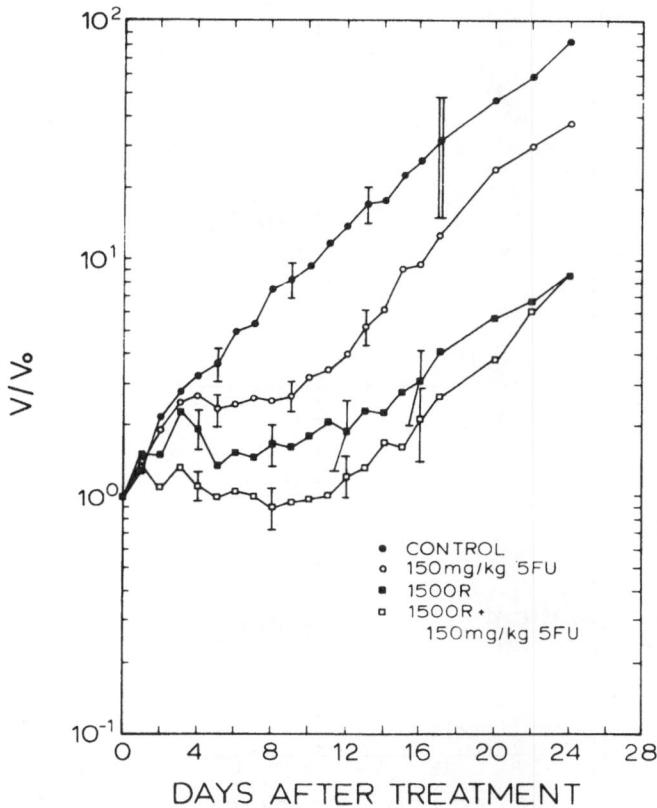

Figure 28
Average volume response to single and combined treatments.
Each point is average of approximately 11 animals; the volumes
have been divided by the average treatment volume at each dose, V_0.
The single error bars are $\pm$ 1 standard error of the mean; the double
error bars are $\pm$ 1 standard deviation.

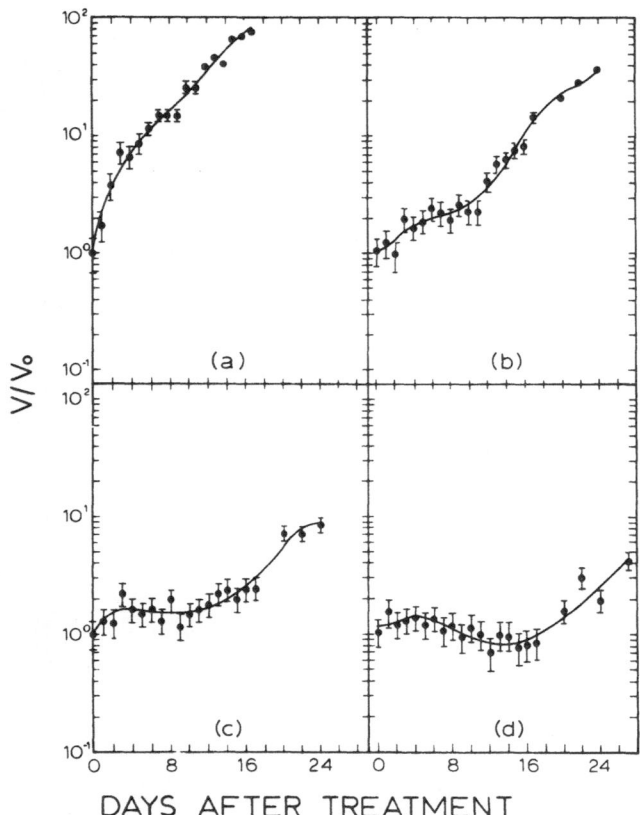

Figure 29

The response of individual animals to various treatments: (a) control; (b) 150 mg/kg of 5-FU; (c) 1500R; (d) 1500R + 100 mg/kg 5-FU. The solid curves are the polynomial fits to logarithm of (V/V_0). The error bars are $\pm$ 1 standard deviation in volume measurement at that particular volume.

They range from 25% at the small volumes (200 mm^3) to 4% at the large volumes (40,000 mm^3) so individual volumes can be known more accurately than can the means of treatment groups. By analyzing each tumor response individually within a treatment group non-uniform responses can be accomodated and volumes can be more accurately known for analysis.

Tabulation of the percentage of tumors which fall into each response class are shown in Fig 30 as dose response histograms (DRH) for 50, 100 and 150 mg/kg of 5-FU as a function of radiation dose. The radiation dose scale has been repeated three times at each 5-FU dose, in order to show the histograms of each class separately. For comparative purposes, Fig 31 illustrates the DRH's from previous experiments in which 5-FU and radiation were administered singly.

A number of important points emerge from the histogram for the combined treatment:

(1) 5-FU used in combination with radiation lowers the radiation dose at which some individual tumors begin to exhibit regression.

(2) The addition of 5-FU greatly reduces the number of tumors which show no volume reduction at all, and seems to move significant numbers of tumors from class III to class II responses at radiation levels above 500R.

(3) The percentage of tumors exhibiting regression (class I) at the highest radiation doses used does not seem to be sensitive to 5-FU, but remains roughly constant.

THE EFFECTS OF COMBINED CHEMOTHERAPY AND IMMUNOTHERAPY (BCG CELL WALLS) ON TUMOR GROWTH AND ANIMAL MORTALITY

The use of BCG or other immunopotentiating agents in combination with radiotherapy or chemotherapy has recently gained in prominence. Combination therapy with BCG and chemotherapy has had varying results. When administered after chemotherapy, BCG appears to aid in the recovery of immunocompetence, providing a beneficial effect upon prognosis. Pearson et al. (28) have reported an increase in animal survival, from 35% to 80-100%, in a murine leukemic system under remission when chemotherapy was combined with BCG. However, Mathe et al. (25) have reported that chemotherapy of the L-1210 leukemia was actually less effective if BCG immunotherapy had preceded treatment. Furthermore, Wepsic et al. (40) have reported that BCG actually enhances growth of a solid tumor. It becomes apparent that few studies have systematically attempted to evaluate how the administration of BCG, BCG cell walls, BCG-like agents, or

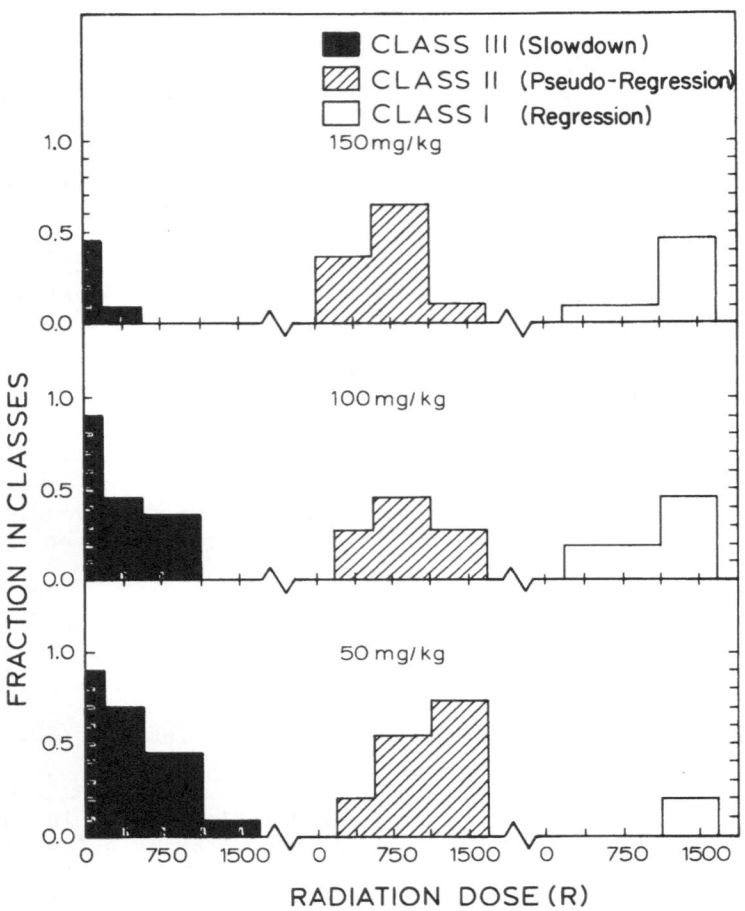

Figure 30
Dose response histogram for combined thearpy. The radiation
axis has been repeated to show each class separately.

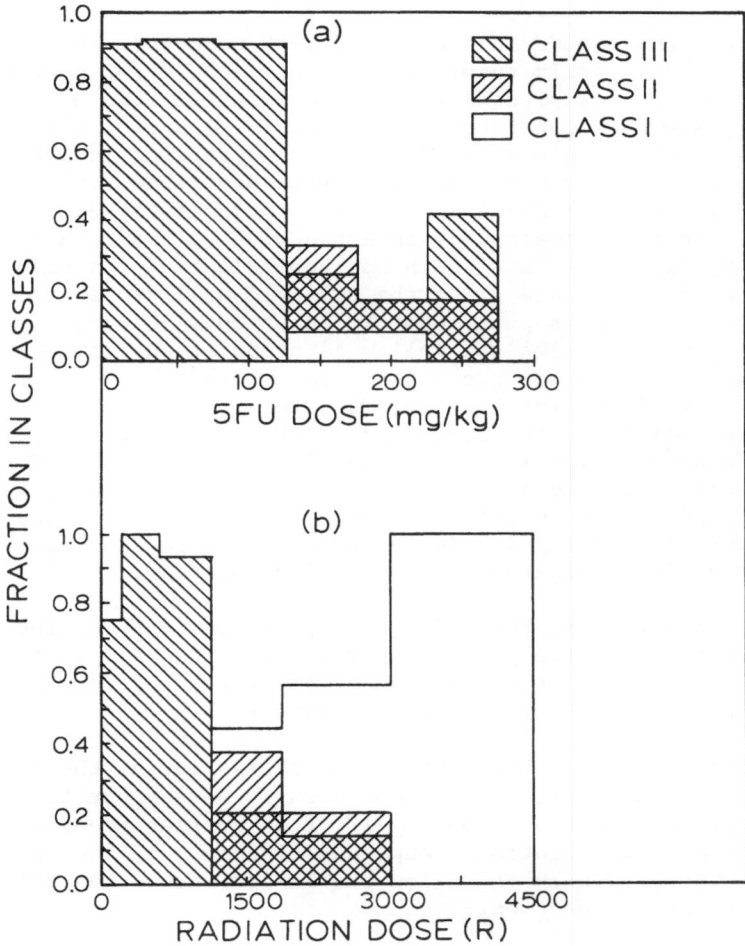

Figure 31
Dose response histogram for single mode therapy: (a) 5-FU;
(b) radiation. Note that the cross-hatching has been left out in
a portion of (a) to show class I response explicitly.

other non-specific stimulants of the reticuloendothelial system
(c. parvum, etc.) can affect the chemotherapy of tumors. It is
presently unknown how these agents protect the host tissue from
chemotherapy injury or if treatment with such immunopotentiating
agents aids in host tissue recovery post-chemotherapy.

Combinations of BCG cell wall and 5-FU were evaluated using
the hepatoma 3924A solid tumor system (See Table 8 for protocol)
(22). The mycobacterial cell walls were obtained from Dr. Edgar
Ribi, Rocky Mountain Laboratory, National Institute of Allergy and
Infectious Diseases, Hamilton, Montana, and prepared in a Drakeol
Between 80 saline suspension as previously described (26). 5-FU
was given by intraperitoneal injection (I.P.) between 8:00 and
8:30 A.M. Control animals were injected with saline. Each group
contained 9, 11, or 12 rats which had been allotted randomly.
Groups B, C, F and G were given the BCG cell wall preparation intraperitoneally (7 days post tumor inoculation). Groups I, J, K
and L were given the same BCG cell wall preparation intralesional-
ly into the tumor. The appropriate dose of 5-FU was then given to
each rat 7 days later (or 14 days after tumor inoculation). Group
H was given saline and the medium in which BCG cell walls were dissolved. This was given intraperitoneally. The analysis of changes
in the growth curves following BCGcw were confined to the groups
which received the BCGcw intraperitoneally. Swelling of the tumors
from the intralesional injection of BCGcw precluded the use of these
tumors for analysis of growth changes (See Table 7).

New information on the effects of BCGcw and 5-FU on tumor
growth were found in two areas. They are (i) the effect of the BCG
on the early growth of the tumor, and (ii) the effect of treating
tumors with the 5-FU following BCG administration.

To determine the effects of BCG on early growth, the control
tumors were compared with those tumors which were first treated with
BCG, then given wither 5-FU on day 12 or no further treatment. There
were 9 tumors in the control groups and 21 tumors in the second
category. The growth curve during the 12 day period was fit with a
simple exponential function,

$$V = V_o e^{bt}$$

where V is the volume, V_o is the volume on day zero (the day of BCG
treatment) and b is the average growth rate over the 12 days. Since
the tumors were not palpable at day zero, the initial volume was de-
ducted from computer derived fits to the data on each tumor. The
relevant results are shown in Table 8.

Those tumors which received BCGcw achieved a higher volume by
day 12 (p $<$ .05). There was a fourfold increase in tumor volumes

Table Seven
Experimental Protocol

	BCG Cell Wall Administration			5-Fluorouracil Admin.
Animal Group	BCG Cell Walls	Route of Admin.	Day Given*	5-FU Dose Given I.P. 7 Days After BCG Cell Walls**
A	None	---	---	100 mg/kg
B	300/µg	(I.P.)+	(Day 7)	100 mg/kg
C	None	---	---	150 mg/kg
D	300/µg	(I.P.)	(Day 7)	150 mg/kg
E	None	---	---	200 mg/kg
F	300/µg	(I.P.)	(Day 7)	200 mg/kg
G	300/µg	(I.P.)	(Day 7)	None
H	None	---	---	None
I	300/µg	(I.L.)++	(Day 7)	None
J	300/µg	(I.L.)	(Day 7)	150 mg/kg
K	300/µg	(I.L.)	(Day 14)	150 mg/kg
L	300/µg	(I.L.)	(Day 14)	None

* The tumor becomes palpable 6-8 days after inoculation. The BCG cell walls were given at 7 days after tumor inoculation.

** 5-FU was given 7 days after BCG cell walls, with the exception of Group K in which the 5-FU and BCG were given on the same day.

+ (I.P.) Intraperitoneal injection of BCG cell walls.

++ (I.L.) Intralesional injection of BCG Cell walls.

Table Eight

	Volume – (mm^3) Day – 12	Volume – (mm^3) Day – 0	b*
Tumors – BCG Treated	339 $\pm$ 155	29.3 $\pm$ 9	.65 $\pm$ .15
Tumors – Controls	84 $\pm$ 36	27.5 $\pm$ 10	.48 $\pm$ .21

* b is the average growth rate.

in BCGcw treated animals compared to control tumors in non-BCGcw treated animals during this period.

To determine whether there was any effect on the BCG after this 12 day period, the control tumors were compared to those tumors that received only BCG (and no 5-FU) from day 12 to day 34. Because the average size of the tumors differ dramatically at day 12, comparison of these two groups is based on their growth rates, rather than on their volumes. The average growth rates during this period were 0.18 $\pm$ 0.02 for the tumors in the BCGcw treated animals and 0.919 $\pm$ 0.04 for the tumors in the control animals. Therefore, BCG has little or no effect after day 12.

It should be emphasized that our present experiment allows us to set this upper limit on the time during which the BCG has an effect on the tumor, but does not allow us to determine whether this time might not, in fact, be shorter than 12 days. For example, a situation in which the BCG affected the tumor for only 6 days would be compatible with our findings. Having established the effect of the BCG on a previously untreated tumor, the question remains: what effect does 5-FU have on a tumor which has been previously treated with BCG? The results of previous studies of this series have established that the effect of 5-FU acting alone is to produce a growth rate minimum about 7 days after treatment, followed by a growth rate maximum about 12 days after treatment. Prior intraperitoneal injections of BCG have a marked effect on this behavior, and, in fact, the order of the maxima and minima is reversed. In other words, when 5-FU is administered to tumors which have been treated with BCG, the tumors exhibit a growth rate maximum within 3 days of the 5-FY injection, followed by a minimum 3-5 days later.

This point is made in Fig 32 where histograms are presented of the number of tumors displaying a maximum in a given 3 day interval for various treatment schedules. The tendency of these tumors receiving the combined treatment to display growth maxima soon after the 5-FU injection is clear.

It is important in interpreting this data to realize that the existence of a growth rate maximum in a volume curve does not necessarily imply that growth is faster than control. In the case of combined 5-FU and BCGcw therapy, the tumors are growing rapidly at the time of 5-FU treatment. Rather than being associated with a more rapid rate of growth, the maxima seem to correspond to slower growth rates than exhibited at the same time by tumors which did not receive 5-FU. In Table 9, the values of the growth rates at day 15 for tumors receiving BCG alone and in combination with 100 and 150 mg/kg 5-FU are presented. The rate of growth 3 days after 5-FU injection seems to fall with increasing dose within wide statistical limits.

Table Nine

5-FU Dose	Average Growth Rate
0	$.29 \pm .05$
100 mg/kg	$.27 \pm .09$
150 mg/kg	$.21 \pm .07$

This is probably a "rebound" from temporarily inhibited growth immediately following injection of 5-FU. Such fine structure in the growth curve would not be detected in this experiment. However, this phenomenon will be examined more closely in future experiments.

Survival data for the different groups are given in Table 10. No animals were lost in 6 groups (C, G, H, I, J and L) and only 1 animal was lost in 3 groups (A, B and D). Major losses occurred in 3 groups (E, F and K). There were 6 out of 9 animals lost in group E which received the highest dose of 5-FU (200 mg/kg) with BCGcw. The group F of animals which received the same dose of 5-FU (200 mg/

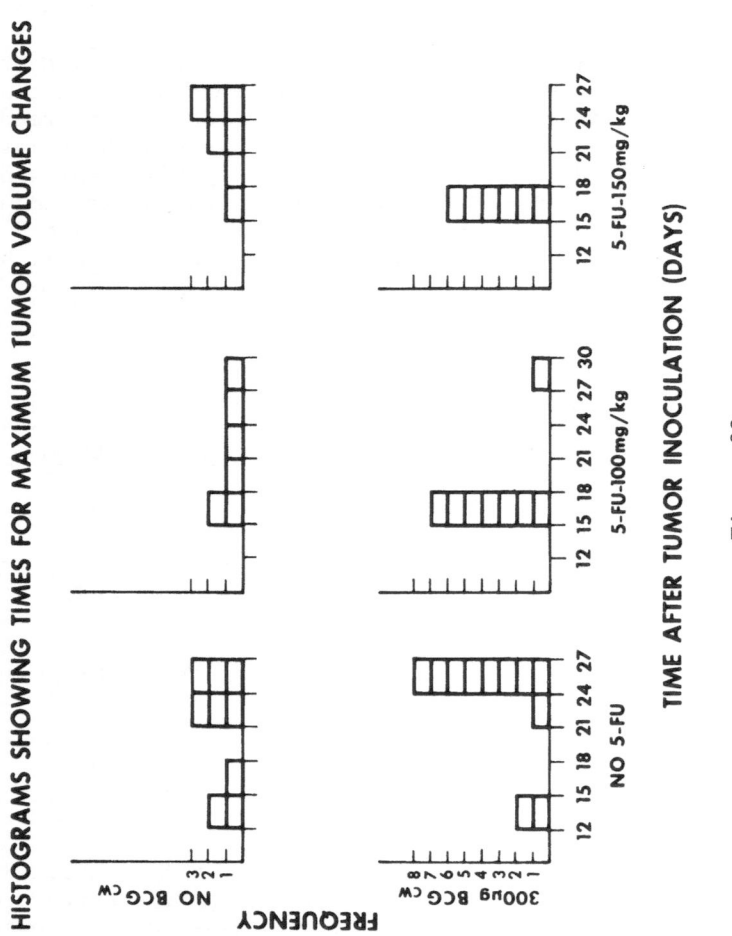

Figure 32

Table Ten

Animal Survival After BCGcw & 5-FU*

Animal Group	mg/kg 5-FU	ug BCG	Number Animals	#Animals Dead	Percent Survival
A	100	None	9	1	89%
B	100	300	11	1	91%
C	150	None	9	0	100%
D	150	300	11	1	91%
E	200	None	9	6	33%
F	200	300	11	4	64%
G	None	300	11	0	100%
H	None	None	9	0	100%

* BCG given intraperitoneally 7 days after tumor inoculation.

5-FU given intraperitoneally 14 days after tumor inoculation.

kg) but had received 300 μg of BCGcw 7 days previously had 4 of
11 animals to die, or 64% survival. A similar survival rate (67%)
occurred in group K in which 150 mg/kg of 5-FU and 300 μg of BCGcw
were given on day 14. No loss of animals occurred in either the
group C in which 150 mg/kg of 5-FU was given without BCGcw or in
group J in which 300 μg of BCGcw was given on day 7 prior to being
given 150 mg/kg of 5-FU on day 14.

These findings are not conclusive, however, they suggest that
BCGcw administration may increase animal survival mitigating against
the effects of chemotherapeutic agents such as 5-FU on the animal
immune mechanism. Other studies have shown that the BCG given
after chemotherapy appears to aid in the recovery of immunocompetence. However, BCGcw given at the same time as 5-FU may reduce
the survival since 4 out of 12 animals were lost when BCGcw was
given at the time of 150 mg/kg of 5-FU (22).

The finding of increased tumor growth following BCGcw administration underscores the complexity of the response of tumors to
non-specific stimulation of the immune mechanism with agents such
as BCG (40). Low tumor specific antigenic response is one possible
explanation for the increased tumor growth. Since a number of
human tumors also have low specific antigenic responses it illustrates the care which should be exercised in the use of these agents
in immunotherapy. Extension of studies such as these in experimental
solid tumors should be helpful in better understanding the conditions
under which non-specific agents such as BCGcw cause increased tumor
growth and conditions under which tumor growth is decreased.

THE SEQUENTIAL UTILIZATION OF CHEMOTHERAPY WITH RADIOTHERAPY

Studies of the effects of 5-FU and radiation on the solid tumor
model hepatoma 3924A indicated that neither radiation alone (375-
1500R) nor 5-FU alone (50-250 mg/kg) would control tumor growth.
Recovery from the toxic effects of a large dose of 5-FU in rats occurs 10-11 days following treatment (10) (Fig 33). The maximum
rate of tumor volume change occurs 12 days after 5-FU (21) (Fig 15).
It has also been demonstrated that the rate of proliferation in the
tumor is at a maximum 11-days after 5-FU (10) (Fig 9). These results suggest that radiation in combination with 5-FU treatment
could in principle transform the management of a chemotherapeutically resistant solid tumor from an untreatable situation to a treatable
situation by the combined modality treatment every 11 days until the
tumor is eradicated (20).

It is feasible to design experiments for the sequential utilization of different treatment modalities which can produce maximum effects on the tumor following recovery of the host. The bone marrow
has been shown to be the critical organ in animal recovery following

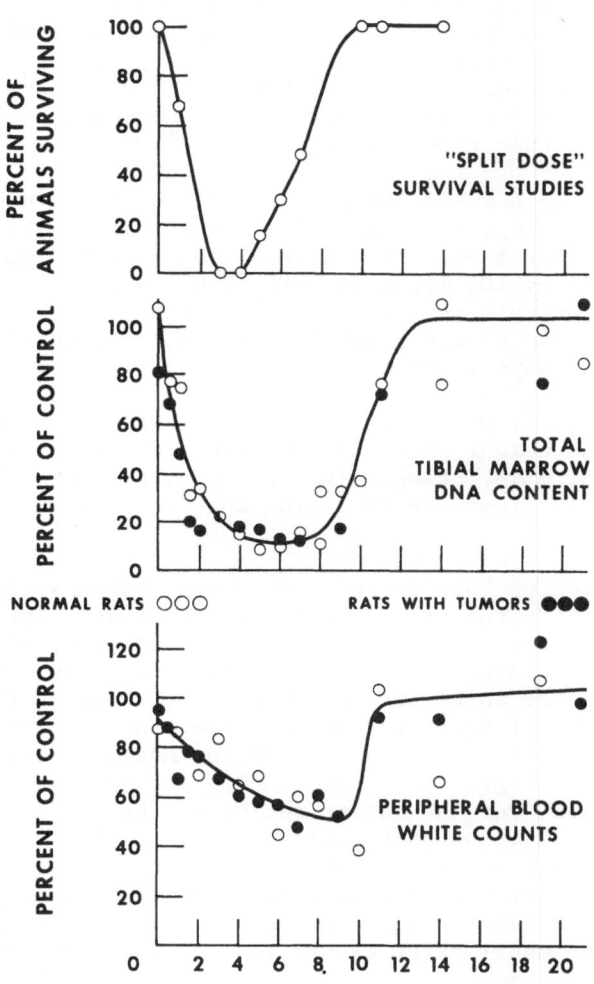

DAYS AFTER 5-FLUROROURACIL ADMINISTRATION

Figure 33
Relative changes in the tibial bone marrow, peripheral white
blood cell concentrations following a large single dose of 5-FU
(150 mg/kg): "split dose" survival studies following 2 doses of
5-FU (150 mg/kg).

5-FU since the intestines recover prior to the recovery of the
bone marrow (10). The therapeutic strategy for the sequential use
of chemotherapy with radiotherapy is diagrammatically represented
in Fig 34 (23). The tumors were locally irradiated according to
the method described in section 5. The 5-FU was given 12 hr after
local tumor irradiation on each of the three 11-day treatment courses
to take advantage of the partial synchrony of the cells by local
tumor irradiation at this time (15) (Fig 26).

Four groups of 15 animals per group were used in this experiment.
The rats in group A received 1500R of local tumor irradiation, group
B received 100 mg/kg of 5-FU, group C received 1500R of local tumor
irradiation followed by 100 mg/kg of 5-FU 12 hr later. Group E acted
as controls. The controls were anesthesized with ether (as were the
irradiated groups A and C) and given 1 ml saline I.P. to simulate the
5-FU injections in groups B and C.

Tumor volumes (mm^3) were calculated (1/2 lxwxh) from measurements
of length, width and height made daily before and after treatment
during the period of major changes in tumor growth rates. Measurements were made three times weekly during the remaining period of the
experiment.

Previous studies of this series have demonstrated variability of
response to treatment within the same treatment group. The divergence
of response is accentuated in this multiple course study of combined
modality therapy given over longer periods of time. The computer derived growth curves for three treated tumors are shown in Fig 35
together with the actual tumor volume measurements to illustrate the
differences in therapeutic response. Combined modality therapy obviously did not control growth of tumor C-2. The tumor volume remains
essentially unchanged over the entire period of therapy for tumor C-12
The tumor volume for C-4 showed a rapid decrease at the end of the 11-
day interval following the first course of combined modality therapy.
The second course of therapy 11 days after the first course resulted
in eradication of the tumor. In some tumors rapid reductions in tumor
volumes were delayed until after the third course of therapy 22 days
after the initial treatment.

The mean tumor volume curve for the group of 15 animals treated
successively with radiation and 5-FU was similar to that of C-12 (Fig
35). The standard error of the mean increased with time after therapy
because of the increasing divergence of the tumor curves as illustrated by the growth curve for C-2. The mean and standard error for the
treated group was $452 + 52$ mm^3 on day 7, 462 ± 129 mm^3 on day 16 and
636 ± 234 mm^3 on day 28. Eleven of the 15 tumors showed regression
(seven regressed completely while four regressed and regrew) (Fig 36).

Analysis of the individual tumor growth curves was made using

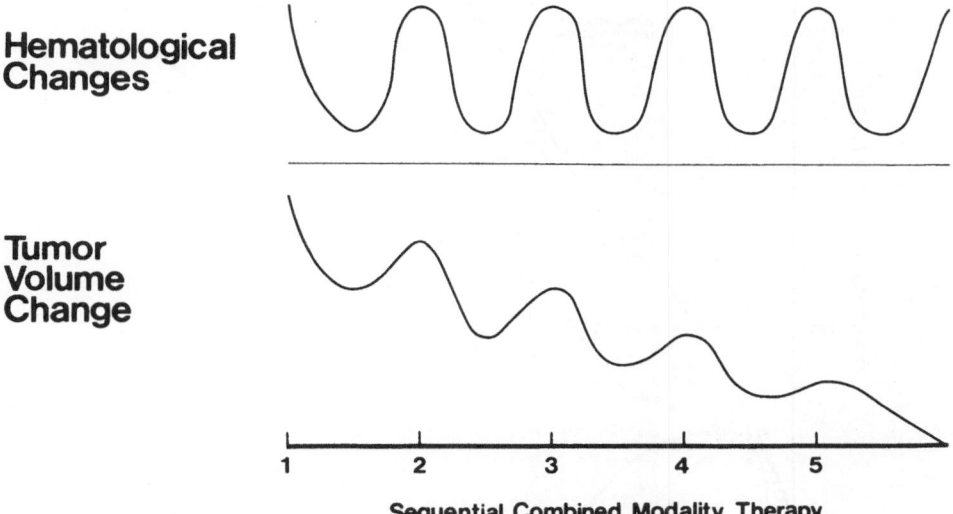

Hematological Changes

Tumor Volume Change

Sequential Combined Modality Therapy

Figure 34

The therapeutic strategy for the sequential use of chemotherapy and radiotherapy. The second and subsequent therapy course are given when the animal recovery for the previous course and at a time when the rate of proliferation in the volume is at a maximum.

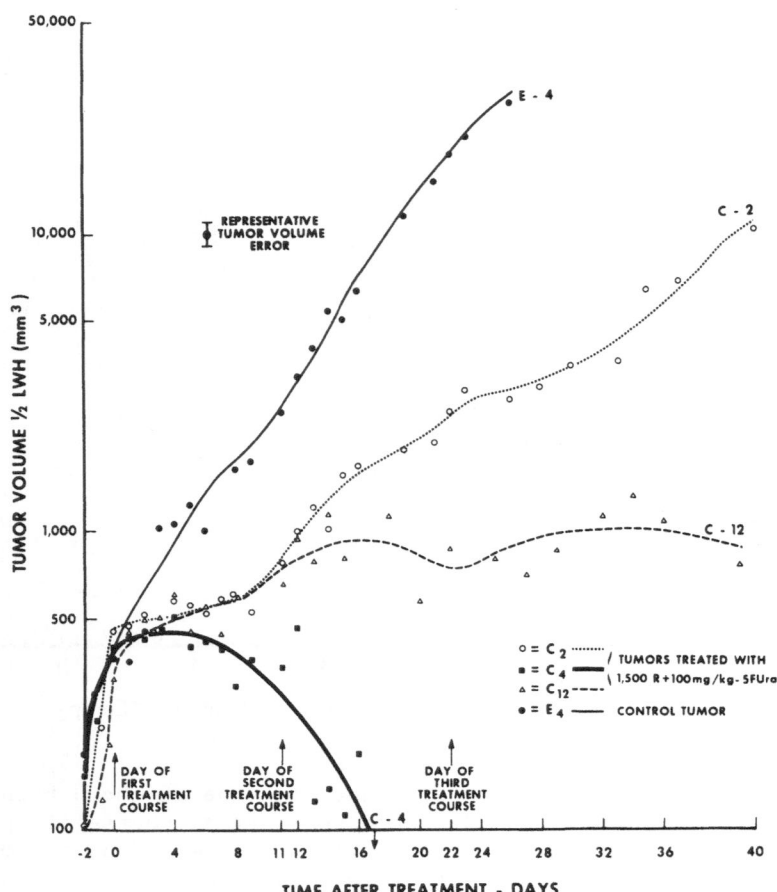

Figure 35
Representative growth curves for one control and three treated
tumors.   The different symbols represent actual tumor measurements.
The lines are computer fitted growth curves for each tumor.   The
representative tumor volume error represents the accuracy with which
the caliper measurement of tumor volume can be made.

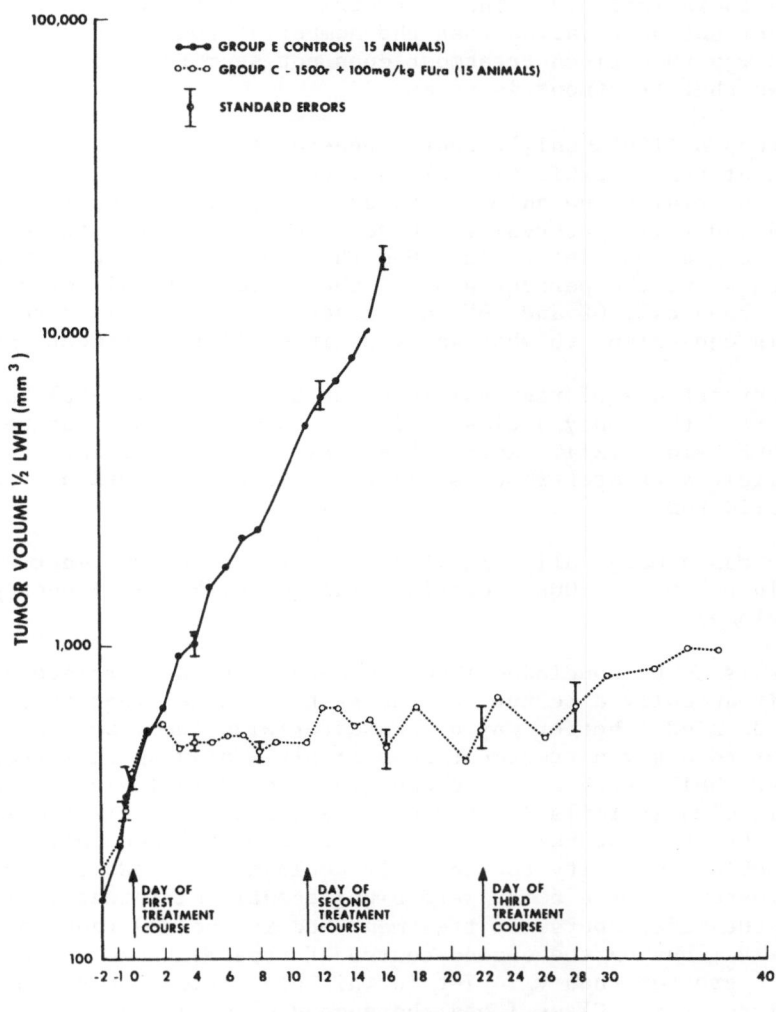

Figure 36

Changes in mean tumor volumes of 15 animals treated with 1500R of radiation and 100 mg/kg 5-FU after radiation. Three successive therapy courses were given 11 days apart. Changes in mean tumor volume of 15 animals in the control group are given for comparison with the treated group (standard errors are shown).

techniques described in section 3. The percentages of the tumors
in each of the three response categories during each treatment period
are tabulated in Table 11. The most striking fact shown in the Table
is the important observation that the number of tumors which respond
in a given way to a given treatment does not seem to change significantly when that treatment is repeated.

In group A (1500R only), there appeared to be a drop in the
percentage of tumors exhibiting Class I responses in the third
treatment interval. One animal died during anesthesia during each of
the second and third intervals. These animals had exhibited Class I
responses in previous intervals. Had they survived and continued this
response pattern, the percentages for the third interval for group A
would have been 64%, 0% and 36% in Classes I, II and III respectively,
and this is equivalent to what was seen in earlier treatment intervals.

The persistence of response in group B (100 mg/kg 5-FU) is related to the fact that only a Class III (slowdown) response can be produced by 5-FU alone (21). Animal toxicity precludes giving enough
5-FU to elicit a greater response in this chemotherapeutically resistant solid tumor.

There was a marginally significant increase in treatment effectiveness in group C (1500R radiation plus 100 mg/kg 5-FU) over group
A (1500R alone).

If it is to be concluded from the data that the persistence of
response is actually a feature of the system, it is clear that it is
necessary to find a better way of characterizing the response of a
given tumor to a given treatment than simply assigning that response
to a class. While such a method can give an overall view of the responses, it clearly fails to characterize the more detailed features
that might be the most helpful in evaluation of the sequential utilization of combined modality therapy. It would not be possible to say
that two responses of a tumor were significantly different for a tumor
which, on the first course of treatment had its volume reduced to
just below V_o, but on the second course of treatment had a minimum
volume just greater than v_o. Yet in this classification scheme, one
would call the first Class I and the second Class II and conclude that
the tumor had responded differently to each treatment.

A more detailed description of tumor response was realized by in-
troducing the concept of treatment efficiency for each class. The
basic idea here is to define a quantity which varies smoothly from
zero to one, with the proviso that the quantity should be zero for the
least effective response for a given class and one for the most effective response.

For example, the treatment efficiency for a Class I (Regression)

Table Eleven

Single or Combined Treatment	Treatment Scheduling Therapy Courses 1, 2, 3	Therapeutic Response Classes (%)		
		Class I	Class II	Class III
Group A 1500R	Course 1	60	13	27
	Course 2	71	0	29
	Course 3	55 (64)*	0	45 (36)*
Group B 100 mg/kg 5-FUra	Course 1	0	0	100
	Course 2	0	0	100
	Course 3	0	0	100
Group C 1500R + 100 mg/kg 5-FUra	Course 1	70	10	20
	Course 2	82	0	18
	Course 3	57	0	43

* percent in different classifications if 2 animals in Class I which died from anesthesia are included.

response could be defined by $\eta_I = 1 - \dfrac{V_{min}}{V_{max}}$ where V_{max} is the maximum volume attained by the tumor following treatment and V_{min} is the minimum. The most effective response for this class would be a complete regression of the tumor, i.e., a situation where V_{min} became zero. In this case $\eta_I = 1$. On the other hand, the least effective Class I response would be one in which the volume following treatment remained near the treatment volume, V_o, and the tumor eventually regrew. In this case, $V_{min} \mathcal{X} V_{max} \mathcal{X} V_o$ and $\eta_I = 0$. The concept of an efficiency takes the analysis one step beyond a simple classification. Saying a response is Class I indicates that the tumor exhibited some regression. Stating the efficiency tells how much regression was seen.

In an analogous way an efficiency appropriate to a Class II response can be introduced as follows:

$$\eta_{II} = 1 - \frac{V_{min} - V_o}{V_{max} - V_o}$$

where V_{min} and V_{max} are the minimum and maximum volumes attained by the tumor following treatment, and V_o is the volume of treatment. This index tells how much decrease in tumor volume is seen relative to V_o.

Finally, an efficiency for Class III response is introduced as

$$\eta_{III} = 1 - \frac{b_{min}}{\langle b \rangle}$$

where b_{min} is the growth rate at the point of minimum growth and $\langle b \rangle$ is the average growth rate of the controls at that point. Clearly, this quantitiy is a measure of how much the growth rate is reduced by the treatment.

An overall treatment efficiency (OTE) can be defined which allows the characterization, in one number, of the effect of a given treatment once these efficiencies have been defined, each one being calculated as appropriate for a given class of response. In this way, simple comparisons of successive treatments can be made by comparing the OTE of a given tumor in different treatment intervals.

The OTE for a given treatment interval is defined as

$$f_i = 3-n + \eta$$

In this equation i represents the treatment interval. For our results, i will be 1, 2 or 3. "n" represents the class into which a particular response is placed and had the value 1 for Class I (Regression), 2 for Class II, and so on. η is then the treatment efficiency for that class as defined in the preceding paragraphs.

This seemingly arbitrary definition of the OTE was chosen for a number of reasons. In the first place, it varies continuously from a value of 3 (for total regression of the tumor) to 0 (for controls). In the second place, it varies uniformly across the boundaries of the three main classes, and assigns roughly an equal OTE to responses which differ only by a small amount but which fall into different categories because of this difference. For example, we discussed above the case of two responses which were very similar, but which overlapped the Class I-Class II boundary. The OTE for each of these responses can be calculated.

The first curve had a Class I response with $V_{max} \approx V_{min} \lesssim V_o$ which gives $\eta_I = 0$. From this formula, we would have $f_I = 3-1+ 0= 2$. On the second course $V_{max} \approx V_{min} \gtrsim V_o$, which gives a Class II response with $\eta_{II} = 1$. In this case $f_2 = 3-2 + 1 = 2$. Thus the OTE does indeed have nearly equal values for similar tumor responses, even when these responses straddle a class boundary. This makes it an appropriate one number characterization of the response.

The main result suggested by Table 12, that responses of tumors tend to be the same in each treatment interval, can now be evaluated by means of the OTE. In Fig 37 the OTE for the tumors are plotted for treatment intervals 1 and 2, Fig 38 gives the same results for intervals 2 and 3. Figs 37 and 38 give confirmation of the hypothesis which has been advanced. The clustering of points inside the dotted squares shows that virtually all of the tumors will continue to exhibit the same response in each treatment interval throughout the experiment. In the case of Class I responses, this means that repeated treatments will eventually destroy the tumor if conditions can be extrapolated.

Once the **persistence** of response is established, one more question can be asked --- whether the treatment becomes more effective or less effective as the repetitions increase. Any consistent trend for the OTE to increase or decrease from interval to interval would answer this question. For example, if the treatment became more effective with repetition, the lower righthand side of the Class I squares in Figs 36 and 37 would contain a preponderance of the points, while if the treatment became less effective, the points would tend to cluster in the upper lefthand corner. From Fig 37, 12 tumors exhibited a higher OTE during the second interval than during the first, while only 3 had decreased OTE. This is a strong indication that the treatment is becoming somewhat more effective as it is repeated.

It has been found in well-defined "split-dose" animal survival studies that rats recover rapidly and reach 100% survival levels when the second dose of 5-FUra is given 10-11 days after the first dose of

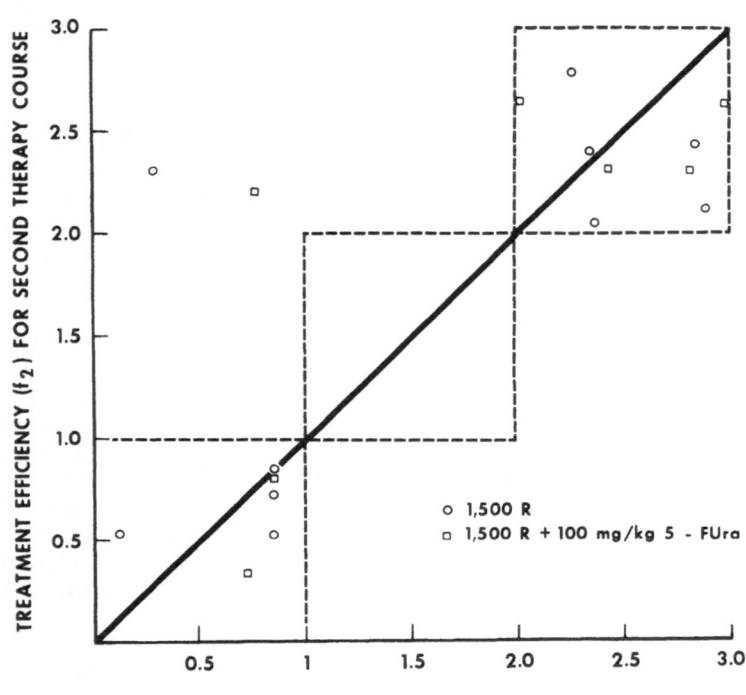

Figure 37
Overall treatment efficiency of the first treatment course
1500R of radiation and 100 mg/kg of 5-FU in relation to the second
treatment course 11 days later.

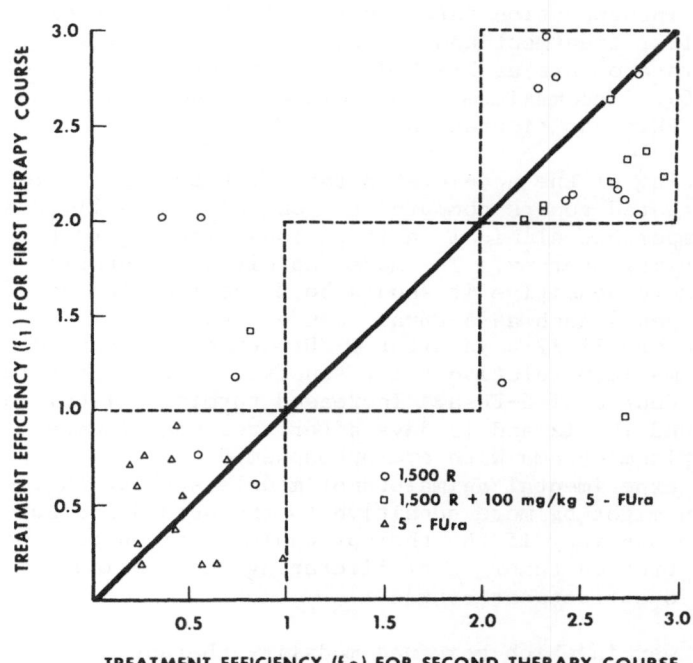

Figure 38
Overall treatment efficiency of the second treatment course of
1500R of radiation and 100 mg/kg 5-FU in relation to the third treatment course given 11 days after the second treatment course and 22
days after the first treatment course.

5-FUra. All animals die when the second dose of 5-FUra is given
3-4 days after the first. This rapid recovery in animal survival
at 10-11 days is also associated with a rapid return to normal
values for total bone marrow DNA and peripheral white blood counts
(10). The epithelium of the gastrointestinal tract recovers earlier
than the hematopoietic system. Thus, treatment of tumors in the rat
with 5-FUra can be carried out every 10-11 days since hematopoietic
tissue recovery occurs within this time frame. Studies on the recovery of the kinetics of tumor cell proliferation have shown that
deoxyuridine incorporation into tumor cell DNA is markedly depressed
for 2 days after treatment and returns to control levels by day 9.
The maximum rate occurs at 11-12 days and returns to control value
by day 21 (10). The maximum tumor volume change also occurred 12
days after 5-FUra administration (21).

        The finding of the accelerated rate of tumor proliferation in
the 5-FUra treated tumors compared to control tumors 11-12 days after
5-FUra has important clinical ramifications with regard to sequential
combined modality therapy. The more rapidly proliferating a tumor
becomes the more sensitive it should be to cell cycle specific chemotherapeutic agents such as 5-FUra. Since the maximum time of proliferation occurs 11-12 days after 5-FUra then this should be the
time for the maximum relative tumor sensitivity to 5-FUra following
the previous course of 5-FUra. Increased thymidine labelling indices
have been found 10, 12 and 15 days after treatment (compared to controls) of a plasmacytoma with cyclophosphamide (34). These findings
in different experimental animal tumor models suggest that solid
tumors in man might be more sensitive to the second and subsequent
course of chemotherapy if the therapy could be given clinically at
the time the treated tumor is proliferating at a maximum rate following the previous treatment course.

        Another way in which combined modality therapy may be more ef-
fectively utilized is to give the second form of therapy at a time
when the maximum number of cells are in the most sensitive stages of
the cell cycle as a result of partial synchrony by the first form of
therapy. Previous studies have shown that a 2-3-fold increase in
numbers of tumor cells in the "S" phase of the cell cycle are present
after a single exposure to 5-FUra or radiation (15, 17). The maximum
cell synchrony occurs 12 hr after a single exposure to radiation and
24 hr after 5-FUra. In these studies 5-FUra was given 12 hr after
radiation. In future studies, radiation would be given 24 hr after
5-FUra to take advantage of the later maximum in cell synchrony after
5-FUra compared to radiation.

        The relationship between changes in tumor cellularity and changes
in tumor volume is complex. Much additional information is needed to
elucidate further the dynamic relationship between tumor cell kill
following chemotherapy and/or radiotherapy, and changes in tumor

volume. In addition to immediate changes in cell viability following radiotherapy and/or chemotherapy, more information is needed
about the kinetic cellular changes and tumor histology over the
entire period between courses of treatment. At present, changes in
tumor volume following treatment provide an index for the net result of all of the complex internal cellular and histological
changes that occur in solid tumors following treatment. In addition
it is one of the more clinically relevant measurements that can be
made to assess therapeutic response. Tumor volume change is one of
the most frequently used clinical methods for evaluating tumor response to different forms of therapy.

Previous studies of this series and the studies of other investigations using different solid tumor models in different animal
species have all demonstrated the variability of response to different forms of treatment in experimental tumors which have been
serially transplanted for many years in inbred hosts (23, 24). This
lack of a uniform response to treatment indicates that conventional
methods of analysis such as mean values mask important experimental
therapeutic results. For example, mean values mask the fact that C-2
(Fig 35) does not respond to therapy and the fact that tumor C-4 is
eradicated after the second course of combined modality therapy.
These findings also underscore the differences in the response to
therapy previously found by single course of treatment in this animal
tumor system as well as animal systems in other species (21, 34).
These differences in tumor response to treatment for the same tumor
in different hosts is analogous to many clinical situations where
the same tumor type varies in therapeutic response from patient to
patient. It is evident that a better understanding of these differences in experimental solid tumor models is needed to better understand similar differences in therapeutic response in the same tumor
type found in patients.

One of the important findings in this study with regard to
clinical relevance is that found in the type of response individual
tumors demonstrate over successive courses of therapy. These findings have shown that a tumor which responds well to the first course
of therapy will respond well to the second and third courses of
therapy. The ability to predict which tumors will respond to treatment has rather obvious clinical ramifications. Future studies designed to better understand why some of these tumors respond to
therapy while others do not should provide information which leads
to better clinical management of patients with solid tumors.

The suggestive evidence of increased efficiency of treatment with
the second and third courses of therapy compared to the first course
needs additional study to determine if this is a consistent finding.
If this can be confirmed then it has obvious ramifications with regard
to the sequential utilization of combined modality therapy. It also

suggests that clinical management might be improved by the more effective sequencing of therapy. Combined chemotherapy and radiotherapy has the added advantage of permitting the chemotherapy to
act prophylactically to prevent the metastatic spread of the cancer
during the series of treatments designed to control the primary
tumor. These results have also demonstrated the validity of the
therapeutic strategy employed in this study since successive combined doses of radiation and 5-FU do result in successively smaller
tumor volumes with eventual eradication in some tumors.

    Supported in part by a public health service (CREG) Research
Emphasis Grant CA-20516 on Experimental Combined Modality (Radio-
therapy-Chemotherapy) Studies (ECMRC) from the National Cancer
Institute.

REFERENCES

1. Ansfield, F.J. In: <u>Chemotherapy of Malignant Neoplasms</u>, Second Edition, Charles C. Thomas, Springfield (1973).

2. Ansfield, F.J. J.A.M.A., 190 (1964) 686.

3. Ansfield, F.J., Mackman, S. and Ramirez, G. Oncology, 26 (1972) 114.

4. Bhuyan, B.K., Day, K.J. and Bono, V. Proc. Am. Assoc. Cancer Res. 16 (1975) 114.

5. Denekamp, J. Eur. J. Cancer, 8 (1972) 335.

6. DiMarco, A., Gaetani, M. and Scarpinato, B. Cancer Chemother. Rep. 53 (1969) 33.

7. Evans, M.J. and Kovacs, C.J. Cell Tissue Kin. (in press).

8. Heidelberger, C., Chaudhuri, N.K., Danneberg, P., Mooren, D., Griesbach, L., Duschinsky, R., Schnitzer, R.J., Pleven, E. and Schneider, J. Nature 179 (1957) 663.

9. Hermens, A.F. and Barendsen, G.W. In: <u>Radiation Research Biochemical, Chemical and Physical Perspectives</u>, O.F. Nygaard, H.I. Adler and W.K. Sinclair (eds). Academic Press, New York (1975) pp. 834-849.

10. Hopkins, H.A., Kovacs, C.J., Looney, W.B. and Wakefield, J.A. Cancer Biochem. Biophys. 1 (1976) 303.

11. Kim, S.H. and Kim, J.H. Cancer Res. 32 (1972) 323.

12. Kitaura, K., Imai, R., Ishihara, Y., Yanai, H. and Takahira, H. J. Antibiotics 25 (1972) 509.

13. Kovacs, C.J., Evans, M.J. and Hopkins, H.A. Cell Tissue Kin. (in press).

14. Kovacs, C.J., Evans, M.J., Wakefield, J.A. and Looney, W.B. Radiat. Res. (in press).

15. Kovacs, C.J., Hopkins, H.A., Evans, M.J. and Looney, W.B. Int. J. Radiat. Biol. 30 (1976) 101.

16. Kovacs, C.J., Evans, M.J., Hopkins, H.A. and Looney, W.B. Radiat. Res. 69 ABS (1977) (in press).

17. Kovacs, C.J., Hopkins, H.A., Simon, R.M. and Looney, W.B.

Br. J. Cancer 32 (1975) 42.

18. Looney, W.B., Mayo, A.A., Allen, P.M., Morrow, J.Y. and Morris, H.P. Br. J. Cancer 27 (1973) 341.

19. Looney, W.B., Mayo, A.A., Kovacs, C.J., Hopkins, H.A., Simon, R. and Morris, H.P. Life Sciences 18 (1976) 377.

20. Looney, W.B., Schaffner, J.G., Trefil, J.S., Kovacs, C.J. and Hopkins, H.A. Br. J. Cancer 34 (1976) 254.

21. Looney, W.B., Trefil, J.S., Schaffner, J.G., Kovacs, C.J. and Hopkins, H.A. Proc. Natl. Acad. Sci. U.S.A. 73 (1976) 818.

22. Looney, W.B., Wpsic, H.T., Trefil, J.S., Schaffner, J.G., Hopkins, H.A., Kovacs, C.J. and Morris, H.P. (in preparation).

23. Looney, W.B., Trefil, J.S., Hopkins, H.A., Kovacs, C.J., Ritenour, R. and Schaffner, J.G. Proc. Natl. Acad. Sci. U.S.A. (1977) (in press).

24. Madoc-Jones, H. and Bruce, W.R. Cancer Res. 28 (1968) 1976.

25. Mathe, G., Halle-Pannenko, O. and Bourut, C. Proc. Am. Assoc. Cancer Res. 15 (1974) 75.

26. Meyer, T.J., Ribi, E.E., Azuma, I. and Zbar, B. J. Natl. Cancer Inst. 52 (1974) 103.

27. Morris, H.P. In: Handbuch der allgem., Pathologie, E. Grundmann (ed). Springer-Verlag, New York Vol. 6 No. 7 (1975) pp. 277-334.

28. Pearson, J.W., Chaparas, S.D. and Chirigos, M.A. Cancer Res. 33 (1973) 1845.

29. Pitot, H.C., Peraino, C., Morse, P.A. and Potter, V.R. Natl. Cancer Inst. Mono. 13 (1964) 443.

30. Regelson, W. In: Cancer Chemotherapy, I. Brodsky, S.B. Kah, and J.H. Moyer (eds). Grune & Stratton, New York II (1972) pp. 117-124.

31. Reuber, M.D. J. Natl. Cancer Inst. 26 (1961) 891.

32. Rockwell, S.C., Kallman, R.F. and Fajardo, L.F. J. Natl. Cancer Inst. 49 (1972) 735.

33. Sandburg, J.S., Howsden, F.L., DiMarco, A. and Goldin, A. Cancer Chemother. Rep. 54 (1970) 1.

34. Schabel, F.M., Jr. In: <u>Cancer Chemotherapy</u>, Nineteenth Annual Clinical Conference on Cancer. M.D. Anderson Hospital and Tumor Institute, Year Book Medical Publishers Inc., Chicago (1974) 323.

35. Terzaghi, M. and Little, J.B. J. Natl. Cancer Inst. 55 (1975) 865.

36. Thomlinson, R.H. Brookhaven Symp. Biol. 14 (1961) 204.

37. Trefil, J.S., Schaffner, J.G., Looney, W.B., Hopkins, H.A. and Kovacs, C.J. Methods in Cancer Res. 14 (1977) (In press).

38. Twentyman, P.R. Br. J. Cancer 35 (1977) 208.

39. Vietti, T., Eggerding, F. and Valeriotte, F. J. Natl. Cancer Inst. 47 (1971) 865.

40. Wepsic, H.T., Harris, S., Sander, J., Alaimo, J. and Morris, H.P. Cancer Res. 36 (1976) 1950.

41. Wepsic, H.T., Nickel, R. and Alaimo, J. Cancer Res. 36 (1976) 246.

42. Wheatley, D.N. In: <u>International Symposium on Adriamycin</u>, S.K. Carter, A. DiMarco, M. Ghione, I.H. Krakoff and G. Mathe (eds). Springer-Verlag, New York (1972) pp. 47-52.

43. Zubrod, C.G. J.A.M.A. 178 (1961) 832.

44. Zunino, F., Gambetta, R., DiMarco, A. and Zaccara, A. Biochim. Biophys. Acta 277 (1972) 489.

SPECIAL BIBLIOGRAPHY OF HEPATOMA
CELL LINES

Compiled by

Joyce E. Becker
McArdle Laboratory
Madison, Wisconsin

1963

Morse, P.A., Jr. Pyrimidine metabolism of rat hepatomas in tissue
culture. Thesis, p. 117-147, 1963.

1964

Pitot, H.C., Peraino, C., Morse, P.A., Jr. and Potter, V.R.
Hepatomas in tissue culture compared with adapting liver
in vivo. Nat. Cancer Institute Monograph 13: 229-245, 1964.

1965

Morris, H.P. Studies on the development, biochemistry, and biology
of experimental hepatomas. Advances in Cancer Res.
9: 227-302, 1965.

1967

Potter, V.R., Watanabe, M., Becker, J.E. and Pitot, H.C. Hormonal
effects on enzyme activities in tissue culture and in
whole animals. Advances in Enzyme Regulation 5: 303-316,
1967, Pergamon Press, Oxford and New York.

Stecher, V.J. and Thorbecke, G.J. Sites of synthesis of serum
proteins. III. Production of βIC, βIE and transferrin by
primate and rodent cell lines. J. Immun. 99: 660-668, 1967.

Pitot, H.C. and Jost, J.P. Control of biochemical expression in
morphologically related cells in vivo and in vitro. Nat.
Cancer Institute Monograph 26: 145-166, 1967.

1968

Dickson, J.A. and Potter, V.R. The use of non-metabolizable amino
acids as an index of cell viability in vitro. In Vitro 4:
161, 1968 (Abstract)

759

Goldberg, B. and Green, H. The synthesis of collagen and proto-
          collagen hydroxylase by fibroblastic and nonfibroblastic
          cell lines. Proc. Nat. Acad. Sci. 59: 1110-1115, 1968.

Grossman, A., Lele, K.P. and Sheldon, J. Response of tyrosine amino-
          transferase (TAT) to cortisol in non-dividing rat hep-
          atoma cells grown in tissue culture. Pharmacologist 10:
          224, 1968 (Abstract).

Kenney, F.T., Reel, J.R., Hager, C.B. and Witliff, J.L. Hormonal
          induction and repression. In: San Pietro, A., Lamborg,
          M.R. and Kenney, F.T., Eds. Regulatory Mechanisms for
          Protein Synthesis in Mammalian Cells. Academic Press,
          New York, p. 119-142, 1968.

Reel, J.R. and Kenney, F.T. "Superinduction" of tyrosine trans-
          aminase in hepatoma cell cultures: differential inhibi-
          tion of synthesis and turnover by actinomycin D.
          Proc. Nat. Acad. Sci. 61: 200-206, 1968.

1969

Borek, C., Higashino, S. and Loewenstein, W.R. Intercellular com-
          munication and tissue growth. IV. Conductance of
          membrane junctions of normal and cancerous cells in
          culture. J. Membrane Biol. 1: 274-293, 1969.

Goldberg, B. and Green, H. Relation between collagen synthesis and
          collagen proline hydroxylase activity in mammalian cells.
          Nature 221: 267-268, 1969.

Mendelson, D., Grossman, A. and Boctor, A. Induction of tyrosine
          aminotransferase by D-glucosamine in rat hepatoma cell
          culture. Biochem. Biophys. Res. Comm. 36: 721-727, 1969.

Ohanian, S.H., Taubman, S.B. and Thorbecke, G.J. Rates of albumin
          and transferrin synthesis in vitro in rat hepatoma-derived
          H4-II-E-C3 cells. J. Nat. Cancer Inst. 43: 397-406, 1969.

1970

Brady, R.O., Mora, P.T., Kolodny, E.H. and Borek, C. Ganglioside
          metabolism in virally transformed and chemically induced
          hepatoma cell lines. Fed. Proc. 29: A410 1970 (Abstract).

Dickson, J.A. The metabolism of hepatoma cell strains in an improved
          filter well apparatus. Cancer Res. 30: 2336-2345, 1970.

Dickson, J.A. Uptake of non-metabolizable amino acids as an index
    of cell viability in vitro. Exp. Cell Res. 61: 235-245,
    1970.

Grossman, A., Mendelson, D. and Boctor, A. Glucose suppression of
    tyrosine aminotransferase in rat hepatoma cells grown in
    culture. Fed. Proc. 29: 883, 1970 (Abstract)

Jackson, J.F. and Morse, P.A. Desulferase activity and chromosome
    analysis of cultured rat hepatoma cells. Rev. Eur.
    Etud. Clin. Biol. 15:906-910, 1970.

Krawitt, E.L., Baril, E.F., Becker, J.E. and Potter, V.R. Amino
    acid transport in cultures of hepatoma cells during
    tyrosine aminotransferase induction. Gastroenterology
    58: 285, 1970 (Abstract).

Krawitt, E.L., Baril, E.F., Becker, J.E. and Potter, V.R. Amino
    acid transport in hepatoma cell cultures during tyrosine
    aminotransferase induction. Science 169: 294-296, 1970.

Lee, K.L. and Kenney, F.T. Induction of alanine transaminase by
    adrenal steroids in cultured hepatoma cells. Biochem.
    Biophys. Res. Comm. 40: 469-475, 1970.

Lee, K.L., Reel, J.R. and Kenney, F.T. Regulation of tyrosine alpha-
    ketoglutarate transaminase in rat liver. 9. Studies of
    mechanisms of hormonal inductions in cultured hepatoma
    cells. J. Biol. Chem. 245: 5806-5812, 1970.

Reel, J.R., Lee, K.L. and Kenney, F.T. Regulation of tyrosine
    alpha-ketoglutarate transamianse in rat liver. 8. Induc-
    tions by hydrocortisone and insulin in cultured hepatoma
    cells. J. Biol. Chem. 245: 5800-5805, 1970.

1971

Barker, K.L., Lee, K.L. and Kenney, F.T. Turnover of tyrosine trans-
    aminase in cultured hepatoma cells after inhibition of
    protein synthesis. Biochem. Biophys. Res. Comm. 43:
    1132-1138, 1971.

Barnett, C.A. and Wicks, W.D. Regulation of phosphoenolpyruvate
    carboxykinase and tyrosine transaminase in hepatoma cell
    cultures. I. Effects of glucocortocoids, N^6, 0^2-dibutryl
    cyclic adenosine 3'-5'-monophosphate and insulin in Reuber
    H35 cells. J. Biol. Chem. 246: 7201-7206, 1971.

Butcher, F.R., Becker, J.E. and Potter, V.R. Induction of tyrosine
        aminotransferase by dibutyryl cyclic-AMP employing hep-
        atoma cells in tissue culture. Exp. Cell Res. 66:
        321-328, 1971.

DeLuca, C., Gioeli, R.P. Transhydrogenase activity in mammalian
        cells in vitro: its possible physiological significance.
        In Vitro 7(1): 13-16, 1971.

Lee, K.L. and Kenney, F.T. Regulation of tyrosine-α-ketoglutarate
        transaminase in rat liver. Regulation by L-leucine
        in cultured hepatoma cells. J. Biol. Chem. 246:
        7595-7601, 1971.

Mendelson, D., Grossman, A. and Boctor, A. D-glucose suppression
        of tyrosine aminotransferase in rat-hepatoma cells
        grown in culture. Eur. J. Biochem. 24: 140-148, 1971.

Sahib, M.K., Jost, Y.C. and Jost, J.P. Role of cyclic adenosine
        3',5'-monophosphate in the induction of hepatic en-
        zymes. III. Interaction of hydrocortisone and $N^6,0^2$-
        dibutyryl cyclic adenosine 3',5'-monophosphate in the
        induction of tyrosine aminotransferase in cultured H-
        4-II-E hepatoma cells. J. Biol. Chem. 246: 4539-4545,
        1971.

Schneider, J.A. and Weiss, M.C. Expression of differentiated func-
        tions in hepatoma cell hybrids. I. Tyrosine amino-
        transferase in hepatoma-fibroblast hybrids. Proc.
        Natl. Acad. Sci. 68: 127-131, 1971.

Weiss, M.C. and Chaplain, M. Expression of differentiated functions
        in hepatoma cell hybrids. 3. Reappearance of tyrosine
        aminotransferase inducibility after loss of chromosomes.
        Proc. Nat. Acad. Sci. 68: 3026-3030, 1971.

1972

Bertolotti, R. and Weiss, M.C. Expression of differentiated functions
        in hepatoma cell hybrids. VI. Extinction and re-
        expression of liver alcohol dehydrogenase. Biochimie
        54: 195-201, 1972.

Bertolotti, R. and Weiss, M.C. Aldolase in hepatoma cell hybrids:
        Extinction of the hepatic form and its reexpression fol-
        lowing loss of chromosomes. In: Harris, R. and Viza, D.
        Eds., Cell Differentiation, Proc. of the 1st Int. Conf.
        on Cell Differentiation, Williams and Wilkins Co., p.
        202-205, 1972.

Bertolotti, R. and Weiss, M.C. Expression of differentiated func-
        tions in hepatoma cell hybrids. II. Aldolase.
        J. Cell. Physiol. 79: 211-224, 1972.

Butcher, F.R., Bushnell, D.E., Becker, J.E. and Potter, V.R.
        Effect of Cordycepin on induction of tyrosine amino-
        transferase employing hepatoma cells in tissue culture.
        Exp. Cell Res. 74: 115-123, 1972.

DeLuca, C. and Gioeli, R.P. Pyridine-adenine dinucleotide trans-
        hydrogenase activity in cells cultured from rat hepatoma.
        Canadian J. Biochem. 50: 447-456, 1972.

DeLuca, C., Massaro, E.J. and Cohen, M.M. Biochemical and cyto-
        genetic characterization of rat hepatoma cell lines in
        vitro. Cancer Res. 32: 2435-2440, 1972.

Granner, D.K. Defective regulation of protein kinase activity in
        three liver-derived tissue culture lines. J. Clin.
        Invest. 51, No. 6: 38a, 1972.

Miller, D.A., Dev, V.G., Borek, C. and Miller, O.J. The quinacrine
        fluorescent and giemsa banding karyotype of the rat,
        Rattus norvegicus, and banded chromosome analysis of
        transformed and malignant rat liver cell lines.
        Cancer Res. 32: 2375-2382, 1972.

Nordquist, R.E., Muragashi, H., Lovig, C.A. and Bottomley, R.H.
        Ultrastructure of the H4-II-E rat hepatoma cell line
        in vivo and in vitro. In Vitro 7: 281-282, 1972
        (Abstract).

Peterson, J.A. and Weiss, M.C. Expression of differentiated func-
        tions in hepatoma cell hybrids. Induction of mouse
        albumin production in rat hepatoma mouse fibroblast
        hybrids. Proc. Nat. Acad. Sci. 69: 571-575, 1972.

Peterson, J.A. and Weiss, M.C. Induction of mouse albumin synthesis
        in hybrids between rat hepatoma and mouse fibroblast
        cells. In: Harris, R. and Viza, D., Eds. Cell Dif-
        ferentiation, Proc. 1st Int. Conf. on Cell Differentia-
        tion, Williams and Wilkins Co., p. 198-201, 1972.

Van Wijk, R., Clay, K. and Wicks, W. D. Effects of derivatives of
        cyclic 3',5'-AMP on the growth, morphology and gene
        expression of cultured hepatoma cells. Fed. Proc. 31:
        439A, 1972. (Abstract)

Van Wijk, R., Wicks, W.D. and Clay, K. Effects of derivatives of
        cyclic 3',5'-adenosine monophosphate on the growth,
        morphology, and gene expression of hepatoma cells in
        culture. Cancer Research 32: 1905-1911, 1972.

Weinstein, I.B., Gebert, R., Stadler, U.C., Orenstein, J. and
        Axel, R. Type C virus from cell cultures of chemical-
        ly induced rat hepatomas. Science 178: 1098-1100,
        1972.

Wicks, W.D. and McKibbin, J.B. Regulation of phosphoenolpyruvate
        carboxykinase and tyrosine transaminase in hepatoma
        cell cultures. 2. Evidence for translational reg-
        ulation of specific enzyme synthesis by $N^6,O^{2'}$-
        dibutyryl cyclic AMP in hepatoma cell cultures.
        Biochem. Biophys. Res. Comm. 48: 205-211, 1972.

1973

Borek, C., Grob, M. and Burger, M.M. Surface alterations in trans-
        formed epithelial and fibroblastic cells in culture:
        a disturbance of membrane degradation versus bio-
        synthesis? Exp. Cell Res. 77: 207-215, 1973.

Corpening, B.J. and Bottomley, R.H. Giemsa banding patterns of
        normal rat and H4-II-E chromosomes. In Vitro 8:
        443, 1973 (Abstract)

Croce, C.M., Bakay, B., Nyhan, W.L. and Koprowski, H. Reexpression
        of the rat hypoxanthine phosphoribosyltransferase
        gene in rat-human hybrids. Proc. Nat. Acad. Sci.
        U.S.A. 70: 2590-2594, 1973.

Croce, C.M., Kieba, I. and Koprowski, H. Unidirectional loss of
        human chromosomes in rat-human hybrids. Exp. Cell
        Res. 79: 461-463, 1973.

Croce, C.M., Litwack, G. and Koprowski, H. Human regulatory gene
        for inducible tyrosine aminotransferase in rat-human
        hybrids. Proc. Nat. Acad. Sci. U.S.A. 70: 1268-1272,
        1973.

Haggerty, D.F., Young, P.L., Popjak, G. and Carnes, W.H. Phenyl-
        alanine hydroxylase in cultured hepatocytes. J.
        Biol. Chem. 248: 4528-4531, 1973.

Kenney, F.T., Lee, K.L., Stiles, C.D. and Fritz, J.E. Further
        evidence against post-transcriptional control of
        inducible tyrosine aminotransferase synthesis in

cultured hepatoma cells. Nature New Biol. 246:
208-210, 1973.

Singer, S., Becker, J.E. and Litwack, G. The principal gluco-
        corticoid binding macromolecule in hepatoma cells
        in culture is similar to corticosteroid binder II
        of rat liver cytosol. Biochem. Biophys, Res. Comm.
        52: 943-950, 1973.

Sparkes, R.S. and Weiss, M.C. Expression of differentiated functions
        in hepatoma cell hybrids: alanine aminotransferase.
        Proc. Nat. Acad. Sci. U.S.A. 70: 377-381, 1973.

van Wijk, R., Wicks, W.D., Bevers, M.M. and van Rijn, J. Rapid
        arrest of DNA synthesis by $N^2,0^2$-dibutyryl cyclic
        adenosine 3',5'-monophosphate in cultured hepatoma
        cells. Cancer Res. 33: 1331-1338, 1973.

1974

Bertolotti, R. and Weiss, M.C. Expression of differentiated func-
        tions in hepatoma cell hybrids v. re-expression of
        aldolase B in vitro and in vivo. Differentiation
        2: 5-17, 1974.

Bushnell, D.E., Becker, J.E. and Potter, V.R. The role of messenger
        RNA in tyrosine aminotransferase superinduction: ef-
        fects of camptothecin on hepatoma cells in culture.
        Biochem. Biophys. Res. Comm. 56: 815-821, 1974.

Bushnell, D.E., Yager, J.D., Becker, J.E. and Potter, V.R.
        Inhibition of messenger RNA accumulation but not
        translation in ultraviolet irradiated hepatoma cells.
        Biochem. Biophys. Res. Comm. 57: 949-956, 1974.

Malawista, S.E. and Weiss, M.C. Expression of differentiated func-
        tions in hepatoma cell hybrids: high frequency of
        induction of mouse albumin production in rat hepatoma-
        mouse lymphoblast hybrids. Proc. Nat. Acad. Sci.
        U.S.A. 71: 927-931, 1974.

Peterson, J.A. Discontinuous variability, in the form of a
        geometric progression of albumin production in hep-
        atoma and hybrid cells. Proc. Nat. Acad. Sci. U.S.A.
        71: 2062-2066, 1974.

Richardson, U.I., Snodgrass, P.J., Nuzum, C.T. and Tashjian, A.H. Jr.
        Establishment of a clonal strain of hepatoma cells
        which maintain in culture the five enzymes of the

urea cycle. J. Cell Physiol. 83: 141-149, 1974.

Szpirer, C. Reactivation of chick erythrocyte nuclei in hetero-
    karyons with rat hepatoma cells. Exp. Cell Res.
    83: 47-54. 1974.

van Rijn, H., Bevers, M.M., van Wijk, R. and Wicks, W.D. Regula-
    tion of phosphoenolpyruvate carboxykinase and tyrosine
    transaminase in hepatoma cell cultures. III. Com-
    parative studies in H35, HTC, MH_1C_1, and RLC cells.
    J. Cell Biol. 60: 181-191, 1974.

Whitlock, J.P., Jr., Miller, H. and Gelboin, H.V. Induction of
    aryl hydrocarbon (benzo[α]pyrene) hydroxylase and
    tyrosine amintransferase in hepatoma cells in culture.
    J. Cell Biol. 63: 136-145, 1974.

Wicks, W.D. Regulation of protein synthesis by cyclic AMP.
    Advances in Cyclic Nucleotide Res. 4: 335-438, 1974.

Wolf, C.F.W., Minkelt, B.E. and Kaighn, M.E. The conjugation of
    bilirubin by rat hepatoma cells in tissue culture.
    Proc. Soc. Exp. Biol. Med. 145: 918-924, 1974.

1975

Borek, C. Studies on normal and neoplastic liver cells in culture:
    contact behavior, cellular communication and trans-
    formation. In: Gene Expression and Carcinogenesis in
    Cultured Liver, L.E. Gerschenson and E. Brad Thompson,
    Eds., Academic Press, New York, pp. 62-93, 1975.

Brown, J.E. and Weiss, M.C. Activation of production of mouse liver
    enzymes in rat hepatoma -- mouse lymphoid cell hybrids.
    Cell 6: 481-494, 1975.

Croce, C.M., Litwack, G. and Koprowski, H. Regulation of the cortico-
    steroid inducbility of tyrosine aminotransferase in
    somatic cell hybrids. In: Gene Expression and Carcino-
    genesis in Cultured Liver. L.E. Gerschenson and E. Brad
    Thompson, Eds., Academic Press, New York, pp. 325-332,
    1975.

Gunn, J.M., Tilghman, S.M., Hanson, R.W., Reshef, L. and Ballard,
    F.J. Effects of cyclic adenosine monophosphate, dexa-
    methasone and insulin on phosphoenolpyruvate carboxykinase
    synthesis in Reuber H-35 hepatoma cells. Biochemistry
    14: 2350-2357, 1975.

Hanson, R., Haggerty, D.F., Young, P.L., Buese, J.V. and Popjak, G.
        Effect of serum on phenylalanine hydroxylase levels in
        cultured hepatoma cells. J. Biol. Chem. 250: 8428, 1975.

McClure, D., Miller, M. and Shiman, R. Correlation of phenylalanine
        hydroxylase activity with cell density in cultured hep-
        atoma cells. Exp. Cell Res. 90: 31-29, 1975.

Owens, I.S., Niwa, A. and Nebert, D.W. Expression of aryl hydro-
        carbon hydroxylase induction in liver and hepatoma
        derived cell cultures. In: Gene Expression and Carcino-
        genesis in Cultured Liver, L.E. Gerschenson and E. Brad
        Thompson, Eds., Academic Press, New York, pp. 378-401,
        1975.

Strunk, R.C., Tashjian, A.H., Jr. and Colten, H.R. Complement bio-
        synthesis in vitro by rat hepatoma cell strains.
        J. Immunol. 114: 331-335, 1975.

Tashjian, A.H., Jr., Richardson, U.I., Strunk, R. and Ofner, P.
        Differentiated functions in clonal strains of hepatoma
        cells. In: Gene Expression and Carcinogenesis in
        Cultured Liver, L.E. Gerschenson and E. Brad Thompson,
        Eds, Academic Press, New York, pp. 168-180, 1975.

Tilghman, S.M., Gunn, J.M., Fisher, L.M. and Hanson, R.W. Deinduc-
        tion of phosphoenolpyruvate carboxykinase (guanosine
        triphosphate) synthesis in Reuber H-35 cells. J. Biol.
        Chem. 250: 3322-2239, 1975.

Wagner, K., Roper, M.D., Leichtling, B.H., Wimalasena, J. and Wicks,
        W.D. Effects of 6- and 8-substituted analogs of adeno-
        sine 3':5'-monophosphate on phosphoenolpyruvate carboxy-
        kinase and tyrosine aminotransferase in hepatoma cell
        cultures. J. Biol. Chem. 250: 231-239, 1975.

Weinstein, I.B., Orenstein, J.M., Gebert, R., Kaighn, M.E. and
        Stadler, U.C. Growth and structural properties of
        epithelial cell cultures established from normal rat
        liver and chemically induced hepatomas. Cancer Res.
        35: 253-263, 1975.

Weinstein, I.B., Yamaguchi, N., Orenstein, J.M.,Gebert, R. and
        Kaighn, M.E. Mechanisms of chemical carcinogenesis
        analyzed in rat liver and hepatoma cell cultures.
        In: Gene Expression and Carcinogenesis in Cultured
        Liver, L.E., Gerschenson and E. Brad Thompson, Eds.,
        Academic Press, New York, pp. 441-459, 1975.

Weiss, M.C.   Extinction, re-expression and induction of liver
          specific functions in hepatoma cell hybrids.   In:
          <u>Gene Expression and Carcinogenesis in Cultured Liver</u>,
          L.E. Gerschenson and E. Brad Thompson, Eds., Academic
          Press, New York, pp. 346-357, ,975.

Wicks, W.D., Wagner, K., Roper, M.D., Leichtling, B.H. and
          Wimalasena, J.   Regulation of specific protein syn-
          thesis in cultured hepatoma cells by analogs of cyclic
          AMP.   In: <u>Gene Expression and Carcinogenesis in
          Cultured Liver</u>, L.E. Gerschenson and E. Brad Thompson,
          Eds., Academic Press, New York, pp. 205-219, 1975.

<u>1976</u>

Clark, J.L. and Fuller, J.L.   Protein inhibitor of ornithine de-
          carboxylase does not account for effect of putrescine
          on 3T3 cells.   Biochem. Biophys. Res. Comm. 73: 785-
          790, 1976.

DeLuca, C. and Matheisz, J.S.   Glucose-6-phosphatase dehydrogenase
          activity in a hepatoma cell line: preliminary evidence
          for negative genetic control.   J. Cellular Physiol.
          87: 101-109, 1976.

Fong, W.F., Heller, J.S. and Canellakis, E.S.   The appearance of an
          ornithine decarboxylase inhibitory protein upon the
          addition of putrescine to cell cultures.   Biochim.
          Biophys. Acta 428: 456-465, 1976.

Gunn, J.M., Ballard, F.J. and Hanson, R.W.   Influence of hormones
          and medium composition on the degradation of phosphoenol-
          pyruvate carboxykinase (GTP) and total protein in Reuber
          H35 cells.   J. Biol. Chem. 251: 3586-3593, 1976.

Gunn, J.M., Williams, G.M. and Shinozuka, H.   Enhancement of pheno-
          typic expression in cultured malignant liver epithelial
          cells by a complex medium.   J. Cellular Physiol. 87(1):
          79-88, 1976.

Haggerty, D.F., Popjak, O. and Young, N.L.   Properties of phenyl-
          alanine hydroxylase of cultured hepatoma cells.   J. Biol.
          Chem. 251: 6901-6908, 1976.

Heller, J.S., Fong, W.F. and Canellakis, E.S.   Induction of a protein
          inhibitor to ornithine decarboxylase by the end product
          of its reaction.   Proc. Nat. Acad. Sci. U.S.A. 73: 1858-
          1862, 1976.

Knowles, S.E. and Ballard, F.J. Selective control of the degradation
    of normal and aberrant proteins in Reuber H35 hepatoma
    cells. Biochem. J. 156: 609-617, 1976.

Miller, M.R., McClure, D. and Shiman, R. Mechanism of inactivation
    of phenylalanine hydroxylase by p-chlorophenolalanine
    in hepatoma cells in culture. Two possible models.
    J. Biol. Chem. 251: 3677-3685, 1976.

Miller, M.R. and Shiman, R. Hydrocortisone induction of phenyl-
    alanine hydroxylase isozymes in cultured hepatoma
    cells. B.B.R.C. 68(3): 740-745, 1976.

Mullen, V.T. and Barnett, C.A. Banded karyotypes of H-4-IIE-C3 rat
    hepatoma cells grown in vitro. In Vitro 12(9): 658-
    664, 1976.

Munns, T.W., Johnson, M.F.M., Liszewski, M.K. and Olson, R.S.
    Vitamin K-dependent synthesis and modification of pre-
    cursor prothrombin in cultured H35 hepatoma cells.
    Proc. Nat. Acad. Sci. U.S.A. 73: 2803-2807, 1976.

Peterson, J.A. Clonal variation in albumin messenger RNA activity
    in hepatoma cells. Proc. Nat. Acad. Sci. U.S.A.
    73: 2056-2060, 1976.

Tourian, A. Control of phenylalanine hydroxylase synthesis in tissue
    culture by serum and insulin. J. Cellular Physiol.
    87(1): 15-24, 1976.

Stiles, C.D., Lee, K.L. and Kenney, F.T. Differential degradation of
    messenger RNAs in mammalian cells. Proc. Nat. Acad.
    Sci. 73(8): 2634-2638, 1976.

Szpirer, C. and Szpirer, J. Extinction, retention and induction of
    serum protein secretion in hepatoma-fibroblast hybrids.
    Differentiation 5: 97-99, 1976.

Szpirer, C., Szpirer, J. and Wiener, F. The expression of differen-
    tiated functions in somatic cell hybrids: retention and
    activation of C3 production. Cell Diff. 5: 139, 1976.

INDEX